GENETICS
OF
DEVELOPMENTAL
DISABILITIES

PEDIATRIC HABILITATION

Series Editor

ALFRED L. SCHERZER
Cornell University Medical Center
New York, New York

ADDITIONAL VOLUMES IN PREPARATION

GENETICS
OF
DEVELOPMENTAL
DISABILITIES

edited by

MERLIN G. BUTLER
Children's Mercy Hospitals and Clinics
University of Missouri–Kansas City School of Medicine
Kansas City, Missouri, U.S.A.

F. JOHN MEANEY
University of Arizona College of Medicine
Tucson, Arizona, U.S.A.

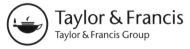

Taylor & Francis
Taylor & Francis Group

Boca Raton   London   New York   Singapore

Published in 2005 by
Taylor & Francis Group
6000 Broken Sound Parkway NW, Suite 300
Boca Raton, FL 33487-2742

International Standard Book Number-10: 0-8247-5813-7 (Hardcover)
International Standard Book Number-13: 978-0-8247-5813-4 (Hardcover)

Library of Congress Cataloging-in-Publication Data

Catalog record is available from the Library of Congress

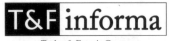

Taylor & Francis Group
is the Academic Division of T&F Informa plc.

Visit the Taylor & Francis Web site at
http://www.taylorandfrancis.com

Preface

Genetics of Developmental Disabilities is written as a textbook and resource for physicians, basic and clinical researchers, and other professionals, students, and health care providers. Those interested in the causes and scientific understanding of developmental disabilities (DD) as well as the care of individuals with these disabilities should find this book useful. Interested individuals involved in the testing, care, and treatment of DD should include special educators, developmental specialists, nurses, occupational/physical therapists, speech pathologists, public health experts, psychologists, psychiatrists, geneticists and genetic counselors, child life experts, ethicists, social workers, and other health professionals. In addition, this book can be used as a resource for parents and other family members of individuals with DD and agencies involved in providing services.

The types and causes of DD are discussed including genetic and environmental factors and the ever-increasing knowledge of their interaction. The chapters are organized into sections to address genetics and related factors pertinent to the area of medical and clinical genetics. Specifically, genetic conditions with developmental disability as a major component will be addressed by different disciplines (neurology, developmental pediatrics, rehabilitation medicine, psychology, epidemiology, public and mental health experts, pharmacology, and ethics). Noted experts are utilized to address diagnostic testing, dual diagnoses, treatment approaches for related health and behavioral problems (e.g., autism, self-injurious behavior, attention deficit hyperactivity), special education, social services, early intervention programs, and counseling.

The opening chapters comprise a section that includes the history of mental retardation specifically addressing historical advances in genetics, patterns of inheritance and our understanding of the causes, diagnosis, and treatment of individuals with DD. The areas of genetics include basic mammalian genetics, multifactorial inheritance, molecular genetics, clinical cytogenetics and biochemical genetics as these areas relate to testing for DD. The Human Genome Project and how it relates to DD and mental retardation is also presented. Finally, examples of animal modeling using transgenic mice for certain disorders and especially Down syndrome are described in a separate chapter.

The second section presents, in separate chapters, examples of conditions with DD, including specific single gene and chromosome syndromes, microdeletion chromosome anomalies, fetal alcohol syndrome and environmental causation, expanded newborn screening and sporadic disorders. Genetic conditions that are classical and often under consideration by the clinical geneticist when evaluating individuals with DD are described including Prader–Willi syndrome, Angelman syndrome, Smith–Magenis syndrome, Williams–Beuren syndrome, 22q deletion syndrome (velo-cardio-facial syndrome), Rett syndrome, Down syndrome, sex chromosome aneuploidy, phenylketonuria, and fragile X syndrome, the most common cause of familial mental retardation.

The final section begins with a chapter that addresses the causes and prevalence of DD and recurrence risks. Chapters discussing aspects of neurogenetic disorders, cerebral palsy, behavioral genetics, and manifestations of certain conditions such as self-injurious behavior, attention deficit-hyperactivity, and autism are presented. The current treatment and diagnostic approach for children with DD are addressed, including the use of early intervention programs, complementary and alternative medical interventions, and use of computers to search for genes causing DD or mental retardation.

This text is intended to be read and used by all individuals interested in DD and the role of genetics in these conditions. References are cited for the reader interested in learning more about the information given and for those interested in pursuing the subject and related topics in more depth.

Merlin G. Butler
F. John Meaney

Contents

CLASSICAL EXAMPLES OF CONDITIONS WITH DEVELOPMENTAL DISABILITIES

8. Fragile X and X-linked Mental Retardation .. *247*
Sebastien Jacquemont, Vincent des Portes, and
Randi Hagerman

Acknowledgments

First, the editors wish to express their appreciation to their colleagues who have contributed chapters to this edition of *Genetics of Developmental Disabilities*. The chapter authors represent an extraordinary knowledge base concerning genetics and developmental disabilities, and we are grateful for each of their contributions to this book. We have benefited immensely from our interactions with each of the authors before and during the production of the book, and we look forward with enthusiasm to the continuation of our association.

Additionally, we would like to express our appreciation to the many mentors and teachers, who through the years have been instrumental in our training as scientists, teachers, and health care providers. We express our deepest gratitude to all who contributed their clinical and genetic expertise to our understanding of both genetics and developmental disabilities. We include as our teachers all the patients and their families with whom we have interacted. We wish to express our special thanks for their participation in clinical investigations and research related to developmental disabilities. Mostly we thank them for teaching us beyond words about their individual lives.

The editors would also like to thank the many individuals who have provided outstanding assistance during the book's production, particularly in the publisher's office. In addition, we are especially grateful to Heather Baroni and Linda Heim at Children's Mercy Hospitals and Clinics for their technical assistance to both of us during the writing of our book chapters and the editing process. We wish to express our appreciation to Kathleen Pettit and Christiane Pretzinger at the University of Arizona for providing assistance with literature searches and other details of the editing process.

Lastly, our deepest thanks go to our respective families for their encouragement and support over all the years of our professional lives, but especially during the many hours that went into the production of this book. We can never thank them enough for their patience and understanding while we are hard at work.

Contributors

Margaret P. Adam   Department of Pediatrics, Division of Medical Genetics, Stanford University School of Medicine, Stanford, California, U.S.A.

Kevin Antshel   Department of Psychiatry and Behavioral Sciences, State University of New York Upstate Medical University, Syracuse, New York, U.S.A.

Michael Begleiter   Section of Medical Genetics and Molecular Medicine, Children's Mercy Hospitals and Clinics, University of Missouri–Kansas City School of Medicine, Kansas City, Missouri, U.S.A.

Thierry Bienvenu   Institut Cochin, INSERM, Paris, France

Coleen A. Boyle   National Center on Birth Defects and Developmental Disabilities, Centers for Disease Control and Prevention, Atlanta, Georgia, U.S.A.

Merlin G. Butler   Section of Medical Genetics and Molecular Medicine, Children's Mercy Hospitals and Clinics, University of Missouri–Kansas City School of Medicine, Kansas City, Missouri, U.S.A.

Nancy J. Carpenter Center for Genetic Testing, Saint Francis Health System, Tulsa, Oklahoma, U.S.A.

William I. Cohen Children's Hospital of Pittsburgh, University of Pittsburgh School of Medicine, Pittsburgh, Pennsylvania, U.S.A.

Linda D. Cooley Section of Medical Genetics and Molecular Medicine, Children's Mercy Hospitals and Clinics, University of Missouri–Kansas City School of Medicine, Kansas City, Missouri, U.S.A.

Melinda F. Davis Department of Pediatrics, University of Arizona College of Medicine, Tucson, Arizona, U.S.A.

Vincent des Portes INSERM, Institut Cochin de Génétique Moléculaire, Paris, France

Melissa A. Doffing University of Oklahoma Health Sciences Center, Child Study Center, Oklahoma City, Oklahoma, U.S.A.

Burris Duncan Department of Pediatrics, University of Arizona College of Medicine, Tucson, Arizona, U.S.A.

Wallace C. Duncan Mood and Anxiety Disorders Program, National Institute of Mental Health, National Institutes of Health, HHS, Bethesda, Maryland, U.S.A.

Kathy Ellerbeck Developmental Disabilities Center, University of Kansas Medical Center, Kansas City, Kansas, U.S.A.

Charles J. Epstein Department of Pediatrics, University of California, San Francisco, California, U.S.A.

Jane A. Evans Departments of Biochemistry and Medical Genetics; Pediatrics and Child Health; and Community Health Sciences, University of Manitoba, Winnipeg, Manitoba, Canada

Wanda Fremont Department of Psychiatry and Behavioral Sciences, State University of New York Upstate Medical University, Syracuse, New York, U.S.A.

Randi Hagerman Department of Pediatrics, University of California, Davis; M.I.N.D. Institute, UC Davis Medical Center, Sacramento, California, U.S.A.

John L. Hamerton Departments of Biochemistry and Medical Genetics; Pediatrics and Child Health, University of Manitoba, Winnipeg, Manitoba, Canada

Richard Hillman Division of Medical Genetics, University of Missouri, Columbia, Missouri, U.S.A.

Edward Hoffman Special Care Pediatrics, P.A., Leawood, Kansas, U.S.A.

H. Eugene Hoyme Department of Pediatrics, Division of Medical Genetics, Stanford University School of Medicine, Stanford, California, U.S.A.

Sebastien Jacquemont M.I.N.D. Institute, UC Davis Medical Center, Sacramento, California, U.S.A.

Chet Johnson Developmental Disabilities Center, University of Kansas Medical Center, Kansas City, Kansas, U.S.A.

Wendy R. Kates Department of Psychiatry and Behavioral Sciences, State University of New York Upstate Medical University, Syracuse, New York, U.S.A.

Cheryl Klaiman Child Study Center, Yale University School of Medicine, New Haven, Connecticut, U.S.A.

Joan H. M. Knoll Section of Medical Genetics and Molecular Medicine, Children's Mercy Hospitals and Clinics, University of Missouri–Kansas City School of Medicine, Kansas City, Missouri, U.S.A.

Shannon Lillis Section of Medical Genetics and Molecular Medicine, Children's Mercy Hospitals and Clinics, University of Missouri–Kansas City School of Medicine, Kansas City, Missouri, U.S.A.

Molly Lund Section of Medical Genetics and Molecular Medicine, Children's Mercy Hospitals and Clinics, University of Missouri–Kansas City School of Medicine, Kansas City, Missouri, U.S.A.

F. John Meaney Department of Pediatrics, University of Arizona College of Medicine, Tucson, Arizona, U.S.A.

Maximilian Muenke   Department of Health and Human
Services, Medical Genetics Branch, National Human Genome
Research Institute, Bethesda, Maryland, U.S.A.

Giovanni Neri   Istituto di Genetica Medica, Facoltà di Medicina e
Chirurgia "A. Gemelli," Università Cattolica del Sacro Cuore,
Rome, Italy

Stephen A. Petrill   Department of Biobehavioral Health,
The Pennsylvania State University, University Park,
Pennsylvania, U.S.A.

Barbara Pober   Department of Pediatrics, MassGeneral
Hospital for Children, and Department of Surgery, Division of
Genetics, Children's Hospital, Boston, Massachusetts, U.S.A.

Nancy Roizen   Department of Pediatrics, State University of
New York Upstate Medical University, Syracuse, New York, U.S.A.

Robert Schultz   Child Study Center, Yale University School of
Medicine, New Haven, Connecticut, U.S.A.

Robert J. Shprintzen   Departments of Pediatrics and
Otolaryngology and Communication Sciences, State University of
New York Upstate Medical University, Syracuse, New York, U.S.A.

Ann C. M. Smith   National Human Genome Research Institute,
National Institutes of Health, HHS, Bethesda, Maryland, and
Department of Oncology, Institute of Molecular and Human
Genetics, Georgetown University School of Medicine, Washington,
D.C., U.S.A.

Francesco D. Tiziano   Istituto di Genetica Medica, Facoltà di
Medicina e Chirurgia "A. Gemelli," Università Cattolica del Sacro
Cuore, Rome, Italy

Kim Van Naarden Braun   Oak Ridge Institute for Science and
Education, United States Department of Energy, Oakridge,
Tennessee, U.S.A.

Gopalrao V. N. Velagaleti Division of Genetics, Departments of Pediatrics and Pathology, University of Texas Medical Branch, Galveston, Texas, U.S.A.

Angela J. Villar Department of Pediatrics, University of California, San Francisco, California, U.S.A.

Daniel J. Wattendorf Department of Health and Human Services, Medical Genetics Branch, National Human Genome Research Institute, Bethesda, Maryland, U.S.A.

Barbara Y. Whitman Department of Pediatrics, Cardinal Glennon Children's Hospital, St. Louis, Missouri, U.S.A.

Charles A. Williams Department of Pediatrics, Division of Genetics, Raymond C. Philips Research and Education Unit, University of Florida, Gainesville, Florida, U.S.A.

Mark L. Wolraich University of Oklahoma Health Sciences Center, Child Study Center, Oklahoma City, Oklahoma, U.S.A.

Marshalyn Yeargin-Allsopp National Center on Birth Defects and Developmental Disabilities, Centers for Disease Control and Prevention, Atlanta, Georgia, U.S.A.

Hui Zhang Department of Genetics, Yale University School of Medicine, New Haven, Connecticut, U.S.A.

1

A History of Mental Retardation

GIOVANNI NERI and FRANCESCO D. TIZIANO
Istituto di Genetica Medica, Facoltà di Medicina e
Chirurgia "A. Gemelli," Università Cattolica del
Sacro Cuore, Rome, Italy

I. INTRODUCTION

Mental retardation (MR) is arbitrarily and conventionally defined by an intelligence quotient (IQ) of less than 70. It would therefore seem logical that a history of mental retardation be preceded by a brief history of mental normality and even of mental superiority, coinciding to a large extent with the emergence and consolidation of the concept of IQ. This implies entering a very controversial and divisive field, in fact a minefield. Because, while a formal, "scientific" measurement of intelligence has served the study of mental retardation well, its application to society at large has had disastrous consequences. The reason why the word "eugenics" still has a sinister ring to it is largely rooted in the misuse of

IQ to measure intelligence and to uphold the idea of its heritability. Much harm was done and much suffering was caused
by the social consequences of this stance, and while the con-
demnation of extremes, such as Nazi eugenics, is universal,
the realization that eugenics was born and largely applied
in respectable societies is too easily forgotten.

II. SIR FRANCIS GALTON AND THE EMERGENCE OF EUGENICS

One of the major and long-lasting contributions Sir Francis
Galton (Fig. 1) made to science was the collection and analysis of pedigrees to study heredity. His *Hereditary Genius*,

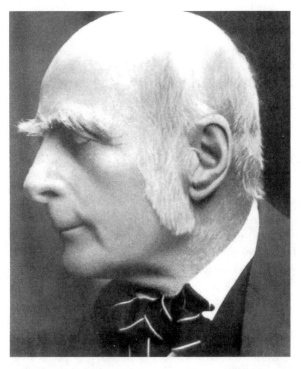

Figure 1   Photograph of Sir Francis Galton (1822–1911) taken in
the 1870s. (Reprinted with permission from "www.galton.org"
edited by Gavin Tredoux.)

published in 1869 (1), was largely based on pedigree analysis, and one wonders whether he may have been influenced by his own membership in a remarkable pedigree. On the maternal side of the family, he and his first cousin, Charles Darwin, both descended from Erasmus Darwin, an expert physician, botanist, and inventor, and a prolific writer. Charles Darwin's mother was Susannah Wedgwood of the famous china manufacturers. The Galtons were businessmen who rose to prominence by amassing a large fortune that allowed Sir Francis to devote himself leisurely to a wide range of scientific pursuits. Interestingly, the most common edition of the famous Galton–Darwin pedigree (Fig. 2) is in fact an abridged version, hiding a number of less achieving family members, who may have marred the proposition that superior talent and intellect was a heritable trait in the family (2).

Hereditary Genius is the cornerstone of eugenics and reflects Galton's conviction that mental ability is determined by nature, much more than by nurture, like any simple

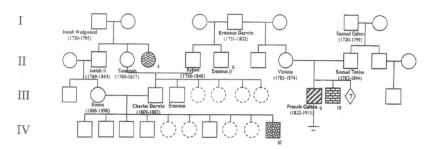

Figure 2 The Wedgewood–Darwin–Galton family pedigree. The most eminent persons in the family are identified by name. Shadowed symbols indicate individuals who were not included in the original published pedigree. Among them, II, 4, died at the age of 8 years for unknown reasons. She was mentally retarded. The last of Charles Darwin's children (IV, 10) was also retarded, and died at 18 months. The mother was 48 years old at the time of his birth and one may suspect that he had Down syndrome (2). II, 6, Erasmus Jr, was probably suffering from psychiatric problems. Francis Galton himself (III, 9) was infertile and his younger brother Darwin (III, 10) was epileptic.

character shaped by evolution and selection. To prove the point, he leaned heavily on pedigree analysis, assuming that a "natural" trait should show a high correlation among first-degree relatives, the correlation fading rapidly in more distant relatives. With genes yet to be discovered and with Darwinism and Mendelism yet to be merged into the mainstream of early genetics, Galton had to turn to whatever tools were available at the time. First he decided that reputation is a reliable measure of mental ability. Next he selected a group of eminent men (English judges) from distinguished families to finally come to the conclusion that 36% of the sons of eminent men, 23% of the brothers, and 26% of the fathers were themselves eminent, an extremely high proportion compared to the prevalence of eminent men in the general English population, calculated by Galton to be approximately 1 in 4000.

The idea that reputation is a fair measure of eminence may seem hilarious within the cultural context of the present day and probably did not sound entirely convincing to Galton either. Galton was an anthropometrist, obsessed by the urge of measuring "every measurable faculty of body and mind" (3), to the point of even trying to measure the efficacy of prayer (4). His work on fingerprints and dermatoglyphics stands as a monumental contribution to the field of anthropometry, securing him long-lasting glory. Other figures that rose to fame in the same field are now either forgotten (Bertillon) or discredited (Lombroso). We can only guess that Galton would have welcomed Binet's work on the measure of intelligence for its quantitative approach and probably adopted it for his own measurements of intellectual eminence. Unfortunately, this work was published only a few years prior to the death of both these great men, in 1911.

Alfred Binet (Fig. 3) was a young psychologist when he went to study at the Hôpital Salpêtrière at a time when the great Charcot was mostly interested in hypnosis and hysteria. The clinical experience he gained in those years and the impression he received from reading John Stuart Mill were key factors influencing his subsequent work when he moved to the Sorbonne. He set out to study intelligence as a classical

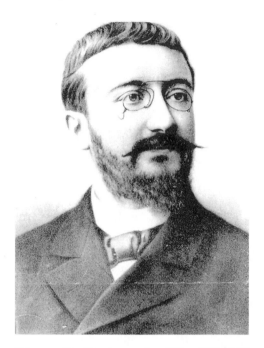

Figure 3   Photograph of Dr. Alfred Binet (1857–1911). (Reprinted with permission from the Archives of the History of American Psychology, University of Akron.)

anthropometrist by measuring heads of schoolchildren, on the assumption that the best students should have head size, as a proxy for brain size, significantly larger than that of the worst students. The results were a huge disappointment and persuaded Binet to take a different course. Therefore, when in 1904 he was appointed by the French Government to a commission in charge of evaluating the problem of mental deficiency among schoolchildren, he chose to proceed by way of an innovative approach. In order to gauge their general mental ability, he asked the students to perform a set of different tasks that, collectively, would result in a grading of their intelligence. Each task was assigned a level of difficulty in relation to a certain age, so that at the end, it should be possible to compare the actual chronological age with the mental age, calculated by the number of tests that were correctly performed. Binet had invented a new scale of intelligence that, deservedly, still goes by his name. In 1912, a year after his death, the German psychologist W. Stern proposed that the results of the Binet test would be best expressed dividing the mental age by the chronological age, formally giving birth to the intelligence quotient, or IQ.

III. EUGENICS AND THE IQ TEST

In that same year of 1912, the First International Congress of Eugenics opened in London with great fanfare and enthusiasm. A vivid account of this event is given by Nicholas Gillham in the epilogue of his excellent biography of Francis Galton. Under the subtitle *Out of Pandora's Box*, Gillham summarizes the dire consequences of eugenics in one chilling sentence "Galton had discovered the mystical box that Darwin [Major Leonard Darwin, one of Charles Darwin's sons, president of the Congress (*authors' note*)] now opened, out of which flapped eugenics accompanied by its courtiers: involuntary segregation, sterilization, and racial intolerance. They would spread a pestilence through Europe, America, and beyond that would rage in its most virulent and hideous form in the Nazi Germany of the 1930s and 40s" (5).

In America, the eugenic movement leaned heavily on the application of Binet's IQ test, imported by H. H. Goddard, director of the Vineland School for the feeble-minded in New Jersey and popularized by Stanford University psychologist Lewis Terman. As noted by Stephen Jay Gould in *The Mismeasure of Man* (6), both men made essentially the same mistakes: (a) asserting the "reification of intelligence as a single, measurable entity" (6, p. 189) and (b) assuming that intelligence could be measured linearly by the IQ test from idiocy, to imbecility to normality, with morons (a new term coined by Goddard) scoring between imbeciles and normals. Intelligence was treated as a simple Mendelian trait becoming, by definition, a heritable character. A substantial contribution to this entirely gratuitous conclusion came from another prominent figure, Charles Spearman, a statistician and psychologist at University College, London. In 1904, he published a famous paper in which the focal assertion was that mental tests measure a real entity, a factor he named *g*, or general intelligence (7). The IQ test, empirically designed by Binet to identify schoolchildren in need of special help was elevated by Spearman to the status of an objective measurement for an extremely complex trait such as human intelligence.

These arguments received further strength in 1909 from another famous paper "Experimental Tests of General Intelligence" published in the *British Journal of Psychology* by Cyril Burt (8), Spearman's successor to the Chair of Psychology at the University College and a strong advocate of the theory of intelligence as an innate, hereditary, and substantially nonmodifiable property. It may be worth recalling here Burt's posthumous disgrace, when evidence was uncovered that he had fabricated data and had tried to give himself credit for Spearman's technique of factor analysis (9).

The practical consequences of those two mistakes were especially felt during the first half of the 20th century, but continued even afterwards and until very recently. If intelligence is a Mendelian trait, the inescapable conclusion is that the more talented people should be encouraged to breed and reproduce, while the morons should be prevented from doing so. This is, in a few words, the quintessence of the eugenic movement of the past century. But how to prevent morons from reproducing? Certainly not by intellectual or moral persuasion, which would be impossible for them to understand. Involuntary sterilization became the tragic, inevitable alternative. Sterilization laws were passed in Europe and North America and sterilization programs widely implemented. The prevailing cultural mood of the time was epitomized by a *cause celèbre*, Buck vs. Bell, argued before the U.S. Supreme Court in 1927 with Harry Laughlin, superintendent of the Eugenics Record Office, as expert witness. The case was that of Carrie Buck, a feeble-minded woman whose mother and illegitimate daughter were also feeble-minded. The majority opinion, written by Justice Oliver Wendell Holmes, upheld the Virginia sterilization law and contained the now famous (or rather infamous) phrase "Three generations of imbeciles are enough."

Not just the cruelty, but also the arbitrariness of decisions like that in Buck vs. Bell are illustrated by other, now seemingly incredible stories. One, vividly told by Gould (6), is the story of the so-called Kallikak family living in the pine barrens of New Jersey. The Kallikak family came under the care of Dr. Goddard. Its members were declared mentally deficient on simple inspection or even by hearsay. Pictures of members of the family, taken by Goddard's field workers, were apparently retouched to give the portrayed individuals an appearance of stupidity. The family was presented as *prima facie* evidence of the hereditarian theory of mental weakness, since its ancestry could be traced to the illicit union of a respectable man with a feeble-minded tavern servant. From his legitimate wife, a well-to-do woman, the same man had only normal descendants. The inescapable conclusion was that feeble-mindedness was a hereditary character transmitted by the mother.

The segregationist furor soon extended from individual cases to entire populations. To the indefatigable Dr. Goddard, the domestic problem of keeping morons from reproducing was already too troublesome to allow other morons to enter the country. Two field workers were dispatched to Ellis Island with the task of administering an IQ test to indigent and culturally deprived immigrants. The results were too much even for Dr. Goddard: on average, 80% of those tested (Jews, Hungarians, Italians, and Russians) had a mental age below 12 years (10). The tragedy took an almost comic turn when mental tests were introduced among the army recruits at the instigation of Robert Yerkes. A psychologist, and later an Army colonel, he pressed the case for taking advantage of the mobilization for World War I to test a large number of subjects, thus building a significant data base from which to derive a reliable definition of mental "normality." At that time, the average mental age of white American males was considered to be 16 years; Yerkes' results were alarmingly lower. In his own words, "It appears that the intelligence of the principal sample of the white draft, when transmuted from Alpha and Beta exams into terms of mental age, is about 13 years (13.08)" (11, p. 785). The embarrassing conclusion was that the average intelligence of white American adults was just above the level of moronity, set at the mental age of 12 years. Needless to say, immigrants from Southern European countries and the American "Negroes" scored even lower. The fallacies within the tests that led to these incredible results would be easy to expose, as cogently discussed by Gould (6). The fact remains that these "mismeasurements," for a very long time, and almost to the present day, continued to provide a subtle justification for the acceptance of a subdivision of the society into predetermined intellectual classes, as well as racial discrimination.

Hernstein and Murray's *The Bell Curve: the Reshaping of American Life by Difference in Intelligence* (12) is the most recent and voluminous defense of the idea that human intelligence is an innate property, a heritable genetic trait set by nature, that nurture cannot modify. The IQ measurements allocate individuals within classes of intelligence and also allow the distinction of ethnic groups, depending on their average scores. The less talented should be cared for compassionately, the more talented should be in charge of serious business. The perspective and hope to move upward from one class to another is virtually nonexistent, given the minimal effect of the environment on the attainable level of intelligence.

IV. MENTAL RETARDATION

At the end of this cursory foray into the history, definition and measurement of human intelligence over the last 150 years, a foray that may have revealed some personal biases on the matter, it is time to go back to the central issue of mental retardation and to ask a crucial question: if the quantification of intellectual talent by the IQ test has caused so much social damage and individual suffering, what consequences should we expect from its application to the study of mental retardation, in a medically defined setting? The reassuring answer brings us back to Binet himself, whose intentions were clear and honest from the outset. He was well aware of the fact that intelligence is not a single and simple entity that can be measured as one would measure the weight of a brain, and that the IQ test is no more than an empirical tool designed to identify the mentally disabled that are in need of special education. Binet strongly believed that these individuals could be helped to improve their intellectual performance by *ad hoc* educational programs. Thus, IQ testing should be seen as an instrument that, like any other instrument, e.g., a kitchen knife, can do good or wrong, depending on how it is used. The brief history that follows should demonstrate that its use has been generally beneficial within the medical specialties that are concerned with the problem of mental retardation and the well-being of the mentally disadvantaged.

Needless to say, we could not even think of being encyclopedic in narrating, although briefly, a history of mental retardation. Therefore, we made choices and decided to illustrate three subjects that can be considered, in a way, prototypic. The first of these is mental retardation in chromosome syndromes, specifically in Down syndrome. The second deals with mental retardation in the inborn errors of metabolism, specifically in phenylketonuria. The third subject is X-linked mental retardation.

V. DOWN SYNDROME

The 19th century produced radical societal changes. In England, but also in other countries, there was a very rapid population increase due to increased life expectancy that was in turn attributable to improvements in medicine, sanitation, quality of health structures, care for pregnant women, and so forth. The coronation of Queen Victoria in 1837 granted England peace, prosperity, and territorial expansion throughout the entire duration of the century. In France, there were the decline of Napoleon, the Restoration, and then the Third Republic, while Germany and Italy achieved national territorial unification. This was the century of the Curies, Roentgen,

Pasteur, and Koch. Addison described the adrenal gland insufficiency and Virchow identified the function of cells. In 1866,
Mendel published the results of his experiments on plants,
founding the scientific study of heredity. "With regard to intellectual functioning and the brain, Santiago Ramon y Cajal and
Camillo Golgi wrote complex histological studies of the nervous system; François Magendie, founder of experimental
physiology, distinguished between the motor and sensory portions of the peripheral nerves; Paul Broca provided an atlas of
the brain; Freud, Charcot, and Kraepelin significantly
advanced the studies of mental illness" (13, p. 52). Charcot's
studies on hysteria and psychopathology of trauma opened
the way to Freud's psychoanalysis. "Intellectually, the single
most epochal and equally controversial publication of the era
was Darwin's *Origin of Species*, 1859. Based on years of observation and study, Darwin's thesis emphasized three points: 1)
organisms do not reproduce identical replicas of their kind, but
rather produce variations, many of which are hereditary; 2)
nature allows the survival of only those organisms that can
adapt to their environment; and 3) all organisms, therefore,
undergo a struggle for existence" (13, p. 52). Darwin's theories,
especially the concept of adaptation and survival, had a profound impact in several fields, including that of psychology,
which modified radically its bases, giving rise to its modern
appearance. "Psychology was certain to become consistently
more biological: mental processes tended more and more to
be stated in terms of functions served in the task of adjusting
to the world" (G. Murphy, *Historical Introduction to Modern
Psychology*, 1949, quoted in Ref. 13, p. 52).

The 19th century was also somewhat of a golden age for
the field of mental retardation studies. At the beginning of
the century, a new discipline was born, destined to influence
both diagnosis and treatment of mental retardation. Phrenol-
ogy (or craniology, as originally named) was conceived by
Franz Joseph Gall and was based on the assumption that
the brain is the seat of mind, that each intellectual faculty
is connected with specific brain areas, and that the size
of each area is directly related with the developmental
level of the associated faculty. It was thought that skull

measurements could allow one to establish the level of individual faculties, since the development of brain areas is strictly related to the bony development (13, p. 53). Many causes of mental retardation were identified during this age, including von Recklinghausen (1863) and Bourneville (1880) diseases, Sturge–Weber syndrome (1879), Tay–Sachs (1881), Gaucher (1882), and Marfan (1896) syndromes. Curling (1860) and Fagge (1870) related cretinism to hypothyroidism; perinatal traumas were recognized as possible causes of mental delay in infants and cerebral palsy was described by Little (as noted in Ref. 13).

Another important revolution in this field, strongly supported by Edouard Séguin (1812–1880) and other scientists, concerned the role of governments in the care of people affected with mental retardation. In fact, this was a conquest of the second half of the century. As reported by Scheerenberger (13, p. 65) "mentally retarded persons on the farm continued to work long hours in poverty with their parents. In the cities, pauper children who could not work in the industrial setting or were not accepted into an apprentice program frequently ran the streets as beggars or thieves. Those who could not be tended at home or who were picked up by the police frequently were placed in almshouses, workhouses, jails, or mental hospitals, where conditions continued to be deplorable by any humane standards [. . .]. Wealthy parents tended to keep their mentally retarded children at home, occasionally providing tutors for their education. According to Down, many of these children were kept in secret and great effort was made to hide them from public view." During the century, many laws were enacted, especially aimed at residential and educational programs for retarded persons, starting in England and spreading throughout Western European countries. In spite of good intentions, the conditions of hospitals for the mentally ill and retarded persons remained inadequate for a long time with respect to hygiene, humanity, and social assistance to patients.

This was the fervent background of an epoch when many classifications of mental retardation were advanced. Esquirol (1845) distinguished the two main categories of "imbeciles" and "idiots," with a high degree of variability inside each category. Imbeciles were defined as "generally well formed, and their organization is nearly normal. They enjoy the use of intellectual and affective facilities, but in less degree than the perfect man, and they can be developed only at a certain extent" (from *Mental Maladies: A Treatise on Insanity*, 1845, as quoted in Ref. 13, p. 54). About idiots, Esquirol wrote: "we have at least reached the utmost limit of human degradation. Here, the intellectual and moral faculties are almost null; not that they have been destroyed, but never developed" (13). Furthermore, Esquirol distinguished "amentia," that is mental retardation, from "dementia," mental illness.

Séguin used the term "idiocy" to refer to mental retardation in general and also to one of the categories of his classification, according to which idiocy was "an infirmity of the nervous system which has for its radical effect the separation of all or part of the child's organs and faculties from the regular control of his will, which frees him to his instincts and separates him from the world. The typical idiot is an individual who knows nothing, thinks of nothing, wills nothing, and each idiot approaches more or less the summum of incapacity." (13, p. 55). Séguin identified four categories: idiocy, including probably moderate to profound retardation; imbecility, comprising mildly retarded patients; backwardness or feeble-mindedness; simpleness, including people not really retarded but just slow in their development.

William Wetherspoon Ireland classified mental retardation into 10 categories, namely: (1) genetous (congenital), (2) microcephalic (head circumference below 17 inches), (3) eclamptic, (4) epileptic, (5) hydrocephalic, (6) paralytic, (7) cretinism, (8) traumatic, (9) inflammatory, (10) by deprivation (13, p. 59).

John Langdon Down's (1828–1896, Fig. 4) ethnical classification can be appropriately inserted in this context. Although the classification was not itself particularly successful, it was expanded in a paper in which "Mongolian idiocy" is described for the first time. As we all know, the definition of "Mongolian" to refer to people affected with this condition, survived until a few decades ago in medical practice and even

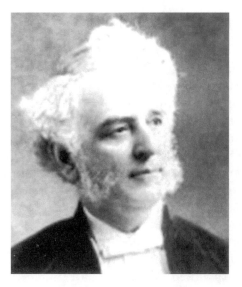

Figure 4 Photograph of Dr. John Langdon Down (1826–1896). (Reprinted with permission from Ref. 14.)

today is still in public use on occasion.* "Those who have given any attention to congenital mental lesions, must have been frequently puzzled how to arrange, in any satisfactory way, the different classes of this defect which may have come under their observation. Nor will the difficulty be lessened by an appeal to what has been written on the subject. The systems of classification are generally so vague and artificial, that, not only do they assist but feebly, in any mental arrangement of the phenomena which are presented, but they completely fail in exerting any practical influence on the subject" (15, reported in Ref. 16, p. 209). This is the *incipit* of the original paper by Down, *Observations on an Ethnic Classification of Idiots*, published in 1866. In this paper, the author attempted a classification of patients with mental retardation based on ethnic characteristics, thus recognizing four categories: the

---

*In 1959, after the discovery of trisomy 21, the Peoples Republic of China asked the World Health Organization to avoid the use of the term "Mongol" to refer to people affected with Down syndrome (14).

Ethiopian variety (characteristic malar bones, prominent eyes, puffy lips, retreating chin, woolly hair); the Malay variety (soft, black, curly hair, prominent upper jaws, large mouths); the American continent variety (shortened foreheads, prominent cheeks, deep-set eyes, slightly apish nose); and the Mongolian variety. It is very interesting to note what Down wrote: "the great Mongolian family has numerous representatives [...]. A very large number of congenital idiots are typical Mongols. So marked is this, that when placed side by side, it is difficult to believe that the specimens compared are not children of the same parents. The number of idiots who arrange themselves around the Mongolian type is so great, and they present such a close resemblance to one another in mental power, that I shall describe an idiot member of this racial division, selected from the large number that have fallen under my observation" (16, p. 210). As to patients affected with "Mongolian idiocy," Down wrote "the hair is not black, as in the real Mongol, but of a brownish colour, straight and scanty. The face is flat and broad, and destitute of prominence. The cheeks are roundish, and extended laterally. The eyes are obliquely placed, and the internal canthi more than normally distant from one another. The palpebral fissure is very narrow. The forehead is wrinkled transversely from the constant assistance which the levatores palpebrarum derive from the occipito-frontalis muscle in the opening of the eyes. The lips are large and thick with transverse fissures. The tongue is long, thick, and is much roughened. The nose is small" (16, p. 210). Down also defined some cognitive aspects of the patients by writing, "they are humorous, and a lively sense of ridiculous often colours their mimicry [...]. They are usually able to speak; the speech is thick and indistinct, but may be improved very greatly by a well-directed scheme of tongue gymnastics. The coordinating faculty is abnormal, but not so defective that it cannot be greatly strengthened" (16, p. 210). Furthermore, "the Mongolian type of idiocy occurs in more than 10% of the cases which are presented to me. They are always congenital idiots, and never result from accident after uterine life"; they derive, "for the most part, [as] instances of degeneracy arising from tuberculosis in the parents"; "the life expectancy, however is far below the average, and the tendency is to tuberculosis" (16, p. 210). In this description, the mix of visionary concepts, like that of rehabilitation, and of old prejudices, like the origin of the syndrome from the degeneracy of parents, is truly amazing. In a later study, *Mental Affections of Children and Youth*, 1887, Down classified idiocy into three etiological categories: congenital (idiots); accidental (idiots and feeble-minded); and developmental (feeble-minded)" (13, p. 56). The use of the term "imbecile" was restricted to mental illness.

But was Dr. J. L. Down really the first to describe the syndrome universally known by his name? In the same year that saw the publication of Down paper, Séguin described the case of a 9-year-old girl affected with a form of "furfuraceous cretinism" resembling Down syndrome (17). He wrote: "other cases of similar but aggravated character have been observed, but the description of their repulsive symptoms would not make us less ignorant of the true nature of their affection. We have not seen enough of this affection to express any opinion upon it, but as a conjecture: and we hazard the hypothesis that is a variety of idiocy connected with some form or hereditary cretinism" (17, reported in Ref. 16, p. 211). The implication is that while Down identified "Mongolism" as a form of idiocy, which is a congenital form of mental retardation, Séguin identified the same condition as caused by cretinism, i.e., mental retardation due to congenital hypothyroidism. Thus, Down was the first to recognize Mongolism as a specific condition with mental retardation and typical facial features.

Since the early 1960s, the question whether Down syndrome existed before Down's age or whether it represents a "modern" disease, has been debated in great length (16,18–22). And, if the former is the case, why was such a common condition never described previously as a specific nosological entity? As hypothesized by Richards (19), the incidence of Down syndrome increased during the 19th century, as a result of at least three characteristics of the English population compared to previous times: (1) larger size; (2) higher mean age and life-span of fertile women; (3) lower infant mortality. However, it is quite likely that some previous descriptive knowledge existed, as can be inferred from the analysis of ancient figurines, paintings, or skeletal remains (16). Recently, Levitas and Reid (21) reported the case of an angel in a Flemish painting from the 16th century who presented a facial appearance markedly different from the other angels depicted, and strongly resembling Down syndrome. But, while Berg and Korossy (16) concluded that "though perhaps being unduly sceptical, we do not feel on the basis of the above survey that there is written and/or visual evidence of unequivocal recognition of Down syndrome before Down's initial report" (16, p. 209), Levitas and Reid (21) hypothesized that "it is possible that those with milder degrees of mental handicap were not recognized as having what we now call mental retardation [...]. In this context, a surviving teen or adult with Down syndrome, no life-threatening malformations, and relatively high intellectual function might not have been recognized as sufficiently different to warrant unusual treatment in a social context" (21, p. 404). Although confirmation of the clinical suspicion of Down syndrome in the reported cases is clearly impossible, there is no reason to think that, even if more rare, Down syndrome did not exist before Down. He probably described this condition for the first time as a result of both the cultural, medical ferment, and social interest in mental retardation during his times and to the higher prevalence of the condition.

The etiology of Down syndrome remained obscure until 1959, when Lejeune et al. demonstrated that it was due to trisomy of chromosome 21 (23). The chromosomal origin had already been hypothesized by others during the 1930s, like Waardenburg or Bleyer (24–26). Before these studies, Down himself related the condition to parental tuberculosis, while the associated congenital heart disease was explained by Garrod's doctrine of fetal endocarditis (27). According to this theory, which was strengthened by the demonstration of the frequent cardiac involvement in rheumatic fever, cardiac malformations were related to an inflammatory process occurring during prenatal life, thus interfering with normal heart development.

Starting from the identification of the aneuploidy responsible for Down syndrome, research had many successes in the definition of the pathophysiology of this condition. Two main explanatory approaches can be identified, which emerged clearly during the symposium on "Trisomy 21" which took place in Rome (Italy) in May 1989, on the occasion of the 30th anniversary of the discovery of trisomy 21. Eminent scientists from all over the world participated to this symposium. Their formal presentations and discussion favored the emergence of two different theories explaining the phenogenesis of Down syndrome. Lejeune and Epstein apparently took a reductionistic approach. The former (28) described intelligence as a "symphony" in which "each musician (the genes) reads a score and follows the tempo of the conductor," and suggested that some of the behavioral and mental aspects of Down syndrome patients could be explained by a single biochemical defect caused by trisomy, like hypothyroidism or purine, pyrimidine, folic acid, biopterine, or methionine metabolism. Lejeune concluded, "it must be precisely stressed that this general model is for the moment strictly speculative. Even if the reasoning is sound, it remains to be seen whether the correction of such troubles will, in the long run, alleviate the mental deficiency."

The position of Epstein (29) derived from his outstanding studies, both clinical and experimental. By analyzing very rare cases of partial trisomy 21 (generally due to familial translocations), he attempted to assign to the different regions of 21q a determining role for the various aspects of Down syndrome phenotype, thus reconstructing a "phenotypic mapping." Epstein asserted that "individual phenotypic anomalies or features can often be assigned or mapped to specific regions of the genome, and conversely, the component manifestation of individual aneuploid states can often be added together to generate the phenotypes of combined aneuploidies" (29, p. 32). Furthermore, "the phenotype of an aneuploid state can be decomposed into a series of sub-phenotypes associated with sub-segments of the overall region of imbalance and, furthermore, that these sub-phenotypes can then be added together or recombined to give the overall phenotype [. . .]. The reconstructions of phenotypes from sub-phenotypes is not without problems, and there is a certain amount of 'noise' in the analysis which extends beyond that expected just from variability of expression" (29, p. 32) Then, Epstein argued that there must exist a direct relationship between the genes involved in the aneuploidy and their effect, thus leading to the specific phenotypic spectrum of a syndrome.

The position of Opitz (30), which we can refer to as organicistic, was somewhat different since he did not emphasize so much the role of specific genes, but rather a generic disturbance of developmental fields due to chromosomal imbalance per se. "Here we should like to emphasize that most malformations in Down syndrome represent *incomplete* development, e.g., oral clefts, AV canal defects, imperforate anus, syndactyly of digits. They rarely represent *abnormal* development such as polydactyly [. . .]. The most astonishing thing about Down syndrome, or for that matter about any one of several thousands of duplication, deletion, polyploidy, or duplication/deficiency syndromes, is not a virtually unlimited repertoire of dysmorphogenetic disasters and novelties, but rather the remarkably limited, one might even say impoverished, repertoire of dysmorphogenetic responses. That is to say, the number and type of anomalies in individual instances of aneuploidy are no different from those encountered in the normal population, but only more common and monotonously similar to what is found in other Mendelian and aneuploidy syndromes in spite of the massive qualitative and quantitative genetic differences imposed by trisomy. The causes are many, but the final common paths to a dysmorphogenetic outcome are very few, an insight not unique to aneuploidy syndromes" (30, p. 41). In conclusion, the correct development of an organism passes through a delicate balance between genetic and epigenetic factors: " . . . it may transpire that a single heterochronous disturbance delaying growth and development and making the whole epigenetic system more vulnerable to stochastic factors and environmental perturbations will be a sufficient explanation of the pathogenesis of Down syndrome. The specific nature of the heterocronous disturbance, its pattern of timing, and its pattern of structural involvement will, to some extent, be determined by the specific time, amount, and location of the genetic material involved" (30, p. 49).

In spite of these intriguing theories, the exact pathophysiology of Down syndrome remains elusive. A great bulk of
studies has been performed more recently in order to define
the regions of chromosome 21 responsible for the single phenotypic characteristics and many animal models of the disease have been constructed (31–34). After these studies,
especially based on mouse models and on the rare segmental
human trisomies, it is now clear that the region around
21q22.3, syntenic to part of murine chromosome 16, is responsible for some of the characteristics of the syndrome, like
craniofacial and limb morphology, duodenal stenosis, hypotonia, and joint hyperlaxity (32). The remaining human
chromosome 21 is syntenic with part of murine chromosome
10 and 17.

According to Epstein, one of the most important lessons
learned from Down syndrome, and that can be virtually
extended to all chromosomal imbalances, is that "...it was
possible to demonstrate specific functional consequences of
the increased dosage of just a single gene. Furthermore, an
analysis of the specificity and reproducibility of the patterns
of abnormalities in the various trisomies and monosomies,
even in the face of individual variability, has convinced me
that the aneuploid phenotypes that are genetically unbalanced when a duplication or deletion is present and are not
the result of some kind of random noise or general loosening
up of developmental homeostasis" (32, p. 304). Detailed physical and genetic maps of human chromosome 21 have been
available for some years (35) as much as the complete
sequence has been available since 2000 (36), but the exact
number of genes it contains, remains unclear. It is appropriate to conclude this necessarily brief overview of Down syndrome with Epstein's own words, presented at the 51st
Annual Meeting of the American Society of Human Genetics
in 2001, as part of the William Allan Award lecture: "Despite
[a] the length of time that Down syndrome has been known as
an entity and studied and [b] the elegance of the methods for
studying the nervous system that have been developed, we
actually know very little about what is abnormal about the
brains and nervous system of people with Down syndrome

[...]. This is not really surprising, because our hands seem to be very much tied when it comes to studying what is happening within the black box of the human cranium" (32, p. 310).

VI.   INBORN ERRORS OF METABOLISM: THE CASE OF PKU

Inborn errors of metabolism gained greater significance as a cause of mental disability once the reduction of neonatal and infantile morbidity due to infectious diseases was achieved through the introduction of antibiotic therapy and other medical treatments. Sir Archibald Garrod, arguably one of the founders of medical genetics and a pioneer in the field of inborn errors of metabolism, identified four classes of metabolic disorders: albinism, alkaptonuria, cystinuria, and pentosuria (37). During the 20th century, the list of these conditions grew enormously. Most of these disorders are transmitted as autosomal or X-linked recessive traits and their incidences vary from rare to very rare (Table 1) (38,39). Inborn errors of metabolism have generally been viewed as typical Mendelian traits. Deeper knowledge of these diseases has led in recent years to a revision of this postulate, as a wide phenotypic heterogeneity, which cannot be explained solely by gene mutations, has emerged. Evidence of this variability is the observation of phenotypic differences in sibs affected with the same disease. The explanation of this phenomenon is partially coming from post genomic/proteomic insights into the metabolic homeostasis of cellular systems and the biochemical effect of different mutations. What is currently emerging is that the mutant gene is not the only factor determining the biochemical phenotype; it should be viewed within the framework of a buffered system which is regulated by at least three mechanisms: (a) genome redundancy for genes with overlapping functions; (b) plasticity of the homeostatic system/ pathway in which a defective protein is involved; and (c) negative feedback regulation (40).

Phenylketonuria is the paradigm of these conditions. It was once considered to be a simple, monogenic trait, but has acquired in the last few years a growing level of complexity.

Table 1 Most Common Inborn Errors of Metabolism Associated
with Mental Retardation

Condition	Transmission	Frequency
Congenital hypothyroidism	AR/sporadic	1:3,500
Phenylketonuria	AR	1:12,000
Sanfilippo syndrome (MPS III, Netherlands)	AR	1:24,000
Metachromatic leuokodistrophy (Sweden)	AR	1:40,000
Fabry disease	XR	1:40,000
Gaucher disease (Ashkenazi Jews)	AR	1:2,500
Tay–Sachs disease	AR	
Ashkenazi Jews		1:5,600
General population		1:500,000
Arginosuccinicaciduria	AR	1:60,000
Hunter syndrome (MPS II)	XR	
Ashkenazi Jews		1:67,500
British Columbia		1:150,000
Galactosemia	AR	1:75,000
Hurler syndrome (MPS I)	AR	1:100,000
Maple syrup urine disease	AR	1:120,000
Homocystinuria	AR	
Ireland		1:40,000
General population		1:200,000

AR, autosomal recessive; XR, X-linked recessive.
Source: Ref. 38.

Furthermore, the story of its discovery is the story of a rare
therapeutic triumph in medical genetics.

If Down syndrome can be considered the para
digmatic example of a chromosomal imbalance, phenylketonuria (PKU, OMIM 261600) is the prototypic example of a
metabolic defect responsible for mental retardation. The discovery of PKU was made by Asbjörn Fölling (1888–1973,
Fig 5), a Norwegian physician, in 1934 (41,42). The story of
this discovery is fascinating, as it tells about the relationship
between a doctor and a family (especially the mother) of two
mentally retarded children, Liv and Dag. As in the majority
of such cases, the parents, Borgny and Harry Egeland, began
to look around for someone who was able to explain why both
of their children were retarded. When Dag was an infant,
they noticed that the urine of both children had a very

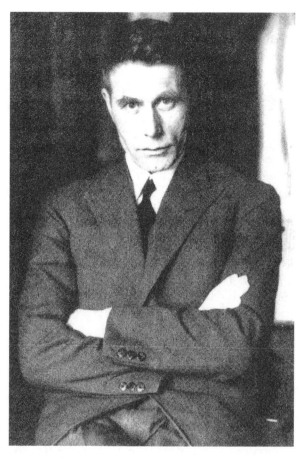

Figure 5 Photograph of Dr. Asbjörn Fölling (1888–1973) taken about the time of the discovery of PKU in 1934. (Reprinted with permission from Ref. 42.)

particular odor and they were wondering whether this could be related to the cause of their retardation. They came to the conclusion that Liv and Dag had the same condition, although Dag was much more severely affected. Harry Egeland took some courses from Professor Fölling at the Dental College in Oslo. After being informed of the odor of the children's urine, Fölling, who had a strong scientific background in chemistry, asked for urine samples from Liv. The profile of urine was normal for blood, albumin, pus, and acidity. However, during an evaluation for ketones, which cause a reddish brown pigmentation after addition of aqueous ferric chloride, the urine turned dark green after a few minutes of time had elapsed. This type of pigmentation had never been observed or described in urine before. Fölling repeated the test on Dag's urine with an identical result. In order to exclude that the pigmentation could be due to the administration of drugs, Fölling asked the mother to repeat the urine collection after one week of wash out from any drug. After verifying the reproducibility of the result, Fölling tested another 430 children, all affected with mental retardation, institutionalized in the Oslo region. He found eight showing the same phenomenon in the urine. After chemical studies, he concluded that the green pigmentation was due to the presence of phenylpyruvic acid, and defined the newly discovered condition "imbecillitas phenylpyruvica" (41). The term "phenylketonuria" was introduced by Lionel Penrose (Fig. 6) (43) for the metabolic marker found in affected patients. The overall incidence of PKU is now indicated to be 1/15,000, with variability among populations for which incidence data are available (39,44).

The cause of PKU is a defect in the metabolism of phenylalanine (Phe), an amino acid accounting for 5% of all dietary protein intake. The defective enzyme phenylalanine hydroxylase (PAH), which converts Phe into tyrosine, was identified in 1947 by George Jervis in hepatocyte cytosol (42). In the 1950s, an effective treatment of PKU was devised by a dietary restriction of Phe (45), which resulted in a virtually normal psychomotor development of PKU children (44,46,47). The first treatment for PKU was undertaken in Birmingham, UK, by Horst Bickel and coworkers (45). Again, the role of a mother was the determining factor: Sheila, a 2-year-old girl, was severely retarded, unable to sit and with no interest in her surroundings. Her mother "awaited me every morning in front of the laboratory asking me impatiently when I would at last find a way to help Sheila. She was very upset and did not accept the fact that at the time no treatment was known for PKU. Couldn't I find one?," Bickel wrote (45, p. S2). Phenylalanine dietary restriction improved

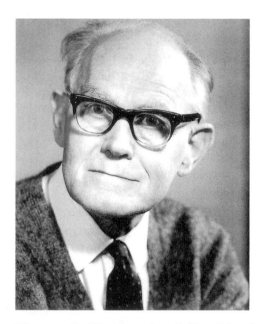

Figure 6 Photograph of Dr. Lionel S. Penrose (1898–1972). (Reprinted with permission from the Genetics Society of America®.)

dramatically Sheila's condition: she learned to walk within a few months.

The possibility of a treatment for PKU increased interest in the idea that a neonatal screening test could be developed to identify infants with PKU and treat them to prevent mental retardation. This screening was made possible by the development of the Guthrie test, a simple and inexpensive test to measure the level of Phe in the infant's blood. Robert Guthrie, a physician, was the father of a mentally retarded child. During a meeting of the New York State Association for Retarded Children, in 1957, he met Dr. Robert Warner, Director of the Children's Rehabilitation Center in Buffalo (48). Dr. Warner told Guthrie about PKU, underlining the need for a rapid test to quantify the blood level of Phe, essential to screen a large population and to monitor the effect of dietary therapy. Guthrie wrote: "It seemed that this might be possible, by modifying the bacterial tests I was using to screen the different substances in the blood of patients who were being treated for cancer. These tests relied on a technique called 'competitive inhibition'. I was able to develop the test for PKU using the same principle. It was very simple: a compound which normally prevents growth of bacteria in culture plates no longer inhibits the growth when large amounts of Phe are present in a blood spot that is added to the plate. The large quantity of Phe in the blood sample 'competes' with the inhibitor compound and overcomes its capacity for stopping bacterial growth. The result is that wherever there is an abnormal amount of Phe in the blood sample, there will be bacterial growth that is easily detected" (48, p. s4).

The gene of PAH was eventually cloned in 1983, by Woo and coworkers (49). Since then, hundreds of mutations have been identified and genotype–phenotype correlations have been established between the residual enzymatic activity and the metabolic phenotype (50). Perhaps surprisingly, no strict correlations were found between metabolic phenotype and cognitive impairment, as measured by IQ, the latter being a quantitative trait determined by the interaction of many different factors (44,46,47).

There are at least two lessons to learn from PKU: the first is that it is one of the very few examples of a human genetic disease which can be treated by a metabolic approach: dietary exclusion of Phe is sufficient to prevent mental impairment. Many studies have been performed on the intellectual outcome of patients with PKU (44,46,47). Although their IQ is on average slightly below the familial target, it is always in the normality range. Furthermore, the earlier the initiation of treatment the better is the outcome of IQ values (44).

Secondly, this Mendelian trait is not so simple after all. There are interfering factors, different from the PAH mutations that contribute to the phenotype (40,50,51). In summarizing his review of the lessons derived from PKU, Scriver asks the questions "Is it any wonder that the so-called monogenic human diseases are indeed complex in their phenotypic manifestations?" and "How should the clinician respond?" (40, p. 505). His answer is as follows: "...Treat patients, not the genome. The patient's 'private' genome is always modulating expression of 'public' allele(s) accounting for the 'monogenic' disease. The disease unfolds from the pathophysiologic features of the phenotype; therefore, treat the patient with the personal phenotype. It is not the same as treating the disease. In practice, it is genetic medicine" (40, p. 505).

VII. X-LINKED MENTAL RETARDATION

An account of the modern history of X-linked mental retardation (XLMR), although brief, deserves a place within a general history of mental retardation. It has been known for quite some time that there is an excess of males among the mentally retarded. In 1938, Penrose published his famous Colchester Survey (52), a milestone in the history of mental retardation, showing a 20% excess of males in a hospital sample of 1280 mentally retarded individuals. He attributed this unexpected observation to ascertainment bias, demonstrating that even the great Penrose could be mistaken, as we shall see in a moment. Again, 25 years later, he wrote in *The Biology of Mental Defect* that " ... in general, the genes on the X chromosome do not play any greater part in the causation of mental defect than might be supposed from the fact that there are 22 autosomes to one sex chromosome in man ... The conclusion may be drawn that there is no outstanding tendency for sex-linked genes to influence the genetics of mental deficiency" (53, p. 127). The statement is more surprising if one considers that at that time Penrose must have been aware of several maternally transmitted XLMR conditions, including the Martin–Bell syndrome (54), which is now considered the archetype of XLMR. Martin and Bell's report of 1943 is of historical value per se and also for the demonstration, almost 40 years later, that surviving members of the family were positive for the fragile X test (55), proving beyond doubt that the Martin–Bell and the fragile X syndrome are one and the same condition. Other families of historical value are described by Allan et al. (56), whose affected members were known as the "limbernecks" of rural North Carolina, and that described by Dr. Renpenning when he was a medical student at the University of Saskatchewan (57). Curiously, the

Renpenning syndrome, which is distinctively characterized by microcephaly and short stature, was considered for a period of time the prototype of XLMR, and, as such, confused with the Martin–Bell syndrome, usually characterized by macrocephaly and tall stature.

In 1965, Reed and Reed published their famous book *Mental Retardation: A Family Study* (58), again missing the opportunity to provide an explanation for the excess of males in their sample of retarded subjects. However, they did make an interesting observation, namely that 9.1% of offspring of mentally retarded males and their mates with normal or unknown intelligence were mentally retarded, whereas this percentage rose to 19.4% in offspring of mentally retarded women mating with males of normal or unknown intelligence. It took almost another decade before Robert Lehrke came up with the correct interpretation of the phenomenon, attributing it to the existence of genes on the X chromosome, the mutation of which causes mental deficit, more likely to be expressed in the hemizygous males than in the heterozygous females (59). As a graduate student of John Opitz, he had access to XLMR families that were studied at the University of Wisconsin, and that also led to the definition of several specific syndromes, such as the FG syndrome (60), the Waisman–Laxova syndrome (61), the W syndrome (62), and others.

In 1969, Lubs (63) reported on a marker X chromosome, characterized by a secondary constriction near the end of the long arm, in the affected males of an XLMR family. Retrospectively, it turned out to be the first example of a chromosome fragile site, and it was destined to identify the most common XLMR condition, the fragile X syndrome. The emergence of this condition, with its relatively high prevalence and peculiar association with a chromosome fragile site, attracted considerable interest in the field, which in turn facilitated the discovery of the responsible gene, *FMR1*, in 1991 (64). This can be considered a significant date in the history of genetics, not only of the genetics of mental retardation, because the mutation of *FMR1* is the first example of an unstable mutation, soon to be followed by several others. Work on other forms of XLMR has also been intense in recent years, leading to the tentative identification of more than 200 genes, several of which have already been cloned (65). A more detailed account of the history of XLMR was recently published by Neri and Opitz (66).

VIII. CONCLUSIONS

Several genes have been identified as responsible for "pure" forms of mental retardation and one may hope that understanding their function at a molecular level may shed light not only on the mechanisms causing mental retardation, but also on those leading to normal intelligence. Whether this prediction will turn out to be true, or not, is anybody's guess. One may have reason to be doubtful in view of the fact that intelligence is too complex a trait to be presently defined in epistemically valid terms, ultimately conducive to its explanation as a heritable character, no matter how complex. Any definition of intelligence, and all methods devised so far for its measurement, are laden by cultural biases. Moreover, we find it generally hazardous to infer the effect of a normal gene from its mutant. This is not like intimating that, in genetic terms, intelligence is impossible to define and therefore to analyze, although one must admit that intelligence would be a very peculiar character, different from other heritable traits in its being heavily conditioned by nurture. If we think for a minute, we must concede that intelligence, as a biological character, can only be understood by the intelligence of those who are devoted to these kinds of studies. In other words, intelligence must understand itself! It is therefore possible that the ultimate definition of human intelligence resides outside the realm of experimental science. However, before we reach that conclusion, there is a long way to go. The path will be punctuated by the discovery of all human genes, the understanding of their integrated functions, and by a clearer picture of the true relationship between genotype and phenotype. At that point, we may still be unable to define intelligence, but at least we shall know whether this fascinating and most peculiarly human trait can be better understood through a reductionist explanation or, as we rather suspect, only by means of an organicistic approach.

REFERENCES

1. Galton F. Hereditary Genius: An Inquiry into its Laws and Consequences. London: Macmillan, 1869.

2. Resta RG. Genetic drift: whispered hints. Am J Med Genet 1995; 59:131–133.

3. Galton F. Memories of My Life. London: Methuen, 1909:244.

4. Galton F. Statistical inquiries into the efficacy of prayer. Fortnightly Rev 1872; 12:125–135.

5. Gillham NW. A Life of Sir Francis Galton. New York: Oxford University Press, 2001:348.

6. Gould SJ. The Mismeasure of Man. New York: WW Norton and Co, 1996.

7. Spearman C. General intelligence objectively determined and measured. Am J Psychol 1904; 15:201–293.

8. Burt C. Experimental tests of general intelligence. Br J Psychol 1909; 3:94–177.

9. Hearnshaw LS. Cyril Burt Psychologist. London: Hodder and Stoughton, 1979.

10. Goddard HH. Mental tests and the immigrant. J Delinquency 1917; 2:243–277.

11. Yerkes RM. ed. Psychological Examining in the United States Army. Memoirs of the National Academic Science. Washington, DC: US. Government Printing Office, 1921; 15:1–890.

12. Hernstein RJ, Murray C. The Bell Curve: The Reshaping of American Life by Difference in Intelligence. New York: Free Press, 1994.

13. Scheerenberger RC. A History of Mental Retardation. Baltimore, London: Paul Brooks Publishing, 1983.

14. Dunn PM. Dr. Langdon Down (1828–1896) and "mongolism". Arch Dis Child 1991; 66:827–828.

15. Down JLH. Observations on an ethnic classification of idiots. London Hospital Rep 1866; 3:259–262.

16. Berg JM, Korossy M. Down syndrome before Down: a retrospect. Am J Med Genet 2001; 102:205–211.

17. Séguin E. Idiocy and Its Treatment by the Physiological Method. New York: William Wood and Co., 1866.

18. Mirkinson AE. Is Down's syndrome a modern disease? Lancet 1968; 2:103.

19. Richards BW. Is Down's syndrome a modern disease? Lancet 1968; 2:353–354.

20. Zellweger H. Is Down's syndrome a modern disease? Lancet 1968; 2:458.

21. Levitas AS, Reid CS. An angel with Down syndrome in a sixteenth century flamish nativity painting. Am J Med Genet 2003; 116A:339–405.

22. Dobson R. Is painting earliest portrayal of Down's syndrome? Br Med J 2003; 326:126.

23. Lejeune J, Gautier M, Turpin R. Études des chromosomes somatiques de neuf enfants mongoliens. C R Acad Sci 1959; 248:1721.

24. Smith GF, Berg J. The biological significance of Mongolism. Br J Psychiat 1974; 125:537–541.

25. Waardenburg PJ. Das menschliche Auge und seine Erbanlagen. The Hauge: Martinus Nijhoff, 1932.

26. Bleyer A. Indications that mongoloid imbecility is a gametic mutation of degenerate type. Am J Dis Child 1934; 47:342.

27. Lubinsky MS. Sir A.E. Garrod, Congential heart disease in Down syndrome, and the doctrine of fetal endocarditis. Am J Med Genet 1991; 40:27–30.

28. Lejeune J. Pathogenesis of mental deficiency in trisomy 21. Am J Med Genet 1990; suppl. 7:20–30.

29. Epstein CJ. The consequences of chromosomal imbalance. Am J Med Genet 1990; suppl. 7:31–37.

30. Opitz JM, Gilbert-Barnes EF. Reflections on the pathogenesis of Down syndrome. Am J Med Genet 1990; suppl. 7:38–52.

31. Epstein CJ. The Consequences of Chromosome Imbalance. Principles, Mechanisms, and Models. Cambridge: Cambridge University Press, 1986.

32. Epstein CJ. 2001 William Allan Award Address: From Down syndrome to the "human" in "Human Genetics". Am J Hum Genet 2002; 70:300–313.

33. Miller RJ. The ups and downs of Down's syndrome. Lancet 2002; 359:275–276.

34. Reeves RH. A complicated genetic insult. The Lancet 2001; 358(suppl):s23.

35. Antonarakis SE. 10 years of *Genomics*, chromosome 21, and Down syndrome. Genomics 1998; 51:1–16.

36. Hattori M, Fujiyama A, Taylor TD, et al. The DNA sequence of human chromosome 21. Nature 2000; 405:311–319.

37. Scriver CR. Garrod's foresight; Our hindsight. J Inherit Metab Dis 2001; 24:93–116.

38. Scheerenberger RC. A History of Mental Retardation: A Quarter Century of Promise. Baltimore, London: Paul Brooks Publishing, 1987.

39. Seymour CA, Thomason MJ, Chalmers RA, et al. Newborn screening for inborn errors of metabolism: a systematic review. Health Technol Assessment 1997; 1(11).

40. Scriver CR. Why mutation analysis does not always predict clinical consequences: explanations in the era of genomics. J Pediat 2002; 140:502–506.

41. Fölling A. Excretion of phenylpyruvic acid in urine as a metabolic anomaly in connection to imbecility. Nord Med Tidskr 1934; 8:1054–1059.

42. Centerwall SA, Centerwall WR. The discovery of phenylketonuria: the story of a young couple, two retarded children, and a scientist. Pediatrics 2000; 105:89–103.

43. Penrose LS. Phenylketonuria—a problem in eugenics. An Hum Genet 1998; 62:193–202 (original paper in: Lancet 1946; 29: 949–953).

44. National Institute of Health Consensus Development Panel. National Institute of Health Consensus Development Conference Statement: Phenylketonuria: screening and management, October 16–18, 2000. Pediatrics 2001; 108:972–982.

45. Bickel H. The first treatment of phenylketonuria. Eur J Pediatr 1996; 155(suppl 1):S2–S3.

46. Weglage J, Fündres B, Ullrich K, et al. Psychosocial aspects in phenylketonuria. Eur J Pediatr 1996; 155(suppl 1):S101–S104.

47. Bugard P, Rupp A, Konecki DS, et al. Phenylalanine hydroxylase genotypes, predicted residual enzyme activity and phenotypic parameters of diagnosis and treatment of phenylketonuria. Eur J Pediatr 1996; 155(suppl 1):s11–s15.

48. Guthrie R. The introduction of newborn screening for phenylketonuria: a personal history. Eur J Pediatr 1996; 155(suppl 1): s4–s5.

49. Woo SLC, Lidsky AS, Güttler F, et al. Cloned human phenylalanine hydroxylase gene allows prenatal detection of classical phenylketonuria. Nature 1983; 306:151–155.

50. Scriver CR, Waters PJ. Monogenic traits are not simple: lessons from phenylketonuria. Trends Genet 1999; 15:267–272.

51. Scriver CR. What ever happened to PKU? Clin Biochem 1995; 28:137–144.

52. Penrose LS. Clinical and Genetic Study of 1,280 Cases of Mental Defect: Special Report Series 229. Medical Research Council. London: Her Majesty's Stationery Office, 1938.

53. Penrose LS. The Biology of Mental Defect. 3rd ed. London: Sidgwick and Jackson Limited, 1963.

54. Martin JP, Bell J. A pedigree of mental defect showing sex linkage. J Neurol Psych 1943; 6:154–157.

55. Richards BW, Sylvester PE, Brooker C. Fragile X-linked mental retardation: The Martin–Bell syndrome. J Ment Defic Res 1981; 4:253–256.

56. Allan W, Herndon CN, Dudley FC. Some examples of the inheritance of mental deficiency: apparently sex-linked idiocy and microcephaly. Am J Ment Defic 1944; 48:325–334.

57. Renpenning H, Gerrard JW, Zaleski WA, Tabata T. Familial sex-linked mental retardation. Can Med Assoc J 1962; 87: 954–956.

58. Reed EW, Reed SC. Mental Retardation: A Family Study. Philadelphia: WB Saunders, 1965.

59. Lehrke RG. X-linked mental retardation and verbal disability. Birth Defects 1974; 10:1–100.

60. Opitz JM, Kaveggia EG. Studies of malformation syndromes in man XXXIII: the FG-syndrome. An X-linked recessive syndrome of multiple congenital anomalies and mental retardation. Z Kinderheilk 1974; 117:1–18.

61. Laxova R, Brown ES, Hogan K, et al. An X-linked recessive basal ganglia disorder with mental retardation. Am J Med Genet 1985; 21:681–689.

62. Pallister PD, Herrmann J, Spranger JW, et al. The W syndrome. Birth Defects 1974; 10:51–60.

63. Lubs HA. A marker X chromosome. Am J Hum Genet 1969; 21:231–244.

64. Verkerk AJMH, Pieretti M, Sutcliffe JS, et al. Identification of a gene (FMR-1) containing a CGG repeat coincident with a breakpoint cluster region exhibiting length variation in fragile X syndrome. Cell 1991; 65:905–914.

65. Chiurazzi P, Hamel BC, Neri G. XLMR genes: update 2000. Eur J Hum Genet 2001; 9:71–81.

66. Neri G, Opitz JM. Sixty years of mental retardation: A historical footnote. Am J Med Genet (Semin Med Genet) 2000; 97:228–233.

2

Patterns of Inheritance: Mendelian and Non-Mendelian

MERLIN G. BUTLER, MICHAEL BEGLEITER, SHANNON LILLIS, and MOLLY LUND

Section of Medical Genetics and Molecular Medicine, Children's Mercy Hospitals and Clinics, University of Missouri–Kansas City School of Medicine, Kansas City, Missouri, U.S.A.

F. JOHN MEANEY

Department of Pediatrics, University of Arizona College of Medicine, Tucson, Arizona, U.S.A.

I. INTRODUCTION AND TERMINOLOGY

The field of medical genetics has as its overall goal the detection and treatment of pathologic genetic variation. In effect, it focuses on genetic disorders and diseases to which genetic factors contribute significantly. Genetic disorders refer to numerous syndromes and single gene conditions, as well as birth defects of known genetic etiology. Genetic diseases refer to common diseases that are known to have significant genetic

35

involvement such as cardiovascular disease, cancer, and diabetes. Hereafter, we will use the phrase "genetic diseases" to address both entities unless there is cause to distinguish between disorders and diseases or we are referring to diseases involving both genetic and environmental risk factors, such as multifactorial diseases.

Genetic diseases contribute significantly to morbidity and mortality at all ages. Since 3% of newborns have major birth defects and about one-third of all pediatric and about 10% of adult hospital admissions are due to genetically related disorders and diseases, physicians are frequently responsible for diagnosis, screening, and genetic counseling. There are three main categories of genetic diseases: single gene, chromosomal, and multifactorial.

To understand the principles by which diseases are inherited, we need to define and clarify several specific terms. For example, a genetic *locus* is a specific position or location on a chromosome frequently referred to as a *gene* which is a unique DNA sequence encoding the message for a protein. *Alleles* are alternative forms of a gene or segment of DNA at a specific locus. When both alleles at a locus are identical, the individual is *homozygous* at that locus. If the alleles are different, he or she is *heterozygous*. Such individuals are *homozygotes* or *heterozygotes*, respectively. An individual with two different mutant alleles at a given locus is referred to as a *compound heterozygote*, while an individual with one mutant allele at each of two different loci is referred to as a *double heterozygote*. The *genotype* is the genetic make-up of a single individual, while the *phenotype* is the observed result or outcome of the interaction of the genotype with the environment.

There are examples in which genes may have more than two allelic forms, referred to as multiple alleles. Multiple alleles may result from a normal gene having mutated into a number of different alleles. An example is the ABO blood group system whereby four alleles exist (A1, A2, B and O). An individual can possess any two of these alleles (e.g., AO, AB, OO, etc.) which results in a specific blood type.

Single gene traits are often called *Mendelian* because of the work carried out by Gregor Mendel on the inheritance of certain traits in garden peas reported in the mid-1800s. Mendel's work led to four major conclusions: (1) genes come in pairs with one member of each pair inherited from each parent; (2) individual genes can have different forms or alleles with the dominant allele exerting its effect over other forms and referred to as the *principle of dominance*. Those characters which are unchanged or received in their entirety during hybridization are termed dominant and those which become latent in the process are called recessive; (3) *principle of segregation* or alleles segregate or separate from others in meiosis or during germ cell development when each gamete receives only one allele from each parent; and (4) *principle of independent assortment* in which the segregation of different pairs of alleles is independent from each other. Although modified slightly from the early studies with garden peas, these principles are useful today in understanding medical genetics and the inheritance of genetic traits and human genetic diseases.

The online version of *Mendelian Inheritance in Man* (OMIM) is continually updated by Dr. Victor McKusick and his staff, and available through the World Wide Web. OMIM lists more than 10,000 genes of which at least 1500 are established as gene loci and mutations found associated with genetic diseases. Of the estimated 30,000–50,000 known human genes, more than 3% have been identified currently as contributing to human disease in a major way. New genes and their mutations leading to diseases are identified daily. Table 1 shows a partial list of genetic diseases categorized by group with approximate prevalence for each disease.

Mendelian diseases are grouped into *autosomal* if they are encoded by genes on one of the 22 pairs of autosomes, or nonsex chromosomes, and *X-linked* if encoded by a mutant gene on the X chromosome, one of the two sex chromosomes. As Mendel described with garden peas, there are two types: *dominant* and *recessive*. *Dominant* refers to those conditions that are expressed in heterozygotes or individuals having one copy of a mutant allele and one copy of a normal, or wild-type allele. *Recessive* refers to those conditions that clinically manifest only in individuals homozygous for the mutant

Table 1   A Partial List of Genetic Diseases

Disease	Approximate Prevalence
Chromosome Abnormalities	
Angelman syndrome	1/20,000
Cri du chat syndrome	1/25,000
DiGeorge/VCFS	1/5,000
Down syndrome	1/1,000
Klinefelter syndrome	1/1,000 males
Prader-Willi syndrome	1/15,000
Trisomy 13	1/15,000
Trisomy 18	1/6,000 (3:1 female to male ratio)
Turner syndrome	1/2,500 females
Williams syndrome	1/10,000
Single-Gene Disorders	
Adenomatous polyposis coli	1/6,000
Adult-polycystic kidney disease	1/1,000
Albinism	1/10,000 to 1/30,000
α-1-Antitrypsin deficiency	1/2,500 to 1/10,000 Caucasians
Charcot-Marie-Tooth disease	1/2,500
Congenital adrenal hyperplasia	1/50,000
Cystic fibrosis	1/2,500 Caucasians
Duchenne muscular dystrophy	1/3,500 males
Familial hypercholesterolemia	1/500
Fragile X syndrome	1/1,500 males; 1/2,500 females
Galactosemia	1/50,000
Hemochromatosis (hereditary; symptomatic)	1/5,000
Hemophilia A	1/10,000 males
Hereditary nonpolyposis colorectal cancer	1/200
Homocystinuria	1/50,000
Huntington disease	1/20,000
Marfan syndrome	1/10,000 to 1/20,000
Myotonic dystrophy	1/20,000
Neurofibromatosis type I	1/3,000 to 1/5,000
Noonan syndrome	1/2,500
Osteogenesis imperfecta	1/5,000 to 1/10,000
Phenylketonuria	1/15,000
Polydactyly	1/1,000 whites; 1/100 African-Americans
Retinitis pigmentosa	1/5,000
Retinoblastoma	1/20,000

(Continued)

Table 1   A Partial List of Genetic Diseases (*Continued*)

Disease	Approximate Prevalence
Retts syndrome	1/15,000
Sickle cell disease	1/400 to 1/600 African-Americans
Tay-Sachs disease	1/3,000 Ashkenazi Jews
Thalassemia	1/50 to 1/100 (Asians and Mediterraneans)
Tuberous sclerosis	1/25,000
Multifactorial Disorders	
Congenital malformations	
Cleft lip with/without cleft palate	1/500 to 1/1,000
Club foot (talipes equinovarus)	1/1,000
Congenital heart defects	1/200
Neural tube defects (spina bifida, anencephaly)	1/500 to 1/1,000
Pyloric stenosis	1/300
Adult diseases	
Alcoholism	1/10 to 1/20
Alzheimer disease	1/10 (Americans over age 65)
Bipolar affective disorder	1/100 to 1/200
Cancer (all types)	1/3
Diabetes (types I and II)	1/10
Heart disease/stroke	1/3 to 1/5
Schizophrenia	1/100
Mitochondrial Diseases	
Kearnes-Sayre disease	Rare
Leber hereditary optic neuropathy (LHON)	Rare
Mitochondrial encephalopathy, lactic acidosis, and stroke-like episodes (MELAS)	Rare
Myoclonic epilepsy and ragged-red fiber disease (MERRF)	Rare
Neuropathy, ataxia, and retinitis pigmentosa (NARP)	Rare

allele and carry a double dose or two copies of the abnormal gene. Most dominant genes code for structural proteins while recessive genes code for enzymes or regulatory proteins. Of the 8000 human phenotypes that are known to be inherited in a Mendelian fashion, more than one-half are classified as autosomal dominant, about one-third are autosomal recessive, and about one-tenth are X-linked.

The patterns of inheritance of most Mendelian traits have been learned through the observation of the segregation of transmission of traits within families. An important reason for studying the pattern of inheritance of conditions within families is to advise members of a particular family through genetic counseling about recurrence risks or the chance that the genetic disease would be passed to their children. Generally, dominant conditions are passed on at a 50% risk while recessive conditions are passed on at a 25% risk.

To apply the principles of medical genetics and in making a genetic diagnosis for accurate genetic counseling, the taking of a family history or pedigree is important. A family history is a shorthand method whereby pertinent information about a family is obtained from a family historian or a member of the family knowledgeable about previous generations, family relationships, and health status of other family members required to obtain and record an accurate pedigree chart. The person bringing the family to medical attention is referred to as the *index case*, or *proband*. The position or location of the proband in the family tree is indicated by an arrow.

The mode of inheritance can often be established as a result of constructing and reviewing the family history and pedigree. There are certain characteristics present when one reviews a pedigree that would indicate a specific mode of inheritance. For example, there are three specific features of an autosomal dominant pedigree: (1) males and females are equally affected; (2) more than one generation identified with affected members giving the impression of a *vertical* transmission of inheritance; and (3) all forms of transmission between sexes are observed, i.e., male to male (which rules out X-linkage), female to female, male to female, or female to male. Three features that may be observed in autosomal recessive inheritance include: males and females equally affected, usually only one generation involved (i.e., brothers and sisters affected) giving a *horizontal* pattern of inheritance, and consanguinity (or inbreeding). Three features seen in X-linked recessive inheritance may include: males are exclusively affected, unaffected carrier females will pass the genetic disease to sons giving a *diagonal* inheritance pattern (i.e., uncles and nephews affected), and affected males cannot transmit the genetic disease to their sons (fathers pass the Y chromosome to their sons and the X chromosome to their daughters). Three features necessary to establish X-linked dominant inheritance include: both males and females affected but the number of affected females in the pedigree may be twice the number of affected males and females are generally less severely affected than males, and affected females can transmit the genetic disease to male and female offspring but affected males can only transmit the disease to their daughters. A more specific and detailed description of these inheritance patterns will be illustrated and discussed later in the chapter.

The three major categories of genetic diseases are single gene diseases (autosomal dominant, autosomal recessive, and X-linked recessive or dominant); chromosomal; and multifactorial. Multifactorial causes (combination of genetic and environment factors) account for about two-thirds to three-fourths of the morbidity and mortality due to genetic diseases and will be discussed in separate chapters. These conditions include, for example, diabetes, hypertension, heart disease, cancer, obesity, and idiopathic mental retardation.

In addition to the typical Mendelian forms of inheritance, non-Mendelian forms of inheritance do occur and are significant causes of morbidity and mortality as well as for developmental delay and mental retardation. There are at least three non-Mendelian forms of inheritance: mitochondrial, genomic imprinting, and trinucleotide repeats. Mitochondrial diseases are due to mutations of the mitochondrial genome found in the cytoplasm and present in every cell. These diseases vary in age of onset and severity. The mitochondrial genome is inherited from the mother, and thus, is maternally transmitted. Mitochondrial DNA mutations are increasingly recognized as playing a role in neurological and muscle dysfunction. The mutations generally impact on energy expenditure and cellular metabolism and individually are rare but collectively account for an increased number of recognized diseases and pathophysiology. Mitochondrial diseases will be discussed in more detail elsewhere.

Genomic imprinting is the differential expression of genetic information depending on the parent of origin. The first examples reported in humans were Prader–Willi and Angelman syndromes, two separate clinical disorders which share the same chromosome 15 anomaly. The most common chromosome defect in these syndromes is a de novo interstitial chromosome 15q deletion (paternally derived in Prader–Willi syndrome and maternally derived in Angelman syndrome). There are several genes that are paternally expressed (maternally imprinted or inactivated) on the 15q11–q13 region, which are candidates for causing Prader–Willi syndrome, while a single maternally expressed (paternally imprinted) gene (i.e., UBE3A) causes Angelman syndrome. Specific genes are under the control of an imprinting center in the 15q11–q13 region that inactivates the genes through methylation. Therefore, instead of both members of the gene pair being active, which is true for most genes, imprinted genes are inactivated on one homologue of the chromosome pair depending on the parent of origin. Therefore, loss of the chromosome region (maternal or paternal) through a deletion process would impact on expression of imprinted genes in the region causing the two separate syndromes. Genomic imprinting also plays a role in other syndromes and in certain malignancies as discussed elsewhere in this chapter.

Several disorders (e.g., fragile X syndrome, Huntington disease, myotonic dystrophy) are due to trinucleotide or triplet repeats. These disorders are caused when the number of repeating units of a trinucleotide in a particular gene expands beyond a certain threshold and interferes with gene expression or function. The size of the repeat may vary from generation to generation in a family. Individuals may have a "premutation" in which there is a moderate expansion of the number of triplet repeats that causes no phenotypic effect. But these individuals are at a risk of the repeats undergoing further expansion in their gamete production leadingto a "full mutation" in the genes in an offspring. Trinucleotide repeat disorders will be described in more detail elsewhere.

II. FAMILY HISTORY AND PEDIGREE

The record of a family history is simplified by sketching a pedigree obtained from an individual knowledgeable about the family history and health status of individuals within the family. It is important to recognize consanguinity, the ethnic backgrounds within the family, and the health status and findings of first-degree relatives (parents, sibs, and offspring) and other members in the family over three generations. Accurate family history information is vital for diagnosis, genetic counseling, and medical management of patients with genetic diseases. Symbols commonly used in drawing pedigrees are shown in Fig. 1.

III. AUTOSOMAL DOMINANT

Autosomal dominant inheritance accounts for the largest number of genetic diseases despite the presence of a normal gene product made from the normal gene allele. Dominant genes generally code for structural protein such as connective tissue (e.g., collagen). In theory, a condition is inherited in an autosomal dominant manner when it is expressed in the same way in both heterozygotes and homozygotes. In practice, any phenotype expressed in the heterozygous state is dominant. There are over 5000 recognized autosomal dominant conditions and some are quite common. For example, adult polycystic kidney disease has a frequency of 1 in 1000 and familial hypercholesterolemia occurs in 1 of every 500 people. Table 2 lists examples of autosomal dominant conditions.

Most commonly, an individual affected with an autosomal dominant trait is the product of a mating between a normal parent and an affected parent. Students beginning their study of genetics learn to draw Punnett squares to help understand the segregation of genes in the egg and sperm. The Punnett square shown in Fig. 2 illustrates the possible results of the mating between a normal parent and an affected parent. The affected parent passes either the normal gene or the dominant disease gene to the offspring. The

Pedigree Symbols

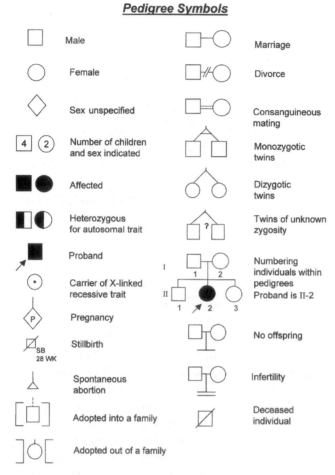

Figure 1 Symbols used for construction of family pedigrees.

unaffected parent passes on a normal gene. Thus, there is a 50% chance of having an unaffected child with a homozygous normal genotype and a 50% chance of having an affected child with a heterozygous disease-causing genotype. When two individuals affected with an autosomal dominant condition conceive a child, there is a 1 in 4 or 25% of having a child who is homozygous for the disease gene. Typically, autosomal dominant conditions are more severe in the less common homozygous state than in the heterozygote state.

Table 2 Examples of Autosomal Dominant Conditions

Autosomal Dominant Disorders	Approximate Prevalence	Chromosome Location	Gene Symbol
Achondroplasia	1/15,000–1/40,000	4p16.3	FGFR3
Craniosynostosis syndromes			
Apert syndrome	1/100,000	10q26	FGFR2
Crouzon syndrome	1/60,000	10q26, 4p16.3	FGFR2, FGFR3
Pfeiffer syndrome	1/100,000	8p11.2–p11.1, 10q26, 4p16.3	FGFR1, FGFR2, FGFR3
Saethre-Chotzen syndrome	~1/100,000	7p21, 10q26, 4p16.3	TWIST, FGFR2, FGFR3
Huntington disease	1/20,000	4p16.3	IT15
Marfan syndrome	1/5,000–1/10,000	15q21.1	FBN1
Noonan syndrome	1/1,000–1/2,500	12q24.1	PTPN11
Neurofibromatosis type 1	1/3,000–1/5,000	17q11.2	NF1
Neurofibromatosis type 2	1/33,000–1/40,000	22q12.2	NF2
Tuberous sclerosis	1/25,000	9q34, 16p13.3	TSC1, TSC2

Affected Father

	Paternal Allele A	Paternal Allele a
Maternal Allele a	Aa	aa
Maternal Allele a	Aa	aa

(Unaffected Mother)

Figure 2   Punnett square illustrating the mating of an unaffected parent (**aa**) with a heterozygous parent affected with an autosomal dominant genetic disease (**Aa**).

For example, in achondroplasia, which is the most common form of dwarfism, most individuals are heterozygous. A homozygous affected child of two parents with achondroplasia is severely affected and often does not survive early infancy. The Punnett square in Fig. 3 shows the possibilities of a mating between two affected individuals in an autosomal dominant condition such as achondroplasia. As mentioned earlier, there is a 25% chance of having a homozygous affected child. There is also a 25% chance of having an unaffected child with homozygosity for the normal gene allele and a 50% chance of having a heterozygous child who will be affected like his or her parents.

There are several important characteristics of autosomal dominant traits that are illustrated in the pedigree shown in Fig. 4. First, autosomal dominant traits follow a vertical transmission pattern meaning that the condition is seen in each successive generation. There are no skipped generations and unaffected individuals do not pass on the condition. Second, each child of an affected parent has a 50% chance to be affected. Third, males and females are equally affected. A final hallmark of autosomal dominant traits is the possibility of male-to-male transmission. This is an important feature

Affected Father

	Paternal Allele A	Paternal Allele a
Maternal Allele A	AA	Aa
Maternal Allele a	Aa	aa

(Affected Mother — left axis label)

Figure 3 Punnett square illustrating the mating of two parents (**Aa**) affected with an autosomal dominant condition. Three of the four children would be affected.

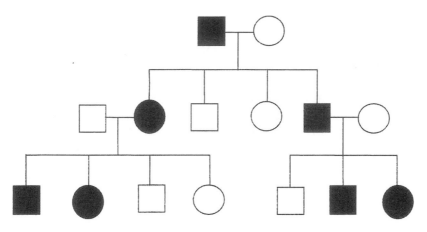

Figure 4 An example of a pedigree representing autosomal dominant inheritance. Note vertical pattern in three generations with affected males and females.

which distinguishes autosomal dominant traits from those that are X-linked.

There are some exceptions to the "rules" of autosomal dominant inheritance mentioned above. Some autosomal dominant genetic diseases do not clearly follow a vertical transmission pattern due to reduced penetrance. *Penetrance* is the probability that a disease gene will have a phenotypic expression. A trait is 100% penetrant if every individual with a disease-causing gene is affected and shows features of the autosomal dominant condition. Achondroplasia is an example of a condition with 100% penetrance. A genetic disease shows reduced penetrance when an individual who has the disease-causing gene does not exhibit the disease phenotype, but can still pass on the disease-causing gene to the next generation. The phenomenon of reduced penetrance is one explanation for a trait that seems to "skip" generations.

Variable expressivity can also cause confusion, because in this scenario the penetrance of a condition may be complete, but the phenotypic expression varies widely between families and family members. For example, tuberous sclerosis is an autosomal dominant condition that occurs in approximately 1 in 25,000 births. The phenotype can vary between a severely affected infant with seizures and mental retardation to an adult who has never had a seizure but has the classical cutaneous and brain imaging findings. Other autosomal dominant conditions that have variable expressivity include neurofibromatosis and osteogenesis imperfecta. Figure 5 shows a patient who has two autosomal dominant conditions (tuberous sclerosis and neurofibromatosis with features of tuberous sclerosis clearly seen in the patient). These genetic diseases also illustrate the concept of *pleiotropy* or when a disease-causing gene causes a wide range or diverse effects on various organ systems. Tuberous sclerosis is a pleiotropic genetic disease because it affects various organs including the brain, heart, kidneys, and skin.

An autosomal dominant condition can also be due to a new mutation or an alteration in the genetic code that disrupts the function of the gene in the sperm or egg which produces a child with an autosomal dominant condition. In this situation,

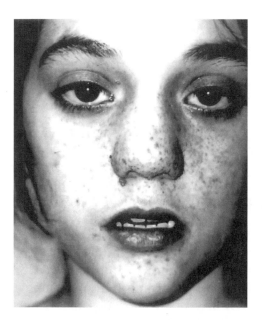

Figure 5 Eleven-year-old female with two autosomal dominant genetic diseases (neurofibromatosis type I and tuberous sclerosis). Note the adenoma sebaceous over her face.

neither parent is affected with the condition and there is no history of affected family members. Once the mutated gene is passed to the offspring, then there will be a 50% risk for the autosomal dominant condition to be passed to the next generation. In some autosomal dominant conditions (e.g., neurofibromatosis, achondroplasia), there is a high probability (e.g., 90% for achondroplasia) of an affected offspring born to unaffected parents due to a new or de novo mutation. There is a correlation with older paternal age and de novo mutations for autosomal dominant conditions to occur in their children.

In some instances, a normal appearing parent can have more than one child affected with an autosomal dominant condition. A possible explanation may be *germline mosaicism* whereby a parent carries the autosomal dominant disease-causing gene in some percentage of their germ cells, but not in their somatic cells. Because the disease-causing gene is only present in the germ cells the parent is not affected with the condition but can pass the condition on to his or her children. Obviously, germline mosaicism has significant implications for recurrence risks in a family and for genetic counseling.

IV. AUTOSOMAL RECESSIVE

One of the classical modes of inheritance for human genetic diseases is autosomal recessive which accounts for over 4000 recognized single gene genetic diseases. Recessive genes generally code for regulatory proteins such as enzymes and frequently produce metabolic or biochemical problems in affected individuals. The term autosomal recessive refers to a pattern of inheritance which requires two copies of the mutant allele in order for an individual to exhibit phenotypic effects. Autosomal recessive inheritance is characterized by the presence of the gene on an autosome (chromosomes 1 through 22) and not on the X or Y or sex chromosome. A horizontal transmission, i.e., affected individuals in only one generation, is frequently observed. There is an equal occurrence in males and females. The parents are unaffected unless the trait is very common. The recurrence risk is 1 in 4 or 25%. In addition, there is increased incidence of consanguinity found for rare recessive traits (i.e., the rarer the recessive condition the more likely the parents are related). A Punnett square demonstrating autosomal recessive inheritance from two unaffected parents in which each carries a recessive allele (**a**) is shown in Fig. 6.

Each pregnancy for this couple (**Aa** × **Aa**) carries a 1 in 4 probability of producing a child who is homozygous dominant (**AA**), a 1 in 2 chance of producing a child who is heterozygous (**Aa**), and a 1 in 4 chance of producing a child who is homozygous recessive (**aa**) and affected with the recessive condition in question. There is a 2/3 chance that an unaffected sibling is a carrier of the recessive gene in the family [the three genetic possibilities for an unaffected sibling would be **AA**, **Aa**, or **Aa** (**aa** would indicate an affected homozygous recessive individual), therefore, two of the three possibilities would be **Aa** or an unaffected (carrier) status for an autosomal recessive genetic disease]. Autosomal recessive inheritance is

Unaffected Father

		Paternal Allele A	Paternal Allele a
Maternal Allele A		AA	Aa
Maternal Allele a		Aa	aa

Figure 6 Punnett square illustrating autosomal recessive inheritance from two unaffected heterozygous parents.

particularly confusing for parents of affected individuals. They frequently will ask, "How can this condition be genetic if my affected child is the only person in the family with this problem?" As demonstrated in the Punnett square, affected individuals are almost always born to unaffected parents. If the condition occurs fairly frequently or the family has multiple instances of inbreeding or consanguineous marriages, one might see other affected individuals in an extended kindred.

Genetic heterogeneity refers to the development of the same or a similar phenotype by different genetic mechanisms and specifically addresses autosomal recessive conditions. For example, the genetics of hearing loss can represent genetic heterogeneity whereby dozens of recessive genes can lead to hearing loss. Additionally, through assortative or nonrandom mating a mate is selected with preference for a particular trait e.g., hearing loss, and genetic heterogeneity may exist. If both parents have the same autosomal recessive gene causing hearing loss, then all of their children would be anticipated to be affected with hearing loss (i.e., each parent would donate a recessive allele). Often hearing loss is not

present in children born to parents with hearing loss even
though the parents have an autosomal recessive form of hearing loss. This scenario can best be explained by both parents
not having the same recessive gene for hearing loss. Thus,
their children are unaffected but are carriers (heterozygous)
for two different recessive genes causing hearing loss.

Pedigrees of autosomal recessive conditions (as previously
noted) demonstrate horizontal transmission. An example of
such a pedigree is shown in Fig. 7. A list of autosomal recessive
conditions is found in Table 3. Figure 8 shows examples of classical oculocutaneous albinism in two children with different
ethnic backgrounds.

A. Consanguinity

The terms "consanguinity" and "inbreeding" are used by
geneticists to describe unions between two individuals who
share at least one ancestor in common. Since all individuals
in the general population carry silent mutant recessive genes
(e.g., on an average about six), which have the potential to
produce problems in the homozygous state, the union of relatives increases the probability that their offspring will be
homozygous by descent. A pedigree demonstrating a consanguineous union is shown in Fig. 9 .

Geneticists frequently calculate a *coefficient of inbreeding* which is the probability that any given gene locus is homozygous by descent from a common ancestor. Table 4 shows
coefficient of inbreeding for various parental relationships.

B. Genetic Counseling

Recently, the National Society of Genetic Counselors published recommendations for genetic counseling and screening
of consanguineous couples and their offspring (1). They estimate that the increased risk for congenital defects (above
the background risk) for the offspring of first cousin unions
is approximately 1.7–2.8%. It was also noted that there is
an approximately 4.4% increased risk for pre-reproductive
mortality (above the background population risk) for these
children. First cousins have 1/8 of their genes in common,

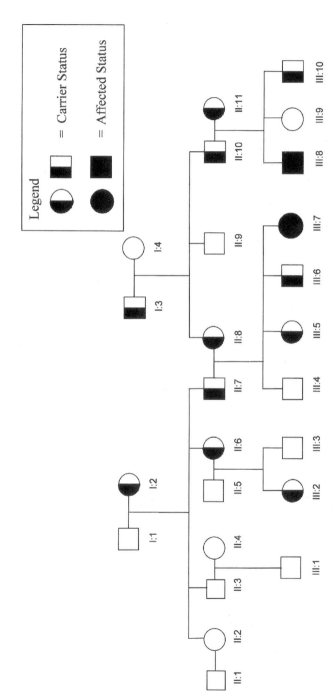

Figure 7 An example of a pedigree representing autosomal recessive inheritance. Note the horizontal pattern with affected males and females in one generation.

Table 3 Examples of Autosomal Recessive Conditions

Condition	Chromosomal Location	Gene Symbol	Incidence	Population Studied
Ataxia-telangiectasia	11q22.3	ATM	1/100,000	Michigan residents, USA
Cystic fibrosis	7q31.2	CFTR	1/2,500	American Whites
Galactosemia	9p13	GALT	1/47,000	American Whites
Gaucher disease	1q21	GBA	1/700	Ashkenazi Jews
Hemochromatosis	6p21.3	HFE	1/333	Utah residents, USA
Hurler syndrome (MPSI)	4p16.3	MPS1	1/100,000	Netherlands
Infantile polycystic kidneys	6p21.1p12	PKHD1	1.4/100,000	Spain
Oculocutaneous albinism (Types I and II)	11q14q21 15q11.2q12	OCA1 OCA2	1/23,500	British Columbia, Canada
Pendred syndrome	7q31	DFNB4	1/15,000	Great Britain
Phenylketonuria	12q24.1	PAH	1/10,000	Northern Europeans
Sickle cell disease	11p15.5	HBB	1/400	African-Americans

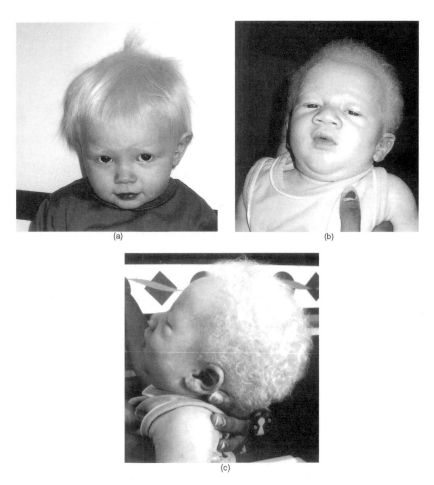

Figure 8 Two infants, ages 9 and 2 months, each affected with an autosomal recessive form of oculocutaneous albinism and from different ethnic backgrounds. (*See color insert.*)

second cousins have 1/32, and third cousins have 1/128. For couples less closely related than second cousins, the risk to their offspring for genetic diseases approaches that of the general population. First cousins may have more than one deleterious recessive gene and with 1/8 of their genes in common, their progeny on an average would then be homozygous at 1/16 of their gene loci. There are many examples of

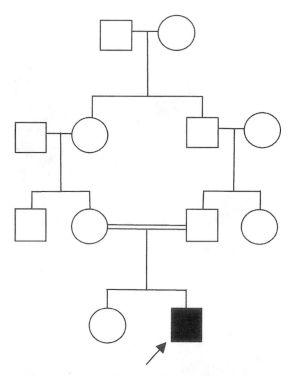

Figure 9 A typical pedigree demonstrating consanguinity or inbreeding from first cousin mating.

rare recessive conditions occurring in isolated genetic groups throughout the world. In Ashkenazi Jews in North America, the gene is very common for Tay–Sachs disease, a neurological degenerative genetic disease due to the absence of a specific lysosomal enzyme (hexoaminidase A). The frequency of this gene is 100 times higher in Ashkenazi Jews (1 in 3600) as compared with other populations (1 in 360,000).

Genetic counseling for consanguineous couples should begin with the collection of a detailed family history (as should all genetic counseling). If there is no history of individuals with genetic conditions, then the above risks are appropriate. If the family history identifies specific diagnoses, then the couple should be offered carrier testing if such testing is available. These couples should also be offered all of the usual

Table 4 Parental Relationships and Coefficient of Inbreeding

Parental Relationship	Coefficient of Inbreeding (F)
Father–daughter	1/4
Uncle–niece	1/8
First cousins	1/16
Second cousins	1/64
Third cousins	1/256

screening tests which are made available to all pregnant women. Consideration should also be given to expanded newborn screening.

V. X-LINKED INHERITANCE

A third inheritance pattern that occurs in genetic diseases is caused by genes on the X chromosome. This group of genetic diseases is referred to as X-linked. There is an unequal distribution of the X chromosomes between the sexes with males possessing one X chromosome (46,XY) and females having two X chromosomes (46,XX). This inequality causes X-linked conditions to have a characteristic sex distribution in families that is readily identifiable in most females when pedigrees are studied. Female carriers are usually unaffected, and males are affected. Table 5 lists several examples of X-linked conditions. Before reviewing the inheritance patterns of X-linked conditions, it is important to understand fundamental concepts related to X-linked inheritance.

Although males have only one copy of an X-linked gene and females have two copies, males and females generally have equal amounts of the proteins encoded for by these genes. In the 1960s, Dr. Mary Lyon proposed a mechanism to explain this "dosage compensation." This principle is known as X inactivation or the "Lyon" hypothesis. This hypothesis states that in females only one X chromosome in each somatic cell is active although recent evidence indicates that part of the inactive X chromosome remains active (2). The other X chromosome is inactivated and appears in interphase

Table 5 Examples of X-linked Disorders

X-linked Disorders	Approximate Prevalence	X-chromosome Location	Gene Symbol
Aarskog syndrome	Rare	Xp11	FDG1
Adrenoleukodystrophy	1/20,000–1/50,000	Xq28	ABCD1
Duchenne muscular dystrophy	1/3,500–1/5,600	Xp21.2	DMD
Fragile X syndrome	1/1,500 males, 1/2,500 females	Xq27.3	FMR1
Hemophilia A	1 in 4,000	Xq28	F8
Hunter syndrome	1 in 111,000	Xq28	IDS
Incontinentia pigmenti	rare	Xq28	IKBKG
Lesch-Nyhan syndrome	1/380,000	Xq26–Xq27.2	HPRT1
Lowe syndrome	1/30,000	Xq26.1	OCRL
Ornithine transcarbamylase (OTC) deficiency	1/10,000–1/15,000 (all urea cycle disorders)	Xp21.1	OTC
Rett syndrome	1/10,000–1/15,000	Xq28	MECP2

cells as a condensed sex chromatin or the "Barr body." Inactivation occurs in the first week of embryonic development. The inactivation process is random with either the paternal or maternal X inactivated. Once an X chromosome is inactivated in a cell, all of the descendents of that cell will have the same inactive X. Therefore, X inactivation is randomly determined but fixed for all future cells. As a result of X inactivation, females have two populations of cells. One population has an active paternal X chromosome and the other has an active maternal X chromosome. Females are "mosaics" for the X chromosome with two populations of cells. Males are not mosaics but are "hemizygous." They have only one X chromosome in each cell and that X remains active.

Because females have two copies of the X chromosome and males are hemizygous, most X-linked conditions are more common in males than females. Geneticists divide X-linked conditions into two categories depending on whether the X-linked gene is dominant or recessive which is based on the affected status of the females. In X-linked recessive conditions, female carriers are usually not affected but in the

X-linked dominant conditions females are consistently affected. Pedigrees for X-linked recessive genetic diseases have characteristics that are clearly distinguishable from autosomal dominant and recessive genetic diseases. These are illustrated by the pedigree in Fig. 10. Since a father can only transmit a Y chromosome to his sons, X-linked genes are not passed from father to son. Thus, male-to-male transmission is never seen in X-linked traits unlike autosomal dominant conditions. An affected father has no affected sons yet all of his daughters will be carriers of the X-linked condition. If a female carrier has a son, there is a 50% chance that he will be affected. If a female carrier has a daughter, there is a 50% that she will be a carrier. An X-linked recessive genetic

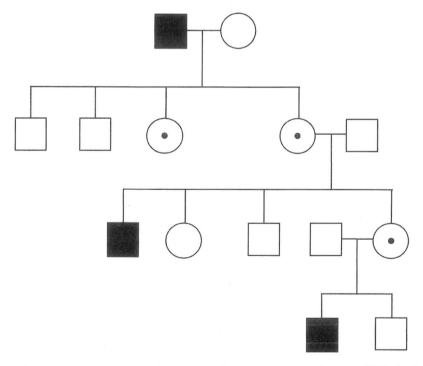

Figure 10 An example of a pedigree representing an X-linked recessive inheritance pattern. Note diagonal pattern (uncle and nephew) with only affected males. Designated carrier females are noted in the pedigree.

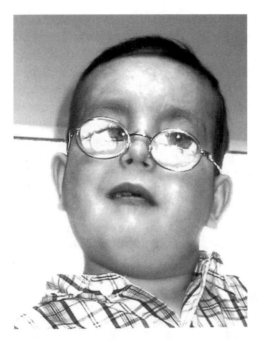

Figure 11 Eight-year-old male with Lowe or oculo-cerebro-renal syndrome, an X-linked recessive condition characterized by cataracts, central nervous system problems, and kidney abnormalities.

disease may be passed through generations of carrier females before it is expressed in a male. Thus, affected males in a family are related through females. Lowe or oculo-cerebro-renal syndrome (Fig. 11) is an example of an X-linked recessive condition which primarily affects the eyes, central nervous system, and kidneys. Affected males have congenital cataracts and impaired vision, and almost all affected males have some degree of intellectual impairment. They also have some degree of proximal tubular renal dysfunction. Lowe syndrome is caused by markedly reduced activity of the enzyme, inositol polyphosphate 5-phosphatase (OCRL-1) which is encoded by the OCRL gene.

A complicating factor in X-linked recessive conditions is the occurrence of manifesting heterozygotes. In some

X-linked conditions including hemophilia A, ornithine trans-carbamylase deficiency, Duchenne muscular dystrophy, and Wiskott–Aldrich syndrome, female carriers actually have some degree of clinical expression of the condition. This variable expression occurs due to "skewed" X inactivation or when the disease gene is located on the active X chromosome and the normal gene is located on the inactive X in all or most cells. The degree of expression by chance in a carrier female depends on the proportion of disease genes on the active X.

Genetic lethals can also result from genetic conditions, i.e., a gene or genetically determined trait that leads to failure to reproduce. A classical genetic lethal condition is Duchenne muscular dystrophy whereby the affected male generally dies from the condition before reproducing. Genetic analysis indicates that one-third of males with genetic lethal X-linked recessive conditions such as Duchenne muscular dystrophy are due to a new or de novo mutation and without a known family history for the genetic disease. If not for new mutations, the gene would not continue to be present in the human population.

As mentioned above, an X-linked condition is described as dominant if it is regularly expressed in female heterozygotes. Figure 12 shows the features of a pedigree with X-linked dominant inheritance. The distinguishing feature of an X-linked dominant condition is that all of the daughters and none of the sons of affected males are affected. If a daughter is unaffected or a male is affected, then the condition must be autosomally inherited. Each child of a female affected with an X-linked dominant condition has a 50% chance of being affected, just like an autosomal dominant trait. In rare X-linked dominant conditions like X-linked hypophosphatemic rickets, there are about twice as many affected females, but the females are usually more mildly affected due to their heterozygous state. Some X-linked dominant conditions like Rett syndrome and incontinentia pigmenti are prenatally lethal in males and only affected females are seen. A further in-depth review and summary of Mendelian causes of genetic diseases can be found elsewhere (3,4).

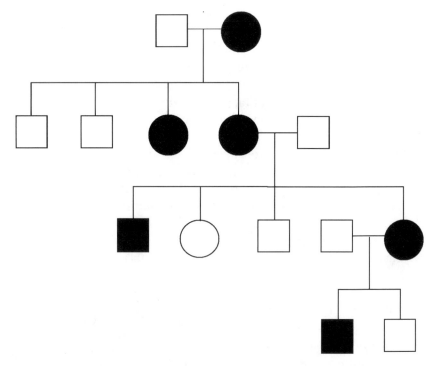

Figure 12 An example of a pedigree representing X-linked dominant inheritance. Note vertical pattern in four generations with
more affected females than males.

VI. NON-MENDELIAN INHERITANCE

A. Mitochondrial Inheritance

Several forms of non-Mendelian inheritance patterns have
been identified during the past decade. One of the most important groups of genetic diseases that do not follow a Mendelian
pattern (single gene inheritance) is mitochondrial. The *mitochondria* are organelles situated in the cytoplasm of every cell
which play a role in cellular respiration. Each mitochondrion
has its own genome, consisting of a small, circular, double
stranded DNA molecule containing 37 genes. This mitochondrial DNA (mtDNA) is separate from the DNA in the nucleus
(nuclear DNA). Each cell contains thousands of copies of
mtDNA and cells that have higher energy requirements, like

brain and muscle, have even more copies. The role of the mitochondria in human diseases is reviewed elsewhere (5,6).

Oocytes also contain thousands of copies of mitochondrial
DNA, while sperm cells have essentially no mitochondria.
Therefore, mitochondria and their DNA are inherited through
the mother, also called mitochondrial or matrilineal inheritance. For genetic conditions that follow a mitochondrial pattern of inheritance, if a mother has a mitochondrial DNA
mutation, all of her children will inherit it. If a father has a
mitochondrial DNA mutation, none of his children will inherit
it. Some proteins working within the mitochondria are
encoded in the nuclear genome and can affect the function
of mitochondria. These nuclear genes would follow the typical
Mendelian patterns of inheritance as previously discussed
and not mitochondrial or non-Mendelian inheritance.

During cell division, the mitochondrial DNA replicates
and sorts randomly among the new mitochondria, which are
then randomly distributed among the new cells. Therefore,
each of the new daughter cells would receive different proportions of mitochondria with normal or mutant mitochondrial
DNA, if present. *Homoplasmy* is a term that refers to cells
that contain a pure population of mitochondria and their
DNA. *Heteroplasmy* refers to a state in which cells contain a
mixture of mitochondria with mutant mtDNA and mitochondria with normal mtDNA. Varying proportions of mitochondria with mutations in their DNA may account for
variability of symptoms and severity seen in mitochondrial
genetic diseases even within the same family.

Mitochondrial genetic diseases generally affect tissues that
have high energy requirements, such as the neuromuscular system and the central nervous system. Common clinical features
include: encephalopathy, seizures, dementia, stroke-like events,
ataxia, spasticity, dementia, myopathy, exercise intolerance,
cardiomyopathy, sensorineural deafness, pigmentary retinopathy, and diabetes mellitus. Symptoms may worsen with stress
as energy requirements increase. A general rule of thumb: if a
disease involves three or more organ systems, consider mitochondrial disease! Table 6 lists common mitochondrial diseases
and mutations in the mitochondrial DNA.

Table 6 Common Mitochondrial Diseases Caused by Mutations in the Mitochondrial DNA

Disorder	Primary Features	Age of Onset	Mutation
MELAS	**M**etabolic **E**ncephalopathy, **L**actic **A**cidosis, **S**troke-like episodes	2–10 years	80% have A3243G mutation in tRNA
MERRF	**M**yoclonic **E**pilepsy with **R**agged **R**ed **F**ibers on muscle biopsy	Late adolescence or early adulthood	80–90% have A8344G mutation in tRNA
Maternally inherited Leigh syndrome	Hypotonia, seizures, myoclonus, developmental delay, optic atrophy	Early childhood	T8993G or T8993C in ATPase 6 gene
NARP	**N**eurogenic weakness, **A**taxia, **R**etinitis **P**igmentosa	Late childhood or early adulthood	T8993G in ATPase 6 gene
LHON (**L**eber's **H**ereditary **O**ptic **N**europathy)	Rapid, bilateral loss of central vision due to optic nerve death	Increased penetrance in males; onset young adults	G11778A, T14484C, G3460A point mutations in respirator chain complex I
CPEO	**C**hronic **P**rogressive **E**xternal **O**phthalmoplegia	Variety of ages of onset according to severity	Large deletions of mtDNA; also various point mutations
Kearns-Sayre syndrome	Progressive external ophthalmoplegia, pigmentary retinal degeneration	Onset prior to age 20 years	mtDNA deletions and duplications

B. Genomic Imprinting

Traditional patterns of inheritance follow the assumption that a mutant allele of an autosomal gene is equally likely to be transmitted from either parent to offspring of either sex. This implies that two working copies of a gene represent the normal state. Advances in genetics have proven, however, that in some genetic diseases expression of the disease phenotype depends on the parent from where the mutant allele was inherited. The first examples in humans of genomic imprinting or differential expression depending on the parent of origin were Prader–Willi and Angelman syndromes (both conditions are described in detail in separate chapters).

Genomic imprinting affects the expression of a gene, but not the DNA sequence. Imprinting is a reversible inactivation of a gene. Imprinting takes place prior to fertilization during the formation of germ cells. During this process certain genes are marked as maternal or paternal. After conception, the imprint acts to suppress expression of a gene in some or all of the tissues. The reversible nature of imprinting is controlled by the imprinting center, which is located within the imprinted region itself.

Several common genetic syndromes show the effects of genomic imprinting. Prader–Willi and Angelman syndromes are two disorders caused by alterations of chromosome 15. Prader–Willi syndrome is characterized by obesity, short stature, hypogonadism, mental deficiency, and food seeking behaviors (7,8) (Fig. 13). Greater than 95% of individuals with Prader–Willi syndrome are caused by a paternally derived deletion of the 15q11–q13 region or from maternal disomy 15 (both 15s from the mother) which results from a trisomy 15 fetus and loss of the paternal chromosome 15 early in the pregnancy. Angelman syndrome is characterized by short stature, severe mental retardation, seizures, lack of speech, ataxia, and distinctive facial features (8,9) (Fig. 14). Greater than 75% of cases of Angelman syndrome are caused by deletions of 15q11–q13 derived from the maternal chromosome 15 or paternal disomy 15 (both 15s from the father). Both of these syndromes can also be caused by a mutation or defect in the imprinting center which controls the activity of genes

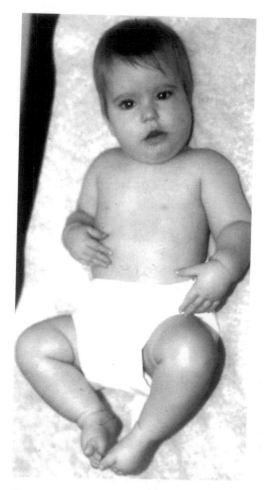

Figure 13   One-year-old white female with Prader–Willi syndrome and a paternally derived 15q11–q13 deletion. Typical features include a narrow bifrontal diameter, down-turned corners of the mouth, a small nose, and small hands and feet.

in the region (10). This results in a failure of the female-to-male or male-to-female switch in imprinting during gametogenesis. A sperm cell with a persistent female imprint would lead to a child with Prader–Willi syndrome and an egg cell with a persistent male imprint would cause Angelman syndrome.

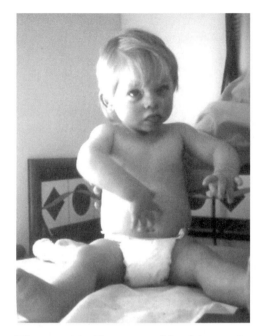

Figure 14 Two-year-old white male with a history of seizures, lack of speech, inappropriate laughter, and developmental delay due to Angelman syndrome and a maternally derived 15q11–q13 deletion. Typical features include blonde hair, a broad appearing head, and hand/arm motion frequently seen in this syndrome.

Imprinting center defects could account for recurrence of Prader–Willi syndrome or Angelman syndrome in some families.

C. Trinucleotide Repeat Mutations

Several genetic conditions are caused by unstable mutations that consist of amplification of triplet repeat sequences (e.g., CGG) within or at a specific gene locus (Table 7). This instability of the triplet repeat sequence may increase the number of repeats outside of a normal range in affected individuals compared to the general population. Triplet repeats below a certain number for each disorder are transmitted accordingly in cell division. Repeats above a certain number, however, become unstable and are typically transmitted with

Table 7 Common Diseases Caused by Trinucleotide Repeat Mutations

Disorder	Symptoms	Trinucleotide Repeat	Inheritance
DRPLA – Dentatorubral Pallidoluysian Atrophy	Occurs predominantly in Japanese population. Ataxia, chorea, dementia. Seizures with juvenile onset.	CAG	Autosomal Dominant
Huntington Disease	Involuntary movements, psychiatric changes. Can have juvenile onset.	CAG	Autosomal Dominant
Spinal and Bulbar Muscular Atrophy (Kennedy's disease)	Progressive muscle weakness and atrophy associated with signs of androgen insensitivity and infertility. Female heterozygotes typically asymptomatic.	CAG	X-linked Recessive
Spinocerebellar Ataxias	An ever-expanding group of disorders (up to 22 separate conditions) generally characterized by ataxia, dysarthria, intention tremor, cerebellar dysfunction and varying other CNS symptoms.	CAG for SCA's 1, 2, 3, 6,7,12,17 CTG in SCA8 Others unknown at this time	Autosomal Dominant
Fragile X Syndrome (FRAXA)	Moderate mental retardation in males, some dysmorphic features. Carrier females may have mild MR.	CGG	X-linked Recessive
FRAXE	Milder mental retardation, no consistent physical features. May have psychiatric problems.	GCC	X-linked Recessive
Freidreich's Ataxia	Progressive ataxia, dysarthria, cardiomyopathy, deafness, optic atrophy, glucose intolerance / diabetes.	GAA	Autosomal Recessive
Myotonic Dystrophy	Mild: mild myotonia, cataracts. Classical: weakness, myotonia, cataracts, balding, cardiac arrhythmia. Congenital: infantile hypotonia, respiratory issues, mental retardation.	CTG	Autosomal Dominant

either an increase or decrease in copy number. For example, in fragile X syndrome, the most common cause of familial mental retardation has an incidence of 1 in 2000–3000 males (11–13). The fragile site occurs at chromosome band Xq27.3. The FMR-1 gene at this site causes the syndrome and is 38 kb in size containing 17 exons. It encodes an RNA-binding protein needed for normal brain development and function. The untranslated first exon of the FMR-1 gene contains a polymorphic CGG triplet which may be unstable but normally varies in size ranging from 6 to 59 repeats. In affected individuals with the fragile X syndrome, the repeat massively expands to hundreds or thousands of CGG triplet repeats. When the expansion exceeds 250 repeats, then the gene becomes hypermethylated, no longer functions, and no protein is produced. Males with this full mutation will be clinically affected with mental retardation, have a long face with prominent ears, large testicles, and joint laxity (11) (Fig. 15). Most females who carry the fragile X syndrome gene

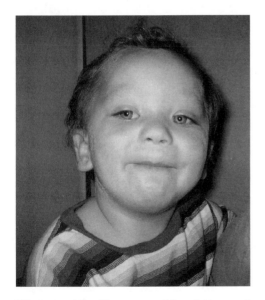

Figure 15 Two-year-old white male with developmental and speech delay due to fragile X syndrome. Note pale blue eyes, flattened nasal bridge, and prominent appearing ears. (*See color insert.*)

have intermediate numbers of the CGG triplet repeats ranging from 60 to 250 and termed a premutation. A detailed description of the clinical and genetic findings of this syndrome will be presented in a separate chapter.

The increase or expansion in copy number of the repeats has been identified as the mechanism responsible for a number of single gene genetic diseases, most neurological in nature. The parent of origin may also affect the likelihood of expansion of the triplet repeat. With triplet repeat genetic diseases, the onset of disease tends to occur at an earlier age or with increasing severity in subsequent generations. This increased severity is termed *genetic anticipation*.anticipation can be due to an expansion in an unstable triplet repeat for specific genes leading to this class of genetic diseases.

VII. MULTIFACTORIAL

Multifactorial diseases are the result of the effects of multiple genes, usually of an undetermined number, environmental exposures throughout life, and the interaction among genes, among environmental factors, and among genes and environmental factors. In other words, they are complex! The underlying hypothesis is that multiple genes contribute to the susceptibility to a given disease and the effects of these genes may be modified through the effects of other genes or environmental exposures.

Multifactorial diseases can be considered dichotomous characters in the sense that they either occur or do not in an individual. For these presence/absence characters, we think of the genetic loci involved as susceptibility genes (14). Dichotomous characters display discontinuous or discrete variation in their expression. Most of the traits we have discussed as governed by Mendelian rules (simple Mendelian traits like blood groups) show discontinuous variation. Each individual in a given population can be assigned to a limited number of discrete phenotypic classes (like A, B, AB, O in the ABO system). For multifactorial diseases, the discrete phenotypic classes would include disease occurs versus disease does not occur. In contrast, quantitative traits showing continuous variation cannot be fit into a finite number of phenotypic classes. When we are dealing with quantitative or continuous characters such as height and skin color, the loci underlying these measured traits are viewed as quantitative trait loci (QTLs). However, our focus in this section is on multifactorial diseases.

Quantitative traits usually approximate the Gaussian or bell-shaped normal distribution curve when you plot on a graph the frequency distribution for the trait. If we take heights in a large population, we can get a frequency distribution curve that approximates the normal distribution illustrated in Fig. 1 of Chapter 21 on Behavioral Genetics and Developmental Disabilities. Some quantitative traits fit this curve better than others. For example, head length closely fits the normal curve. We will return to the normal distribution curve when genetic liability to disease is discussed below.

The vast majority of diseases are multifactorial. They include the common adult diseases such as diabetes, hypertension, heart disease, and schizophrenia. However, they also include common developmental disabilities such as autism spectrum disorders. Table 8 lists some examples of multifactorial diseases, as well as examples of quantitative traits, the latter for the sake of completeness in presenting multifactorial characters. Many quantitative traits are of interest in medical genetics, especially in the clinical evaluation of physical growth (anthropometry) and of behavioral traits and disorders.

The term polygenic refers to the situation where multiple loci, each of small effect individually, influence the expression of the phenotype. This term, however, only describes the role of genetics. In general, most of the aforementioned dichotomous and continuous characters are considered to be polygenic.

During the late 19th century, Sir Francis Galton studied quantitative traits such as intellectual functioning and height in humans. He developed quantitative methods for dealing with such traits, but never an adequate theory of the inheritance of these traits. Galton's methods were further elaborated and refined by the scientists who became known as

Table 8 Examples of Multifactorial Conditions and Traits

Category	Examples
Diseases/disorders	*Birth defects*: orofacial clefts, neural tube defects, clubfoot
	Cancer
	Cardiovascular: heart disease, hypertension
	Developmental disabilities: autism, epilepsy, mental retardation
	Diabetes
	Obesity
	Schizophrenia
	Scoliosis
Traits	*Anthropometric*: head circumference, height, weight
	Intellectual functioning: IQ
	Pigmentation: eyes, hair, skin
	Dermatoglyphic patterns

biometricians for their early applications of quantitative methods to the study of biological variation. It took the rediscovery of Mendel's research and the brilliant work of Sir Ronald Fisher in the early part of the 20th century to produce an adequate theoretical basis for the inheritance of quantitative traits. What Fisher accomplished was the reconciliation of the statistical approaches to quantitative traits of the biometricians with Mendelian genetics by considering the multiple effects of single genetic loci. In doing so, he founded the subfield of quantitative genetics that through the years has focused on the genetics of quantitative traits.

How do we get from the Mendelian genetics approach to that of quantitative genetics? We might ask first whether systems of multiple alleles could account for the continuous variation we observe in quantitative traits. At a single locus, four alleles and no more can be supplied by two parents: $A^1A^2 \times A^3A^4$. These parents will produce the following four genotypes: A^1A^3, A^1A^4, A^2A^3, and A^2A^4. If the phenotypes correspond with the genotypes, then a maximum of four phenotypes could be produced among the offspring. If multiple loci are involved, it should be clear that many more than four phenotypes could occur even in one family for traits like height and hair color.

To see how polygenic inheritance works, consider a hypothetical example with three pairs of genes (three loci) responsible for height. The letters A, B, and C represent the three loci. First consider an individual with the genotype AABBCC. This person's phenotypic expression for height is assumed to be 60 in. Assume there are no effects of dominance in our model and no effects of environmental factors such as diet. Letters shown with a prime (A′) will represent an allele that adds 1 in. to the height of an individual. The effect of an allele adding a measurable amount to the phenotype is called an additive effect. In this model, the genotype A′A′B′BCC would then be 63 in. in height and A′A′B′B′C′C′ would be 66 in. If the two extreme genotypes (AABBCC and A′A′B′B′C′C′) in this example had offspring, they would all be A′AB′BC′C and 63 in. in height. If many individuals of this same genotype (A′AB′BC′C) then produced offspring, the distribution of heights would be as shown in Table 9 .

In this case, 1/64 would be as tall as the original tall parent (A′A′B′B′C′C′). If four loci had been hypothesized, the proportion of offspring of two individuals heterozygous at each of the loci who had one of the extreme heights would be 1/256. Table 10 shows how to estimate the number of offspring that would have the extreme phenotypic expression.

Table 9 Distribution of Height Depending on Genotype

No. Alleles with Primes in Genotype	Phenotype (Height in inches)	Frequency
6	66	1/64
5	65	6/64
4	64	15/64
3	63	20/64
2	62	15/64
1	61	6/64
0	60	1/64

Table 10   Estimate of the Frequency of Offspring at the Extremes
of Phenotypic Expression

Number of Loci	1	2	3	4	N
Fraction of offspring at extremes of phenotypic distribution	1/4	1/16	1/64	1/256	$(1/4)^N$

The previous example illustrates how polygenic inheritance influences continuous characters like height, but how
is it viewed with respect to dichotomous or discontinuous
characters like presence or absence of a disease? David
Falconer extended the theory of polygenic inheritance to disease by postulating the underlying continuous variable of
genetic susceptibility (14). According to this model, an individual either has or does not have a particular multifactorial
disease, but early in development, the individual had a certain susceptibility to the disease. The susceptibility itself is
polygenic, and for any individual, it could be high or low.
In a population, susceptibility in theory is considered to be
distributed normally.

Falconer also introduced the concept of threshold. The
threshold theory holds that individuals whose susceptibility
is greater than a critical threshold value will develop the disease in question, while those below this value will not. Extending the polygenic model used previously for height, consider
the situation where three loci confer susceptibility to a given
disease. This time the alleles with primes signify increased
susceptibility to the disease. If the threshold value is the existence of five or more alleles with primes in a person's genetic
make-up, then according to the distribution of genotypes
in Table 9, approximately seven of every 64 individuals in
the population will develop the disease. This model addresses
only the genetic liability to disease in the population and does
not take into account the environmental factors that are
associated with the occurrence of all multifactorial diseases.

The threshold theory explains how the recurrence risks
for multifactorial disease will vary among families (14).

Individuals who have the disease have genotypes with many high susceptibility alleles (five or more in our example). Relatives of these affected individuals share more genes in common and therefore have an elevated genetic liability, i.e., they have a greater chance than unrelated individuals of falling above the threshold value. This has important implications with respect to genetic counseling for multifactorial diseases.

For multifactorial diseases, the theory of polygenic inheritance is not used to compute recurrence risks in families. Recurrence risk estimates are derived from empirical data collected on many families in which multifactorial diseases such as spina bifida have occurred. As Strachan and Read (14) emphasize, this is the fundamental difference between multifactorial and Mendelian genetic diseases. In the latter, the risks are determined by theory. For a recessive condition, the risk of an affected child in any pregnancy for a couple in which both mother and father are carriers is 1 in 4. The recurrence risk for a couple that has had one previous child with a multifactorial disease generally is 3–5%, but the data vary among populations. In addition, the risk increases if more than one person in the family is affected, for example, if the couple has previously had two affected children.

For consistency with the previous sections of this chapter, we thought it would be helpful to include a pedigree for a multifactorial disease, namely diabetes. Figure 16 shows a family pedigree for diabetes.

The patterns for multifactorial diseases can be quite different than those observed for Mendelian conditions. Note that neither parent of the proband is affected. The male parent lived up to age 88 years and the female parent is alive and 93 years of age at the time of this writing. Although neither parent is affected, susceptibility genes for diabetes exist on both sides of the family, with both grandfathers having been diagnosed with diabetes as well as sibs of both the proband's parents. Family histories like these can be useful tools with respect to the prevention of many multifactorial diseases, especially the more common ones such as diabetes. An initiative by the Centers for Disease Control and Prevention is

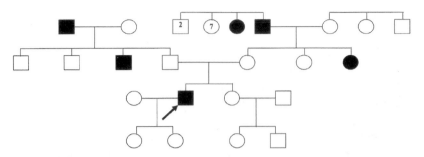

Figure 16 Pedigree of coeditor's (FJM) family for diabetes, a multifactorial disease.

promoting the use of family histories in disease prevention (15). Increased efforts will be needed to educate physicians and other health care providers about the importance and utility of family histories.

Methods have been developed to enable geneticists to estimate the influence of genetic factors in multifactorial diseases. In certain situations it is possible to hold genotype "constant," such as in cases of identical twins. Twin studies to examine the differences between monozygotic twins (same genotype) versus dizygotic (different genotypes) with respect to quantitative traits or disease expression serve the purpose of assessing the possible role of genetics. Table 11 shows the genetic relationships between some relatives typically used in studies of polygenic traits and diseases.

A method for evaluating the role of genetics in a multifactorial disease is to examine concordance among twins.

Table 11 Genetic Relationships Among Relatives

Relationship	Proportion of Genes in Common	Expected Correlation
Identical twins	1	1.00
Dizygotic twins, parent–child, sibs	1/2	0.50
Grandparent–grandchild	1/4	0.25

Concordance is the percentage of twins in which the disease occurs in both members of the pair. A high rate of concordance suggests the influence of genetic factors in a particular disease. Low concordance suggests that environmental factors play a large role in the disease. Concordance can be viewed as a screening method for the detection of genetic influences and can signal the need for more definitive genetic studies.

More detailed methods to detect the influence of genes in multifactorial traits and diseases are presented in Chapter 21 on Behavioral Genetics and Developmental Disabilities. In addition, Chapter 19 applies both genetic and epidemiological methods to the detection of genetic and environmental factors contributing to the cause of autism and mental retardation. A review and perspective concerning genetic and environmental factors in mental retardation is also provided in Meaney (16). Although we have not dealt with the topic herein, research on multifactorial conditions will increasingly be focused on the search for evidence of gene–environment interactions. For example, Dyer-Friedman et al. (17) have provided a model approach to the study of genetic and environmental factors that predict cognitive outcomes such as IQ in fragile X syndrome. The search for the interactions among genes and among genes, environmental exposures, and interventions is very likely to emerge as a major focus of future research in developmental disabilities.

ACKNOWLEDGMENTS

We thank Deborah Moore, Linda Heim, and Heather Baroni for expert preparation of the manuscript and figures. We would also like to thank Chris Cunniff, M.D., for his editorial comments on the section about multifactorial inheritance. This work was partially supported by Children's Mercy Hospital's Physician Scientist Award (GL01.4871), the Missouri State Contract for Genetic Services (GL01.3612), and grant #90DD0532 from the Administration on Developmental Disabilities.

REFERENCES

1. Bennett RL, Motulsky AG, Bittles A, Hudgins L, Uhrich S, Doyle D, Silvey K, Scott CR, Cheng E, McGillivray B, Steiner RD, Olson D. Genetic counseling and screening of consanguineous couples and their offspring: Recommendations of the National Society of Genetic Counselors. J Genet Couns 2002; 11(2):97–119.

2. Brown CJ, Greally JM. A stain upon the silence: genes escaping X inactivation. Trends Genet 2003; 19(8):432–438.

3. Cook J, Lam W, Mueller RF. Mendelian inheritance. In: Rimoin DL, Connor JM, Pyeritz RE, Korf BR, eds. Principles and Practice of Medical Genetics. 4th ed. Edinburgh: Churchill Livingston, 2002:104–124.

4. Jimenez-Sanchez G, Childs B, Valle D. The effect of Mendelian disease in human health. In: Scriver CR, Beaudet AL, Sly WS, Valle D, Childs B, Kinzler KW, Vogelstein B, eds. The Metabolic Molecular Bases of Inherited Disease. 8th ed. NewYork: McGraw Hill Medical Publishing Division, 2001: 167–174.

5. Wallace DC, Lott MT, Brown MD, Kerstann K. Mitochondria and neuro-ophthalmological diseases. In: Scriver CR, Beaudet AL, Sly WS, Valle D, Childs B, Kinzler KW, Vogelstein B, eds. The Metabolic and Molecular Bases of Inherited Disease. 8th ed. NewYork: McGraw Hill Medical Publishing Division, 2001:2425–2512.

6. Wallace DC, Lott MT. Mitochondrial genes in degenerative diseases, cancer and aging. In: Rimoin DL, Connor JM, Pyeritz RE, Korf BR, eds. Principles and Practice of Medical Genetics. 4th ed. Edinburgh: Churchill Livingston, 2002:299–409.

7. Butler MG, Thompson T. Prader–Willi syndrome: clinical and genetic findings. Endocrinol 2000; 10:3S–16S.

8. Cassidy SB, Dykens E, Williams CA. Prader–Willi syndrome: sister imprinted disorders. Am J Med Genet 2000; 97(2):136–146.

9. Williams CA, Lossie A, Driscoll D. Angelman syndrome: mimicking conditions and phenotypes. Am J Med Genet 2001; 104(4): 345–346.

10. Sapienza C, Hall JG. Genome imprinting in human disease. In: Scriver CR, Beaudet AL, Sly WS, Valle D, Childs B, Kinzler KW, Vogelstein B, eds. The Metabolic and Molecular Bases of Inherited Disease. 8th ed. New York: McGraw Hill Medical Publishing Division, 2001:417–432.

11. Hagerman RJ, Hagerman PJ. In: Hagerman RJ, Hagerman PJ, eds. Fragile X Syndrome: Diagnosis, and Treatment Research. 3rd ed. Baltimore: The John Hopkins University Press, 2003:3–527.

12. Warren ST, Sherman SL. The fragile X syndrome. In: Scriver CR, Beaudet AL, Sly WS, Valle D, Childs B, Kinzler KW, Vogelstein B, eds. The Metabolic Molecular Bases of Inherited Disease. 8th ed. NewYork: McGraw Hill Medical Publishing Division, 2001:1250–1290.

13. Sutherland GR, Gecz J, Mulley JC. Fragile X syndrome and other causes of X-linked mental handicap. In: Rimoin DL, Connor JM, Pyeritz RE, Korf BR, eds. Principles and Practice of Medical Genetics. 4th ed. Edinburgh: Churchill Livingston, 2002:2801–2826.

14. Strachan T, Read AP. Human Molecular Genetics. 3rd ed. New York: Garland Science, 2004:101–119.

15. Centers for Disease Control and Prevention. Genetics and Genomics: Family History and Genetics [accessed August 15, 2004. http://www.cdc.gov/genomics/fHix.htm].

16. Meaney FJ. Mental retardation. In: Ember CR, Ember M, eds. Encyclopedia of Medical Anthropology: Health and Illness in the World's Cultures. Vol. 1. Kluwer/Plenum, 2004:1: 493–505.

17. Dyer-Friedman J, Glaser B, Hessl D, Johnston C, Huffman LC, Taylor A, Wisbeck J, Reiss AL. Genetic and environmental influences on the cognitive outcomes of children with fragile X syndrome. J Am Acad Child Adolesc Psychiatry 2002; 41: 237–244.

3

Clinical Cytogenetics and Testing for Developmental Disabilities

JOAN H. M. KNOLL and LINDA D. COOLEY

Section of Medical Genetics and Molecular Medicine, Children's Mercy Hospitals and Clinics, University of Missouri–Kansas City, School of Medicine, Missouri, U.S.A.

I. INTRODUCTION

Developmental delay (DD)/mental retardation (MR) has many different causes and is estimated to occur in up to 10% of the population (1). Parents generally want to know the cause of such a disorder in their child, including whether it is genetic (i.e., chromosomal, biochemical, and single gene) or environmental; what can be done about it; whether they will have other children with the same problem; and whether their normal children are at risk for having similar children. To answer these questions and to better understand the clinical symptoms of the patient, the healthcare professional must recognize the cause of the DD/MR.

Understanding the cause of the disorder can direct both the type of treatment and the timing of therapy, which could include surgery, medication, dietary changes, behavior modification, or some combination of these. Well-characterized genetic disorders often have a predictable clinical course. Genetic imbalances cannot be corrected simply by the introduction of new genes, making this an unrealistic approach for treatment in the near future. Therefore, clinical management of genetic disease is currently the only medically accepted approach for improving the quality of life in children with these disorders. Only by recognizing the cause of DD/MR is the healthcare professional able to predict how the child will develop, guide appropriate laboratory testing, initiate appropriate treatment or intervention, and determine recurrence risks. The American College of Medical Genetics has established guidelines regarding the evaluation of individuals with MR and these guidelines include the diagnostic utility of cytogenetic testing (2). This chapter will describe the field of cytogenetics and the available testing for individuals with DD/MR.

II. HISTORY

In 1956, Tijo and Levan (3) discovered that human cells contain 46 chromosomes. Ford and Hamerton (4) confirmed this finding when they reported 23 bivalents in spermatocytes. Soon after in 1959, Lejeune reported that trisomy was associated with "mongolism". This opened a new field of medicine—medical cytogenetics (5). The medical and scientific communities responded by investigating unusual looking children and quickly discovered other congenital autosomal and sex chromosome anomalies as causes of physical and mental deficiencies. In 1970, Caspersson et al. (6) discovered Q-banding, a method using fluorescent staining to bring out bands on chromosomes allowing unambiguous identification of individual chromosomes (7). Amniocentesis, first used in the 1970s, and chorionic villus sampling in the 1980s, were shown to be safe and accurate methods for prenatal diagnosis of chromosome anomalies in the fetus (8). The field of cytogenetics continues to progress rapidly and new chromosome anomalies, e.g., microdeletions, are found to account for syndromes whose etiology has not previously been defined. Microdeletion syndromes will be discussed in a separate chapter.

The alignment of the chromosome pairs according to size and banding pattern called a karyotype, is the standard and basic method for examining the integrity of all chromosomes in a cell. The 46 human chromosomes constitute 23 pairs; 22 pairs of autosomes and one pair of sex chromosomes (XX in females and XY in males) (Fig. 1). Chromosomes are paired and arranged in the karyotype from largest to smallest in size and according to placement of the centromere or primary constriction. Human chromosomes are classified by centromere position into three types: metacentric chromosomes have centrally positioned centromeres, submetacentric chromosomes have an off-center centromere with chromosome arms of different lengths, and acrocentric chromosomes which have the centromere near one end of the chromosome. The short arm of a chromosome is always placed upward in the karyotype and referred to as the "p" arm for "petite"; the long arm is the "q" arm. Chromosomes 1, 3, 16, 19, and 20 are metacentric chromosomes, chromosomes 13–15, 21, and 22 are acrocen-tric chromosomes, and all other human chromosomes are submetacentric.

Each chromosome contains unique, single-copy DNA, repetitive dispersed DNA sequences, and satellite highly repeated DNA sequences. The centromeres of each chromosome and the majority of the chromosome Y long arm contain heterochromatin, a repetitive DNA that is transcriptionally inactive. The acrocentric chromosome short arms are comprised of stalks which contain genes for ribosomal RNA and satellites which contain highly repetitive DNA sequences. The ends of chromosomes contain short telomere-specific repeat DNA sequences that function to cap and protect the ends of the chromosome. Repetitive DNA may be visualized by special cytogenetic staining procedures: C-bands stain heterochromatin and silver (Ag) staining enhances the stalk regions or nucleolar organizer

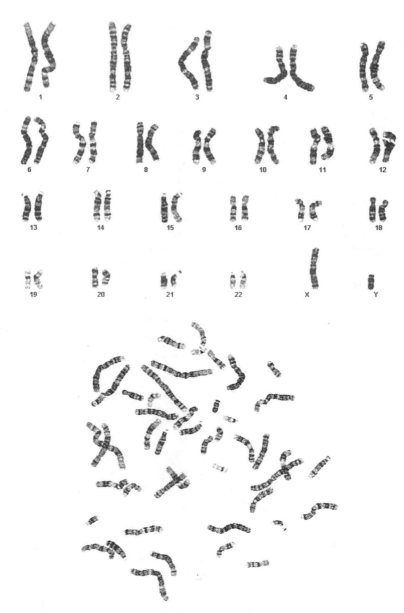

Figure 1 Representative Giemsa (GTG)-banded chromosomes of a normal male cell arranged to form a karyotype (46,XY). The metaphase chromosome spread from the same cell.

regions (NORs) of the acrocentric chromosomes. Fluorescence in situ hybridization (FISH) using DNA probes detects specific unique single-copy or repetitive sequences (Table 1). Chromosome anomalies identified by karyotyping are described using a nomenclature which is designed to communicate the specifics of the abnormality to other cytogeneticists and those interested in knowing about the chromosome findings. The International System for Cytogenetic Nomenclature (ISCN), first introduced in 1975, has undergone several revisions with the 1995 version in current usage around the world (9). Table 2 summarizes forms of nomenclature used to describe common chromosome anomalies. The ISCN also provides a reference for chromosome band resolution. When treated with trypsin and stained with Giemsa stain, each chromosome has a characteristic banded pattern that uniquely identifies that chromosome. Chromosomes captured at different times of the cell cycle, i.e., metaphase vs. prometaphase, results in chromosomes with more or fewer visible bands. The ISCN defines three different levels of band resolution by the number

Table 1 Cytogenetic Stains and Special Procedures

Stains

G-banding—most widely used; chromosomes treated with trypsin and stained with Giemsa to demonstrate the characteristic light and dark bands of each chromosome

Q-banding—stain with quinicrine mustard or derivative and observed with fluorescence microscopy

R-banding—heat pretreatment before Giemsa staining produces dark and light bands that are the reverse of those obtained with G- and Q-banding

Special procedures

C-banding—stains the heterochromatin at the centromeres and the Y chromosome long arm

NOR staining—stains the stalk region of the acrocentric chromosomes

High resolution banding—uses specific chemicals to capture chromosomes in the prometaphase stage

Fluorescence in situ hybridization (FISH)—uses heat to denature chromosomes followed by application of specific fluorochrome-tagged DNA sequence probes that are allowed to anneal with homologous sequences on the denatured chromosomes and then observed with fluorescence microscopy

Table 2   Cytogenetic Nomenclature

Nomenclature usage and abbreviations
47,XY,+21 indicates 47 chromosomes, a male, and an extra copy
   of chromosome 21
   XX, female
   XY, male
   + or − sign, gain or loss of chromosome noted
46,XX,del(5) (p11.2p14) indicates 46 chromosomes, a female, and
   an interstitial deletion of chromosome 5 between the short arm bands
   p11.2 and p14
   "p" designates the short arm of a chromosome
   "q" designates the long arm of a chromosome
46,XY,t(11;22) (q23;q12) indicates 46 chromosomes, a male, and a reciprocal translocation between the long arms of chromosomes 11 and 22
   t, translocation
   First set of parenthesis (11;22), chromosomes involved
   Second set of parenthesis (q23;q12), breakpoints of chromosomes
      involved
   q23, breakpoint of chromosome 11
   q12, breakpoint of chromosome 22
Other common abbreviations
   dup, duplication
   inv, inversion
   add, added unidentified material
   mar, marker; unidentified chromosome
   ish, in situ hybridization
   r, ring

---

of visible bands: 400, 550, and 850 bands per haploid karyotype.
A typical high-resolution cytogenetic study will have a band
resolution of at least 550 bands. In addition to karyotyping, special stains and methods, e.g., C-bands and FISH, are utilized by
the laboratory to investigate chromosome anomalies to best
define chromosomal losses, gains, and rearrangements that
impact patient management and genetic counseling.

III.   TYPES OF CHROMOSOME
ABNORMALITIES

Chromosomal abnormalities occur in about 1 in 200 of all live
births. Physical and developmental anomalies are commonly

associated with chromosomal abnormalities. Chromosome abnormalities occur in ~30% of liveborn children with anomalies and in 5% of phenotypically normal stillbirths. Chromosomal abnormalities involve changes in either chromosomal number or structure. These abnormalities are referred to as constitutional because the child is born with congenital anomalies rather than acquired through a disease process such as cancer. While some chromosomal abnormalities occur more frequently, the number of abnormal chromosome possibilities is almost infinite. Indications and specimen types for chromosome studies are given in Table 3.

A. Numerical

The most common numerical abnormalities with corresponding clinical features observed in live births are presented in Table 4. As a rule, chromosomal loss (i.e., monosomy) is more detrimental than chromosomal gain (i.e., trisomy); and a change in the number of autosomes is more serious than a change in the number of sex chromosomes. The majority of the conceptuses having the numerical abnormalities listed in Table 4 are lost during pregnancy, and only the most fit survive to birth. Additionally, numerical abnormalities for all other chromosomes have been observed in early pregnancy losses. Triploidy (69 chromosomes with trisomy for all chromosomes) also occurs but most conceptuses are lost early in gestation due to the gross genetic imbalance.

B. Structural

Structural chromosome abnormalities involve changes in the structure (and resulting banding pattern) of one or more chromosomes. These structural abnormalities can be balanced (no net loss and/or gain of genetic information) or unbalanced (net loss and/or gain of genetic information). The most common types of structural abnormalities include deletions, duplications, inversions, translocations, markers, or extra structurally abnormal chromosomes (ESACs). Less common abnormalities include isochromosomes, dicentric chromosomes, insertions, and ring chromosomes, although other

Table 3   Indications and Specimen Types for Chromosome Studies

I. Indications for cytogenetic analysis
Prenatal
   Pregnancies at risk for aneuploidy (e.g., maternal age, family history)
   Parent is a known carrier of a balanced rearrangement
Postnatal
   Confirm or exclude suspected chromosome syndrome
   Unexplained mental or developmental retardation
   Ambiguous genitalia
   Abnormal sexual development
   Infertility
   Recurrent miscarriage or stillbirths
High-resolution study
   Suspected microdeletion syndrome
   To further characterize a chromosome anomaly
II. Indications for FISH analysis
Prenatal
   Late gestation pregnancy at risk for aneuploidy
Postnatal
   Confirm or exclude microdeletion syndrome
   Clarify and characterize chromosome anomalies detected by routine
      cytogenetic analysis
   Detect chromosome mosaicism
III. Specimen types suitable for cytogenetic analysis
Prenatal
   Amniocytes
   Chorionic villus
   Percutaneous blood sample
Postnatal
   Peripheral blood
   Skin
   Other tissues (cells must have a nucleus and undergo division)

abnormalities do exist. The more common types of structural abnormalities (with examples) will be discussed, and diagrams showing different types of structural rearrangements are presented in Fig. 2.

1. Deletions

Deletions involve loss of material from a single chromosome which results in haploinsufficiency of the region. The deletions can be terminal (excluding the telomeric region) or

Table 4 Most Common Numerical Chromosome Abnormalities Observed in Live Births

Chromosome abnormality	Primary clinical findings
Trisomy 8[a]	Mild-to-severe MR, facial dysmorphology, cleft palate, variable growth
Trisomy 9[a]	Severe MR, joint and cardiac anomalies, growth deficiency, craniofacial anomalies
Trisomy 13	Patau syndrome—severe MR and CNS anomaly, cleft lip and palate, polydactyly
Trisomy 18	Edward syndrome—severe MR and CNS anomaly, cardiac anomalies, rocker bottom feet
Trisomy 21	Down syndrome—mild-to-moderate MR, characteristic facial appearance, hypotonia, increased incidence of leukemia and Alzheimer disease
Monosomy X	Turner syndrome—short stature, infertility, lack of secondary sexual characteristics
Additional X[b]	XXX (Triple-X syndrome)—learning disabilities XXY (Klinefelter syndrome)—learning disabilities, infertility, tall stature, small testes Learning problems increase as the number of Xs increase from XX and XY
Additional Y	XYY—learning/behavior problems in some individuals

MR, mental retardation; CNS, central nervous system
[a]Trisomy 8 and trisomy 9 exist in mosaic state with normal cells, the other chromosome abnormalities are observed in mosaic and non-mosaic states.
[b]Learning problems increase as the number of X chromosomes increase from 46, XX and 46,XY.

interstitial. Subtle deletions are observed in most of the microdeletion syndromes and often require confirmation by FISH (Fig. 3). The most common and well-recognized microdeletion syndromes are included in Table 5. The typical deletions in these syndromes include multiple genes that span several million base pairs of DNA. Recent studies for chromosomes 15q11.2q13, 17p11.2, and 22q11.2 have demonstrated that most interstitial deletions and corresponding duplications originate de novo through recombination errors between low copy repetitive sequences (10–16). Terminal deletions can

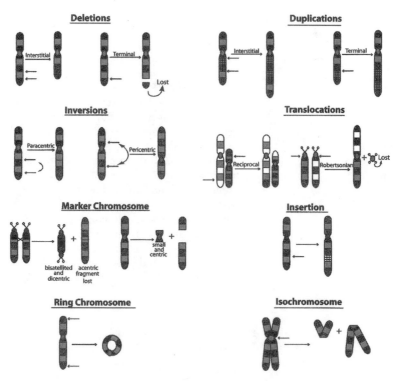

Figure 2 Diagram showing different types of structural chromosome abnormalities.

also occur by de novo mechanisms other than interstitial deletions or they can occur from errors in chromosomal segregation during the formation of gametes in parents who carry a balanced reciprocal translocation.

2. Duplications

Duplications involve gain of material from the same chromosome (intrachromosomal) or between homologs (interchromosomal), which results in an extra copy of the duplicated region. Interstitial duplications are often viewed as the reciprocal product of the process leading to deletion chromosomes. As described above, those deletions and duplications on chromosomes 15, 17, and 22 result from recombination errors in meiosis between repetitive DNA

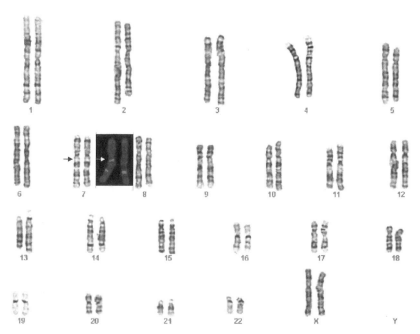

Figure 3 GTG-banded karyotype of a cell from a female with Williams syndrome (WS). An interstitial deletion of one chromosome 7q11.23 is evident by FISH (colored inset) where the WS critical region DNA probe (red color, white arrow) is absent. The chromosome 7s appear normal by GTG banding. Chromosome 7q11.23 is indicated by arrows. (*See color insert.*)

sequences flanking the region that becomes either duplicated or deleted. The resulting phenotype from the duplicated region is dependent upon the function of the genes that are duplicated. In the case of chromosome region 15q11.2q13, the phenotypic effect of the duplication is also dependent upon whether it is derived from the maternally inherited chromosome 15 or from the paternally inherited chromosome 15, as this region is genetically imprinted (i.e., the genes are expressed differently depending upon the parent of origin). Individuals with duplications of maternal origin have autistic behavior, hypotonia, and varying degrees of mental retardation (17), whereas those with paternally derived duplications are likely to have a milder phenotypic effect (18).

Table 5 Autosomal Contiguous Gene Syndromes Associated with DD/MR

Disorder	Chromosome region	Detectable by GTG banding[a]	Detectable by FISH[b]
Monosomy 1p36	del(1)(p36.3)	Occasionally	Yes
Wolf–Hirshhorn	del(4)(p16)	Usually	Yes
Cri-du-chat	del(5)(p15)	Usually	Yes
Williams	del(7)(q11.23q11.23)	No	Yes
Langer–Gideon	del(8)(q24.1q24.1)	Occasionally	Yes
WAGR[c]	del(11)(p13p13)	Occasionally	Yes
Prader–Willi	del(15)(q11.2q13)pat	Usually	Yes
Angelman	del(15)(q11.2q13)mat	Usually	Yes
Rubinstein–Taybi	del(16)(p13.3)	No	Yes
Miller–Dieker	del(17)(p13.3)	Occasionally	Yes
Smith–Magenis	del(17)(p11.2p11.2)	Occasionally	Yes
Alagille	del(20)(p11.23p11.23)	No	Yes
DiGeorge/Velo-cardio-facial [VCF]	del(22)(q11.2q11.2)	Rarely	Yes

[a] Ability to detect by GTG-banding is dependent upon factors that include the resolution of the chromosomes, the condensation of the chromosomal region in question and the size of the deleted region which can vary between individuals with the same disorder.
[b] Not all patients within each disorder have a deletion; depending upon the syndrome some may have mutations, uniparental inheritance, or other etiologies. Such patients often require DNA testing to determine the etiology.
[c] Wilm's tumor/aniridia/genitourinary/growth retardation malformation.

3. Inversions

Inversions involve two breaks within a single chromosome where the broken segment inverts or rotates and reunites to form a structurally abnormal chromosome. If both breaks occur in the same chromosomal arm, the inversion is termed "paracentric"; if the breaks occur in different chromosomal arms, the inversion is termed "pericentric." An individual who carries an inherited inversion generally has minimal clinical risk, whereas a de novo inversion carries an increased risk because disrupting an important gene is possible. Balanced inversion carriers, while phenotypically normal, are at risk for producing unbalanced gametes due to meiotic recombination events within the inverted segment (for review, see Ref. 19). In general, the greater the chromosomal imbalance resulting from recombination within the inverted segment, the less likely the pregnancy will continue. However, with a small chromosomal imbalance, the pregnancy is likely to continue and result in a live birth with clinical abnormalities.

A pericentric inversion of chromosome 9 at region p11q12 is the most common inversion in the general population. This inversion is a common variant and is not of clinical significance (20,21). When this inversion is detected, no additional studies in the individual or his or her family are recommended. Pericentric inversions of chromosome 2 at p11q13 (22) and chromosome 10 at p11.2q21.2 (23) are also relatively common and have been suggested to be without phenotypic effect to offspring of carriers. However, since the phenotypic effect (or lack of it) remains unclear in the published literature, the observation of chromosomes 2 and 10 inversions prompts most cytogenetic laboratories to perform chromosomal studies on parental samples to determine if the abnormality is inherited or de novo.

4. Translocations

Translocations involve exchange of material between two or more chromosomes and can be either balanced or unbalanced, inherited or de novo. A specialized type of translocation is the Robertsonian translocation, which involves a break and reunion of material in the centromeric regions of the acrocentric chromosomes (i.e., chromosomes 13, 14, 15, 21, and 22). Carriers of Robertsonian translocations are at risk for producing abnormal gametes that could result in trisomic offspring or offspring with clinically significant uniparental disomy if a chromosome with an imprinted region (i.e., chromosome 14 or 15) is involved in the translocation. Carriers of the other form of chromosome translocations (i.e., reciprocal translocations) are also at risk for producing abnormal gametes that could result in partial chromosomal monosomies and trisomies rather than entire chromosomal trisomies. Transmission of inherited balanced translocations to offspring generally has a low risk for clinical abnormality, but recent studies have suggested rearrangement or loss of DNA at the regions of exchange in abnormal offspring with "balanced" translocations (24,25).

The most common non-Robertsonian translocation is the reciprocal translocation found in the general population involving chromosomes 11 and 22 and designated as t(11;22) (q23;q11.2). The shared sequence homology in the regions that exchange in this translocation is likely to account for its frequency (26–28). Carriers of this translocation are at risk of having chromosomally unbalanced children who have an additional small chromosome derived from chromosome 22. Children with this chromosomal imbalance have findings that overlap with the findings of children that have the cat-eye syndrome and who are tetrasomic (four copies) for part of chromosome 22q. This additional chromosome originates in the carrier parent due to aberrant chromosomal segregation during gametogenesis.

Detection of cryptic translocations involving subtelomeric regions is relatively new in the cytogenetics laboratory and requires the use of molecular cytogenetic methods (29). Translocations are often present in an unbalanced form resulting in both partial monosomy and partial trisomy of chromosomal segments. These translocations can be either inherited or de novo and are often detectable in selected DD/MR patient populations by FISH using subtelomeric probes (30) as the majority of G-banded chromosomes end with light staining regions difficult to detect with routine cytogenetic studies.

In patients with idiopathic *mild* mental retardation and a normal high-resolution karyotype (i.e., >550 band level), the detection rate of terminal chromosomal imbalances is <0.5% (31). The detection rate for terminal chromosome imbalances in individuals with moderate-to-severe idiopathic mental retardation and a normal high-resolution karyotype ranges from 0% to 7% with an average of 3–4% (30–33). The best clinical indicators for the higher detection rates currently are moderate-to-severe mental retardation with a positive family history, growth retardation detected prenatally and/or postnatally, at least one dysmorphic facial feature, and at least one dysmorphic nonfacial abnormality including cardiac defects (34). It is possible that the frequency of chromosomal telomeric abnormalities in this population will increase as the clinical indicators become better defined and the DNA probes for detecting these abnormalities are refined and located closer to the chromosomal ends.

5. Marker Chromosomes

Marker chromosomes are chromosomes whose origin cannot be recognized by their GTG-banding pattern and are some-times referred to as ESACs. These chromosomes are generally small and have a centromere. Their effect on the phenotype is dependent upon their genetic composition. In the initial laboratory work-up to identify the chromosomal origin or com-position of a marker chromosome, C-banding and NOR stain-ing are generally performed to determine if the marker is comprised of heterochromatin and/or active ribosomal genes (or satellites or NORs) from the acrocentric chromosomes, respectively. Markers that are comprised only of heterochro-matin, repetitive noncoding DNA, or active ribosomal genes are without phenotypic effect. However, those containing euchromatin often have an adverse effect on the phenotype (35). Fluorescence in situ hybridization is useful in identifying the chromosomal origin of the marker chromosome (36,37) and, in some instances, determining the precise source of the marker chromosome.

Marker chromosomes derived from either chromosome 15 or 22 are the most common. They are often bisatellited (see Fig. 2, marker chromosomes) as detected by NOR staining. Those derived from chromosome 15 (often referred to as inverted duplicated chromosome 15s) have little or no effect on phenotype if they do not include the Angelman/Prader–Willi syndrome chromosome region (38). They may result in an abnormal phenotype if the Angelman/Prader–Willi syndrome region is present (39). Distinction between these two classes of chromosome 15 markers can be determined by FISH, with probes for genes that localize to the Angelman/ Prader–Willi syndrome region. Similarly, markers derived from chromosome 22 can be distinguished by size and location to identify those that have an effect from those that do not (40). For most other marker chromosomes of known chromosomal origin, the correlation between genotype and phenotype is limited (36,37) and in most cases will need more precise characterization for gene content of that particular marker chromosome.

IV. CHROMOSOMAL VARIATION

Variation (often referred to as a chromosomal heteromorphism or polymorphism) is observed in certain chromosomal regions between homologs of normal chromosomes. It is important to distinguish between normal variation and chromosomal abnormalities. There are two major regions of variation: the first includes size, location, and staining of heterochromatin (genetically inactive chromatin), which is concentrated in distal Yq and the centromeric regions of the other chromosomes, and the second is the morphology of acrocentric short arms, which have varying amounts of repetitive DNA and copy numbers and activity of ribosomal genes. Additional techniques are utilized to characterize these regions as variants or abnormalities, such as C-banding, which stains heterochromatin, NOR staining, which recognizes active ribosomal genes, and FISH with chromosome-specific centromeric heterochromatin probes or acrocentric short arm probes.

As mentioned earlier, the most common variants for nonacrocentric chromosomes include changes in the amount of heterochromatin on chromosomes 1q, 9q, 16q, and Yq and the position of the heterochromatin on the pericentric inversion of chromosome 9. Variation in staining characteristics as well as the amount of heterochromatin in centromeric regions also varies to a lesser extent for the remaining chromosomes. The most common variants for the acrocentrics are changes in short arm morphology and length that result from increases or decreases in heterochromatin (which stains C-band positive or FISH positive with repetitive sequence short arm probes such as *acro-p*) and/or copy number of active ribosomal genes (which are NOR stain positive). Parental chromosomal studies are usually requested when deviations in the expected staining properties of suspected common variants occur.

Other less common variations, such as fragile sites, additional G-bands near centromeres, and differential condensation between homologous chromosome regions require family studies to assist in interpreting whether the finding represents a true abnormality or a family-specific variant. Differential chromosome condensation between homologues poses a particular dilemma if the region involves a known microdeletion or duplication syndrome such as those that occur on chromosome 15q11.2q13 in the Angelman/Prader–Willi syndrome region. A summary of how to distinguish true abnormalities in the Angelman/Prader–Willi syndrome region on chromosome 15q11–q13 from potential variants is presented in Table 6.

V. MOSAICISM

Individuals occasionally have more than one cell line (one normal and one abnormal) present in their tissues. If one cell line is derived from the other, the individual is referred to as a mosaic. If the cell lines are derived from different zygotes (i.e., 46,XX/46,XY), the individual is referred to as a chimera. In most instances of mosaicism, the abnormal cell line has a numerical abnormality (i.e., 46,XX/47,XX,+8). Mosaicism is rare for structural abnormalities. The degree to which a mosaic individual is clinically affected usually depends upon the tissues that are affected and to a lesser degree on the

Table 6 Distinguishing Chromosome 15q11–q13 Abnormalities from Variants

---

(1) Deletions
(a) May be detectable by routine GTG-banded chromosome analysis, confirmed by FISH
(b) Clinically significant, result in either AS or PWS
(2) Duplications of PWS/AS region
(a) Identified by routine GTG-banded chromosome analysis and confirmed by FISH
(b) Clinically significant with findings that include autistic-like features, dysmorphology, and developmental delay
(3) Variants
(a) Identified by routine GTG-banded chromosome analysis and not duplicated in the AS/PWS region by FISH
(b) Not clinically significant

Parental studies are requested on individuals with potential duplications or variants of chromosome 15q11–q13 to distinguish between the two possibilities.
Angelman (AS) and Prader–Willi (PWS) syndromes—they are clinically distinct syndromes that localize to chromosome 15q11.2q13. Angelman syndrome is characterized by lack of speech, ataxia, seizures, hypopigmentation, inappropriate laughter, and developmental delays. Prader-Willi syndrome is characterized by hypotonia, short stature, small hands and feet, hyperphagia and obesity, hypopigmentation, and developmental delays. Maternal genetic information is absent in AS (55) and paternal genetic information is absent in PWS (56). The population frequency for AS and PWS is 1/10,000–1/20,000. The population frequency of duplications of the AS/PWS region is unknown but is likely to be under ascertained due to milder clinical findings (17,18).

frequency of abnormal cells within a specific tissue. A routine cytogenetic analysis of 20 cells in a single tissue sample typically excludes ~20% mosaicism with 99% confidence (41).

VI. NON-MENDELIAN PHENOTYPES DUE TO CHROMOSOMAL EFFECTS

A. X Chromosome Inactivation

X chromosome inactivation refers to the process whereby many genes on one X chromosome are inactivated to equalize the X-linked gene expression in males and females. As a general rule, there is only one active X per cell regardless of the number of X chromosomes and in the case of X/autosome translocations, the normal X is generally inactivated to prevent spread of inactivation into autosomal genes. The inactive X can be detected by its late replication and dense compaction (42,43). A more comprehensive description of X inactivation is presented elsewhere in this textbook.

B. Genomic Imprinting

This refers to the process whereby genes are marked or modified differently depending upon whether they have passed through male gametogenesis or female gametogenesis. The expression of imprinted genes is determined by the parent who contributed them. To date, the best-characterized imprinted regions are on chromosomes 11p (Beckwith–Weidemann region) and 15q (Angelman/Prader–Willi region), but other chromosomes (such as 7, 14, and 20) also have proven imprinted regions, and several other chromosomes are suspected to contain imprinted genes that contribute to congenital disease (for a review, see Ref. 44). The finding of an imprinted chromosome or chromosomal region involved in an abnormality prompts additional investigation at the molecular level by FISH or DNA testing. As previously described in Table 6, FISH is useful for distinguishing abnormal chromosomes from variant chromosomes for these regions.

In addition to conventional FISH, which detects the large deletions, FISH has been used to detect very small deletions (45) of the element that controls the imprinting process, known as the imprinting center, where the recurrence risk in other offspring may be as high as 50% (46). Fluorescence in situ hybridization can also distinguish uniparental from biparental inheritance through differences in allele-specific replication of imprinted regions on interphase cells (47,48).

VII. DIAGNOSTIC ADVANCES IN CYTOGENETICS BASED ON THE HUMAN GENOME PROJECT

The human genome project has provided a comprehensive set of chromosomally mapped recombinant BAC, PAC, and PI clones (49). However, clone density varies from 0.3 to 5 per Mb, which means that some regions of the genome are much more sparsely covered than others. The best covered chromosomes are 1, 6, 20, 22, and X, whereas the lowest coverage is found on chromosomes 2, 17, 18, 19, and Y. Due to the high frequency of segmental duplication revealed by the genome sequence, many of these clones cross-hybridize to other genomic locations on the same and/or different chromosomes. These low copy duplications are particularly evident on chromosomes 1, 7, 11, 16, the X and Y chromosome pseudoautosomal region (49), and at sites of the olfactory receptor gene family (50).

In addition to uneven chromosomal coverage and cross-hybridization, probe length and lack of available sequences on some BAC, PAC, and P1 clones, including commercial ones, limit the precision in defining chromosome rearrangements. These recombinant probes are large (on average 100–300 kb in length) and often span more than one gene locus. The commercially available clones are generally useful for detecting the more common abnormalities: FISH detection or characterization of rare chromosomal abnormalities or family-specific abnormalities relies on the availability of clones from research laboratories.

The availability of the human genome sequence (51,52) has overcome many of these limitations, as we have readily developed FISH probes from single-copy (sc) intervals of the human genome (53) for over 30 different chromosomal regions and can develop additional probes for almost any region as warranted (45). This technique, referred to as scFISH or single-copy FISH, utilizes probes that are much smaller (1500–3500 bp; i.e., 1–3 orders of magnitude) and have a greater genomic density (average of 1 per 20 kb for chromosomes 21 and 22) than recombinant ones, thereby enabling detection of common and rare chromosomal rearrangements with greater precision than is currently possible. Such precision will be useful in phenotype–genotype characterization of contiguous gene syndromes and other disorders.

The human genome project has spawned a number of other exciting new molecular technologies for simultaneous comprehensive genome analysis [i.e., comparative genomic hybridization (CGH) microarrays]. However, the diagnostic information produced by FISH and conventional cytogenetics will remain the gold standard for some time to come. While both molecular genetic and cytogenetic studies can detect abnormalities, only conventional chromosome and FISH metaphase studies can reveal the chromosomal context of such abnormalities or detect mosaicism, balanced transloca-tions, or rearrangements within a chromosome. While CGH microarray studies have the advantage of being automated, the results of those studies currently demonstrate a high degree of variability among laboratories and internal repro-ducibility is not reliable (54). Furthermore, they are techni-cally challenging and require complex statistical methods that have not been standardized to interpret results. All of the above reasons indicate that recognition of chromosome abnormalities by trained cytogeneticists will not be replaced by CGH array or similar methods.

REFERENCES

1. Battaglia A, Carey JC. Diagnostic evaluation of developmental delay/mental retardation: an overview. Am J Med Genet 2003; 117C:3–14.

2. Curry CJ, Stevenson RE, Aughton D, Byrne J, Carey JC, Cassidy SB, Cunniff C, Graham JM Jr, Jones MC, Kaback MM, Moeschler J, Schaefer BG, Schwartz S, Tarleton J, Opitz J. Evaluation of mental retardation: Recommendations of a Consensus Conference: American College of Medical Genet-ics. Am J Med Genet 1997; 72:468–477.

3. Tijo JH, Levan A. The chromosome number in man. Hereditas 1956; 42:1.

4. Ford CE, Hamerton JL. The chromosomes of man. Nature 1956; 10(178):1020–1023.

5. Lejeune J. Le mongolisme. Premier exemple d'aberration autosomique humaine. Ann Genet Sem Hop 1959; 1:41.

6. Caspersson T, Zech L, Johansson C. Analysis of the human metaphase chromosome by aid of DNA-binding fluorescent agents. Exp Cell Res 1970; 62:490.

7. Hsu TC. Human and Mammalian Cytogenetics: An Historical Perspective. New York: Springer-Verlag, 1979.

8. Canadian Collaborative CVS–Amniocentesis Clinical Trial Group. Multicentre randomised clinical trial of chorion villus sampling and amniocentesis: first report. Lancet 1989; 1:1–6.

9. ISCN. An International System for Human Cytogenetic Nomenclature. In: F Mitelman, ed. Basel: S. Karger, 1995.

10. Robinson WP, Dutly F, Nicholls RD, Bernasconi F, Penaherrera M, Michaelis RC, Abeliovich D, Schinzel AA. The mechanisms involved in formation of deletions and duplications of 15q11–13. J Med Genet 1998; 35:130–136.

11. Amos-Landgraf JM, Ji Y, Gottlief W, Depinet T, Wandstrat AE, Cassidy SB, Driscoll DJ, Rogan PK, Schwartz S, Nicholls RD. Chromosome breakage in the Prader–Willi and Angelman syndromes involved recombination between large, transcribed repeats at proximal and distal breakpoints. Am J Hum Genet 1999; 65:370–386.

12. Potocki L, Chen KS, Park SS, Osterholm DE, Withers MA, Kimonis V, Summers AM, Meschino WS, Anyane-Yeboa K, Kashork CD, Shaffer LG, Lupski JR. Molecular mechanism for duplication 17p11.2—the homologous recombination reciprocal of the Smith–Magenis microdeletion. Nat Genet 2000; 24:84–87.

13. Shaikh TH, Kurahashi H, Saitta SC, O'Hare AM, Hu P, Roe BA, Driscoll DA, McDonald-McGinn DM, Zackai EF, Budarf ML, Emanuel BS. Chromosome 22-specific low copy repeats and the 22q11.2 deletion syndrome: genomic organization and deletion endpoint analysis. Hum Mol Genet 2000; 9:489–501.

14. Nicholls RD, Knepper JL. Genome organization, function and imprinting in Prader–Willi and Angelman syndromes. Ann Rev Genomics Hum Genet 2001; 2:153–175.

15. Shaikh TH, Kurahashi H, Emanuel BS. Evolutionarily conserved low copy repeats (LCRs) in 22q11 mediate deletions,

duplications, translocations, and genomic instability: an update and literature review. Genet Med 2001; 3:6–13.

16. Shaw CJ, Bi W, Lupski JR. Genetic proof of unequal meiotic crossovers in reciprocal deletion and duplication of 17p11.2. Am J Hum Genet 2002; 71:1072–1081.

17. Repetto GM, White LM, Bader PJ, Johnson D, Knoll JH. Interstitial duplications of chromosome region 15q11q13: clinical and molecular characterization. Am J Med Genet 1998; 79:82–89.

18. Bolton PF, Dennis NR, Browne CE, Thomas NS, Veltman MW, Thompsons RJ, Jacobs P. The phenotypic manifestations of interstitial duplications of proximal 15q with special reference to the autistic spectrum disorders. Am J Med Genet 2001; 105:675–685.

19. Gardner RJM, Sutherland GR. Inversions [Chapter 8]. In: Chromosome Abnormalities and Genetic Counseling. 3rd ed. Oxford University Press, 2004:142–162.

20. Vine DT, Yarkoni S, Cohen MM. Inversion homozygosity of chromosome no.9 in a highly inbred kindred. Am J Hum Genet 1976; 28:203–207.

21. Park JP, Wojiski SA, Apellman RA, Rhodes CH, Mohandas TK. Human chromosome 9 pericentric homologies: implications for chromosome 9 heteromorphisms. Cytogenet Cell Genet 1998; 82:192–194.

22. Gelman-Kohan Z, Rosensaft J, Ben-Cohen RN, Chemke J. Homozygosity for inversion (2) (p12q14). Hum Genet 1993; 92:427.

23. Collinson MN, Fisher AM, Walker J, Currie J, Williams L, Roberts P. Inv(10) (p11.2q21.2), a variant chromosome. Hum Genet 1997; 101:175–180.

24. Wenger SL, Steele MW, Boone LY, Lenkey SG, Cummins JH, Chen XQ. "Balanced" karyotypes in six abnormal offspring of balanced reciprocal translocation normal carrier parents. Am J Med Genet 1995; 55:47–52.

25. Bugge M, Bruun-Petersen G, Brondum-Nielsen K, Friedrich U, Hansen J, Jensen G, Jensen PK, Kristoffersson U, Lundsteen C, Niebuhr E, Rasmussen KR, Rasmussen K, Tommerup N. Disease associated balanced chromosome rearrangements: a

resource for large scale genotype–phenotype delineation in man. J Med Genet 2000; 37:858–865.

26. Hill AS, Foot NJ, Chaplin TL, Yound BD. The most frequent constitutional translocation in humans, the t(11;22)(q23;q11) is due to a highly specific Alu-mediated recombination. Hum Mol Genet 2000; 9:1525–1532.

27. Kurahashi H, Emanuel BS. Long AT-rich palindromes and the constitutional t(11;22) breakpoint. Hum Mol Genet 2001; 10:2605–2617.

28. Spiteri E, Babcock M, Kashork CD, Wakui K, Gogineni S, Lewis DA, Williams KM, Minoshima S, Sasaki T, Shimizu N, Potocki L, Pulijaal V, Shanske A, Shaffer LG, Morrow BE. Frequent translocations occur between low copy repeats on chromosome 22q11.2 (LCR22s) and telomeric bands of partner chromosomes. Hum Mol Genet 2003; 12:1823–1837.

29. Xu J, Chen Z. Advances in molecular cytogenetics for the evaluation of mental retardation. Am J Med Genet 2003; 117C:15–24.

30. Knight SJL, Lese CM, Precht KS, Kuc J, Ning Y, Lucas S, Regan R, Brenan M, Nicod A, Lawrie NM, Cardy DLN, Nguyen H, Hudson TJ, Riethman HC, Ledbetter DH, Flint J. An optimized set of human telomere clones for studying telomere integrity and architecture. Am J Hum Genet 2000; 67: 320–332.

31. Knight SJL, Flint J. Perfect endings: a review of subtelomeric probes and their use in clinical diagnosis. J Med Genet 2000; 37:401–409.

32. Joyce CA, Dennis NR, Cooper S, Browne CE. Subtelomeric rearrangements: results from a study of selected and unselected probands with idiopathic mental retardation and control individuals by using high resolution G-banding and FISH. Hum Genet 2001; 109:440–451.

33. Rossi E, Piccini R, Zollino M, Neri G, Caselli D, Tenconi R, Castellan C, Carrozzo R, Danesino C, Zuffardi O, Ragusa A, Castigilia L, Galesi O, Greco D, Romano C, Pierluigi M, Perfumo C, DiRocco M, Faravelli F, Dagna Bricarelli F, Bonaglia MC, Bedeschi MR, Borgatti R. Cryptic telomeric rearrangements in subjects with mental retardation associated

with dysmorphism and congenital malformations. J Med Genet 2001; 38:417–420.

34. de Vries BBA, White SM, Knight SLJ, Regan R, Homfray T, Young ID, Super M, McKeown C, Splitt M, Quarrell OWJ, Trainer AH, Niermeijer MF, Malcolm S, Flint J, Hurst JA, Winter RM. Clinical studies on submicroscopic subtelomeric rearrangements: a checklist. J Med Genet 2001; 38:145–150.

35. Warburton D. De novo balanced chromosome rearrangements and extra marker chromosomes identified at prenatal diagnosis: clinical significance and distribution of breakpoints. Am J Hum Genet 1991; 49:995–1013.

36. Crolla JA. FISH and molecular studies of autosomal supernumerary marker chromosomes excluding those derived from chromosome 15: II Review of the literature. Am J Med Genet 1998; 75:367–381.

37. Crolla JA, Long F, Rivera H, Dennis NR. FISH and molecular study of autosomal supernumerary marker chromosomes excluding those derived from chromosomes 15 and 22: I Results of 26 new cases. Am J Med Genet 1998; 75:355–366.

38. Leana-Cox J, Jenkins L, Palmer CG, Plattner R, Sheppard L, Flejter WL, Zackowski J, Tsien F, Schwartz S. Molecular cytogenetic analysis of inv dup(15) chromosomes, using probes specific for the Prader–Willi/Angelman syndrome region: clinical implications. Am J Hum Genet 1994; 54:748–756.

39. Cheng SD, Spinner NB, Zackai EF, Knoll JH. Cytogenetic and molecular characterization of inverted duplicated chromosomes 15 from 11 patients. Am J Hum Genet 1994; 55: 753–759.

40. Rosias PR, Sijstermans JM, Theunissen PM, Pulles-Heintzberger CF, Die-Smulders CR, Engelen JJ, Van Der Meer SB. Phenotypic variability of the cat eye syndrome. Case report and review of the literature. Genet Couns 2001; 12: 273–282.

41. Hook EB. Models and assumptions in calculating the probabilities of detecting chromosomal mosaicism. Hum Genet 1978; 40:235–239.

42. Latt SA, Willard HG, Gerald PS. BrdU-33258 Hoechst analysis of DNA replication in human lymphocytes with supernumerary or structurally abnormal X chromosomes. Chromosoma 1976; 57:135–153.

43. Torchia BS, Call LM, Migeon BR. DNA replication analysis of FMR1, XIST and factor 8C loci by FISH shows nontranscribed X-linked genes replicate late. Am J Hum Genet 1994; 55: 96–104.

44. Engel E, Antonarakis SE. Genomic imprinting and uniparental disomy. Medicine: Clinical and Molecular Aspects. New York: Wiley-Liss, 2002.

45. Knoll JHM, Rogan PK. Sequence-based, *in situ* detection of chromosomal abnormalities at high resolution. Am J Med Genet 2003; 121A(3):245–257.

46. Saitoh S, Buiting K, Rogan PK, Buxton JL, Driscoll DJ, Arnemann J, Konig R, Malcolm S, Horsthemke B, Nicholls RD. Minimal definition of the imprinting center and fixation of chromosome 15q11–q13 epigenotype by imprinting mutations. Proc Natl Acad Sci USA 1996; 93(15):7811–7815.

47. Knoll JH, Cheng SD, Lalande M. Allele specificity of DNA replication timing in the Angelman/Prader–Willi syndrome imprinted chromosomal region. Nat Genet 1994; 6:41–46.

48. White LM, Rogan PK, Nicholls RD, Wu BL, Korf B, Knoll JH. Allele-specific replication of 15q11–q13 loci: a diagnostic test for detection of uniparental disomy. Am J Hum Genet 1996; 59:423–430.

49. Cheung VG, Nowak N, Jang W, Kirsch IR, Zhao S. Integration of cytogenetic landmarks into the draft sequence of the human genome. Nature 2001; 409(6822):953–958.

50. Trask BJ, Massa H, Brand-Arpon V, Chan K, Friedman C, Nguyen OT, Eichler E, van den Engh G, Rouquier S, Shizuya H, Giorgi D. Large multi-chromosomal duplications encompass many members of the olfactory receptor gene family in the human genome. Hum Mol Genet 1998; 7:2007–2020.

51. International Human Genome Sequencing Consortium. Initial sequencing and analysis of the human genome. Nature 2001; 409(6822):860–921.

52. Venter JC, Adams MD, Meyers EW, Li PW, Mural RJ. The sequence of the human genome. Science 2001; 291(5507): 1304–1351.

53. Rogan PK, Cazcarro PM, Knoll JHM. Sequence-based design of single-copy genomic DNA probes for fluorescence in situ hybridization. Genome Res 2001; 11:1086–1094.

54. Carter NP, Fiegler H, Piper J. Comparative analysis of comparative genomic hybridization microarray technologies: report of a workshop sponsored by the Wellcome Trust. Cytometry 2002; 49:43–48.

55. Knoll JH, Nicholls RD, Magenis RE, Graham JM Jr, Lalande M, Latt SA. Angelman and Prader–Willi syndromes share a common chromosome 15 deletion but differ in parental origin of the deletion. Am J Med Genet 1989; 32:285–290.

56. Butler MG, Palmer CG. Parental origin of chromosome 15 deletion in Prader–Willi syndrome. Lancet 1983; 1(8336): 1285–1286.

4

Molecular Genetics and Diagnostic Testing

NANCY J. CARPENTER

Center for Genetic Testing, Saint Francis Health
System, Tulsa, Oklahoma, U.S.A.

I. INTRODUCTION

Advances in molecular biology promise to enhance our
understanding of the genetic basis of many disorders associated with developmental disabilities. The development of
new technologies, such as polymerase chain reaction (PCR)
and automated deoxyribonucleic acid (DNA) sequencing,
and the extraordinary outcome of the Human Genome Project
in identifying ~35,000 genes in the human genome will allow
the study of many of these disorders in more detail at the
molecular level. Ultimately, understanding the molecular
basis of these disorders may result in improved therapies
directed toward the basic molecular defects that cause them.

This chapter reviews molecular genetic approaches to the study of conditions with developmental disabilities. It provides a review of basic molecular genetics including DNA and RNA structure, DNA replication, transcription, translation, gene structure, and mutations. In addition, there is a discussion of molecular techniques currently in use in diagnostic laboratories, indications for diagnostic testing, and selection of methods for detection of various types of disease-causing mutations.

II. BASICS OF MOLECULAR GENETICS

A. DNA Structure

Genes are made of DNA consisting of two strands of nucleotides that form a double helix by hydrogen bonding between the bases (Fig. 1). Each nucleotide is composed of a nitrogen base attached to a deoxyribose sugar and a phosphate. Hydrogen bonding occurs between the bases—adenine (A) pairs with thymine (T) and guanine (G) pairs with cytosine (C). At one end of a DNA strand is a free phosphate group (5') and at the other end, a free hydroxyl group (3'). The two strands run in opposite directions; one strand runs in the 5' to 3' direction and the other runs in 3' to 5' direction (1).

B. DNA Replication

DNA replication produces identical copies of the DNA molecule in each of the two daughter cells during cell division, thus preserving the genetic information. During the process, the DNA strands unwind with the use of an enzyme, DNA polymerase, and each strand serves as a template for the synthesis of a complementary strand. Consequently, two new double-stranded DNA molecules are formed, each with one of the original strands and a new daughter strand.

C. Transcription

Genetic information is encoded by the sequences of bases along the DNA molecule. In order to preserve the coded information

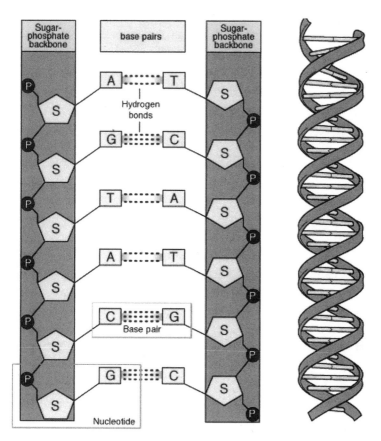

Figure 1 The DNA molecule showing the component nucleotides and base pairing (left) and the double helical structure of DNA (right). (Reprinted from Access Excellence with permission from the Office of Education, National Human Genome Research Institute.)

in each cell, the genes are transcribed into RNA molecules. RNA has a nucleotide structure that is similar to DNA; however, it is single-stranded, contains the ribose as its sugar, and has the base uracil (U) instead of thymine (T). During transcription, DNA unwinds and one of the strands serves as a template for the synthesis of messenger RNA (mRNA). RNA polymerase, the enzyme required for synthesis, binds to the promoter located on the 5′ end of genes. Transcription

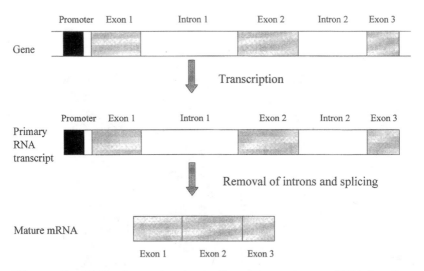

Figure 2   RNA processing to produce the mature mRNA involves cleavage and removal of intronic RNA segments from the primary transcript and splicing of exonic RNA segments.

factors are proteins that determine whether transcription occurs for any given gene and the level of transcription.

Genes are composed of sequences coding for proteins (exons) interspersed with noncoding sequences (introns). During transcription, the exons are spliced together from a larger precursor RNA to form the mature mRNA (Fig. 2). There are invariant sequences at the beginning and end of introns termed splice donor (GT) and acceptor (AT) sequences that facilitate correct splicing.

D. Translation

After splicing and the addition of a polyadenine (poly A) tail, the mature mRNA moves from the nucleus of the cell to the cytoplasm and attaches to ribosomes. At the site of protein synthesis, ribosomes are composed of ribosomal RNA and protein. The mRNA is scanned until a specific sequence is reached. Initiation of protein synthesis occurs with the first AUG sequence of bases (the start codon) and the mRNA is

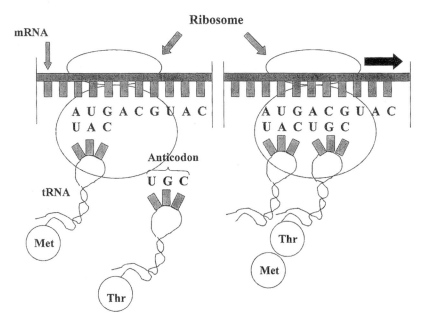

Figure 3   The sequence of bases in the mRNA is translated into protein on the ribosome. Transfer RNAs with amino acids attached are matched by codon–anticodon pairing and result in the synthesis of an amino acid chain (protein).

read in groups of three bases (codons). As shown in Fig. 3, transfer RNA (tRNA) molecules bind in the ribosome to the mRNA through codon–anticodon pairing during translation. Every tRNA has an anticodon and is attached to an amino acid specified by the anticodon. Amino acids are linked by peptide bonds, as they are brought into the ribosome by the appropriate tRNA. The mRNA sequence of codons is translated until one of the three stop codons (UAA, UAG, UGA) is encountered at which point protein synthesis is terminated.

Additional protein processings including glycosylation, hydroxylation, proteolytic cleavage, and phosphorylation may occur after synthesis. Proteins are then either localized to a particular cellular compartment or extruded into the extracellular space.

E. Types of Mutations

Changes in the base sequence in coding regions of the DNA may have significant effects on cell structure and metabolism. These disease-causing mutations can be classified on the basis of the type and scale of the genetic change that is produced. There are mutations that produce small changes in DNA structure, such as single nucleotide substitutions, small deletions, insertions, inversions, and duplications. There are also those that cause a significant change in gene structure, such as expansions of the nucleotide repeats and large deletions, insertions, inversions, and duplications.

1.   The simplest and most frequent mutations are single nucleotide substitutions referred to as point mutations. Most occur during DNA replication when an incorrect base is inserted into the daughter strand. Point mutations that result in the wrong amino acid being inserted in the protein are termed missense mutations, whereas those that produce stop codons and consequently cause the translation of proteins to halt prematurely are termed nonsense mutations (Fig. 4).

2.   Frame shift mutations result from deletion or insertion of a few nucleotides that are not a multiple of three bases. This type of alteration changes the reading frame of the codons in genes and usually results in a stop codon that is not normally placed. The result is a protein that is truncated or elongated and has the wrong amino acid sequence starting from the site of the frame shift.

3.   Other types of small mutations include: (i) exon deletions when some or all of an exon or exons are lost resulting in loss of a significant portion of amino acids from the protein, (ii) exon duplications in which an exon or exons are repeated in tandem leading to repetition of a segment of amino acids in a protein, and (iii) exon inversion in which the order of an exon or several exons is inverted causing the

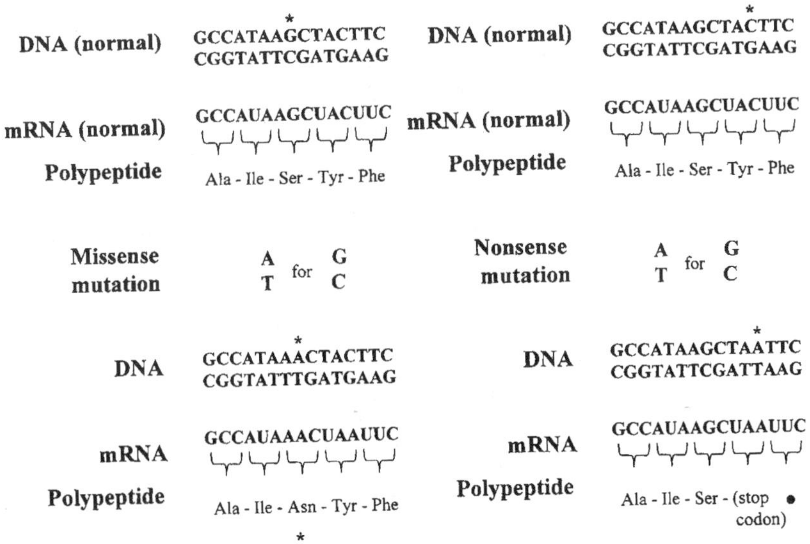

Figure 4 A missense mutation (left) produces a change in a codon that, in turn, results in a change in a single amino acid of the protein. A nonsense mutation (right) produces a stop codon in the mRNA that prematurely terminates translation of the protein. (Reprinted from Medical Genetics, by Jorde, Carey, White, 1995, with permission from Elsevier.)

order of a segment of the amino acids in the protein to be disturbed.

4. Single base substitutions and small deletions and duplications that occur at specific sites outside of the coding regions may also have considerable effect on the gene product. For example, the loss of the exon–intron boundary by elimination of a splice-site sequence results in the reduction or absence of normally spliced mRNA. Consequently, there is exon skipping and loss of amino acids from the protein. Utilization of a cryptic splice site leads to the production of an abnormal mRNA with premature stop codons or to the inclusion of additional amino acids from the reading of intron sequences. Other examples are mutations occurring in promoter regions that alter the transcription level of genes

and mutations preventing the addition of the poly A tail that reduce the stability of the mRNA.

5. Another type of mutation is the instability of certain trinucleotide repeats and their expansion in affected genes. This type of mutation was first described in Fragile X syndrome (2) and now has been reported in at least 30 other disorders such as Huntington disease and myotonic dystrophy (3,4). The precise mechanism for expansion of these repeats is unknown, but the progression of DNA polymerase during replication is known to be blocked by certain repeats, and the resulting slippage may lead to repeat expansions. In some disorders, there are a certain number of repeats (premutation) that exhibit a high probability of further expansion to yield an even larger number of repeats (full mutation) associated with disease.

6. Large deletions or duplications of a single gene or contiguous genes are common causes of certain disorders. A considerable number of these alterations are generated by mispairing of homologous sequences in the genome (low-copy repeats) followed by unequal crossing over (5). Examples of such disorders are the deletion 22q syndrome (DiGeorge/VCFS) and Prader–Willi and Angelman syndromes.

Overall, missense mutations are by far the most frequent mutation type followed by small deletions, nonsense mutations, and splice-site mutations. However, the frequency of different mutations is not the same for every gene. The characteristics of the DNA sequence and the presence of unstable repeats or homologous sequences (low-copy repeats) largely determine the type of mutation that is most common for a given gene. Some genes exhibit mainly missense or nonsense mutations, whereas others manifest a special type of lesion such as an inversion or an expansion of trinucleotide repeats. A review of many types of mutations is given by Antonarakis et al. (6).

III. MOLECULAR TECHNIQUES

A. Characteristics of DNA

Two characteristics that are particularly important for DNA analysis are: (i) its linearity that allows the ordering of the bases within genes and genes on the chromosomes, and (ii) the complementary nature of the two DNA strands. The two strands can be denatured (separated) by heating to a certain temperature. A single-stranded sequence of DNA or RNA will only recognize and bind (hybridize) to the complementary sequence of DNA. Therefore, purified DNA sequences can be used as probes to detect the complementary sequence in a mixture of DNA molecules.

B. Restriction Enzymes

One of the major factors in the development of techniques to analyze DNA was the discovery of proteins that cut DNA at specific base sequences called restriction enzymes. Each enzyme recognizes a different sequence and cuts the DNA into fragments of about 10^3–10^4 bases. For example, the enzyme *Eco*RI cuts at the sequence GAATTC, whereas *Hind*III cuts at AAGCTT. Variations in DNA sequence among individuals in a population that can be observed by digestion with restriction enzymes are termed restriction fragment length polymorphisms (RFLPs). RFLPs were very useful for early gene mapping studies but have been supplanted by microsatellite polymorphisms that are variations in small repeat sequences such as dinucleotide repeats, (CA)n.

C. Southern Blotting

This technique was devised by Southern in 1975 (7) as a method for transferring DNA fragments to a membrane, so that they may be hybridized to specific DNA probes. The DNA is first digested using restriction enzymes to produce a large number of fragments of different sizes ranging from ~1 to 25 kb. The DNA that is being targeted for investigation will be present in only one or a few specific fragments. As shown in Fig. 5, the DNA fragments are then separated by

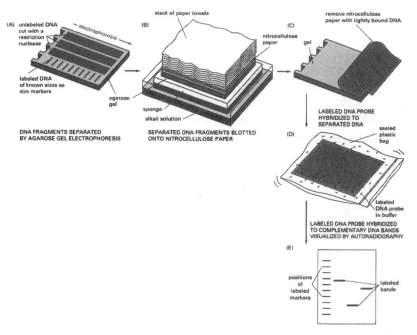

Figure 5 Southern blot procedure showing transfer of the DNA digested with a restriction enzyme to a membrane, then hybridized with a labeled DNA probe, and visualized by autoradiography. (Reprinted from Essential Cell Biology by Alberts, Bray, Johnson, Lewis, Raff, Roberts, and Walter, 1998, with permission from Taylor & Francis Books, Inc.)

electrophoresis through an agarose gel (A). Denaturation with alkali into single strands of DNA follows, and these strands are transferred to a membrane of nitrocellulose or modified nylon by capillary action (B). The membrane or "blot" retains the same arrangement of the fragments that was produced by electrophoresis (C). The blot is exposed to a chemically or radioactively labeled DNA probe that hybridizes to its complementary sequence in the single-stranded DNA (D). Detection of the DNA fragment(s) that corresponds to the probe is performed by chemiluminescence or autoradiography. The sizes of the targeted DNA fragments are determined by comparing to fragments of known size that are separated by electrophoresis.

The Southern blotting technique is most useful for assessment of large segments of DNA measuring several kilobases in size. The technique was initially used to detect RFLPs for linkage analysis in gene mapping and for parentage and forensic testing. It is currently used in diagnostic laboratories to detect large alterations in gene structure, such as large expansions of trinucleotide repeats and large inversions and deletions.

D. Polymerase Chain Reaction

Developed by Mullis in 1985 (8,9), the PCR technique was designed to amplify DNA, i.e., to increase the number of molecules of a targeted region of DNA. As shown in Fig. 6, initially the double-stranded DNA (template) is denatured or separated into single strands at high temperature (94°C). These strands are cooled to around 55°C to allow two short synthetic nucleotides to hybridize to their complementary sequences, one on each strand flanking the region of interest in the template DNA. These short nucleotides serve as primers to start DNA synthesis by a thermostable DNA polymerase (*Taq* polymerase) at 72°C. The cycle is repeated 25–30 times and during each cycle, DNA synthesis terminates at the end of the template corresponding to the primer sequences. The product is a fixed length of DNA that corresponds to the interval between and including the two primers. To visualize the PCR product, the DNA may be separated by electrophoresis on an agarose or polyacrylamide gel and stained with the fluorescent dye, ethidium bromide. Primers may be fluorescently labeled allowing the product to be detected by laser-equipped instruments. Radioactively labeled PCR products are detected by autoradiography.

The PCR process increases the number of copies of a specific DNA region by 100 million times in 3–4 hr. Therefore, the technique is capable of amplifying a minute amount of DNA to produce a large amount in a short period of time. The *Taq* polymerase is highly reliable, so that the sequence of the PCR product is an exact copy of the target region and may be analyzed for specific mutations or for polymorphic alleles for linkage.

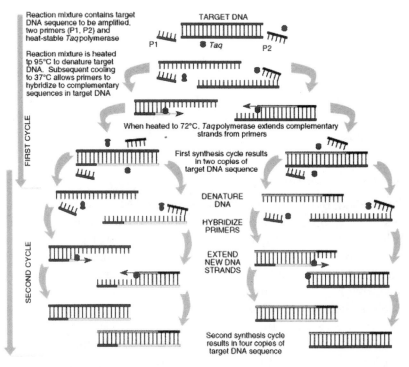

Figure 6 DNA amplification using PCR. In the first cycle (top), target DNA is denatured at high temperature and then cooled to allow two primers (P1 and P2) to attach to the single strands. *Taq* polymerase, a heat stable enzyme, facilitates the synthesis of complementary DNA strands resulting in two copies of the target DNA. During subsequent cycles of heating and cooling (bottom), the target DNA amplifies exponentially as each new double strand denatures to become two templates for further synthesis. (Human Genome Program, U.S. Department of Energy, *Primer on Molecular Genetics*, Washington, DC, 1992.)

E. Mutation Scanning Techniques

Searching for disease-causing mutations in a gene may require identification of a single nucleotide or a few nucleotides in a coding sequence composed of thousands of nucleotides. To avoid sequencing large amounts of DNA, strategies have been developed to rapidly scan genes for small mutations. The techniques use PCR to amplify the gene or gene segment to be scanned and, ultimately, each method leads to sequencing of the region shown to contain a mutation.

1. Single-strand conformational polymorphism analysis is based on the conformational change in DNA resulting in an alteration in electrophoretic mobility that is produced by some mutations.
2. Mismatch heteroduplex analysis is a method in which the PCR products are denatured and allowed to renature forming heteroduplexes, if a mismatch (mutation) is present. The heteroduplexes can be distinguished because they move more slowly on nondenaturing polyacrylamide gels than do homoduplexes.
3. Denaturing gradient gel electrophoresis and denaturing high-performance liquid chromatography are methods that are based on the differences in mobility of heteroduplex and homoduplex molecules when they are heated to temperatures just below the melting temperature of the homoduplexes.

F. DNA Sequencing

Determining the order of the nucleotide bases in DNA is typically done by the dideoxy method (chain-termination of Sanger method) (10). DNA polymerase proceeds to synthesize DNA strands of various lengths, stopping DNA replication at one of four bases and determining the resulting fragment lengths. In addition to the DNA template and the enzyme, sequencing reactions contain a primer to bind to the DNA, four deoxynucleotides to be incorporated into the new DNA strand, one labeled deoxynucleotide (using radioactivity or fluorescent dye), and one dideoxynucleotide that terminates the strand wherever it is incorporated. The concentration of the nucleotides is adjusted, so that dideoxynucleotides are incorporated into each position in which that nucleotide occurs producing a collection of DNA fragments, each with a dideoxynucelotide at the end. The fragments are separated by electrophoresis and the positions of the nucleotides visualized by autoradiography or by an automated laser-equipped instrument to determine the sequence (Fig. 7).

1. Sequencing reactions loaded
   onto polyacrylamide gel for
   fragment separation

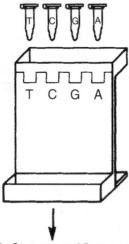

2. Sequence read (bottom to top)
   from gel autoradiogram

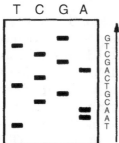

Figure 7 Sequencing of DNA by the chain termination or Sanger method. A template DNA is replicated using the four nucleotides and one dideoxy nucleotide (T, C, G, or A) in each of the sequen Scing reactions. The dideoxy nucleotide terminates the synthesis wherever it is incorporated, producing DNA fragments of varying length. The fragments are separated by electrophoresis (1) and the positions of the nucleotide are analyzed to determine the sequence reading from smallest to largest (2). (Human Genome Program, U.S. Department of Energy, *Primer on Molecular Genetics*, Washington, DC, 1992.)

Sequencing may be directed to a certain area of a gene with a known mutation such as the single-base substitution in the β-globin gene in sickle cell anemia or an entire gene may be sequenced if the mutations are known to be heterogeneous such as the MeCP2 gene in Rett syndrome.

G. DNA Microarrays

DNA microarrays are the most rapidly developing innovations of molecular technology. Thousands of different DNA molecules can be attached to small regions of glass microscope slides. The patient DNA is usually labeled with a fluorescent dye and allowed to hybridize to complementary DNA on the array. Automated detection of the fluorescent hybridization signals allows thousands of sequences to be analyzed simultaneously. Among many applications, microarrays can be used to detect heterogeneous mutations and to assess levels of transcription of genes. Although this technology is currently used for research purposes, it may soon have widespread clinical use.

IV. MOLECULAR GENETIC TESTING

A. Specimens for Testing

Because genetic disorders are due to inherited mutations in the germline, DNA tests in most cases can be performed on any accessible body fluid or tissue. Blood collected in EDTA or ACD tubes is the most common specimen although dried blood spots, buccal swabs, and cultured cells can also be used. Amniotic fluid cells and chorionic villus specimens (CVS) are collected for prenatal testing.

The amount of the specimen is determined by the molecular technique necessary for testing. PCR amplification of DNA allows testing to be performed on minute samples of tissue, whereas the Southern blotting method requires substantially more blood or cultured cells. Tests that use mRNA as the starting material for analysis require a sample of the tissue in which the gene is expressed.

B. Indications for Testing

1. Diagnostic Tests

Diagnostic tests performed on symptomatic patients are the most straightforward and common form of molecular tests. The circumstances in which such tests are ordered are usually to confirm a diagnosis made from a clinical impression or to assist in differential diagnosis. Some diagnostic assays are able to identify most or all mutations for a given disorder, whereas other tests are designed for specific mutation types and may not be able to detect all mutations in a gene or critical region of a chromosome. Molecular assays designed for detection of mutations in one gene will not detect mutations in other genes that cause closely related disorders. For a diagnostic test, a positive result in a proband will often lead to testing of the parents and other family members who are at risk of carrying the mutation.

2. Carrier Testing

Carrier testing is defined as the detection of recessive mutations in healthy persons (usually a parent or other relative) when the mutation causing the disorder has already been identified in the proband. The identification of carrier status is essential for genetic counseling to evaluate the risk of recurrence of the disease in the family.

3. Prenatal Diagnosis

DNA obtained from amniocytes or CVS can be tested when there is a risk of recurrence of the disorder and the exact mutation causing the disease is known from previous testing of the proband. A recent variation of prenatal diagnosis, preimplantation genetic diagnosis (PGD), involves PCR amplification and mutation analysis of DNA from a single blastomere from an embryo produced by in vitro fertilization (IVF) (11). This technique also requires knowing the exact identity of the familial mutation(s). PGD is reserved for couples who are adverse to terminating an *in utero* pregnancy or who are already undergoing IVF for other reasons.

4. Predisposition and Presymptomatic Testing

Predictive DNA testing is for individuals with strong family histories of autosomal dominant disorders with adult onset. Most patients have a 50% risk of inheriting the mutation from a parent. Testing of children under 18 years of age is only justified for disorders with onset in childhood, such as the hereditary cancer syndromes, familial adenomatous polyposis coli (APC gene), and multiple endocrine neoplasia type 2 (RET oncogene), where increased surveillance of mutation carriers and decreased surveillance of noncarriers are desirable.

5. Carrier Screening

Carrier screening, like carrier testing, is for detection of recessive mutations in healthy individuals. However, screening is performed for individuals who are at risk, not because of family history, but by virtue of belonging to an ethnic group in which the frequency of certain mutations is particularly high. Because carrier screening assays involve large numbers of patients and must be cost-effective, they are designed to test the most common mutations and may not necessarily detect all mutations known for a specific gene. For example, for cystic fibrosis, couples are screened for the 32 most common mutations in the CFTR gene, whereas more than 500 different mutations have been identified. The goal of screening tests is to allow couples at risk to make informed decisions about reproduction and to offer prenatal diagnosis.

V. SELECTION OF MOLECULAR TECHNIQUES

The choice of technique depends on the size and complexity of the gene being studied, the type of mutation to be detected, and, to some extent, the type and condition of the specimen. PCR-based methods are required for extremely small, fixed, or degraded tissues. Once the DNA is amplified, it is amenable to further methods such as restriction digestion or sequencing. On the other hand, Southern blotting requires larger amounts of purified DNA of high molecular weight that can be digested with enzymes and produce reproducible patterns on gel electrophoresis.

VI. DETECTION OF SPECIFIC MUTATION TYPES

A. Known Point Mutations, Small Deletions, and Duplications

For the detection of known point mutations, small deletions, and duplications, PCR-amplified DNA samples can be hybridized with allele-specific oligonucleotide (ASO) probes containing either the normal or the mutant sequence. The ASO probes can distinguish between single nucleotide differences in DNA sequence and hybridize to the exact complementary sequences in patient DNA. Used in pairs, the probes can identify homozygotes and heterozygotes for normal and mutant alleles.

A cutting site for a restriction enzyme may be created or destroyed by a mutation making it possible to digest a PCR-amplified DNA product with a specific enzyme and analyze the cleavage fragments by gel electrophoresis to distinguish between the normal and the mutant alleles (Fig. 8).

B. Unknown and Heterogeneous Mutations

For some disorders, a wide range of point mutations or small deletions and duplications have been reported. In such cases, it is not possible to assay one or a few mutant alleles for diagnostic testing. Instead, the entire gene must be evaluated for mutations. One strategy is to use mutation scanning techniques to find a region of the gene likely to harbor a mutation and to confirm the mutations by sequencing the region identified. Mutation scanning methods are not 100% sensitive; so, some mutations may be missed. Alternatively, sequencing of the entire coding region of a gene can be performed. Even then, some mutations may be missed because they may be located at some distance from the gene, for example, in a promoter region.

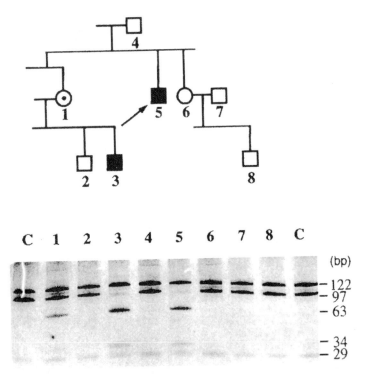

Figure 8 The detection of a mutation in the L1CAM gene is shown in a family with X-linked hydrocephalus. The mutation creates a site for the restriction enzyme *Bso*F1 resulting in cleavage of a 97 bp band into fragments of 63 and 34 bp. The smaller fragments are observed in a carrier female (lane 1) and two affected males (lanes 3 and 5) but are not seen in controls (C) and other family members without the mutation (lanes 2, 4, 6, 7, and 8). (From Jouet et al. New domains of neural cell adhesion molecule L1 implicated in X-linked hydrocephalus and MASA syndrome. Am J Hum Genet 1995; 56(6):1304–1314.)

C. Detection of Trinucleotide Repeat Expansions

Accurate sizing of trinucleotide repeats is important for detecting the expansions that are characteristic of certain diseases. For expansions of moderate length (a few hundred bases), PCR amplification and sizing of products by denaturing gel or capillary gel electrophoresis are adequate.

If the expansion is large and difficult to amplify, such as the CGG repeat in Fragile X syndrome or the CTG repeat in myotonic dystrophy, sizing by Southern blotting is required.

D. Detection of Large Deletions and Inversions

Large deletions and inversions are usually detected by Southern blotting and are represented by the absence of bands for the expected DNA fragments. PCR amplification can be used if primers are designed such that there is a failure to produce a PCR product, because the primers do not hybridize to the patient DNA owing to deletion or inversion (Fig. 9). Extremely large rearrangements require very high molecular weight DNA and the technique of pulsed-field gel electrophoresis for detection.

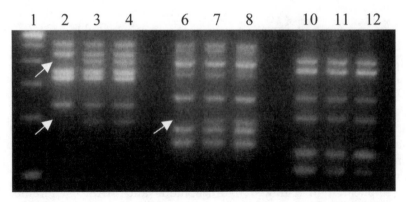

Figure 9 Multiplex PCR analysis of the dystrophin gene in Duchene Muscular Dystrophy using primers for amplification of 21 exons from two affected male patients (male patient 1 in lanes 2, 6, and 10; male patient 2 in lanes 3, 7, and 11) and a male control (in lanes 4, 8, and 12). Lane 1 is a size marker. Lanes 2–4 show PCR results for seven exons, lanes 6–8 show results for eight exons, and lanes 10–12 show results for six exons. Deletions (indicated by arrows) are detected in lane 2 (two exons) and lane 6 (one exon). The affected male patient 2 did not show a deletion-type mutation.

E. Detection of Altered Methylation

Certain restriction enzymes are sensitive (will not cut) to methylated DNA sequences allowing distinction between methylated and unmethylated fragments. Digestion combined with Southern blotting is useful in determining methylation status of Fragile X mutations, distinguishing between maternal and paternal alleles for imprinted genes in Prader–Willi and Angelman syndromes and for determining the pattern of X-inactivation in females (Fig. 10). Methylation PCR techniques involving bisulfite treatment of DNA or sequence-specific primers have also been developed for the purpose of detecting alterations in methylation.

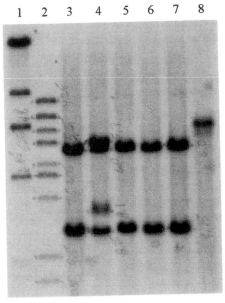

Figure 10 Southern blot analysis of the Fragile X (FMR1) gene mutation is shown using probe StB12.3. Lanes 1 and 2 are size markers. The normal females (lanes 3, 5, 6, and 7) have two DNA bands, lower ~2.8 kb (active X chromosome) and upper 5.2 kb (inactive X chromosome) bands. A carrier female with a premutation (lane 4) has additional bands slightly larger than the normal bands. An affected male (lane 8) has a full mutation with a smear of bands much larger than the 2.8 kb or 5.2 kb bands.

F. Linkage Analysis

The analysis of polymorphisms is useful in certain circumstances. One of these is a disease-causing gene has been localized to a region of a chromosome but has not been isolated as in the case of many of the X-linked mental retardation syndromes. This analysis is also helpful for carrier testing when a mutation cannot be identified in the DNA sequence in a proband. Polymorphic loci that are known to be located within the critical chromosomal region or that are extremely close to the gene in question are said to be linked because they are inherited together. Previously, RFLPs were used for linkage analysis, but variations in small repeats (microsatellites) are now used predominantly.

VII. RESOURCES

1. Online Mendelian Inheritance in Man (OMIM) is a comprehensive catalog of over 10,000 human genetic disorders, which includes information on clinical presentation, inheritance pattern, and molecular pathology (www.ncbi. nlm.nih.gov/omim).
2. GeneReviews has expert-written material for over 200 human genetic disorders that are subject to molecular testing. The reviews include information on clinical diagnosis, molecular genetic pathology, and genetic counseling issues (www.genetests.org).
3. GeneTests is the primary international listing of genetic testing laboratories (www.genetests.org).
4. Human Gene Mutation Database is a comprehensive listing of mutations in over 1000 genes (uwcmml1s.uwcm. ac.uk/uwcm/mg/hgmd0.html).
5. Gene Cards has entries for human genes, their proteins, and their expression in human tissues (http:// bioinformatics.weizmann.ac.il/cards).
6. The Genome Database has entries for many genes and comprehensive maps of the genome (www.gdb.org/ gdb/).

REFERENCES

1. Strachan T, Read AP. DNA structure and function. In: Human Molecular Genetics. 2d ed. New York: John Wiley & Sons, Inc, 2001:1–31.

2. Yu S, Pritchard M, Kremer E, Lynch M, Nancarrow J, Baker E, Holman K, Mulley JC, Warren ST, Schlessinger D, Sutherland GR, Richards RI. Fragile X genotype characterized by an unstable region of DNA. Science 1991; 252:1179–1181.

3. Huntington's Disease Collaborative Research Group. A novel gene containing a trinucleotide repeat that is expanded and unstable on Huntington's disease chromosomes. Cell 1993; 72: 971–983.

4. Mahadevan M, Tsilfidis C, Sabourin L, Shutler G, Amemiya C, Jansen G, Neville C, Narang M, Barcelo J, O'Hoy K, Leblond S, Earle-MacDonald J, De Jong PJ, Wieringa B, Korneluk RG. Myotonic dystrophy mutation: an unstable CTG repeat in the 3′ untranslated region of the gene. Science 1992; 255: 1253–1258.

5. Inoue K, Lupski JR. Molecular mechanisms for genomic disorders. Annu Rev Genomics Hum Genet 2002; 3:199–242.

6. Antonarakis SE, Krawczak M, Cooper DN. Mutations in human disease: nature and consequences. In: Rimoin DL, Connor JM, Pyeritz RE, Korf BR, eds. Principles and Practice of Medical Genetics. 4th ed. London: Churchill Livingstone, 2002: 83–103.

7. Southern EM. Detection of specific sequences among DNA fragments separated by gel electrophoresis. J Mol Biol 1975; 98:503–517.

8. Saiki RK, Scharf S, Faloona F, Mullis KB, Horn GT, Erlich HA, Arnheim N. Enzymatic amplification of beta-globin genomic sequences and restriction site analysis for diagnosis of sickle cell anemia. Science 1985; 230:1350–1354.

9. Mullis KB, Faloona F. Specific synthesis of DNA in vitro via a polymerase-catalyzed chain reaction. Methods Enzymol 1987; 155:335–350.

10. Sanger F, Nicklen S, Coulson AR. DNA sequencing with chain-terminating inhibitors. Proc Natl Acad Sci USA 1977; 74: 5463–5467.

11. Thornhill AR, Snow K. Molecular diagnostics in preimplantation genetic diagnosis. J Mol Diagn 2002; 4:11–29.

5

The Human Genome Project and Its Impact on Understanding Developmental Disabilities

DANIEL J. WATTENDORF and
MAXIMILIAN MUENKE

Department of Health and Human Services,
Medical Genetics Branch, National Human
Genome Research Institute, Bethesda,
Maryland, U.S.A.

I. INTRODUCTION

The sequence of the human genome has been the most visible goal of the Human Genome Project (HGP) since its initiation in 1990. However, during the past decade the medical community has reaped the most tangible benefits from the accomplishments of specific and quantifiable goals defined prospectively as part of the process itself (1). The construction of physical and genetic maps, the mapping and sequencing of model organisms, the development of readily accessible public databases, and the rapid gains in technology allowable only by the scale of investment from a "big science" project has provided key research opportunities (2). A new and more comprehensive understanding of developmental disabilities has coincided with the 50th anniversary of the discovery of the double helix (3) and the completion of sequencing the human genome in 2003. The medical research community is now straddled between the phases of cataloging these diseases and understanding the pathophysiology of the developmental processes gone awry. While most developmental disabilities can be included under the spectrum of genetic disease, the inherited components have only recently been revealed for some. The transition from identifying and describing developmental disabilities to understanding and treatment has begun. A century of progress, which began with the clinical insights of Bateson and Garrod (4,5), will be enriched by the results of the HGP. The latest successes of those that have studied or cared for people with developmental disabilities best demonstrate the primary purpose of the HGP—medical care. Furthermore, new research opportunities and forecasts for the genomics of developmental diseases are continually updated as accomplishments made during the last decade provide new insights into the underlying causes.

The clinical approach to the child with a developmental disability is a complex problem and one of the reasons to have clinical genetics as a recognized specialty. The meticulous investigation and documentation of specific developmental disabilities over the past century has provided a foundation for their study through the application of methodologies used as part of the HGP. The most common disorders associated with developmental delay or mental retardation seen by clinical geneticists are listed in Table 1 and described in more detail in other chapters. Selected photographs of children with specific genetic syndromes are shown in Fig. 1. Some of these disorders were chosen as examples to provide a perspective on the opportunities created by methodological advances over the past decade and to lay out potential clinical strategies that may aid in the care of a patient with a developmental disability.

Table 1 Inherited Disorders with a Frequency of > 1/100,000

Mental Retardation in Most Affected Individuals	
Monogenic[a]	Cytogenetic/Polygenic
Tuberous Sclerosis	Trisomy 21
Fragile X syndrome	Trisomy 18
Holoprosencephaly	Trisomy 13
NTD/Hydrocephalus?	Williams syndrome
CHARGE association	Prader-Willi syndrome
Angelman syndrome	Smith-Magenis syndrome
Rett syndrome	5p deletion
ATXR	4p deletion
Opitz syndrome	Tetrasomy 12p (Pallister-Killian syndrome)
FraXE	1p36 deletion
Lissencephalies	Submicroscopic deletions/duplications

Smith-Lemli-Opitz syndrome
Zellweger syndrome
Kabuki syndrome
Rubenstein-Taybi syndrome
Cornelia de Lange syndrome
Mild/Borderline Mental Retardation in Most Affected Individuals
22q11.2 deletion
Sotos syndrome
Mild/Borderline Mental Retardation in Some Affected Individuals
Noonan syndrome
Triple X syndrome
Mild/Borderline Mental Retardation in Rare Affected Individuals
Neurofibromatosis 1
Russell-Silver syndrome
Beckwith-Wiedemann syndrome
Aarskog syndrome
Mild (Specific) Learning Disabilities
Klinefelter syndrome
Turner syndrome

[a]May be heterogenous, syndrome listed here unless known to be polygenic.

II. GENETIC MAPS AND A POSITIONAL CLONING APPROACH

In 1980, a theoretical plan of identifying DNA sequence variations across the genome at regular intervals was defined

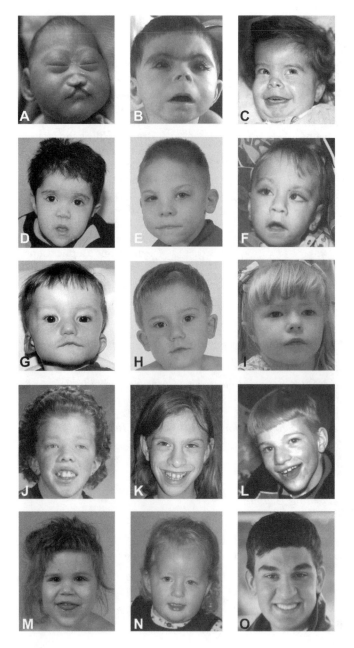

Figure 1 (*Caption on facing page*)

Figure 1 (*Facing page*) Characteristic facial photographs of children with selected developmental disabilities commonly seen in the geneticist's office. (A) *Holoprosencephaly* (CNS findings of alobar, semilobar, or lobar holoprosencephaly, microcephaly and structural midline defects including closely spaced eyes, midfacial agenesis with midline cleft of the lip and palate). (B) *Cornelia de Lange syndrome* (multisystem disorder with microcephaly, characteristic synophrys and long eyelashes, low-set ears, depressed nasal bridge, anteverted nostrils, thin upper lip, downturned corners of mouth, and low posterior and anterior hairline). (C) *Miller–Dieker syndrome* (lissencephaly with microcephaly, bitemporal narrowing, low-set ears, small nose with upturned nares, flat philtrum and thin vermillion border of upper lip). (D) *Chromosome 1p36 deletion syndrome* (multisystem deletion syndrome with brachycephaly, deep-set eyes, flat nasal bridge, asymmetric ears, pointed chin). (E) *Smith–Lemli–Opitz syndrome* (multisystem disorder with microcephaly, bitemporal narrowing, hypertelorism, ptosis, strabism, epicanthal folds, posteriorly rotated, low-set ears, broad, flat nasal bridge, anteverted nostrils, and micrognathia). (F) *Kabuki syndrome* (multisystem disorder with microcephaly and long palpebral fissures, eversion of lateral third of lower eyelids, broad, arched, and sparse eyebrows, large prominent, low-set ears, depressed nasal tip, short nasal columella, and characteristic trapezoid philtrum). (G) *CHARGE association* (multisystem disorder with *c*oloboma of the iris and other structures of the eye, *h*eart defects, *a*tresia of choanae, *r*etarded growth, *g*enital hypoplasia, and *e*ar anomalies). (H) *Smith–Magenis syndrome* (multisystem deletion syndrome with brachycephaly, broad face, broad nasal bridge, and protruding ears). (I) *Chromosome 22q11 deletion syndrome* (multisystem deletion syndrome with micrognathia, low-set ears, hypertelorism, short palpebral fissures, prominent nose with narrow alar base, and short philtrum). (J) *Noonan syndrome* (multisystem disorder with hypertelorism, down-slanting palpebral fissures, epicanthal folds, blue-green irides, low-set, posteriorly rotated ears, dental malocclusin, and micrognathia). (K) *Williams–Beuren syndrome* (multisystem disorder with medial eyebrow flare, periorbital fullness, epicanthal folds, stellate pattern of iris, thick lips, and hypodontia). (L) *Angelman syndrome* (multisystem disorder with microbrachycephaly, decreased pigmentation of iris, prognathia, and hypopigmentation of skin). (M) *Beckwith–Wiedemann syndrome* (multisystem disorder with macrosomia, macroglossia, omphalocele, ear creases, and organomegaly). (N) *Prader–Willi syndrome* (mulitsystem disorder due to genomic imprinting with infantile hypotonia, hypogonadism, hyperphagia and early onset childhood obesity, developmental delay, and small hands and feet). (O) *Fragile X syndrome* (multisystem disorder with mental retardation, macroorchidism, large ears, long narrow face, and prominent nose and chin). (*See color insert.*)

(6). These variants, or markers, could then be linked to a disease phenotype and followed through large families. Analysis of polymorphic markers located throughout the genome could identify linkage of a given disease to an interval on a specific chromosome. If the size of the interval is small enough (<0.5–1 cM), then mutations found in a candidate gene located within this critical region would likely identify the disease-causing gene. By 1983, *Huntington's disease* became the first disorder affecting cognition to be found by this process (7). However, a genome-wide search for a disease gene proved cumbersome without multiple markers mapped across the genome. With so few markers available, many research teams created their own genetic maps. Less than 40 genes were isolated by positional cloning methods from the limited genetic maps available prior to 1994. Then in 1994, building on earlier success (8), a dense genetic map was published (9) achieving one of the first goals of the HGP.

The availability of thousands of markers mapped to the human genome led not only to an increased rate of identification of genes that cause developmental disabilities, but also revealed the complexity of human disease. Positional cloning efforts have demonstrated concepts such as genetic heterogeneity (i.e., different mutations causing the same trait or pattern of traits (phenotype), locus heterogeneity (i.e., more than one mutated gene causing the same phenotype), allelic heterogeneity (i.e., more than one mutation within a gene causing the same phenotype), pleiotropy (i.e., one mutated gene having multiple phenotypes), and even digenic inheritance (i.e., the necessity of mutations at two loci causing a specific phenotype). All of these concepts are exemplified by the study of one disease, *Bardet–Biedl syndrome* (BBS). BBS is characterized primarily by mental retardation, obesity, pigmentary retinopathy, polydactyly, renal malformations, and hypogenitalism (10). The multiple, seemingly unrelated, effects in multiple organ systems due to one altered gene demonstrate pleiotropy. Some of the phenotypic features are common to many disorders and may make accurate diagnosis in early childhood difficult even for the experienced clinician. Early efforts at positional cloning showed linkage to chromosomes 3, 11, 15, 16 (11–14). By 2000, 10 years after the start of the HGP, six loci had been mapped (15–17). Careful assessment of the involved pedigrees showed that despite the significant variation of phenotypic features (expressivity) within the families used for linkage, the characteristic features were present across studies involving different chromosomes, demonstrating locus heterogeneity. All of the mapped loci fit an autosomal recessive pattern of inheritance. Two mutations at the given locus being evaluated in a particular family or genetic isolate segregated with the phenotype.

In 2000, another subset of BBS patients (representing the sixth of currently eight known loci for this disease, BBS1–BBS8) was found to have mutations in a gene known to cause another disease, *McKusick–Kaufman syndrome* (18,19). McKusick–Kaufman syndrome is characterized primarily by congenital heart defects, postaxial polydactlyly, and hydrometrocolpos (i.e., accumulation of fluids in the uterus and vagina) in affected females (20), but is caused by mutation in the same gene. In other words, different alleles of this gene can cause two entirely different disease phenotypes. The success of positional cloning and the acquisition of the sequence of the clones allowed more comprehensive analysis of inheritance mechanisms and illustrated even more diverse mechanisms of inheritance. Evaluation of pedigrees that contained mutations in BBS6 showed affected individuals that contained only one mutant allele. Molecular testing of another cloned gene, BBS2, in the same pedigrees identified cases with two mutant alleles. Further analysis of pedigrees segregating with BBS2 showed affected individuals with a single BBS2 mutant allele and two BBS6 mutant alleles. Multiple alleles at different loci appeared to cause BBS in these families. Furthermore, individuals were found within these pedigrees that had two mutant alleles at one locus and two wild-type (i.e., normal) alleles at the other locus, yet were unaffected (15). This representation of digenic inheritance causing a developmental disorder would not have been feasible if all of these families were grouped together as part of a large positional cloning study that was typically required prior to the availability of dense genetic maps provided by the HGP. Even more complex positional cloning efforts are now possible.

III.   PHYSICAL MAPS AND UTILIZATION
OF BACTERIAL ARTIFICIAL
CHROMOSOMES (BACs)

The development of bacterial artificial chromosomes was in
response to one of the earliest goals of the HGP: to obtain a
map prior to sequencing (21). This map was to contain
guideposts for future sequenced fragments. Polymerase chain
reaction (PCR) developed in the mid-1980s (22) had an amplification limit of hundreds of base pairs and assembly was dependent on knowing the specific chromosomal position of the
fragments. In the 1980s, there were no clear starting points
to sequencing; furthermore, there were not a significant
number of mapped positions on which to place sequenced fragments. The solution was to partially digest a genome with
restriction endonucleases into fragments (23). While different
methods were used to make copies of the fragments in a hybrid
cell (somatic cell genetics), a prevalent method was to digest the
genome into pieces of approximately 150,000–170,000 base
pairs. Then, with molecular manipulation, these fragments
were inserted into BACs. The bacteria replicated the DNA
and produced multiple identical copies of the unique insert in
a short time. This "clone" was then digested by restriction endonucleases. A characteristic pattern of sizes of fragments was
created specific to each clone. This became the "fingerprint" of
each clone. Analysis of the fingerprint patterns of each clone
compared to one another distinguished which BACs contained
overlapping sequence and, when multiple BACs were tiled
across, created a contig (i.e., a large contiguous stretch of
DNA sequence). A complete set of overlapping BACs is a physical map (24). Finally, the clones were restriction digested into
subclones that were small enough to sequence and then
reassembled within the BACs. Later, the location of overlapping BACs on each chromosome was used to rapidly reassemble
many sequenced subclones. This approach, termed hierarchi-
cal shotgun assembly, is what differentiated the public from
the private projects (25).

The acquisition of the BAC (26) and its mapping to human
chromosomes provided uses other than a step towards sequence

fidelity (27). Many developmental disabilities can now be diagnosed by fluorescent in situ hybridization (FISH) originally developed in 1980 (28). The most common probe used in FISH experiments is a BAC that has been labeled with a fluorescent molecule (Fig. 2). Specific BACs that have been used as part of the HGP can now be used as probes to identify specific causes

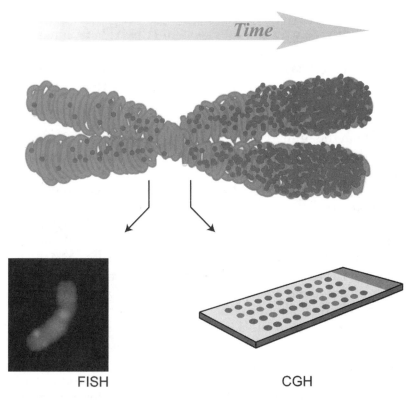

FISH   CGH

Figure 2 Bacterial artificial chromosomes (BACs) mapped to a human chromosome. Over time, the development of BACs has served as guideposts for the Human Genome Project and has been invaluable as tools for diagnosing and understanding developmental disabilities. A single BAC may be used to probe for losses or gains of a gene(s) or region(s) of a chromosome that is involved in a particular disease or, more recently, bound to a slide in an array of BACs to perform many experiments at once (comparative genomic hybridization; CGH array). (*See color insert.*)

of developmental disability and are especially useful for screening for deletions. For example, contiguous gene deletions at 7q11.23 cause *Williams–Beuren syndrome*, a neurodevelopmental disorder characterized by auditory and language strengths with severe visuospatial deficits, characteristic facial dysmorphism, elastin arteriopathy, and a stereotypic behavioral profile of overfriendliness, anxiety, and decreased attention (29) (Fig. 1K). Gene duplications may also be detected by FISH. *Pelizaeus–Merzbacher disease* is a disorder of dysmyelination of the central nervous system (CNS). It is caused by mutations or duplications of the proteolipid protein (PLP) gene at Xq22. A duplication of a FISH probe containing PLP can be seen in interphase cells (30). Or, in a patient with developmental delay of unknown cause found to have a balanced translocation by routine chromosome analysis, the selection of a series of BACs from the human genome databases may be used to probe across the translocation breakpoint and potentially clone a gene disrupted by this breakpoint. This has recently been demonstrated by the isolation of the NSD1 gene as a cause of *Sotos syndrome* (31).

If there is no cytogenetic abnormality detectable by high-resolution chromosome banding in a child with mental retardation of unknown cause, then the gene-rich subtelomeric regions at the ends of the chromosomes can be tested (32). Fluorescent probes again prove effective (33). The high rate of recombination between subtelomeric regions raised the possibility of *cryptic unbalanced translocations* (typically less than 2–3 Mb) that usually cannot be detected by high-resolution chromosome banding. Multiple BACs obtained from subtelomeric regions that, with few exceptions, are unique to particular chromosomes can now be batched as a panel of probes to screen for a submicroscopic subtelomeric rearrangement. By using various clinical selection criteria that generally include developmental delay or mental retardation, the yield of identifying a subtelomeric chromosome rearrangement has typically been near 5%. Eleven studies published in 2001–2002 alone utilized FISH methodology (34–44). A recent review of the frequency of specific subtelomeric deletions and a preliminary characterization of the phenotypic features observed has been published (44).

Limitations of these studies that only screen for subtelomeric alterations can now be overcome by an extension of technology known as comparative genomic hybridization or CGH (45,46). Labeling the patient's DNA in one color and normal control DNA in a different color, followed by cohybridization onto a BAC array will allow detection of losses or gains of DNA at the BAC target site   (Fig. 2). This technology, originally developed for detecting abnormal chromosome copy number in tumors, can now be used as a genomic screen for cryptic unbalanced chromosomal rearrangements. CGH arrays have been predicted to become an inexpensive and readily available screening tool (47).

A recent demonstration of CGH is its application to a constitutional deletion of the distal short arm of chromosome 1. This *1p36 deletion* occurs in approximately 1 in 5000 births (48) and is characterized by mental and growth retardation, seizures, hearing loss, and characteristic dysmorphic features (49–51) (Fig. 1D). Given the difficulty in detecting deletions or rearrangements of chromosomes that involve less than 10 Mb with traditional cytogenetics, the CGH array offers a rapid, high-resolution tool for the diagnosis of developmental disabilities. The use of BACs as a guideposts for sequence assembly and targeting to chromosome regions has been supplemented by its use as a functional probe for detecting specific developmental disorders or as a screen for cryptic chromosome rearrangements.

IV. UTILIZATION OF COMPARATIVE ORGANISMS AND FUNCTIONAL ANALYSIS

Another area providing new insights into the genetic underpinnings of developmental disabilities is comparative genomics. Comparative genomics refers to interspecies genetic analysis vs. intraspecies analysis comparing variation among humans. Mapping model organisms had been a priority of the HGP from the beginning and now sequencing of many model organisms has been completed. Genomes of model organisms are of particular interest because of the ease of use in scientific experiments (e.g., mouse) or for phylogenetic similarity (e.g., chimpanzee). The sequence of the mouse is nearing completion (52) and an initial comparative map of the human genome to the chimpanzee has been published (53) (Fig. 3).

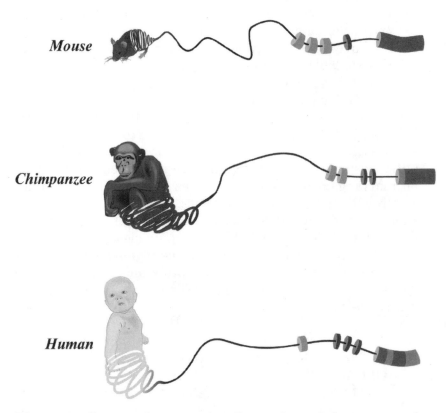

Figure 3 Comparative genomics. Comparison of the mouse and chimpanzee genomes with the human genome has identified a similar number of genes. However, large variations are created by duplicated genes and/or chromosomal segments. In addition, differences are also seen in the way genes are processed: alternative splicing leads to different exon use that results in different proteins from the same genetic sequence. These variations lead to new insight into human gene function and dysfunction. (*See color insert.*)

Comparative genomics has aided in the identification of the first gene involved in *speech and language pathology*, FOXP2, a member of the *forkhead* family of transcription factors. This gene was identified by the genetic analysis of a family and an unrelated boy with a chromosome rearrangement with both a specific speech deficit that impairs fine facial movements as well as a neural processing language deficit that interferes with the mental process of forming words (54). The ability to compare human sequence with DNA sequence from primates allowed the recognition that the specific sequence of the human variations of the FOXP2 gene were found at a frequency higher than expected by chance and fit with a model of natural selection. Thus, by finding sequence variations in patients with rare developmental disabilities and comparing these variations to sequences from model organisms, the genetic pathways defining human cognition may eventually be revealed.

The most common monogenic disorder associated with mental retardation is *fragile X syndrome*. Pleiotropic somatic and behavioral features include facial dysmorphism with a long narrow face and prominent ears, unusual growth patterns, macroorchidism, developmental delay with mental retardation, hyperactivity, and autistic-like behaviors (55). Caused by a mutated allele of FMR1, fragile X syndrome is transmitted as an X-linked dominant disorder that is due to a trinucleotide repeat (CGG) that expands during meiosis from a premutation size to a full mutation. This increase in size of the CGG-repeat leads to excessive methylation extending from the site of the repeat in the 5'UTR to the adjacent promoter with subsequent loss of expression of its protein, FMRP. While the phenotypic effects are attributed to the absence, and thus, loss of function of FMRP, there may be detrimental effects associated with a premutant allele (i.e., an expanded CGG-repeat, but without methylation induced gene silencing) due to a gain-of-function. For example, premutation females may have premature ovarian failure (56).

FMR1 was identified by positional cloning efforts in 1991 (57) and the molecular biology of the involved mutations has been extensively analyzed in the past decade. A contribution of genomics is demonstrated by studies of FMRP function using comparative model organisms and techniques for functional analysis. Fragile X syndrome is an ideal disease process to examine in a model organism because not only is it monogenic and characterized by loss-of-function in humans, but in several model organisms there is a single homolog of the human FMR1. Experiments can be designed to study the function of a disease gene by examining associated proteins in a model organism and then using sequence databases to identify human homologs. Alternatively, the gene/protein can be turned off (knock-out) or turned on, or overexpressed (knock-in) in a model organism. Both of these methods were successful for studying FMRP and its targets in the brain.

In the brain, FMRP is found in the dendrites of neurons. In the cytoplasm, FMRP is found bound to polyribosomes engaged in protein translation. The FMRP associated mRNAs were unknown until the utilization of microarrays. Antibodies to FMRP (isolated from Fmr1 knock-out mice) were used to coimmunoprecipitate FMRP–mRNA complexes from mice brain or from lymphoblastoid polyribosomes from fragile X patients. Then, thousands of cDNA fragments labeled to a slide (the microarray) were used as a screen to identify the mRNA bound to FMRP by fluorescence patterns when hybridization occurs (58). This was possible because the cDNA from the mouse and human genome was mapped and sequenced. Messenger RNA that bound FMRP was found to share a common structure termed intramolecular "G quartets". The availability of sequence databases (Unigene/TIGR) and algorithms for determining protein conformation allowed researchers to identify predicted human sequences that would also form G quartets. When tested, the mRNAs created from the predicted sequences were found to be targets of FMRP. These mRNAs were subsequently demonstrated to be involved in dendritic growth or synaptic function, thus are compelling targets for a gene known to cause mental retardation (59).

Even the fruit fly, *Drosophila melanogaster* has been used as a model organism to study the effects of the fragile

X mutation (60). The ability to conduct these experiments relied on the ability to move from the human to the mouse genome database or the fly to the human genome database. The identification of target mRNAs under control of FMRP in *Drosophila* and murine models and the ability to compare consensus sequences and regulatory mechanisms will yield advances in understanding brain development and offer avenues for treatment of fragile X syndrome. As demonstrated, comparative organisms provide a rapid search for genes and their regulation. However, limitations include examples of individual proteins with radically different function in different tissues and/or species.

V. SEQUENCE AND UTILIZATION OF PUBLIC DATABASES

In 1959, Lejeune and colleagues described trisomy 21 in patients with *Down syndrome* (DS). Since then, DS has become the prototypic and most common genetic cause of mental retardation. The phenotype has been well characterized and includes characteristic dysmorphism, hypotonia, frequent congenital heart disease, gastrointestinal malformations, and a predisposition to leukemia and Alzheimer-like dementia. However, despite intensive investigation over the past decades the pathophysiology is still not fully understood and treatment other than surgical management has been largely unsuccessful. The creation of a physical map of chromosome 21, obtaining and annotating the sequence, functional studies of the involved genes, and the elucidation of regulatory mechanisms and epigenetic factors derived from comparative organisms all contribute towards understanding and treating this confounding disease. Much of this research can now be performed in silico because of the early completion of the sequence of chromosome 21 and creation of annotated public databases.

Most of the successes of treatment of genetic disease have been in the area of classical inborn errors of metabolism. The diseases have been monogenic and the loss of protein product or accumulation of substrate has been defined. This has allowed an obvious choice of treatment. Unlike the inherited metabolic defects that cause complete or near-complete loss of a single protein, the notion of DS as a polygenic syndrome requires the molecular imbalances of each gene and its metabolic pathway to be defined (61). The definition of a minimal critical region of the long arm of chromosome 21 that contains the genes whose products in triplicate cause all of the phenotypic features of DS was considered in 1993 (62). In 1994, a phenotypic map of 25 features with molecular boundaries assigned for each phenotype was defined using a physical map of chromosome 21 (63); thus, creating a physical map of DS (61). The cloning of the individual genes involved in these regions would be cumbersome without known sequence data. With the completion of the HGP, experimentation and gene prediction have been possible using the public databases (64,65). The current state-of-the-art has been to refine the algorithms that extract putative genes from public databases. Nineteen new transcripts from chromosome 21, in addition to the 127 previously characterized by 2000, have been defined solely by improving on in silico methodology (66). Chromosome 21 will likely be the first to be completely annotated and the research methods and successes will foreshadow opportunities across the genome. New technologies such as serial analysis of gene function (SAGE) will allow gene expression to be measured within tissues and offer insight into developmental perturbations that may be modified with treatment. With immediate access to annotated sequence, investigators can now screen specific genes from model organisms that have phenotypic features similar to DS and determine if the involved gene has a human homolog that maps to the critical region(s) for DS. Then, the human homolog can be tested in a transgenic animal model (most frequently in the mouse) to study gene function and thus lead to a better understanding of this gene's involvement in DS (67,68). The utility of public databases and the ability to manipulate experimentation back and forth between human and model organism sequences offers immediate benefit towards a functional understanding of developmental disease.

VI. COMPLEX DISEASES AND HAPLOTYPE ANALYSIS

The success of large-scale sequencing and the mapping of an extensive collection of variants allows the discovery of the inherited components of developmental disorders to be expanded from the rare single gene disorders to the common and complex disorders. Research has now begun to measure the relationship of sequence variations to phenotypes, a phase that has described this as "the end of the beginning" (69). Diseases such as *autism* and *attention deficit-hyperactivity disorder* (ADHD) can now be studied from an extensive survey of the genome for association of all of the pieces of chromosomes inherited together through a family. While our genome is 99.9% identical between any two people, the 0.01% difference includes both variations that are inconsequential to human disease (i.e., polymorphisms) and variations that are associated or even causal of disease. Linkage is the finding that some of these variable DNA sequences are inherited together because of their close physical proximity to one another. A commonly used variation is a single nucleotide polymorphism (SNP). Linkage disequilibrium is the inheritance of two SNPs more frequently than predicted by chance alone. One of the intriguing findings of the HGP has been that relatively long stretches of DNA, longer than predicted by chance, share identical SNPs (Fig. 4). This finding allows investigators to scan a whole genome for variations by looking at a smaller set of variations across the genome each representing a commonly inherited block of DNA. This haplotype analysis (or HapMap) is a recent initiative evolved from the HGP. The International HapMap project seeks to record the SNPs within the genome and further define the size and location of these haplotype blocks. Once available, genome-wide scans for associations between complex disorders and susceptibility genes/loci can be obtained by screening only thousands rather than millions of SNPs (70).

While twin studies have been successful for ADHD, autism and other complex disorders by demonstrating a heritable contribution, positional cloning, and positional candidate

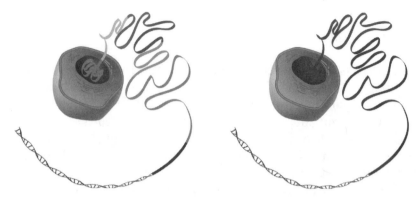

Figure 4 Haplotype blocks across the genome. Variation across the genome has been conserved through evolution in large, shared lengths of DNA referred to as "haplotype blocks." The discovery that sequence variation occurs in large units, rather than randomly across the genome, allows large-scale association studies to screen for fewer variations by identifying the shared haplotype blocks. Complex diseases such as developmental disabilities may be studied by tracking these blocks with specific phenotypes. (*See color insert.*)

strategies have been unsuccessful. The success of association studies of these disorders utilizing haplotype analysis will depend in part on a clear definition of diagnostic criteria in disorders such as ADHD. Alternatively, the identification of quantifiable risk factors or "endophenotypes" in ADHD families may be used in the future for large-scale association studies by haplotype analysis. To date, three endophenotypes have been defined for ADHD (71). The number and frequency of genes contributing to the endophenotypes will determine the success of such studies (72). However, even if the contribution of susceptibility genes to complex developmental disorders is small, the elucidation of the developmental pathway may offer insight into drug therapy (73).

VII. THE FUTURE

The first "Grand Challenge" of the future of genomics research (74) is to "elucidate the structure and function of genomes."

The first phase that has been initiated is the Encyclopedia of DNA Elements (ENCODE) Project (www.genomegov/Pages/Research/ENCODE). This project will closely analyze approximately 1% of the genome for the function of nonprotein-coding genes, chromosomal functional elements, high repeat sequences, and unique sequences that are not noncoding. The knowledge derived from ENCODE will certainly help our understanding of developmental disabilities. For example, the finding of a "positional effect" of chromosomal translocation breakpoints near known *holoprosencephaly* (Fig. 1A) genes contributing to the varying phenotype is likely to be due to these undiscovered functional elements.

However, the ultimate goal is the transformation of medical treatment based on our knowledge derived from the HGP (75). Even though a catalogue of approximately 20,000 genes is available, the number of gene products and, more specifically, documentation of therapeutic targets is in its infancy. The pharmaceutical industry has achieved therapeutics from genomic information by generating recombinant proteins that replace a deficient protein (e.g., insulin and erythropoietin) (Fig. 5). To date, drug companies have not targeted many of the developmental disabilities. A large scale, high-throughput approach, in the academic sector is needed. The ability to determine protein folding based on sequence and computer modeling will allow thousands of proteins to be considered as drug targets (Fig. 5). Using a similar organization (and funding mechanisms) as the HGP, screening for therapeutic targets with small molecules may achieve the fastest way towards translating genomic sequence to therapeutics (76). This effort will, at the same time, define the functions of genes concomitant with drug discovery. A government led effort is especially important to keep research efforts directed to include "orphan" diseases so often overlooked. These are bold plans, but the tools of the HGP make these realizable goals. Since its inception, the human genome project has been about "big science." As the HGP evolves into new arenas, the objective is still to implement new technologies with broad reach and to translate this into improved resources for clinical research. The HapMap project, ENCODE, the development of chemical libraries and

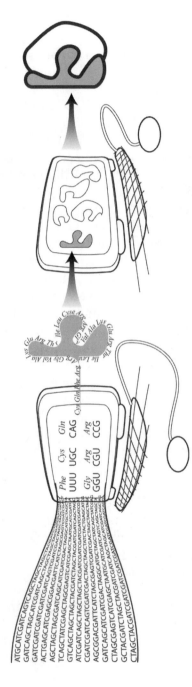

Figure 5 Computational genomics and public databases. Sequence data derived from the human genome project enable a computer to model the shape of proteins. Additional computer modeling can screen thousands of proteins, termed "biologics" in the pharmaceutical industry for matching proteins that may bind and alter the protein's activity in a therapeutic manner. In addition, small molecules can now be screened with high-throughput techniques to find potential drugs. The current forecast for the human genome project targets these investigations to the study of development disabilities.

Table 2   Research Opportunities and Forecast: Genomics of Developmental Disabilities

Key Research Opportunities	Forecast
Define complete list of all genes affecting developmental disability	Accelerate research into improved diagnostics, prevention, and therapeutics
Define all common variants of these genes and determine hereditary factors	Precise personalized risk assessment and determination of critical gene-environment interactions
Provide low cost genotyping	Employ preventative measures by genetic counseling, *in utero* therapies, or early intervention
Determine regulatory signals affecting expression in normal or abnormal state	Drug therapy based on modifying aberrant signaling or modifying normal signaling to ameliorate condition
Determine structure of all proteins affecting cognition	Drug therapy based on precise 3-dimensional information about target protein
Develop safe and effective gene-transfer vectors for many different tissues, including the brain	Gene therapy for single-gene disorders and complex traits
Vigorously explore the ethical, legal, and social implications of genome research	Legal safeguards against genetic discrimination and breaches of privacy
	Effective oversight of clinical application of genetic testing, and robust human subjects protections
	Mainstreaming of genetics into the practice of medicine with achievement of "Genetic Literacy" among clinicians and patients

Source: Modified from Ref. 2.

participation in the NIH Roadmap for Medical Research—
which involves the plan to aid the high-throughput identification of protein structures—should create and accelerate
understanding of the etiology of developmental disabilities
and offer new opportunities for treatment (Table 2).

ACKNOWLEDGMENTS

We are grateful to our patients for allowing us to reproduce
their photographs. We express thanks to the following collea-
gues for providing us with photographs: Dr. Joseph Wagstaff
(Angelman syndrome), Dr. Rosanna Weksberg (Beckwith–
Wiedemann syndrome), Dr. Ian Krantz (Cornelia de Lange
syndrome), Dr. Lisa Shaffer (deletion 1p36), Dr. Elaine H.
Zackai and Dr. Donna McDonald-McGinn (deletion 22q11),
Dr. Jeffrey E. Ming (Kabuki syndrome), Dr. William Dobyns
(Miller–Dieker syndrome), Dr. Judith Allanson (Noonan
syndrome), Dr. Suzanne Cassidy (Prader-Willi syndrome),
Dr. D. Forbes Porter (Smith–Lemli–Opitz syndrome),
Dr. Ann C.M. Smith (Smith–Magenis syndrome), Dr. Colleen
Morris (Williams syndrome), National Fragile X Foundation,
and the CHARGE Syndrome Foundation, Inc.. We are also
grateful to Daryl Leja and Michael Cichanowski for developing the figures. We are indebted to Dr. Francis Collins for
his continued support and the permission to use a modified
version of Table 2.

REFERENCES

1. Collins FS, Patrinos A, Jordan E, Chakravarti A, Gesteland R,
    Walters L. New goals for the U.S. human genome project:
    1998–2003. Science 1998; 282(5389):682–689.

2. Collins FS, McKusick VA. Implications of the human genome
    project for medical science. JAMA 2001; 285(5):540–544.

3. Watson JD, Crick FHC. Molecular structure of nucleic acids: a
    structure for deoxyribose nucleic acid. Nature 1953; 171:737–738.

4. Bateson W. Problems of heredity as a subject for horticultural investigation. J R Hortic Soc 1900; 25:54–61.

5. Garrod AE. The incidence of alkaptonuria: a study in chemical individuality. Lancet 1902; 2:1616–1620.

6. Botstein D, White RL, Skolnick M, Davis RW. Construction of a genetic linkage map in man using restriction fragment length polymorphisms. Am J Hum Genet 1980; 32(3):314–331.

7. Gusella JF, Wexler NS, Conneally PM, Naylor SL, Anderson MA, Tanzi RE, et al. A polymorphic DNA marker genetically linked to Huntington's disease. Nature 1983; 306(5940):234–238.

8. Donis-Keller H, Green P, Helms C, Cartinhour S, Weiffenbach B, Stephens K, et al. A genetic linkage map of the human genome. Cell 1987; 51(2):319–337.

9. Murray JC, Buetow KH, Weber JL, Ludwigsen S, Scherpbier-Heddema T, Manion F, et al. A comprehensive human linkage map with centimorgan density. Cooperative Human Linkage Center (CHLC). Science 1994; 265(5181):2049–2054.

10. Green JS, Parfrey PS, Harnett JD, Farid NR, Cramer BC, Johnson G, et al. The cardinal manifestations of Bardet–Biedl syndrome, a form of Laurence–Moon–Biedl syndrome. N Engl J Med 1989; 321(15):1002–1009.

11. Carmi R, Rokhlina T, Kwitek-Black AE, Elbedour K, Nishimura D, Stone EM, et al. Use of a DNA pooling strategy to identify a human obesity syndrome locus on chromosome 15. Hum Mol Genet 1995; 4(1):9–13.

12. Kwitek-Black AE, Carmi R, Duyk GM, Buetow KH, Elbedour K, Parvari R, et al. Linkage of Bardet–Biedl syndrome to chromosome 16q and evidence for non-allelic genetic heterogeneity. Nat Genet 1993; 5(4):392–396.

13. Leppert M, Baird L, Anderson KL, Otterud B, Lupski JR, Lewis RA. Bardet–Biedl syndrome is linked to DNA markers on chromosome 11q and is genetically heterogeneous. Nat Genet 1994; 7(1):108–112.

14. Sheffield VC, Carmi R, Kwitek-Black A, Rokhlina T, Nishimura D, Duyk GM, et al. Identification of a Bardet–Biedl syndrome locus on chromosome 3 and evaluation of an efficient approach to homozygosity mapping. Hum Mol Genet 1994; 3(8):1331–1335.

15. Katsanis N, Ansley SJ, Badano JL, Eichers ER, Lewis RA, Hoskins BE, et al. Triallelic inheritance in Bardet–Biedl syndrome, a Mendelian recessive disorder. Science 2001; 293(5538):2256–2259.

16. Slavotinek AM, Stone EM, Mykytyn K, Heckenlively JR, Green JS, Heon E, et al. Mutations in MKKS cause Bardet–Biedl syndrome. Nat Genet 2000; 26(1):15–16.

17. Young TL, Penney L, Woods MO, Parfrey PS, Green JS, Hefferton D, et al. A fifth locus for Bardet–Biedl syndrome maps to chromosome 2q31. Am J Hum Genet 1999; 64(3):900–904.

18. Katsanis N, Beales PL, Woods MO, Lewis RA, Green JS, Parfrey PS, et al. Mutations in MKKS cause obesity, retinal dystrophy and renal malformations associated with Bardet–Biedl syndrome. Nat Genet 2000; 26(1):67–70.

19. Slavotinek A, Rosenberg M, Knight S, Gaunt L, Fergusson W, Killoran C, et al. Screening for submicroscopic chromosome rearrangements in children with idiopathic mental retardation using microsatellite markers for the chromosome telomeres. J Med Genet 1999; 36(5):405–411.

20. Robinow M, Shaw A. The McKusick–Kaufman syndrome: recessively inherited vaginal atresia, hydrometrocolpos, uterovaginal duplications, anorectal anomalies, postaxial polydactyly, and congenital heart disease. J Pediatr 1979; 94(5):776–778.

21. Watson JD, Cook-Deegan RM. Origins of the Human Genome Project. FASEB J 1991; 5(1):8–11.

22. Mullis K, Faloona F, Scharf S, Saiki R, Horn G, Erlich H. Specific enzymatic amplification of DNA in vitro: the polymerase chain reaction. Cold Spring Harb Symp Quant Biol 1986; 51(Pt 1): 263–273.

23. White R, Lalouel JM. Chromosome mapping with DNA markers. Sci Am 1988; 258(2):40–48.

24. Olson MV. The human genome project: a player's perspective. J Mol Biol 2002; 319(4):931–942.

25. Waterston RH, Lander ES, Sulston JE. On the sequencing of the human genome. Proc Natl Acad Sci USA 2002; 99(6): 3712–3716.

26. Shizuya H, Birren B, Kim UJ, Mancino V, Slepak T, Tachiiri Y, et al. Cloning and stable maintenance of 300-kilobase-pair fragments of human DNA in *Escherichia coli* using an F-factor-based vector. Proc Natl Acad Sci USA 1992; 89(18): 8794–8797.

27. Cheung VG, Nowak N, Jang W, Kirsch IR, Zhao S, Chen XN, et al. Integration of cytogenetic landmarks into the draft sequence of the human genome. Nature 2001; 409(6822):953–958.

28. Bauman JG, Wiegant J, Van Duijn P, Lubsen NH, Sondermeijer PJ, Henning W, et al. Rapid and high resolution detection of in situ hybridisation to polytene chromosomes using fluorochrome-labeled RNA. Chromosoma 1982; 84(1):1–18.

29. Morris CA, Mervis CB. Williams syndrome and related disorders. Annu Rev Genomics Hum Genet 2000; 1:461–484.

30. Woodward K, Kendall E, Vetrie D, Malcolm S. Pelizaeus–Merzbacher disease: identification of Xq22 proteolipid–protein duplications and characterization of breakpoints by interphase FISH. Am J Hum Genet 1998; 63(1):207–217.

31. Kurotaki N, Imaizumi K, Harada N, Masuno M, Kondoh T, Nagai T, et al. Haploinsufficiency of NSD1 causes Sotos syndrome. Nat Genet 2002; 30(4):365–366.

32. Wilkie AO. Detection of cryptic chromosomal abnormalities in unexplained mental retardation: a general strategy using hypervariable subtelomeric DNA polymorphisms. Am J Hum Genet 1993; 53(3):688–701.

33. Flint J, Wilkie AO, Buckle VJ, Winter RM, Holland AJ, McDermid HE. The detection of subtelomeric chromosomal rearrangements in idiopathic mental retardation. Nat Genet 1995; 9(2):132–140.

34. Anderlid BM, Schoumans J, Anneren G, Sahlen S, Kyllerman M, Vujic M, et al. Subtelomeric rearrangements detected in patients with idiopathic mental retardation. Am J Med Genet 2002; 107(4):275–284.

35. Baker E, Hinton L, Callen DF, Altree M, Dobbie A, Eyre HJ, et al. Study of 250 children with idiopathic mental retardation reveals nine cryptic and diverse subtelomeric chromosome anomalies. Am J Med Genet 2002; 107(4):285–293.

36. Brown J, Saracoglu K, Uhrig S, Speicher MR, Elils R, Kearnie L. Subtelomeric chromosome rearrangements are detected using an innovative 12-color FISH assay (M-TEL). Nat Med 2001; 7(4):497–501.

37. Clarkson B, Pavenski K, Dupuis L, Kennedy S, Meyn S, Nezarati MM, et al. Detecting rearrangements in children using subtelomeric FISH and SKY. Am J Med Genet 2002; 107(4):267–274.

38. Fan YS, Zhang Y, Speevak M, Farrel S, Jung JH, Siu VM. Detection of submicroscopic aberrations in patients with unexplained mental retardation by fluorescence in situ hybridization using multiple subtelomeric probes. Genet Med 2001; 3(6):416–421.

39. Helias-Rodzewicz Z, Bocian E, Stankiewicz P, Obersztyn E, Kostyk E, Jakubow-Durska K. Subtelomeric rearrangements detected by FISH in three of 33 families with idiopathic mental retardation and minor physical anomalies. J Med Genet 2002; 39(9):e53.

40. Joyce CA, Dennis NR, Cooper S, Browne CE. Subtelomeric rearrangements: results from a study of selected and unselected probands with idiopathic mental retardation and control individuals by using high-resolution G-banding and FISH. Hum Genet 2001; 109(4):440–451.

41. Pettenati MJ, Jackle B, Bobby P, Stewart W, Von Kap-Herr C, Mowrey P, et al. Unexpected retention and concomitant loss of subtelomeric regions in balanced chromosome anomalies by FISH. Am J Med Genet 2002; 111(1):48–53.

42. Popp S, Schulze B, Granzow M, Keller M, Holtgrove-Grez H, Schoell B, et al. Study of 30 patients with unexplained developmental delay and dysmorphic features or congenital abnormalities using conventional cytogenetics and multiplex FISH telomere (M-TEL) integrity assay. Hum Genet 2002; 111(1):31–39.

43. Sismani C, Armour JA, Flint J, Girgalli C, Regan R, Patsalis PC. Screening for subtelomeric chromosome abnormalities in children with idiopathic mental retardation using multiprobe telomeric FISH and the new MAPH telomeric assay. Eur J Hum Genet 2001; 9(7):527–532.

44. De Vries BB, Winter R, Schinzel A, van Ravenswaaij-Arts C. Telomeres: a diagnosis at the end of chromosomes. J Med Genet 2003; 40:385–398.

45. Snijders AM, Nowak N, Segraves R, Blackwood S, Brown N, Conroy J, et al. Assembly of microarrays for genome-wide measurement of DNA copy number. Nat Genet 2001; 29(3): 263–264.

46. Kallioniemi A, Kallioniemi OP, Sudar D, Rutovitz D, Gray JW, Waldman F, et al. Comparative genomic hybridization for molecular cytogenetic analysis of solid tumors. Science 1992; 258(5083):818–821.

47. van Karnebeek CD, Koevoets C, Sluijter S, Bijlsma EK, Smeets DF, Redecker EJ, et al. Prospective screening for subtelomeric rearrangements in children with mental retardation of unknown aetiology: the Amsterdam experience. J Med Genet 2002; 39(8):546–553.

48. Antonarakis SE. BACking up the promises. Nat Genet 2001; 27(3):230–232.

49. Shaffer LG, Lupski JR. Molecular mechanisms for constitutional chromosomal rearrangements in humans. Annu Rev Genet 2000; 34:297–329.

50. Shapira SK, McCaskill C, Northrump H, Spikes AS, Elder FF, Sutton VR, et al. Chromosome 1p36 deletions: the clinical phenotype and molecular characterization of a common newly delineated syndrome. Am J Hum Genet 1997; 61(3):642–650.

51. Yu W, Ballif BC, Kashork CD, Heilstedt HA, Howard LA, Cai WW, et al. Development of a comparative genomic hybridization microarray and demonstration of its utility with 25 well-characterized 1p36 deletions. Hum Mol Genet 2003; 12(17):2145–2152.

52. Waterston RH, Lindblad-Toh K, Birney E, Rogers J, Abril JF, Agarwal P, et al. Initial sequencing and comparative analysis of the mouse genome. Nature 2002; 420:385–398.

53. Fujiyama A, Watanabe H, Toyoda A, Taylor TD, Itoh T, Tsai SF, et al. Construction and analysis of a human-chimpanzee comparative clone map. Science 2002; 295:131–134.

54. Lai CS, Fisher SE, Hurst JA, Vargha-Khadem F, Monaco AP. A forkhead-domain gene is mutated in a severe speech and language disorder. Nature 2001; 413:519–523.

55. Hagerman RJ, Staley LW, O'Conner R, Lugenbeel K, Nelson D, McLean SD, et al. Learning-disabled males with a fragile X CGG expansion in the upper premutation size range. Pediatrics 1996; 97(1):122–126.

56. Hagerman RJ, Hagerman PJ. The fragile X premutation: into the phenotypic fold. Curr Opin Genet Dev 2002; 12(3):278–283.

57. Verkerk AJ, Pieretti M, Sutcliffe JS, Fu YH, Kuhl DP, Pizzuti A, et al. Identification of a gene (FMR-1) containing a CGG repeat coincident with a breakpoint cluster region exhibiting length variation in fragile X syndrome. Cell 1991; 65(5):905–914.

58. Brown V, Jin P, Ceman S, Darnell JC, O'Donnell WT, Tenenbaum SA, et al. Microarray identification of FMRP-associated brain mRNAs and altered mRNA translational profiles in fragile X syndrome. Cell 2001; 107(4):477–487.

59. Darnell JC, Jensen KB, Jin P, Brown V, Warren ST, Darnell RB. Fragile X mental retardation protein targets G quartet mRNAs important for neuronal function. Cell 2001; 107(4):489–499.

60. Zhang YQ, Bailey AM, Matthies HJ, Renden RB, Smith MA, Speese SD, et al. Drosophila fragile X-related gene regulates the MAP1B homolog Futsch to control synaptic structure and function. Cell 2001; 107(5):591–603.

61. Korenberg JR, Chen XN, Schipper R, Sun Z, Gonsky R, Gerwehr S, et al. Down syndrome phenotypes: the consequences of chromosomal imbalance. Proc Natl Acad Sci USA 1994; 91(11):4997–5001.

62. Delabar JM, Creau N, Sinet PM, Ritter O, Antonarakis SE, Burmeister M, et al. Report of the Fourth International Workshop on Human Chromosome 21. Genomics 1993; 18(3):735–745.

63. Chumakov I, Rigault P, Guillou S, Ougen P, Billaut A, Guasconi G, et al. Continuum of overlapping clones spanning the entire human chromosome 21q. Nature 1992; 359(6394):380–387.

64. Onodera K, Patterson D. Structure of human chromosome 21—for an understanding of genetic diseases including Down's syndrome. Biosci Biotechnol Biochem 1997; 61(3):403–409.

65. Antonarakis SE. Chromosome 21: from sequence to applications. Curr Opin Genet Dev 2001; 11(3):241–246.

66. Reymond A, Camargo AA, Deutsch S, Stevenson BJ, Parmigiani RB, Ucla C, et al. Nineteen additional unpredicted transcripts from human chromosome 21. Genomics 2002; 79(6): 824–832.

67. Agarwala KL, Ganesh S, Tsutsumi Y, Suzuki T, Amano K, Yamakawa K. Cloning and functional characterization of DSCAML1, a novel DSCAM-like cell adhesion molecule that mediates homophilic intercellular adhesion. Biochem Biophys Res Commun 2001; 285(3):760–772.

68. Barlow GM, Micales B, Chen XN, Lyons GE, Korenberg JR. Mammalian DSCAMs: roles in the development of the spinal cord, cortex, and cerebellum? Biochem Biophys Res Commun 2002; 293(3):881–891.

69. Collins FS. Contemplating the end of the beginning. Genome Res 2001; 11(5):641–643.

70. Ruddle F. Hundred-year search for the human genome. Annu Rev Genomics Hum Genet 2001; 2:1–8.

71. Castellanos FX, Tannock R. Neuroscience of attention-deficit/ hyperactivity disorder: the search for endophenotypes. Nat Rev Neurosci 2002; 3(8):617–628.

72. Monaco AP, Bailey AJ. Autism. The search for susceptibility genes. Lancet 2001; 358(suppl):S3.

73. Collins FS, Guttmacher AE. Genetics moves into the medical mainstream. JAMA 2001; 286(18):2322–2324.

74. Collins FS, Green ED, Guttmacher AE, Guyer MS. A vision for the future of genomics research. Nature 2003; 422(6934): 835–847.

75. Bell JI. The double helix in clinical practice. Nature 2003; 421:414–416.

76. Austin CP. The completed human genome: implications for chemical biology. Curr Opin Chem Biol 2003; 7(4): 511–515.

6

Animal Models of Down Syndrome and Other Genetic Diseases Associated with Mental Retardation

ANGELA J. VILLAR and CHARLES J. EPSTEIN

Department of Pediatrics, University of California,
San Francisco, California, U.S.A.

I. INTRODUCTION

The creation and analysis of genetically modified mice is currently the most commonly used approach to investigate the role of specific genetic alterations in the causation of mental retardation (MR) and to model the pathogenesis of the abnormalities that result (reviewed in Refs. 1–5). In addition to providing insight into the aberrations that lead to alterations in brain development and function, the investigation of disorders in genetically modified mice also advances our

163

knowledge of the roles that selected genes play in regulating normal aspects of learning and memory.

Over the past two decades, the mouse has emerged as the pre-eminent model organism for four principal reasons. First, the physiology of the mouse is quite similar to that of humans. Although the anatomical differences between humans and mice appear striking, these differences principally represent alterations in size and shape. Detailed analyses of organs, tissues, and cells reveal many similarities that extend to organ systems, physiological homeostasis, reproduction, behavior, and disease. The ability to use the whole animal becomes increasingly important when attempting to investigate the basis of a human condition as complex as MR.

Second, there is an enormous wealth of genetic information known about the mouse. Both mice and humans have about 30,000 genes and have a common ancestor that lived between 75 and 125 million years ago. The human and mouse genomes are about the same size (approximately 3.1 billion base pairs), and they share virtually the same set of genes (6). Only 300 genes are unique to either organism, and most of the genes unique to the mouse are linked with reproduction and with the mouse's highly developed sense of smell (7). Furthermore, despite considerable rearrangement of the mammalian genome, sizable chromosomal regions carry many genes remaining intact (syntenic) and are structurally similar in both humans and mice (8). Therefore, the DNA sequence of the mouse has become an essential tool to identify and study the functions of human genes.

Third, mice breed frequently, produce large litters, and can be genetically and environmentally manipulated in ways not possible in other higher organisms. Transgenes with well-characterized promoters can be expressed, specific mutations can be "knocked-in," and genes can be "knocked-out," in both the whole animal and in a tissue-specific manner. Putative therapies can be investigated under controlled conditions in preclinical trials.

Fourth, laboratory mice are available on many defined inbred genetic backgrounds. To model a human condition accurately, whether in developmental or functional terms, it is advisable to study the effects of genetic manipulations in pure inbred strains to avoid potentially confounding background effects. Many neurobehavioral phenotypes are sensitive to genetic background differences, probably because they are regulated or affected by many genes (9–11). In some cases, phenotypic variability on different background strains can be striking. For example, transgenic mice overexpressing mutant β-amyloid precursor protein (*APP*) on a FVB/N background suffer from lethality, even though the APP protein expression levels are similar to those known to produce amyloid plaques in outbred strains (12). In addition, FVB/N mice are inherently hyperactive and visually impaired because of the *rd* mutation, which causes retinal degeneration (13). Therefore, they are not useful for studying retinal phenotypes in genetically engineered mice, nor are they suitable for assessing cognitive function with certain methods, such as the Morris water maze task, in which mice need to use visual cues (14).

In addition to its effects on the phenotypic expression of genetic modifications, genetic background can directly alter functional processes in nongenetically altered mice in such a way as to affect the interpretation of the effects of genetic changes. Thus, defective learning of CBA/J mice in the Morris water maze makes them less than ideal for studying spatial learning, and both the DBA/2J and CBA/J strains display deficient long-term memory in contextual and cued fear conditioning tests. These findings provide strong support for a genetic basis for some forms of synaptic plasticity that are linked to behavioral long-term memory (15). Unfortunately, in many cases, it is difficult to foresee the effect of genetic background on a particular phenotype.

Skepticism deriving from the expectation that specific symptoms will have the same physical manifestation across species has been expressed towards the idea that human cognitive impairment can be modeled in the mouse. However, elementary forms of learning are common to all animals with an evolved nervous system, suggesting that there are conserved features in the mechanisms of learning at the cell and molecular level that can be studied effectively even in simple invertebrate animals (reviewed in Ref. 16). For example, the cellular and molecular strategies used in *aplysia* for storing short- and long-term memory are conserved in mammals and the same molecular strategies are employed in both implicit and explicit memory storage (17). Furthermore, mice have a medial temporal lobe system, including a hippocampus, that resembles that of humans, and they use their hippocampus much as humans do to store memories of places and objects (reviewed in Ref. 18). Therefore, we believe that the mouse is a legitimate model for learning and memory in humans and that the modeling of human-like symptoms in animals should be based primarily on an expectation of functional similarity of the displayed behavioral strategy, rather than on one of behavior equivalency. However, any animal model of human disease is of little value without standardized characterization and accurate phenotypic evaluation (19). To this end, the SHIRPA protocol (20), which consists of different sets of tests covering mouse neurological, behavioral, biochemical, and histopathological aspects (http://www.mgu.har.ac.uk/) designed to compare new and existing animal models using the same criteria, was developed.

II. DOWN SYNDROME

To study the mechanisms underlying the development of abnormalities associated with a condition such as Down's syndrome (DS), a comprehensive explanation of the phenotype should consider the developmental consequences of aneuploidy on both pre- and postnatal somatic and neurological development. Such an analysis cannot be completed successfully by studying humans. For the reasons just enumerated (and discussed in detail in Refs. 21, 22), the mouse is the most appropriate experimental mammal for this purpose. Although trisomic primates with the genetic and clinical equivalent of DS have been observed, they do not offer any advantages over mice for investigational purposes. Therefore, various mouse models have been generated and studied with a view of gaining insight into the molecular, genetic, and/or developmental mechanisms that underlie the morphological, histological, biochemical, and immunological abnormalities that occur in DS. As was noted earlier, regulation of orthologous genes in development is likely to be similar among mammals, and the primary effects of gene-dosage imbalance on conserved genetic pathways are expected to be analogous in mice and humans. Although we might expect to see species-specific differences, the underlying assumptions in using mouse models of DS are that many of the genetic pathways are conserved and that the phenotypes that are most likely to be recapitulated are those that are highly conserved across vertebrate evolution. Those phenotypes that have been assessed quantitatively in DS individuals will provide a reliable basis for comparison in different species.

A. Trisomic Models

Human chromosome 21 (HSA21) is orthologous to segments of three mouse chromosomes, and there is no example in which a human gene does not have a mouse ortholog. About 30 Mb from 21cen to 21qter, with approximately 150 loci, is orthologous to distal mouse chromosome 16 (MMU16) and ~75 loci are orthologous to genes on 2 Mb each of MMU10 and MMU17 (Fig. 1). Therefore, the trisomy 16 (Ts16) mouse overexpresses the orthologs of many of the genes located on HSA21. However, MMU16 also has segments orthologous to other human chromosomes, principally HSA3, but also HSA8, 16, and 22 (23) (http://www.informatics.jax.org). Therefore, Ts16 mice are not trisomic for some HSA21 genes and are at a dosage imbalance for other genes that are not implicated in the pathogenesis of DS. Consequently, the Ts16 mouse is an imperfect genetic model of human trisomy 21 (Ts21), and mice with "segmental" trisomy provide a better experimental basis for the investigation of the developmental and functional processes disrupted in humans with DS.

The segmental trisomies, Ts65Dn (24), Ts1Cje, and Ms1CjeTs65Dn (25), each possess a partial copy of distal MMU16, a region that shares orthology to the critical DS region of HSA21 (Fig. 2). The first segmental trisomy model

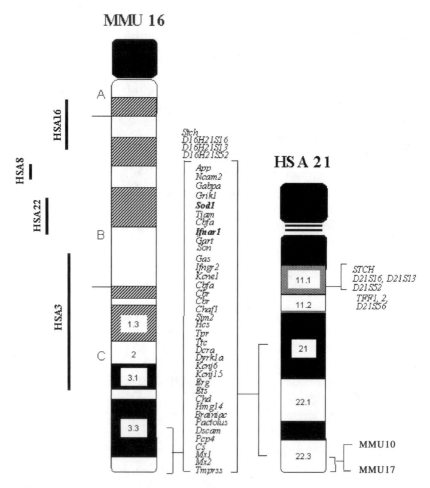

Figure 1 Comparative genetic maps demonstrate significant homology between HSA21 and MMU16. Distal MMU16 shares conserved synteny with HSA21 from *APP* to *MX*. Other chromosomal regions of conserved synteny are also indicated.

developed, Ts65Dn, has an extra marker chromosome composed of the centromere of MMU17 and a portion of MMU16 containing the HSA21-homologous genes from *App* to the telomere beyond *Mx*. The second model, Ts1Cje, which is the result of a chromosome rearrangement in which a portion of MMU16 has been translocated onto MMU12,

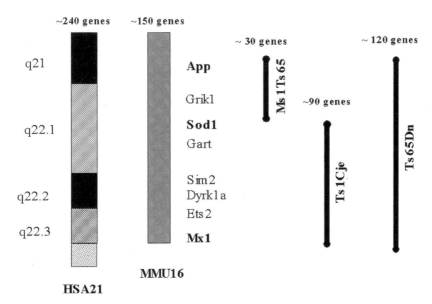

Figure 2 A schematic representation of the MMU16 regions that are triplicated in the different segmental trisomy mouse models of Down syndrome.

is functionally trisomic for a smaller region of MMU16 distal to *Sod1*. The third segmental trisomy, Ms1CjeTs65Dn, is derived by breeding Ts65Dn females with balanced T(12;16) 1Cje males to produce a mouse that is segmentally trisomic for the region that represents the difference between Ts65Dn and Ts1Cje. These mouse models of DS exhibit many of the morphological, biochemical, and immunological features of DS and have provided insight into the molecular, genetic, and developmental mechanisms underlying the various abnormalities.

1. Ts16

Ts16, carries three full copies of MMU16 in its genome (26) and was the original trisomic model of DS. Although a significant proportion of trisomic human fetuses (22) are live born, Ts16 mice rarely survive to term and, when they do, they die shortly after birth. It is unclear whether such differences in survival are based on a species difference or whether they are attributable to a dosage imbalance of a gene(s) that are not on HSA21 but are present on MMU16. It is also possible that some features of DS may be missing from the Ts16 model because of the lack of dosage perturbation of the HSA21 genes that are on MMU17 and/or 10. Furthermore, the inability of the Ts16 mice to survive beyond birth is obviously a major limitation because many of the features that occur as part of the DS phenotype occur postnatally and sometimes even much later in life.

The main features of Ts16 are moderate hypoplasia, slight developmental retardation, thymic hypoplasia, and cardiovascular anomalies (endocardial cushion defects and vascular anomalies). At E14.5, all Ts16 fetuses have edema, ranging from mild to severe, an increased volume of amniotic fluid, and a thickened neck, and small thymus. By E17.5, Ts16 fetuses exhibit two distinct phenotypes, one with an edematous morphology and the other runt-like. Severe cardio vascular malformation is possibly one of the factors responsible for late fetal or neonatal death in some cases. Another possible factor contributing to Ts16 fetal mortality is insufficiency of placental function resulting from hypoplasia of the fetal vasculature of this organ (27–29). Altered development of the Ts16 placenta may also be relevant to understanding some of the phenotypic variation associated with fetal development and Ts21.

Significant and complex alterations are observed in the morphogenesis and neurochemistry of the brain as well as in the properties of cultured neurons (30,31). Alterations have also been described in the development of the cerebellum, hippocampus, cortical plate, and ocular structures (32). In Ts16, there is accelerated neuronal death, altered regulation of neural progenitor cell proliferation, and a dysregulation of Ca^{2+} in both astrocytes and neurons (33–37). Finally, morphogenetic abnormalities have been described during embryonic development of the Ts16 neocortex (33). These abnormalities are caused by a delay in the generation of neocortical neurons and by a deficit in founder cells. Many of the features described are qualitatively similar to those appearing in individuals with DS.

2. Ts65Dn

a. Genetics

Ts65Dn mice are at a dosage imbalance for genes corresponding to those on human chromosome 21q21–22.3, which includes the so-called DS "critical region" (24). A small translocation chromosome, symbolized Ts(17^{16}) 65Dn, contains the HSA21-orthologous region of MMU16 from *App* to the telomere in combination with the centromere and a small portion (~5%) of MMU17. The distal MMU16 segment in Ts65Dn mice corresponds to a portion of HSA21 that spans 15.6 Mb and contains about 120 HSA21 gene orthologs (38). Ts65Dn mice transmit the extra, freely segregating chromosome through the female germline (39,40). However, males are infertile, probably because spermatogenesis arrests in metaphase I owing to the presence of the extra chromosome. Ts65Dn mice are not inbred—indeed, they do not reproduce if inbred—and are maintained by mating female carriers of the 17^{16} chromosome (B6C3H-Ts65Dn) to B6EiC3HF1 hybrid male mice obtained from crossing C57BL/6Ei × C3H/HeSnJ. The fact that the Ts65Dn are on a segregating background involving two inbred strains adds variability to the phenotype. Nevertheless, the behavioral effects observed in these mice have been quite robust, and findings across laboratories show considerable agreement.

The serial analysis of gene expression (SAGE) technique has been applied to study the differences in the global gene expression profiles induced by the aneuploidy in brains of normal and Ts65Dn adult male mice (41). The vast majority of transcripts are expressed at the same or similar levels between Ts65Dn and controls. However, 330 RNA TAGs demonstrated statistically significant differences in expression. Interestingly, approximately half of the differentially expressed TAGs were underexpressed and half were overexpressed in Ts65Dn male brains. Among the differentially expressed TAGs matching known genes, several candidate genes with a potential pathogenic role in both the developmental and neurodegenerative aspects of DS have been identified (41). Microarray experiments to assess gene expression differences in both human DS and mouse models of DS (Ts65Dn) are currently underway.

b. General Phenotype

The Ts65Dn mouse has advantages over the Ts16 model because it more closely resembles human Ts21 genetically (even though some important differences still exist) and it facilitates the study of features that occur in DS postnatally. Postnatal survival is also a distinct advantage for the development of therapies aimed at one or more of the pathologies that occur in DS. Ts65Dn mice display a variety of phenotypic abnormalities that are similar to human DS, including early developmental delay and reduced birth weight. They are ~17% smaller than wild-type littermates prior to weaning, and this smaller size persists throughout life (23,39,42). Ts65Dn mice, like *ETS2* transgenic mice (43) develop hydrocephalus at some time in their lives (23,39). They also display muscular tremors (44), and seizures have been reported in some older mice (23).

Ts65Dn thymuses exhibit greater apoptotic activity than controls, and the thymocytes are highly susceptible to programmed cell death induced by apoptotic drugs (45). However, Ts65Dn mice do not show many of the gross abnormalities frequently observed in DS, such as cardiac valvular congenital abnormalities (42), but they do exhibit analogous effects on craniofacial structures (46). Analysis of the craniofacial skeleton of Ts65Dn mice using three-dimensional morphometric methods demonstrates remarkable parallels between Ts65Dn and DS craniofacial dysmorphology, a distinctive and highly penetrant phenotype of DS. The disruption of development that causes the skull phenotype occurs prenatally, affects the size of all skull elements, and produces localized changes in the shape of specific skull regions. These results reveal a strong conservation of the evolved developmental genetic program that underlies mammalian skull morphology (46).

c. Behavior and Learning

Ts65Dn mice have been studied extensively for altered behavior and/or learning. Ts65Dn pups, assessed before weaning, exhibit hyperactivity and a significant delay in the emergence of adult-like responses and developmental abnormalities and age-related neurodegeneration (42). These findings parallel what is observed in infants and children with DS (47). Ultrasonic vocalization, a communication behavior aimed at eliciting maternal care, is delayed and Ts65Dn pups display abnormal homing, possibly because of poor motor co-ordination or an inability to detect olfactory signals. Despite delays, both Ts65Dn and control mice reach neurobehavioral maturation for these responses before weaning. Similarly, DS children achieve developmental sensorimotor milestones, albeit later than normal (48). As in DS, cognitive deficits have been consistently demonstrated in the adult Ts65Dn model, including hippocampal-dependent spatial learning that requires the integration of visual and spatial information (40,42,49,50), as well as working memory and long-term memory (51,52), which require a functionally competent prefrontal cortex. Tasks that require both of these regions, such as the reversal of spatial learning in the reverse probe tests, are espe-cially impaired. In addition, Ts65Dn mice show consistent hyperactivity, which can be interpreted as a failure of inhibi-tory control or reduced attention levels (40,42,49,50).

No sensorimotor deficits appear in Ts65Dn mice (49,53). However, they do exhibit significant levels of stereotypic behavior compared to littermate controls, and the existence of stereotypy is associated with other aspects of the animal's functioning, such as eating and sleeping (54). Interestingly, stereotypic behavior, a phenotype that is found in approxi-mately one-third of DS patients (55), is observed in only a sub-set of the Ts65Dn mice. This observation can potentially be accounted for by the fact that, as has already been noted, the mice are maintained on a segregating genetic back-ground, which results in a variable genetic background.

d. The Brain

As in DS, high-resolution three-dimensional magnetic resonance imaging has demonstrated that the Ts65Dn cerebellum is reduced relative to the volume of the total brain (46,56). Area measurements of histological sections demonstrate that the internal granule layer and molecular layer are both reduced. The density of granule cells and Purkinje cells is significantly lower in Ts65Dn mice, and the lower granule cell density correctly predicts a corresponding reduction in the DS cerebellum (56). Reduction in cerebellar volume is invariant in individuals with DS, and this completely penetrant phenotype of DS is accurately recapitulated in the Ts65Dn mouse model.

Stereological morphometric studies of young and old Ts65Dn mice have demonstrated minor irregularities in some regions of the hippocampus of Ts65Dn mice, including reductions in the volume of CA2 and in the mean neuron number in the dentate gyrus (57). Microinjection of Lucifer yellow revealed the presence of "giant" spines on the dendrites of dentate gyrus and CA1 neurons which are present as early as postnatal day 21, as well as in mature animals (58). Interestingly, abnormal spines have also been described in the brains of children with DS (59). In addition, long-term potentiation (LTP) could not be elicited in Ts65Dn mice, presumably as a result of the influence of abnormal synaptic contacts on synaptic function (58,60,61). However, when inhibitory inputs were blocked with picrotoxin, LTP was restored. Long-term depression was also increased (60,61). These findings are indicative of abnormal synaptic plasticity in Ts65Dn (61).

There is convincing evidence to suggest a strong relationship between synapse number and cerebral function. Kurt et al. (62) have demonstrated that synaptic deficits in the Ts65Dn mouse temporal cortex are confined to asymmetric synapses (40,42,49,51,53). Aged Ts65Dn mice possess significantly fewer (30%) asymmetric synapses in their temporal cortex without difference in symmetric synapses. However, the mean synaptic apposition lengths of both asymmetric (15%) and symmetric (11%) synapses is significantly larger in Ts65Dn mice, suggesting that excitatory synapses are preferentially affected in Ts65Dn mice and that there is an attempt to compensate for the deficit of asymmetry by increasing the contact zone area of existing synapses (62).

Observations on cultured neurons from Ts65Dn fetuses, as well as from human Ts21 fetuses, have been interpreted as suggesting that the reduced functional connections in the trisomic brain arise from abnormal neuronal electrical and biochemical properties that are evident even during fetal development (63). These include abnormalities in the duration of the action potential and its rates of depolarization and repolarization, altered kinetics of active Na^+, Ca^{2+}, and K^+ currents, and altered membrane densities of Na^+ and Ca^{2+} channels (63). Furthermore, evidence suggests that the abnormalities in the trisomy mouse models are related to defective signal transduction pathways involving the phosphoinositide cycle, protein kinase A, and protein kinase C (63).

Neurochemical studies have revealed functional abnormalities in the adenyl cyclase signaling pathways in the Ts65Dn cerebral cortex and hippocampus but not in the cerebellum. In these regions, basal as well as stimulated production of cyclic AMP (cAMP) is reduced (64–66). Interestingly, adenyl cyclase and phospholipase C signaling pathways are also severely disturbed in the brains of persons with DS and AD, further validating this aneuploid mouse model for DS and AD.

e. Cholinergic Neurons and Alzheimer Disease

During development, the number and size of basal forebrain cholinergic neurons (BFCNs) are similar in Ts65Dn and control littermates. These data suggest that the neurogenesis and early development and differentiation of BFCNs are not affected (67). However, with age, Ts65Dn mice exhibit reduction in BFCN size and number and regressive changes in the hippocampal terminal fields of these neurons (68). Granholm et al. (69) showed that these neurons were normal up to 4 months of age but were significantly reduced in number and size by 6 months and thereafter. In addition, a decline in performance on a spatial reversal task corresponded to the loss of the cholinergic phenotype in medial septal neurons. This age-related cholinergic cell loss in Ts65Dn mice occurs much earlier than normal age-related cholinergic loss, which is observed around 24 months of age in nontrisomic mice (70).

Survival and functional maintenance of cholinergic neurons are dependent upon neurotrophic factors (71). Cooper et al. (68) found that retrograde transport of radiolabeled

nerve growth factor (NGF) from the hippocampus to the basal
forebrain was markedly decreased in Ts65Dn mice even
before degenerative changes were detected. The basis for
the transport defect appears to arise within cholinergic axons
because there is no decrease in either NGF binding or inter-
nalization in synaptosomes prepared from the hippocampus
of Ts65Dn mice. In addition, intraventricular NGF infusion
(68,69) reverses the abnormalities in BFCN size and number
and restores the deficit in cholinergic innervation. The effects
of NGF treatment are most plausibly interpreted as a reversal
of phenotype in surviving BFCNs and are evidence that these
neurons do not actually die in Ts65Dn mice. Instead, the
reduction in the number of immunohistochemically detected
BFCNs in Ts65Dn mice appears to represent a dynamic
down-regulation of phenotypic markers. Therefore, age-related
cholinergic neurodegeneration may be a treatable disorder of
failed retrograde NGF signaling (68,72).

All individuals with DS eventually develop the neuropathology of Alzheimer disease (AD), which is characterized
by a premature loss of BFCN. Such morphological anomalies
are in accordance with human DS individuals in their third or
fourth decade of life (73,74), as well as AD patients (75).
Because Ts65Dn mice show a marked loss of BFCN, they have
been considered an animal model of AD as well as of DS (42).

Early endosomal alterations are the earliest known
pathology in DS and sporadic AD (SAD) (76). Endosomal
pathology in DS occurs as early as 28 weeks gestation, decades
before β-amyloid is deposited in significant amounts (77).
In AD, the appearance of abnormal endosomes develop before
β-amyloid deposition and as soluble β-amyloid (Aβ) peptide
levels first rise (78). Endosomal alterations in DS and AD
develop in otherwise normal appearing neurons of regions that
become the most severely affected in the disease (76,77), including hippocampus, neocortex, and basal forebrain.

Ts65 mice develop age-related endosomal enlargement
and altered expression and distribution of early endosome
markers, which strongly resemble the neuronal endosomal
pathology in DS and SAD (79). Interestingly, Ts65Dn/
App$^{+/+/-}$ mice, which have two copies of *App*, show normal

endosomal morphology in the basal forebrain in contrast to Ts65Dn mice (79). Transgenic mice overexpressing *App* alone, however, exhibit normal expression and distribution of early endosomal markers indicating that increased *App* gene dosage is necessary for endosome pathology to develop in Ts65Dn, but is not sufficient (79). Thus, endosomal pathology in Ts65Dn mice is dependent on triplication of the *App* gene and requires the participation of one or more genes within the trisomic region of MMU16 to alter endosome function.

Similar to what has been described in Ts16 (40,80,81), it appears that for some genes, gene copy number and gene expression are directly correlated in the young adult Ts65Dn brain. This has been shown for *Sod1*, located on the trisomic MMU16 segment, and for *trkB* and *Gap-43*, which are located on nontrisomic segments. However, for other genes, such as *App* (MMU16) and *apoE* (MMU7), gene expression is greater than predicted on the basis of gene dose. It has been postulated that overexpression of *APP* in DS leads to Aβ deposition (82). However, over a 2-year lifespan, *App* overexpression does not lead to Aβ deposition in Ts65Dn. In fact, the only reports to date showing extensive Aβ deposition in the brains of mice are in animals in which a mutant form of human *APP* has been expressed (83) (see below, Tg*APP*). Data showing that overexpression of normal human *APP* in mice also fail to result in plaque formation (84) suggesting that the occurrence of AD pathology in DS may be due to greater overexpression of *APP*.

f. Pain Perception

Although individuals with DS are not insensitive to pain, they do express pain or discomfort more slowly and less precisely than the general population (85). Pain research has found that patients with DS exhibit longer pain latencies and are less accurate in their ability to locate cold stimuli. This elevated sensory threshold and a decreased ability to localize stimuli could be due to a combination of factors, including, delayed pain transmission, a delay in the pain integration process and delayed motor response (verbal or pointing). As in DS, Ts65Dn mice also show reduced responsiveness to painful stimuli (86,87). During tonic pain, Martinez-Cue et al. (86) reported that Ts65Dn mice showed less licking in the early and late phase after subcutaneous formalin injection compared with control littermates. Latency in the tail-flick was increased in Ts65Dn animals after cumulative doses of morphine, indicating an increase in a nociceptive threshold. In contrast, Cao et al. (87) found no differences in tail-flick latency and formalin test responses between Ts65Dn and controls. However, the Ts65Dn mice showed significantly increased latency in the hot plate and tail clip tests (87). Interestingly, the magnitude of their response did not differ from controls suggesting that, like DS individuals, Ts65Dn mice are not insensitive to pain sensation. The authors suggest that altered sensitivity to pain reflects either diminished peripheral nociceptor responsiveness and/or decreased central processing of nociceptive signals. Overexpression of *Grik1*, encoding the GluR5 subunit of the kainate receptor, has been shown to participate in pain transmission (88) and may play a role in reduced pain sensitivity.

3. Ts1Cje

The second partial Ts16 mouse model, termed Ts1je (89) is trisomic for a smaller region of MMU16, from *Sod1* to *Mx1*, corresponding to a HSA21 region that spans 9.8 Mb and contains ~80 genes. The development of this model, with a lesser degree of trisomy, has made it possible to apply a subtractive approach to the analysis of the learning, behavioral, and neurological abnormalities found in Ts65Dn.

Ts1Cje, arose as a fortuitous translocation between MMU16 proximal to *Sod1* and the very distal region of MMU12 in a transgenic mouse line (89). Carriers for the balanced translocation designated T(12;16) 1Cje have one normal MMU12 and MMU16 in addition to the 12^{16} and 16^{12} translocation chromosomes. The Ts1Cje mouse is generated when a gamete carrying $MMU12^{16}$, and MMU16 combines with a normal gamete carrying MMU12 and MMU16. Although this model is trisomic for genes corresponding to the 21q22 region, Ts1Cje animals are not functionally trisomic for *Sod1* because it is disrupted by the neomycin resistance sequence. Ts1Cje mice survive up to adulthood, and, contrary to Ts65Dn, both sexes are fertile.

Ts1Cje mice are growth retarded during the postnatal period and already show some behavioral and learning defects. They exhibit subtle differences from Ts65Dn in their learning and behavioral abnormalities. Ts1Cje mice do not show stereotypic behavior or hyperactivity, but, rather, are hypoactive. Tests of learning in the Morris water maze and assessment of spontaneous locomotor activity reveal distinct learning and behavioral abnormalities, some of which are indicative of hippocampal dysfunction. Except in the reverse probe tests, the learning deficits of Ts1Cje mice in the Morris water maze are similar to those of Ts65Dn. They have an indication of altered exploratory behavior, display an impairment of spatial learning in the hidden platform and probe tasks and deficit in learning flexibility in the reverse platform task (25,89). These findings indicate that an important gene(s) involved in these deficits lies in the region of overlap between these mice, the region from *Sod1* to the telomere.

Ts1Cje mice do not exhibit differences relative to control mice in the number or size of BFCNs at 18 months of age, and there is no significant defect in NGF retrograde transport (72,89). The absence of BFCN degeneration, which is observed in Ts65Dn, suggests that the region from *App* to *Sod1* is required for this neuropathological trait. Several known genes map to this region, including *App*, associated with AD, and *Grik*, whose product, the GluR5 kainate receptor regulates synaptic transmission.

4. Ms1CjeTs65Dn

To assess the contribution of the segment of MMU16 from proximal to *App* to *Sod1*, a segmental trisomic model called Ms1CjeTs65Dn was generated (25). Ms1CjeTs65Dn is derived by breeding Ts65Dn females with T(12;16)1Cje males to produce a mouse that is segmentally trisomic for the region that represents the difference between Ts65Dn and Ts1Cje. Since the impact of mouse strain on the effects of a transgene or a segmental trisomy can be substantial, Ts65Dn, Ts1Cje, and Ms1CjeTs65Dn are generated as littermates to directly compare and assess the phenotypic contribution of the region of difference between them.

Ms1CjeTs65Dn mice present a much less severe phenotypic impact than the longer segmental trisomies. Through subtractive analysis, it might be inferred that the genes involved in producing hyperactivity in the Ts65Dn mice are in the region between *App* and *Sod1*, as Ts1Cje mice are hypoactive. Ms1Ts65 mice, however, are not significantly above normal in activity, indicating that genes in the *Sod1–App* region must interact with others in the Ts65Dn region to produce hyperactivity in the Ts65Dn mice (25). Ms1Ts65 mice show statistically significant deficits compared with controls in the latencies of the visible, hidden, and reverse hidden platform tests, but not in path length nor any of the probe tests (25). Pairwise comparison between Ms1Ts65 and Ts65Dn demonstrates that the deficits of Ms1Ts65 mice in the Morris water maze are significantly less severe than those of Ts65Dn (Fig. 3). Therefore, it can be concluded that, whereas triplication of the region from *Sod1* to *Mx1* plays the major role in causing the abnormalities of Ts65Dn in the Morris water maze, imbalance of the region from *App* to *Sod1* also contributes to the poor performance.

5. Summary

The development and analysis of segmental mouse models are proving to be quite promising in meeting the challenge to understand the role of individual genes in the pathogenesis of the neurological and behavioral phenotype of DS. By comparing the neurological and behavioral differences between Ts65Dn, Ts1Cje, and Ms1CjeTs65Dn, each with varying degrees of segmental trisomy, particular features of the DS phenotype have been assigned to specific regions of MMU16 (Table 1). For example, the age-related loss of BFCNs is specific to the Ts65Dn model, implying that the gene(s) responsible for the BFCN phenotype maps to the set of approximately 30 genes between *App* and *Sod1*. Comparative

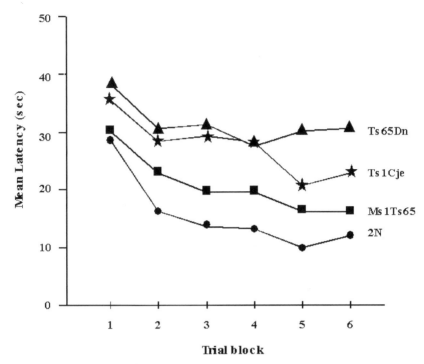

Figure 3   The performance of segmental trisomy mouse models of Down syndrome in the reverse hidden platform phases of the Morris water maze. Performance, as measured by latency (time to reach the hidden platform), improved as the trials were repeated. Although the overall performances of Ms1CjeTs65Dn, Ts1Cje, and Ts65Dn were all impaired compared to controls, Ts65Dn was the most severely impaired and Ms1CjeTs65Dn the least. (Modified from Ref. 25.)

analysis of segmental mouse models with smaller and smaller regions of imbalance holds the potential for producing a "phenotypic map" of MMU16 and ultimately for defining the genes that are responsible for particular DS abnormalities.

B.   Transgenic Models

Although overexpressing a single gene will not in itself model DS, the value of single gene transgenesis is to identify genes related to specific pathophysiological features (Table 2). The

Table 1 Quantifiable Abnormalities Associated with Segmental Trisomic Models of Down Syndrome

---

Abnormalities that are similar to abnormalities observed in DS
Large and fewer dendritic spines	Ts65Dn[a]
Impaired spatial learning (Morris maze)	Ts65Dn > Ts1Cje
Enlarged early neuronal endosomes	Ts65Dn; not in Ts1Cje
Decreased density of cerebellar neurons	Ts65Dn > Ts1Cje
Diminished sensitivity to pain	Ts65Dn[a]
Abnormal craniofacial morphogenesis	Ts65Dn = Ts1Cje

Additional abnormalities that may be relevant to DS
Inhibition of long-term potentiation in hippocampus	Ts65Dn[a]
Atrophy of basal forebrain cholinergic neurons	Ts65Dn; not in Ts1Cje
Decreased NGF retrograde transport from hippocampus	Ts65Dn; not in Ts1Cje

---

[a]Only model investigated.

gene-dosage effects hypothesis of the pathogenesis of DS lends itself to testing by the transgenic approach, which can directly evaluate the phenotype/genotype relationships of individual HSA21 genes (3). This hypothesis proposes that DS phenotypes may result directly from the cumulative effect of dosage imbalance of a specific individual gene or small group of genes from HSA21 and/or indirectly through the interaction of these HSA21 gene products with the whole genome, transciptome, or proteome (90,91). An implicit assumption of this hypothesis, which is not currently supported by any clinical or experimental observation, is that three copies of a reasonably small number of genes on an otherwise diploid background would produce the relevant feature of DS.

There are some serious limitations inherent in the approaches directed at dissecting individual gene function. The random site of integration and the variability of copy number can affect the quantitative expression of the transgene. Other concerns are the possible disruption of an endogenous gene by a transgenic insertion event, which can result in a mutant phenotype as a consequence of a disruption, deletion, or translocation, rather than as a consequence

Table 2 Transgenic Overexpression Models of Down Syndrome

Model	Gene product	DS-like phenotype
Tg*SOD1*	Cu/Zn-superoxide dismutase	Neuromuscular junctions abnormalities; ↓ prostaglandin E_2 and D_2 biosynthesis; deficient spatial learning; diminished LTP; thymic hypoplasia
Tg*APP*	β-Amyloid precusor protein	Cognitive deficits; plaques (with mutated *APP*); premature death
Tg*Dyrk1A*	Serine–threonine kinase	Altered neuromotor development; hyperactivity; impaired learning and memory
Tg*Sim2*	Basic helix–loop–helix protein	Mild cognitive deficit; defect in context-dependent fear conditioning
Tg*SIM2*		Reduced exploratory behavior and sensitivity to pain
Tg*PFKL*	Phosphofructokinase	Altered liver glycolysis (↑ rate of cerebral glucose metabolism)
Tg*S100β*	Acidic calcium binding protein	Behavioral and learning defects; astrocytosis; abnormal dendritic development
Tg*ETS2*	E26 transformation-specific transcription factor	Craniofacial dysmorphology; brachycephaly; skeletal/bone defects

of transgenesis. Finally, whereas genes under control of their natural promoters are expected to recapitulate the cell-type- and stage-specific expression of the endogenous genes, reflecting the genetic situation in DS, the use of heterologous promoters that may allow the generation of inducible transgenic models can lead to nonphysiological effects. Therefore, the best way to produce a transgenic mouse is to introduce the gene under the transcriptional control of its own promoter. In addition, when selecting a candidate gene for the making of a transgenic mouse, knowledge of the functions of the protein that the transgene encodes and of its spatiotemporal pattern of expression should be considered.

1. Tg*SOD1*

Transgenic mice that express the gene *SOD1* for human Cu/Zn-superoxide dismutase (*CuZnSOD, SOD1*) provide one of the best studied models of DS (92). Virtually, all individuals with DS have an extra copy of this locus, even though the DS phenotype, including mental retardation can occur without triplication of *SOD1* (93). A number of studies have demonstrated that CuZnSOD levels are elevated by 50% in a variety of cell types and organs in DS. CuZnSOD, a key enzyme in the metabolism of oxygen free radicals, catalyzes the dismutation of superoxide anion into hydrogen peroxide, which is then converted to water by catalase or glutathione peroxidase. *SOD1* is generally regarded as a protective enzyme. However, in DS, where there is not a corresponding increase in catalase or glutathione peroxidase, increased expression of *CuZnSOD* is suggested to lead to accumulation of hydrogen peroxide, which is toxic by itself or gives rise to the more noxious hydroxyl (OH) radical. Lack of such an adaptive response renders cells vulnerable to oxidative stress, which accounts for the early onset of apoptotic cell loss and activation of proapoptotic genes in the brain of individuals with DS (94).

Evidence from animal models supports the pathogenic role of increased CuZnSOD activity in neurodevelopmental abnormalities and neurodegeneration. Gross anatomy is normal, but specific effects of increased activity of CuZnSOD that resemble changes found in persons with DS have been found (95). For example, the neuromuscular junctions of the transgenic tongue muscles are abnormal, with atrophy, degeneration, withdrawal and destruction of terminal axons; development of multiple small terminals; decreased ratio of terminal axon area to postsynaptic membrane; and hyperplastic secondary folds. Transgenic mice also have reduced prostaglandin E_2 and prostaglandin D_2 biosynthesis in primary fetal cells and in the cerebellum and hippocampus. Tg*SOD1* are deficient in spatial learning, and hippocampal LTP is impaired (96), giving rise to the suggestion that elevated CuZnSOD leads to an increase in tetanic stimulation-evoked formulation of H_2O_2 which leads to diminished LTP and to cognitive defects. It has also been observed that cultured neurons of transgenic mice are more susceptible to kainic acid-induced apoptotic cell death (97).

The early success in recapitulating DS characters in mice overexpressing *CuZnSOD* encouraged the transgenic mouse approach, and especially the approach using genes under control of their natural promoters.

2. Tg*APP*

β-Amyloid precursor protein (*APP*) enhances survival of cultured neurons and regulates the effect of NGF on neurite outgrowth and cell adhesion (98). As has already been noted, individuals with DS over the age of 35 exhibit neuropathological changes (reviewed in Ref. 99) associated with the appearance of cortical amyloid plaques that are very similar to those seen in AD disease (100,101). *APP*, the first gene to be directly implicated in AD, showed gene dosage-related increases in mRNA in human fetal and (93,102,103) and adult (104) DS brain.

Transgenic mice overexpressing *APP* or related peptides show some but not all of the features of AD (105,106). Evidence implicates a central role for β-amyloid (Aβ) peptides in the pathophysiology of AD (107). Processing of *APP* to form Aβ peptides occurs at multiple locations within the cell and leads to the production of two pools of β-amyloid, a secreted (extracellular) pool of Aβ40 and an intracellular pool of Aβ42, a form more likely to be neurotoxic (108). In transgenic mice carrying the mutant form of *APP* associated with autosomal dominant forms of familial AD, increased population of the Aβ42 form leads to prominent deficits in synaptic transmission in the hippocampus of young mice, well before the emergence of amyloid deposits. This suggests a neurotoxic effect of Aβ that is independent of later plaque formation and appears early in development (109,110). The implications of these findings are appealing since they offer the possibility that *APP* overexpression also might account for early appearing deficits in mental processing. However, despite the numerous attempts focusing on transgenic expression of human *APP* to obtain valid models, only mice that express mutant forms of the *APP* protein develop brain deposits, characteristics of AD (83,84,111,112).

Recently, a homolog of β-site amyloid precursor protein cleaving enzyme (*BACE*), a transmembrane aspartic protease that possesses all the known characteristics of the β-secretase involved in AD has been identified in 21q22.3 (113). Thus, concurrent overexpression of *BACE2* and *APP* in mice should help to understand the pathogenic mechanism underlying AD neuropathology in the brains of DS patients.

3. Tg*Dyrk1A*

DYRK1A, the human homolog of the *Drosophila minibrain* gene, maps to the DS critical region of HSA21 and is overexpressed in DS fetal brain. *DYRK1A* encodes a serine–threonine kinase, probably involved in neuroblast proliferation. Mutant Drosophila minibrain flies have a reduction in both optic lobes and central brain, showing learning deficits and hypoactivity (114,115). Transgenic mice (Tg*Dyrk1A*) overexpressing the full-length cDNA of *Dyrk1A* (116) exhibit delayed craniocaudal maturation with functional consequences in neuromotor development. *Dyrk1A* mice also show altered motor skill acquisition and hyperactivity, which is maintained up to adulthood. In the Morris water maze, Tg*Dyrk1A* mice show a significant impairment in spatial learning and cognitive flexibility, indicative of hippocampal and prefrontal cortex dysfunction. In the more complex repeated reversal-learning paradigm, this defect is specifically related to reference memory, whereas working memory is almost unimpaired. The authors suggest a causative role of *DYRK1A* in mental retardation and in motor anomalies of DS (see the section on YAC Transgenic Models).

4. Tg*Sim2*

The mouse genome contains two *Sim* genes, *Sim1* and *Sim2*. They are presumed to be important for central nervous system (CNS) development because they are orthologous to the *Drosophila single-minded* (*Sim*) gene, mutations of which cause a complete loss of CNS midline cells (117). Mice overexpressing mouse *Sim2* under the control of the beta-actin promoter have normal skeletal brain and heart structures, but they exhibit a moderate defect in context-dependent fear conditioning and a mild defect in the Morris water maze test. Mice with an extra copy of human *SIM2* display reduced exploratory behavior and sensitivity to pain (118). Taken together, overexpression of the *Sim2* gene results in abnormalities involving spatial exploration, social interactions, and reduced nociception and may be important for the pathogenesis of DS, especially mental retardation (119).

5. Tg*PFKL*

Tg*PFKL* mice show an increase in activity of phosphofructokinase, a key glycolytic enzyme, in blood and brain, but the rate of glucose metabolism is differentially affected, being slower in blood but faster in brain (120). The faster utilization of glucose in Tg*PFKL* brain is similar to the increased rate of cerebral glucose metabolism found in the brain of young adults with DS (121).

6. Tg*S100β*

S100β encodes a small acidic calcium binding protein not found on MMU16 but found on HSA21 (122). *S100β*, a neurotrophic factor released by astroglial cells, is of particular interest because it is synthesized and released by astrocytes in the brain and functions as a neurotrophic factor for selected neurons as well as a gliotrophic factor, including mitosis and morphogenesis of astrocytes. The number of astrocytes expressing S100β protein in DS is reported to be significantly higher than in controls at all ages (123,124). Astrocytic changes are seen in newborns with DS decades before the appearance of neuritic plaques and neurofibrillary tangles suggesting a potential role for *S100β* in dystrophic neurite formation, and evolution of plaques and neurofibrillary tangle changes (125).

Tg*S100β* mice that overexpress the human gene, *S100β*, tend to be less efficient in some hippocampal-dependent learning and in some prefrontal-dependent behavioral tasks (126) and females present some behavioral alterations (127). Overexpression of *S100β* leads to astrocytosis (128) and abnormal dendritic development with an excess of hippocampal dendrites in younger animals followed by premature loss of dendrites (129).

7. Tg*ETS2*

ETS2, a gene that encodes the E26 transformation-specific transcription factor located on 21q22.3, is ubiquitously expressed and involved in organogenesis, and has been reported to be overexpressed in brain and fibroblasts from subjects with DS (130). Transgenic mice overexpressing *Ets2* develop skeletal/bone defects reminiscent of those seen in DS and particularly those that involve the craniofacial region (43), suggesting that *Ets2* overexpression may be responsible for the genesis of these pathophysiological features. However, that the theory that *ETS2* is overexpressed in DS has been challenged (131).

C. YAC Transgenic Models

Proper gene regulation can be difficult to obtain in conventional transgenesis because the full extent of normal regulatory elements of a gene is usually not defined. YACs are cloning vectors that can carry large pieces of DNA up to 2 Mb in length and allow stable propagation in yeast (132). This means that multiple genes or intact large genes, along with their regulatory sequences can be cloned in one YAC. The ability to introduce large, well-defined genomic regions into transgenic mice has led to the development of random panel of HSA21-derived YACs to localize genes responsible for a particular DS feature. Two groups have reported the construction of such panels (133,134). Smith et al. (135) created a set of transgenic mice, each with all or part of a YAC from a set of four clones spanning more than 2 Mb of HSA21. Since the presence of learning deficits and mental retardation is a characteristic feature of DS, these mice were subjected to behavioral and learning tests. In the Morris water maze, YAC152F7tel transgenic mice were mildly impaired in probe test crossings and severely impaired in the reverse versions of the tasks, which assess learning flexibility. The only gene subsequently found to map to this genomic fragment was *DYRK1A* (136). Smith et al. (135) concluded that the phenotype was most likely due to the mice having three functional copies (two mouse, one human) of the gene, *DYRK1A/Dyrk1a* (135). In the future, it should be possible to test this hypothesis further by ablating one of the three *Dyrk1a* genes in these mice and determining whether the wild-type phenotype is restored.

D. HSA21 Transgenics

Chimeric mice carrying HSA21 as a freely segregating extra chromosome have been reported (137,138). Whereas the contribution ratio of embryonic stem (ES) cells containing HSA21 in chimeras was about 50% in adult heart, it was more than 90% in other organs such as brain, liver, and lung (137). Chimeric mice showed a high correlation between retention of HSA21-containing ES cells in the brain and impairment in learning or emotional behavior by open field, contextual fear conditioning, and forced swim tests (139). A considerable number of fetuses with a high degree of chimerism also exhibited hypoplastic thymus and cardiac defects, reflecting maldevelopment of structures with a substantial input of neural crest.

E. New Models of DS

Mouse models of Ts21 provide the substance for identifying corresponding consequences of gene-dosage imbalance in mouse and human. Transgenic models with a multiple, yet well-defined set of HSA21 genes (double and triple transgenic) offer opportunities to explore how several genes interact in the development of certain features and represent a significant step closer to the goal of reconstructing the full scenario of gene-dosage effects of HSA21 genes. By crossing mice that carry different HSA21–YACs, it may even be feasible to build up a library of mice, each carrying an increasing number of HSA21 genomic fragments, in an attempt to reconstruct the entire DS phenotype.

The availability of mouse ES cells and gene targeting systems allow for the creation of mice carrying an additional copy of a particular gene by using a special form of gap-repair gene targeting that can tandemly duplicate a gene or region of interest (140). Using this approach, Yu et al. (141) propose to recapitulate HSA21 trisomy by engineering a mouse with triple hemizygous duplications of the conserved regions on MMU16, 10, and 17. This model would accurately represent Ts21 and provide the most relevant mouse model of DS to date.

Although the existing segmental models of DS have provided an initial glimpse into the molecular mechanisms that underlie the physical and developmental abnormalities in DS individuals, our ability to assign a particular feature of DS to a specific region of HSA21, referred to as phenotypic mapping, is limited. Overcoming this limitation will require the systematic creation of smaller and smaller segmental trisomics and dissection of the phenotypes. A minimal reduction in trisomy can be achieved by breeding segmental trisomy models (Ts65Dn or Ts1Cje) with mice carrying a disrupted gene(s). Progeny that are on a trisomic background but disomic for the gene(s) of interest subsequently can be evaluated for the absence of the DS phenotype(s) seen in the intact trisomic mice. A "DS critical region" (DSCR) of HSA21 has been proposed based on determining the smallest region in common among partially trisomic individuals who display the same DS feature. Most reports include a region of about 5 Mb (~15% of HSA21) in band q22.2-3 containing approximately 30 genes. Using Cre–LoxP chromosomal engineering, mice have been generated that are monosomic and trisomic for the DSCR (142). Evaluation of these mice to determine whether they exhibit phenotypes with exact parallels to those in DS will directly test the DSCR hypothesis.

The use of antisense oligodeoxynucleotides to decrease targeted protein levels is becoming an increasingly accepted approach and may be valuable in dissecting the contribution of a particular gene or gene subset to the overall DS phenotype. Moreover, evidence strongly supports the proposal that antisense methodology has the potential to be used as a powerful tool not only for the study of the molecular basis of behavior but also for the treatment of associated disorders (143,144).

With the development in recent years of mouse models of DS, the completion of the chromosome 21 (HSA21) sequence, and the development of tools to measure global gene expression it is likely that in the near future we will gain a greater insight into the underlying molecular basis of DS. Ultimately, the value of new and existing models of DS lies in the potential development of diagnostic tests for defined features and therapeutic strategies to eliminate or treat specific features that occur as part of the DS pathogenesis.

III. OTHER DISORDERS

A. Disorders of Genomic Imprinting

Genomic imprinting is the epigenetic process that causes a reversible gamete-of-origin specific marking or an "imprinting" of the genome that is replicated faithfully in somatic cells and ultimately results in mono-allelic gene expression or the inactivation of either the maternal or paternal allele of a particular locus. Although the mechanism of imprinting not fully understood, one modification that is believed to play a role is the reversible addition of methyl groups to specific cytosine residues within the DNA sequence, a process that occurs differently in the production of the egg and the sperm (145). Within the past decade, mutations of imprinted genes on several different chromosomes have been found to cause a wide range of phenotypic effects. This genetic mechanism underlies two well-known genetic disorders, namely, Prader–Willi and Angelman syndromes, the first disorders recognized as occurring because of genomic imprinting (146).

1. Angelman Syndrome

Angelman syndrome (AS) is a disorder characterized by microcephaly, severe mental retardation, minimal or absent speech, hyperactivity, sleep disturbance, seizures, hyperto-nia, gait ataxia, hand flapping, and a happy disposition with frequent inappropriate outbursts of laughter (147,148). The majority of patients (70%) with AS have $\sim$4 Mb interstitial deletions of the maternal HSA15 (q11.2–q13) (149). Although several genes have been located in this region, loss-of-function mutations in *UBE3A*, a gene encoding a ubiquitin protein ligase, found in clinically typical AS patients indicate that the main aspects of the phenotype are attributable to mater-nal deficiency for this locus (150,151). *UBE3A* is expressed only from the maternally inherited HSA15 and is imprinted within the brain (152,153). Therefore, inheritance of a *UBE3A* mutation from the mother causes AS, but inheritance from the father has no detectable effect on the child. Other genetic causes of AS are paternal uniparental disomy (UPD) (in 2–3% of cases), in which the child inherits both copies of HSA15 from the father, and an "imprinting defect" (in 3–5% of cases) in which the allele inherited from the mother func-tions in the same way that a paternal HSA15 should function and is not active. Some AS individuals with imprinting defects have very small deletions of a region called the AS-imprinting center (IC) (154,155) which regulates the activity of *UBE3A* from a distant location by an unknown mechanism.

To model AS in mice and to clarify the relationship between imprinting and *UBE3A* functions, two groups created mice with a null mutation for *Ube3a* (156,157). Whereas mice with paternal deficiency of *Ube3a* were essentially similar to wild-type mice, the phenotype of mice with maternal deficiency resembled that of human AS. They exhibited motor dysfunction, inducible seizures, and a context-dependent learning deficit (156,157). The absence of detectable expression of *Ube3a* in hippocampal neurons and Purkinje cells in mice with maternal deficiency correlated with neurological and cognitive impairments, and LTP in the hippocampus was severely impaired. In addition, the cytoplasmic abundance of p53 was found to be greatly increased in Purkinje cells and in a subset of hippocampal neurons in mice with maternal deficiency, as it was in a deceased AS patient. Jiang et al. (156) suggest that failure of *Ube3a* to ubiquitinate target proteins and to promote their degradation could be a key aspect of the pathogenesis of AS.

2. Prader–Willi Syndrome

Prader–Willi syndrome (PWS) is characterized by neonatal hypotonia and failure to thrive, followed by early childhood-onset hyperphagia and resultant obesity, short stature, typical facial features, small hands and feet, and hypogonadotropic hypogonadism (158). Mild mental retardation or learning disabilities are present, as is a characteristic neurobehavioral profile with temper tantrums, obsessive–compulsive disorder, and occasionally psychosis. Hypothalamic dysfunction is thought to underlie many of the major features of this disorder.

Approximately, 70% of cases of PWS are associated with a deletion of the paternal 15q11–q13 chromosome region (158,159) and about 28% with maternal uniparental disomy in which affected individuals inherit both copies of HSA15 from their mother and none from their father. In the remaining cases (2%) of PWS, there is an intrinsic abnormality in the imprinting mechanism and both the maternal and paternal copies of HSA15 have a maternal imprint. This sometimes involves a chromosomal translocation or a detectable mutation in the IC and can be inherited in an autosomal dominant manner. As a result, there is a lack of expression of the paternally inherited genes. In such situations, it appears that the imprint from the paternal grandmother cannot be erased in the paternal germline.

Within 15q11–q13, there is a cluster of imprinted genes. Ten of these genes are expressed only from the paternally inherited chromosome and are known to be positively regulated by the PWS imprinting center (PWS-IC) located upstream of the *SNRPN* gene. (http://www.mgu.har.mrc.a c.uk/imprinting). To understand PWS and the function of the IC, which maps in part to the promoter and first exon of the *SNRPN* gene, Yang et al. (160) created two deletion mutations in mice. Mice with an intragenic deletion of *Snrpn* were phenotypically normal, suggesting that mutations of *Snrpn* are not sufficient to induce PWS. Mice with a larger deletion involving both *Snrpn* and the putative PWS-IC lacked expression of the imprinted genes *Zfp127* (mouse homolog of *ZNF12*), *Ndn*, and *ipw*, and manifested several PWS phenotypes. These data established that both the position of the IC and its role in the co-ordinate expression of genes are functionally conserved between mouse and human and that the mouse is a suitable model system in which to investigate the molecular mechanisms of imprinting in this region of the genome.

Gabriel et al. (161) reported the characterization of a transgene insertion into mouse chromosome 7C that completely deleted the PWS/AS orthologous region but not the flanking loci. Paternal transmission of the transgene resulted in failure to thrive and early postnatal lethality, a phenotype shared by other PWS models. Maternal transmission yielded viable mice representing AS. Although not tested, these mice are expected to display the mild neurological and behavioral phenotype associated with *Ube3a*-null mutants (156).

Muscatelli et al. (162) produced mice deficient for *necdin* (*Ndn*), a gene expressed in postmitotic neurons that possibly plays a role in cell cycle arrest in terminally differentiated neurons. Viable *Ndn* mutants showed a reduction in both oxytocin-producing and luteinizing hormone-releasing hormone (LHRH)-producing neurons in hypothalamus representing the first evidence of a hypothalamic deficiency in a mouse model of PWS. Although behavioral responses related to motor co-ordination, exploratory activity, anxiety and stress appear unaffected, the mice demonstrated skin scraping activity in the open field test, reminiscent of the skin picking behavior described in PWS patients (162). One of the characteristic strengths of the PWS phenotype is enhanced visual–spatial integration and visual memory, behavioral responses measured by the Morris water maze test. Not surprisingly, *Ndn*-deficient mice demonstrated improved performance in the Morris water maze suggesting that necdin deficiency may improve cognitive function through changes in neuropeptide levels and/or neurotransmitter activity (162).

Studies examining the fate of androgenetic (Ag; duplicated paternal genome) and parthenogenetic/gynogenetic (Pg/Gg; duplicated maternal genome) ES cells in chimeric mouse embryos (163) have shed interesting light on the effects of imprinted genes on brain development and indirectly, the pathogenesis of the distinctive neuropsychological features of PWS and AS. Striking cell-autonomous differences in the role of the two types of uniparental cells in brain development were observed. Whereas Ag cells contributed substantially to the hypothalamic structures and not the cerebral cortex, Pg/Gg cells contributed substantially to the cortex, striatum, and hippocampus but not to the hypothalamic structures. Furthermore, growth of the brain was enhanced by Pg/Gg and retarded by Ag cells.

3. Rett Syndrome

Classic Rett syndrome (RTT) is a neurodevelopmental disorder found almost solely in females, with prevalence of 1:10,000–20,000 (164). The classic RTT patient shows apparently normal development for 6–18 months but then fails to acquire new skills and enters a period of regression in which motor and language skills are lost (164). Clinical characteristics of the syndrome include abnormal motor gait, stereotypic hand wringing movements, and autistic-like behavior. Affected girls also exhibit speech abnormalities and severe cognitive deficits in most cases (165). In addition to classic RTT, there is an extraordinary range of phenotypes in females as a result of differences in X-chromosome inactivation (XCI) patterns and in the specific mutations that are present in the disease-causing gene, *MECP2* (166). This gene encodes the methyl-CpG binding protein 2 (MeCP2) which is thought to be a general transcriptional repressor. In males, different *MECP2* mutations can produce phenotypes ranging from a severe neonatal encephalopathy and infantile death to early-onset psychosis (167).

A unifying hypothesis proposes (168) that the major effect of the *MECP2* mutations could be to disrupt synaptic proliferation and pruning, resulting in the disruption of multiple neurotransmitters, brain regions, and behavioral processes, each with different developmental time courses (169) coinciding with the peak of synaptic proliferation in the cerebral cortex (7–18 months in humans, and the first weeks of life in the mouse). This would suggest that aberrations in neuronal maturation are a primary cause of the behavioral phenotype in RTT.

Mice deficient in *Mecp2* have been generated, and the initial manifestations of abnormal behavior, including nervousness, body trembling, piloerection, and occasional hard respiration, develop at 5 weeks of age (170). A significant portion of mutant mice become overweight, and most exhibit signs of physical deterioration by 8 weeks of age. At late stages of the disease, the mutants are hypoactive, tremble when handled, and often begin to lose weight. Most mutants die at approximately 10 weeks of age. Female mice heterozygous for the null allele are mosaic for *Mecp2* expression as a result of XCI. These mice survive, and about half of them develop hypoactivity by the age of 9 months. Brain-specific deletion of *Mecp2* results in a phenotype that is similar to that of *Mecp2*-null mice, indicating that the main features of the *Mecp2*-null phenotype are caused by loss of *Mecp2* in the CNS (170).

Using similar methods, Guy et al. (171) replaced exons 3 and 4 of *Mecp2*. Although the *Mecp2*-null mutation gives rise to animals with behavioral defects, the brain shows no unusual features of cortical lamination, ectopias, or other abnormalities. Variable progression of symptoms leads ultimately to rapid weight loss and death at approximately 54 days. After several months, heterozygous female mice also showed behavioral symptoms. The relative similar delays before symptom onset in humans and mice, despite their profoundly different rates of development, raises the possibility that stability of brain function, not brain development per se, is compromised by the absence of *MECP2* (171).

Although the female mice that carry a null allele are technically a model for the human disease (because many patients are heterozygous for early truncating mutations), the confounding effect of variable XCI in the mice might render the study of these mice challenging. To circumvent the XCI problem, a male mouse model of classic RTT expressing a truncated MeCP2 protein similar to those found in RTT patients has been created (172). These mice live for up to 15 months and develop a progressive neurological disease at the age of 6 weeks with tremors, motor impairment, hypoactivity, increased anxiety-related behavior, seizures, kyphosis, and stereotypic forelimb motions.

The involvement of the *Mecp2* gene product in methylation-specific transcriptional repression suggests that RTT may be a result of global misregulation of gene expression. Tudor et al. (173) tested this hypothesis by performing global transcriptional profiling of brain tissue from *Mecp2* wild-type and mutant (170) mice by using oligonucleotide microarrays, and found that, despite striking physiological consequences, the mutant brains have few, if any, genes that are significantly changed in expression level when considered singly. These data suggest that *Mecp2* deficiency does not lead to global alterations in transcription but instead leads to subtle changes of gene expression that are only detectable by sensitive statistical analysis of relatively large datasets. Nevertheless, there are transcriptional alterations in the brains of *Mecp2* mutant mice, and the question of their potential biological significance remains the subject of further study.

4. Fragile X Syndrome

Fragile X syndrome (FRAXA) is the most common form of inherited mental retardation, and is characterized by mental retardation, developmental delay, mildly dysmorphic features and, in males, macro-orchidism. It is caused by the absence of the fragile X mental retardation 1 protein (FMRP). In normal individuals, the *FMR1* gene is transmitted stably from parent to child. However, in FRAXA individuals, there is an amplification of a CGG repeat in the 5′ untranslated region of the gene. Normal individuals have 6–50 trinucleotide repeats, whereas individuals with FRAXA have more than 230 (174). The mutation results in the hypermethylation of the *FMR1* promoter and loss of expression of the FMRP (175,176). This protein is a member of a family of RNA-binding proteins that appears to play a central role in brain development, in particular during synaptogenesis (177,178).

As the expression patterns and the amino acid sequence of FMRP are conserved between human and mouse, the knockout animal was predicted to provide an accurate model for the human condition. Consequently, *Fmr1*-knockout mice have been generated. Although the mice do not develop dysmorphic facial features, > 90% of them develop macro-orchidism. More importantly, the mice show behavioral abnormalities, including hyperactivity that is manifested as increased activity in the open field test and decreased anxiety-related response (179,180). Immature, long, tortuous dendritic spine morphology, the most profound finding on autopsy in FRAXA patients (181,182), is also present in *Fmr1*-null mice (183,184). The finding that dendritic spine abnormalities similar to those exhibited by humans are found in FraX mice suggests that these mice are a viable model for the study for fragile-X syndrome.

To investigate whether restoring FMRP function would rescue the phenotypic features of null mutants, an intact copy of the *FMR1* gene was introduced into the knockout mouse (180). Although macro-orchidism was absent in the knockout mice in which human *FMRP* was expressed, these mice still showed abnormal behavioral responses that sometimes were the opposite to those observed in the null mutant (180), i.e., the "rescued" transgenic mice were hypoactive and had high levels of anxiety. These results indicate that the correct level of *FMR1* is as important as proper spatial and temporal regulation.

5. FRAXE (Nonspecific XLMR)

Mutations in the X-linked *FMR2* gene cause FRAXE, a nonspecific form of X-linked MR with an incidence of 1:50,000 (185). Methylation of an expanded CCG trinucleotide repeat located in exon 1 of the gene results in transcriptional silencing and lack of its product, the FMR2 protein. This protein has been hypothesized to be a transcriptional activator (186). *Fmr2* knockout mice (187) display a delay-dependent deficit in contextual fear conditioning, indicating dysfunction of the hippocampus and amygdala (188,189), a slight deficit in spatial learning in a Morris water maze task, and increased sensitivity to the heat source in the hot plate test. Surprisingly, LTP was found to be enhanced in hippocampal slices of *Fmr2* knockouts as compared to control littermate. Although a number of studies have suggested that diminished LTP is associated with memory impairment (60,61), these data suggest that increased LTP also may be as detrimental to the cognitive processes as diminished LTP (187).

6. Wolf–Hirschhorn Syndrome

The Wolf–Hirschhorn syndrome (WHS) is a malformation syndrome associated with a segmental deletion of the distal short arm of chromosome 4 (4p16.3). Children with Wolf–Hirschhorn syndrome are born with specific facial malformations, including a prominent forehead and widely spaced eyes (also known as "Greek helmet"), and have severe mental retardation, growth retardation, and, in many cases, defects of the heart and midline of the body (e.g., cleft palate).

The WHS critical region (*WHSCR*) is approximately 165 kb long and lies between the Huntington's disease gene, *HD*, and *FGFR3* on chromosome 5 in a region of conserved synteny with human 4p16.3 (190). The amount of material deleted may range from about 50% of the short arm to a small break that is not detectable by normal chromosome analysis.

The Wolf–Hirschhorn syndrome candidate 1 gene (*WHSC1*) is ubiquitously expressed in early development, especially in rapidly growing embryonic tissues in a pattern corresponding to affected organs in WHS patients. To derive mouse models of WHS and map genes responsible for subphenotypes of the syndrome, five mouse lines bearing radiation-induced deletions spanning the WHSCR syntenic region were generated and characterized (191). Similar to WHS patients, these animals were growth-retarded and susceptible to seizures. Other phenotypes include cerebellar hypoplasia and a shortened cerebral cortex. Expression of WHS-like traits was variable and influenced by the deletion size suggesting that nested deletions spanning the WHSCR syntenic region will be useful for mapping and identifying loci responsible for the various subphenotypes of WHS (191).

7. Smith–Lemli–Opitz Syndrome

Smith–Lemli–Opitz (SLO) syndrome, which is caused by mutations in the sterol delta-7-reductase gene (*DHCR7*), is a serious inherited disorder that results in an inability to synthesize enough cholesterol to support normal growth and development. This results in mental retardation and physical abnormalities such as, microcephaly, growth retardation, hypoplastic external genitalia, characteristic facies with micrognathia and anteverted nostrils.

Dhcr7(–/–) knockout mice, which survive for only one day after birth, have a marked reduction of serum and tissue cholesterol levels and display intrauterine growth retardation, poor feeding with an unco-ordinated suck, hypotonia, decreased movement, neurological deficits, and variable craniofacial abnormalities including cleft palate (192). Although the response of frontal cortex neurons to the neurotransmitter, gamma-amino-*n*-butyric acid, is normal, the response of these same neurons to the antiproliferative actions of glutamate is significantly impaired.

8. Smith–Magenis syndrome

Smith–Magenis syndrome (SMS), a contiguous gene syndrome caused by haploinsufficiency of one or more genes associated with a deletion in 17p11.2. Phenotypic abnormalities include dysmorphic facies, major and minor congenital malformations, selfinjurious behavior, sleep disturbances, and mental retardation (193). The reciprocal duplication syndrome results in mild to borderline mental retardation and behavioral difficulties. Recently, Walz et al. (194) created chromosomes carrying a deletion [Df(11) 17] or duplication [Dp(11) 17] of the orthologous region on MMU11 spanning the region commonly deleted in SMS patients. Mice heterozygous for the deletion were overweight and exhibited craniofacial abnormalities with complete penetrance. However, only 20% presented with seizures (194).

IV. CONCLUSION

The mouse is the major laboratory species for understanding the biology of mammals and often acts as surrogate for human studies in genetics and development, immunology and pharmacology, cancer and heart disease, as well as behavior, learning, memory, and psychiatric disorders (195,196). The animal models described in this chapter have provided valuable insights into the pathogenesis of many human conditions in which MR is a major component. No animal model can fully recapitulate all of the features observed in the corresponding human disorder. However, with improvements in genome manipulation and the availability of the complete genome sequence, the mouse promises to be a valuable resource for scientific research well into the 21st century.

ACKNOWLEDGMENT

The preparation of this chapter was supported by grant HD-31498 from the National Institute of Child and Human Development.

REFERENCES

1. Branchi I, Bichler Z, Berger-Sweeney J, Ricceri L. Animal models of mental retardation: from gene to cognitive function. Neurosci Biobehav Rev 2003; 27(1–2):141–153.

2. Dierssen M, Fillat C, Crnic L, Arbones M, Florez J, Estivill X. Murine models for Down syndrome. Physiol Behav 2001; 73(5):859–871.

3. Kola PJ, Herzog I. Down syndrome and mouse models. Curr Opin Genet Dev 1998; 8:316–321.

4. Reeves RH, Baxter LL, Richtsmeier JT. Too much of a good thing: mechanisms of gene action in Down syndrome. Trends Genet 2001; 17(2):83–88.

5. Watase HY, Zoghbi K. Modelling brain diseases in mice: the challenges of design and analysis. Nat Rev Genet 2003; 4(4):296–307.

6. Zdobnov EM, Zody MC, Lander ES. Mouse genome sequencing consortium. Initial sequencing and comparative analysis of the mouse genome. Nature 2002; 420(6915):520–562.

7. Boguski MS. Comparative genomics: the mouse that roared. Nature 2002; 420(6915):515–516.

8. Bradley A. Mining the mouse genome. Nature 2002; 420(6915):512–514.

9. Mathis C, Paul SM, Crawley JN. Characterization of benzodiazepine-sensitive behaviors in the A/J and C57BL/6J inbred strains of mice. Behav Genet 1994; 24(2):171–180.

10. Gerlai R. Gene-targeting studies of mammalian behavior: is it the mutation or the background genotype? Trends Neurosci 1996; 19(5):177–181

11. Gerlai R. Contextual learning and cue association in fear conditioning in mice: a strain comparison and a lesion study. Behav Brain Res 1998; 95(2):191–203.

12. Carlson GA, Borchelt DR, Dake A, Turner S, Danielson V, Coffin JD, Eckman C, Meiners J, Nilsen SP, Younkin SG, Hsiao KK. Genetic modification of the phenotypes produced

by amyloid precursor protein overexpression in transgenic mice. Hum Mol Genet 1997; 6(11):1951–1959.

13. Taketo M, Schroeder AC, Mobraaten LE, Gunning KB, Hanten G, Fox RR, Roderick TH, Stewart CL, Lilly F, Hansen CT, et al. FVB/N: an inbred mouse strain preferable for transgenic analyses. Proc Natl Acad Sci USA 1991; 88(6): 2065–2069.

14. Mineur YS, Crusio WE. Behavioral and neuroanatomical characterization of FVB/N inbred mice. Brain Res Bull 2002; 57(1):41–47.

15. Nguyen PV, Abel T, Kandel ER, Bourtchouladze R. Strain-dependent differences in LTP and hippocampus-dependent memory in inbred mice. Learn Mem 2000; 7(3):170–179.

16. Kandel ER. The molecular biology of memory storage: a dialogue between genes and synapses. Science 2001; 294(5544): 1030–1038.

17. Bailey CH, Alberini C, Ghirardi M, Kandel ER. Molecular and structural changes underlying long-term memory storage in aplysia. Adv Second Messenger Phosphoprotein Res 1994; 29:529–544.

18. Tonegawa S, Nakazawa K, Wilson MA. Genetic neuroscience of mammalian learning and memory. Philos Trans R Soc Lond B Biol Sci 2003; 358(1432):787–795.

19. Crawley JN, Paylor R. A proposed test battery and constellations of specific behavioral paradigms to investigate the behavioral phenotypes of transgenic and knockout mice. Horm Behav 1997; 31(3):197–211.

20. Rogers DC, Fisher EM, Brown SD, Peters J, Hunter AJ, Martin JE. Behavioral and functional analysis of mouse phenotype: SHIRPA, a proposed protocol for comprehensive phenotype assessment. Mamm Genome 1997; 8(10): 711–713.

21. Epstein CJ. Animal models for human trisomy. In: de la Cruz FF, Gerald PS, eds. Trisomy 21 (Down Syndrome) Research Perspectives. Baltimore, MD: University Park Press, 1981:263–273.

22. Epstein CJ. The mouse trisomies: experimental systems for the study of aneuploidy. In: Kalter H, ed. Issues and Reviews in Teratology. Vol. 3. New York, NY: Plenum, 1985:177–217.

23. Davisson MT, Costa AC. Mouse models of Down syndrome. In: Popko B, ed. Mouse Models of Human Genetic Neurological Diseases. New York: Plenum Publishing Corporation, 1999:297–327.

24. Davisson MT, Schmidt C, Akeson EC. Segmental trisomy of murine chromosome 16: a new model system for studying Down syndrome. Prog Clin Biol Res 1990; 360:263–280.

25. Sago H, Carlson EJ, Smith DJ, Rubin EM, Crnic LS, Huang TT, Epstein CJ. Genetic dissection of region associated with behavioral abnormalities in mouse models for Down syndrome. Pediatr Res 2000; 48(5):606–613.

26. Gropp A, Kolbus U, Giers D. Systematic approach to the study of trisomy in the mouse. II. Cytogenet Cell Genet 1975; 14(1):42–62.

27. Miyabara S, Gropp A, Winking H. Trisomy 16 in the mouse fetus associated with generalized edema and cardiovascular and urinary tract anomalies. Teratology 1982; 25(3):369–380.

28. Bersu ET, Mossman HW, Kornguth SE. Altered placental morphology associated with murine trisomy 16 and murine trisomy 19. Teratology 1989; 40(5):513–523.

29. Villar AJ, Kim J, de Blank P, Gillespie AM, Kozy HM, Ursell PC, Epstein CJ. Effect of genetic background on cardiovascular anomalies in the Ts16 mouse. Dev Dyn 2005; 232(1):131–139 .

30. Coyle JT, Oster-Granite ML, Reeves R, Hohmann C, Corsi P, Gearhart JP. Down syndrome and the trisomy 16 mouse: impact of gene imbalance on brain development and aging. In: McHughs PR, McKusick VA, eds. Genes, Brain and Behavior. New York: Raven Press, 1991:85–99.

31. Oster-Granite ML, Lacey-Casem ML. Neurotransmitter alterations in the trisomy 16 mouse: a genetic model system for the studies of Down syndrome. Ment Retard Dev Dis Res Rev 1995; 1:227–236.

32. Grausz H, Richtsmeier JT, Oster-Granite ML. Morphogenesis of the brain and craniofacial complex in trisomy 16 mice.

In: Epstein CJ, ed. The Morphogenesis of Down syndrome. New York: Wiley-Liss, 1991:169–188.

33. Haydar TF, Blue ME, Molliver ME, Krueger BK, Yarowsky PJ. Consequences of trisomy 16 for mouse brain development: corticogenesis in a model of Down syndrome. J Neurosci 1996; 16(19):6175–6182.

34. Haydar TF, Nowakowski RS, Yarowsky PJ, Krueger BK. Role of founder cell deficit and delayed neurogenesis in microencephaly of the trisomy 16 mouse. J Neurosci 2000; 20(11): 4156–4164.

35. Bambrick LL, Golovina VA, Blaustein MP, Yarowsky PJ, Krueger BK. Abnormal calcium homeostasis in astrocytes from the trisomy 16 mouse. Glia 1997; 19:352–358.

36. Muller W, Heinemann U, Schuchmann S. Impaired Ca-signaling in astrocytes from the Ts16 mouse model of Down syndrome. Neurosci Lett 1997; 223:81–84.

37. Schuchmann S, Muller W, Heinemann U. Altered Ca^{2+} signaling and mitochondrial deficiencies in hippocampal neurons of trisomy 16 mice: a model of Down's syndrome. J Neurosci 1998; 18:7216–7231.

38. Hattori M, Fujiyama A, Taylor TD, Watanabe H, Yada T, Park HS, Toyoda A, Ishii K, Totoki Y, Choi DK, Groner Y, Soeda E, Ohki M, Takagi T, Sakaki Y, Taudien S, Blechschmidt K, Polley A, Menzel U, Delabar J, Kumpf K, Lehmann R, Patterson D, Reichwald K, Rump A, Schillhabel M, Schudy A, Zimmermann W, Rosenthal A, Kudoh J, Schibuya K, Kawasaki K, Asakawa S, Shintani A, Sasaki T, Nagamine K, Mitsuyama S, Antonarakis SE, Minoshima S, Shimizu N, Nordsiek G, Hornischer K, Brant P, Scharfe M, Schon O, Desario A, Reichelt J, Kauer G, Blocker H, Ramser J, Beck A, Klages S, Hennig S, Riesselmann L L, Dagand E, Haaf T, Wehrmeyer S, Borzym K, Gardiner K, Nizetic D, Frais F, Lehrach H, Reinhardt R, Yaspo ML. Chromosome 21 mapping and sequencing consortium. The DNA sequence of human chromosome 21. Nature 2000; 405(6784):311–319.

39. Davisson MT, Schmidt C, Reeves RH, Irving NG, Akeson EC, Harris BS, Bronson RT. Segmental trisomy as a model for Down syndrome. In: Epstein CJ, ed. The Phenotypic Mapping

of Down Syndrome and Other Aneuploid Conditions. Vol. 384. New York: Wiley-Liss, 1993:117–133.

40. Reeves RH, Irving NG, Moran TH, Wohn A, Kitt C, Sisodia SS, Schmidt C, Bronson RT, Davisson MT. A mouse model for Down syndrome exhibits learning and behavioral deficits. Nat Genet 1995; 11:177–184.

41. Antonarakis SE, Lyle R, Chrast R, Scott HS. Differential gene expression studies to explore the molecular pathophysiology of Down syndrome. Brain Res Brain Res Rev 2001; 36(2–3):265–274.

42. Holtzman DM, Santucci D, Kilbridge J, Chua-Couzens J, Fontana DJ, Daniels SE, Johnson RM, Chen K, Sun Y, Carlson EJ, Alleva E, Epstein CJ, Mobley WC. Developmental abnormalities and age-related neurodegeneration in a mouse model of Down syndrome. Proc Natl Acad Sci USA 1996; 93(23):13333–13338.

43. Sumarsono SH, Wilson TJ, Tymms MJ, Venter DJ, Corrick CM, Kola R, Lahoud MH, Papas TS, Seth A, Kola I. I. Down syndrome-like skeletal abnormalities in Ets2 transgenic mice. Nature 1996; 379:534–537.

44. Davisson MT, Schmidt C, Escorihuela RM, Fernandez-Teruel A, Vallina IF, Baamonde L, Lumbreras MA, Dierssen M, Tobena A, Florez J. A behavioral assessment of Ts65Dn mice: a putative Down syndrome model. Neurosci Lett 1995; 199: 143–146.

45. Paz-Miguel JE, Flores R, Sanchez-Velasco P, Ocejo-Vinyals G, Escribano de Diego J, Lopez de Rego J, Leyva-Cobian F. Reactive oxygen intermediates during programmed cell death induced in the thymus of the Ts(17:16)65Dn mouse, a murine model for human Down's syndrome. J Immunol 1999; 163(10):5399–5410.

46. Richtsmeier JT, Baxter LL, Reeves RH. Parallels of craniofacial maldevelopment in Down syndrome and Ts65Dn mice. Dev Dyn 2000; 217:137–145.

47. Epstein CJ. Consequences of Chromosome Imbalance: Principles, Mechanisms, and Models. Cambridge University Press, 1986.

48. Wishart JG. Early learning in infants and young children with Down syndrome In: Nadel L, ed. Cambridge, MA: MIT Press, 1988:7–50.

49. Escorihuela RM, Fernandez-Teruel A, Vallina IF, Baamonde C, Lumbreras MA, Dierssen M, Tobena A, Florez J. A behavioral assessment of Ts65Dn mice: a putative Down syndrome model. Neurosci Lett 1995; 199(2):143–146.

50. Coussons-Read ME, Crnic LS. Behavioral assessment of the Ts65Dn mouse, a model for Down syndrome: altered behavior in the elevated plus maze and open field. Behav Genet 1996; 26(1):7–13.

51. Escorihuela RM, Vallina IF, Martinez-Cue C, Baamonde C, Dierssen M, Tobena A, Florez J, Fernandez-Teruel A. Impaired short- and long-term memory in Ts65Dn mice, a model for Down syndrome. Neurosci Lett 1998; 247(2–3): 171–174.

52. Bimonte-Nelson HA, Hunter CL, Nelson ME, Granholm AC. Frontal cortex BDNF levels correlate with working memory in an animal model of Down syndrome. Behav Brain Res 2003; 139(1–2):47–57.

53. Hyde LA, Crnic LS, Pollock A, Bickford PC. Motor learning in Ts65Dn mice, a model for Down syndrome. Dev Psychobiol 2001; 38(1):33–45.

54. Turner CA, Presti MF, Newman HA, Bugenhagen P, Crnic L, Lewis MH. Spontaneous stereotypy in an animal model of Down syndrome: Ts65Dn mice. Behav Genet 2001; 31(4): 393–400.

55. Haw CM, Barnes TR, Clark K, Crichton P, Kohen D. Movement disorder in Down's syndrome: a possible marker of the severity of mental handicap. Mov Disord 1996; 11(4):395–403.

56. Baxter LL, Moran TH, Richtsmeier JT, Troncoso J, Reeves RH. Discovery and genetic localization of Down syndrome cerebellar phenotypes using the Ts65Dn mouse. Hum Mol Genet 2000; 9(2):195–202.

57. Insausti AM, Megias M, Crespo D, Cruz-Orive LM, Dierssen M, Vallina IF, Insausti R, Florez J, Vallina TF. Hippocampal volume and neuronal number in Ts65Dn mice: a murine

model of Down syndrome. Neurosci Lett 1998; 253(3): 175–178.

58. Epstein CJ, Kleschevnikov AM, Belichenko PV, Masliah E, Basu SB, Villar AJ, Malenka R, Mobley W. Increased inhibition in the dentate gyrus of Ts65Dn mice [abstr]. The 10th International Meeting of Molecular Biology of Chromosome 21 and Down Syndrome. 19 Suppl, Sitges, Spain, Sep 26–29, 2002.

59. Kaufmann WE, Moser HW. Dendritic anomalies in disorders associated with mental retardation. Cereb Cortex 2000; 10: 981–991.

60. Siarey RJ, Stoll J, Rapoport SI, Galdzicki Z. Altered long-term potentiation in the young and old Ts65Dn mouse, a model for Down syndrome. Neuropharmacology 1997; 36(11–12):1549–1554.

61. Siarey RJ, Carlson EJ, Epstein CJ, Balbo A, Rapoport SI, Galdzicki Z. Increased synaptic depression in the Ts65Dn mouse, a model for mental retardation in Down syndrome. Neuropharmacology 1999; 38(12):1917–1920.

62. Kurt MA, Davies DC, Kidd M, Dierssen M, Florez J. Synaptic deficit in the temporal cortex of partial trisomy 16 (Ts65Dn) mice. Brain Res 2000; 858(1):191–197.

63. Klein SL, Kriegsfeld LJ, Hairston JE, Rau V, Nelson RJ, Yarowsky PJ. Characterization of sensorimotor performance, reproductive and aggressive behaviors in segmental trisomic 16 (Ts65Dn) mice. Physiol Behav 1996; 60(4): 1159–1164.

64. Galdzicki Z, Siarey R, Pearce R, Stoll J, Rapoport SI. On the cause of mental retardation in Down syndrome: extrapolation from full and segmental trisomy 16 mouse models. Brain Res Brain Res Rev 2001; 35(2):115–145.

65. Dierssen M, Vallina IF, Baamonde C, Lumbreras MA, Martinez-Cue C, Calatayud SG, Florez J. Impaired cyclic AMP production in the hippocampus of a Down syndrome murine model. Brain Res Dev Brain Res 1996; 95(1):122–124.

66. Dierssen M, Vallina IF, Baamonde C, Garcia-Calatayud S, Lumbreras MA, Florez J. Alterations of central noradrenergic

transmission in Ts65Dn mouse, a model for Down syndrome. Brain Res 1997; 749(2):238–244.

67. Li Y, Holtzman DM, Kromer LF, Kaplan DR, Chua-Couzens J, Clary DO, Knusel B, Mobley WC. Regulation of TrkA and ChAT expression in developing rat basal forebrain: evidence that both exogenous and endogenous NGF regulate differentiation of cholinergic neurons. J Neurosci 1995; 15(4): 2888–2905.

68. Cooper JD, Salehi A, Delcroix JD, Howe CL, Belichenko PV, Chua-Couzens J, Kilbridge JF, Carlson EJ, Epstein CJ, Mobley WC. Failed retrograde transport of NGF in a mouse model of Down's syndrome: reversal of cholinergic neurodegenerative phenotypes following NGF infusion. Proc Natl Acad Sci USA 2001; 98(18):10439–10444.

69. Granholm AC, Sanders LA, Crnic LS. Loss of cholinergic phenotype in basal forebrain coincides with cognitive decline in a mouse model of Down's syndrome. Exp Neurol 2000; 161(2):647–663.

70. Coyle JT, Singer H, McKinney M, Price D. Neurotransmitter specific alterations in dementing disorders: insights from animal models. J Psychiatr Res 1984; 18(4):501–512.

71. Davies AM. The neurotrophic hypothesis: where does it stand? Philos Trans R Soc Lond B Biol Sci 1996; 351(1338): 389–394

72. Mobley WC, Salehi A. J-D Delcroix, Belichenko P, Klesch A. Defining the genetic and cellular basis for degeneration of basal forebrain cholinergic neurons in Down syndrome [abstr]. The 10th International Meeting of Molecular Biology of Chromosome 21 and Down Syndrome. 19 Suppl, Sitges, Spain, Sep 26–29, 2002.

73. Casanova MF, Walker LC, Whitehouse PJ, Price DL. Abnormalities of the nucleus basalis in Down's syndrome. Ann Neurol 1985; 18(3):310–313.

74. Mann DM, Esiri MM. The pattern of acquisition of plaques and tangles in the brains of patients under 50 years of age with Down's syndrome. J Neurol Sci 1989; 89(2–3): 169–179.

75. Lawrence AD, Sahakian BJ. The cognitive psychopharmacology of Alzheimer's disease: focus on cholinergic systems. Neurochem Res 1998; 23(5):787–794.

76. Cataldo AM, Barnett JL, Pieroni C, Nixon RA. Increased neuronal endocytosis and protease delivery to early endosomes in sporadic Alzheimer's disease: neuropathologic evidence for a mechanism of increased beta-amyloidogenesis. J Neurosci 1997; 17(16):6142–6151.

77. Cataldo AM, Peterhoff CM, Troncoso JC, Gomez-Isla T, Hyman BT, Nixon RA. Endocytic pathway abnormalities precede amyloid beta deposition in sporadic Alzheimer's disease and Down syndrome: differential effects of APOE genotype and presenilin mutations. Am J Pathol 2000; 157(1):277–286.

78. Cataldo AM, Nixon RA, Troncoso JC, Durham R, Buxbaum J, Epstein CJ, Carlson EJ, Peterhoff C. Endocytic alterations in human preclinical Alzheimer's disease and a trisomic mouse model of Down syndrome: implications for β-amyloidogensis. Neurobiol Aging 2000; 21:S65.

79. Cataldo AM, Petanceska S, Peterhoff CM, Terio NB, Epstein CJ, Villar AJ, Carlson EJ, Staufenbiel M. App gene dosage modulates endosomal abnormalities of Alzheimer's disease in a segmental trisomy 16 mouse model of Down syndrome. J Neurosci 2003; 23(17):6788–6792.

80. Coyle JT, Oster-Granite ML, Reeves RH, Gearhart JD. Down syndrome, Alzheimer's disease and the trisomy 16 mouse. Trends Neurosci 1988; 11(9):390–394.

81. Holtzman DM, Bayney RM, Li YW, Khosrovi H, Berger CN, Epstein CJ, Mobley WC. Dysregulation of gene expression in mouse trisomy 16, an animal model of Down syndrome. EMBO J 1992; 11(2):619–627.

82. Rumble B, Retallack R, Hilbich C, Simms G, Multhaup G, Martins R, Hockey A, Montgomery P, Beyreuther K, Masters CL. Amyloid A4 protein and its precursor in Down's syndrome and Alzheimer's disease. N Engl J Med 1989; 320(22):1446–1452.

83. Games D, Adams D, Alessandrini R, Barbour R, Berthelette P, Blackwell C, Carr T, Clemens J, Donaldson T, Gillespie F, et al. Alzheimer-type neuropathology in transgenic mice

overexpressing V717F beta-amyloid precursor protein. Nature 1995; 373(6514):523–527.

84. Lamb BT, Sisodia SS, Lawler AM, Slunt HH, Kitt CA, Kearns WG, Pearson PL, Price DL, Gearhart JD. Introduction and expression of the 400 kilobase amyloid precursor protein gene in transgenic mice. Nat Genet 1993; 5(1):22–30.

85. Hennequin M, Morin C, Feine JS. Pain expression and stimulus localisation in individuals with Down's syndrome. Lancet 2000; 356(9245):1882–1887.

86. Martinez-Cue C, Baamonde C, Lumbreras MA, Vallina IF, Dierssen M, Florez J. A murine model for Down syndrome shows reduced responsiveness to pain. Neuroreport 1999; 10(5):1119–1122.

87. Cao YQ, Carlson EJ, Epstein CJ, Basbaum AI. Acute thermal and mechanical nociceptive responses in Ts65Dn mice, a mouse model for Down syndrome. Ninth World Congress on Pain, Vienna, 1999.

88. Simmons RM, Li DL, Hoo KH, Deverill M, Ornstein PL, Iyengar S. Kainate GluR5 receptor subtype mediates the nociceptive response to formalin in the rat. Neuropharmacology 1998; 37(1):25–36.

89. Sago H, Carlson EJ, Smith DJ, Kilbridge J, Rubin EM, Mobley WC, Epstein CJ, Huang TT. Ts1Cje, a partial trisomy 16 mouse model for Down syndrome, exhibits learning and behavioral abnormalities. Proc Natl Acad Sci USA 1998; 95(11):6256–6261.

90. Korenberg R, et al. Molecular definition of a region of chromosome 21 that causes features of Down syndrome phenotype. Am J Hum Genet 1990; 47:236–246.

91. Gearhart JD, Oster-Granite ML, Reeves RH, Coyle JT. Developmental consequences of autosomal aneuploidy in mammals. Dev Genet 1987; 8(4):249–265.

92. Epstein CJ, Avraham KB, Lovett M, Smith S, Elroy-Stein O, Rotman G, Bry C, Groner Y. Transgenic mice with increased Cu/Zn-superoxide dismutase activity: animal model of dosage effects in Down syndrome. Proc Natl Acad Sci USA 1987; 84(22):8044–8048.

93. Epstein CJ. Down Syndrome. In: Scriver CR, Beaudet AL, Sly WS, Valle D, eds. The Metabolic and Molecular Bases of Inherited Disease. 8th ed. New York: McGraw-Hill, 2001: 1223–1256.

94. de la Monte S. Molecular abnormalities of the brain in Down syndrome: relevance to Alzheimer's neurodegeneration. J Neural Transm Suppl 1999; 57:1–20.

95. Groner Y. Transgenic models for chromosome 21 gene dosage effects. Prog Clin Biol Res 1995; 393:193–212.

96. Gahtan E, Auerbach JM, Groner Y, Segal M. Reversible impairment of long-term potentiation in transgenic CuZn-SOD mice. Eur J Neurosci 1998; 10:538–544.

97. Schwartz PJ, Reaume A, Scott R, Coyle JT. Effects of over- and under-expression of Cu,Zn-superoxide dismutase on the toxicity of glutamate analogs in transgenic mouse striatum. Brain Res 1998; 789(1):32–39.

98. Mrak RE, Sheng JG, Griffin WS. Glial cytokines in Alzheimer's disease: review and pathogenic implications. Hum Pathol 1995; 26(8):816–823.

99. Pueschel SM. Phenotypic characteristics. In: Pueschel SM, Pueschel JK, eds. Biomedical Concerns in Persons with Down Syndrome. Baltimore: Paul H. Brookes Publishing, 1992: 1–12.

100. Mann DM. The pathological association between Down syndrome and Alzheimer disease. Mech Aging Dev 1988; 43(2):99–136.

101. Wisniewski KE, Wisniewski HM, Wen GY. Occurrence of neuropathological changes and dementia of Alzheimer's disease in Down's syndrome. Ann Neurol 1985; 17:278–282.

102. Epstein CJ. Down syndrome. In: Sciver CR, Beaudet AL, Sly WS, Valle D, eds. The Metabolic and Molecular Basis of Inherited Disease. 7th ed. New York: McGraw Hill, 1995: 1223–1256.

103. Tanzi RE, McClatchey AI, Lamperti ED, Villa-Komaroff L, Gusella JF, Neve RL. Protease inhibitor domain encoded by an amyloid protein precursor mRNA associated with Alzheimer's disease. Nature 1988; 331(6156):528–530.

104. Oyama F, Cairns NJ, Shimada H, Oyama R, Titani K, Ihara Y. Down's syndrome: up-regulation of beta-amyloid protein precursor and tau mRNAs and their defective coordination. J Neurochem 1994; 62(3):1062–1066.

105. Lendon CL, Ashall F, Goate AM. Exploring the etiology of Alzheimer disease using molecular genetics. J Am Med Assoc 1997; 227:25–31.

106. Johnson-Wood K, Lee M, Motter R, Hu K, Gordon G, Barbour R, Khan K, Gordon M, Tan H, Games D, Lieberburg I, Schenk D, Acubert P, McConlogue L. Amyloid precursor protein processing and A bets42 deposition in a transgenic mouse model of Alzheimer disease. Proc Natl Acad Sci USA 1997; 94:1550–1555.

107. Hsiao K, Chapman P, Nilsen S, Eckman C, Harigaya Y, Younkin S, Yang F, Cole G. Correlative memory deficits, abeta elevation, and amyloid plaques in transgenic mice. Science 1996; 274(5284):99–102.

108. Storey E, Cappai R. The amyloid precursor protein of Alzheimer's disease and the abeta peptide. Neuropathol Appl Neurobiol 1999; 25(2):81–97.

109. Hsia AY, Masliah E, McConlogue L, Yu GQ, Tatsuno G, Hu K, Kholodenko D, Malenka RC, Nicoll RA, Mucke L. Plaque-independent disruption of neural circuits in Alzheimer's disease mouse models. Proc Natl Acad Sci USA 1999; 96(6):3228–3233.

110. Moechars D, Dewachter I, Lorent K, Reverse D, Baekelandt V, Naidu A, Tesseur I, Spittaels K, Haute CV, Checler F, Godaux E, Cordell B, Van Leuven F. Early phenotypic changes in transgenic mice that overexpress different mutants of amyloid precursor protein in brain. J Biol Chem 1999; 274(10):6483–6492.

111. Lamb BT, Call LM, Slunt HH, Bardel KA, Lawler AM, Eckman CB, Younkin SG, Holtz G, Wagner SL, Price DL, Sisodia SS, Gearhart JD. Altered metabolism of familial Alzheimer's disease-linked amyloid precursor protein variants in yeast artificial chromosome transgenic mice. Hum Mol Genet 1997; 6(9):1535–1541.

112. Sturchler-Pierrat C, Abramowski D, Duke M, Wiederhold KH, Mistl C, Rothacher S, Ledermann B, Burki K, Frey P,

Paganetti PA, Waridel C, Calhoun ME, Jucker M, Probst A, Staufenbiel M, Sommer B. Two amyloid precursor protein transgenic mouse models with Alzheimer disease-like pathology. Proc Natl Acad Sci USA 1997; 94(24):13287–13292.

113. Solans A, Estivill X, de La Luna S. A new aspartyl protease on 21q22 A.3, BACE2, is highly similar to Alzheimer's amyloid precursor protein beta-secretase. Cytogenet Cell Genet 2000; 89(3–4):177–184.

114. Heisenberg M, Borst A, Wagner S, Byers D. Drosophila mushroom body mutants are deficient in olfactory learning. J Neurogenet 1985; 2(1):1–30.

115. Tejedor F, Zhu XR, Kaltenbach E, Ackermann A, Baumann A, Canal I, Heisenberg M, Fischbach KF, Pongs O. Minibrain: a new protein kinase family involved in postembryonic neurogenesis in Drosophila. Neuron 1995; 14(2):287–301.

116. Altafaj X, Dierssen M, Baamonde C, Marti E, Visa J, Guimera J, Oset M, Gonzalez JR, Florez J, Fillat C, Estivill X. Neurodevelopmental delay, motor abnormalities and cognitive deficits in transgenic mice overexpressing Dyrk1A (minibrain), a murine model of Down's syndrome. Hum Mol Genet 2001; 10(18):1915–1923.

117. Fan CM, Kuwana E, Bulfone A, Fletcher CF, Copeland NG, Jenkins NA, Crews S, Martinez S, Puelles L, Rubenstein JL, Tessier-Lavigne M. Expression patterns of two murine homologs of Drosophila single-minded suggest possible roles in embryonic patterning and in the pathogenesis of Down syndrome. Mol Cell Neurosci 1996; 7(1):1–16.

118. Chrast R, Scott HS, Madani R, Huber L, Wolfer DP, Prinz M, Aguzzi A, Lipp HP, Antonarakis SE. Mice trisomic for a bacterial artificial chromosome with the single-minded 2 gene (Sim2) show phenotypes similar to some of those present in the partial trisomy 16 mouse models of Down syndrome. Hum Mol Genet 2000; 9(12):1853–1864.

119. Ema M, Ikegami S, Hosoya T, Mimura J, Ohtani H, Nakao K, Inokuchi K, Katsuki M, Fujii-Kuriyama Y. Mild impairment of learning and memory in mice overexpressing the mSim2 gene located on chromosome 16: an animal model of Down's syndrome. Hum Mol Genet 1999; 8(8):1409–1415.

120. Elson A, Levanon D, Weiss Y, Groner Y. Overexpression of liver-type phosphofructokinase (PFKL) in transgenic PFKL mice: implications for dosage in trisomy 21. Biochem J 1994; 299:409–415.

121. Peled-Kamar M, Degani H, Bendel P, Margalit R, Groner Y. Altered brain glucose metabolism in transgenic-PFKL mice with elevated L-phosphofructokinase: in vivo NMR studies. Brain Res 1998; 810(1–2):138–145.

122. Allore R, O'Hanlon D, Price R, Neilson K, Willard HF, Cox DR, Marks A, Dunn RJ. Gene encoding the beta subunit of S100 protein is on chromosome 21: implications for Down syndrome. Science 1988; 239(4845):1311–1313.

123. Griffin WS, Sheng JG, McKenzie JE, Royston MC, Gentleman SM, Brumback RA, Cork LC, Del Bigio MR, Roberts GW, Mrak RE. Life-long overexpression of S100beta in Down's syndrome: implications for Alzheimer pathogenesis. Neurobiol Aging 1998; 19(5):401–405.

124. Griffin WS, Stanley LC, Ling C, White L, MacLeod V, Perrot LJ, White CL III, Araoz C. Brain interleukin 1 and S-100 immunoreactivity are elevated in Down syndrome and Alzheimer disease. Proc Natl Acad Sci USA 1989; 86(19): 7611–7615.

125. Sheng JG, Mrak RE, Griffin WS. Glial–neuronal interactions in Alzheimer disease: progressive association of IL-1alpha+ microglia and S100beta+ astrocytes with neurofibrillary tangle stages. J Neuropathol Exp Neurol 1997; 56(3): 285–290.

126. Gerlai R, Roder J. Female specific hyperactivity in S100 beta transgenic mice does not habituate in open-field. Behav Brain Res 1993; 59(1–2):119–124.

127. Gerlai R, Roder J. Spatial and nonspatial learning in mice: effects of S100 beta overexpression and age. Neurobiol Learn Mem 1996; 66(2):143–154.

128. Reeves RH, Yao J, Crowley MR, Buck S, Zhang X, Yarowsky P, Gearhart JD, Hilt DC. Astrocytosis and axonal proliferation in the hippocampus of S100β transgenic mice. Proc Natl Acad Sci USA 1994; 91:5359–5363.

129. Whitaker-Azmitia PM, Wingate M, Borella A, Gerlai R, Roder J, Azmitia EC. Transgenic mice overexpressing the neurotrophic factor S-100 beta show neuronal cytoskeletal and behavioral signs of altered aging processes: implications for Alzheimer's disease and Down's syndrome. Brain Res 1997; 776(1–2):51–60.

130. Baffico M, Perroni L, Rasore-Quartino A, Scartezzini P. Expression of the human ETS-2 oncogene in normal fetal tissues and in the brain of a fetus with trisomy 21. Hum Genet 1989; 83(3):295–296.

131. Greber-Platzer S, Schatzmann-Turhani D, Wollenek G, Lubec G. Evidence against the current hypothesis of "gene dosage effects" of trisomy 21: ets-2, encoded on chromosome 21 is not overexpressed in hearts of patients with Down syndrome. Biochem Biophys Res Commun 1999; 254(2): 395–399.

132. Burke DT, Carle GF, Olson MV. Cloning of large segments of exogenous DNA into yeast by means of artificial chromosome vectors. Science 1987; 236(4803):806–812.

133. Cabin DE, Hawkins A, Griffin C, Reeves RH. YAC transgenic mice in the study of the genetic basis of Down syndrome. Prog Clin Biol Res 1995; 393:213–226.

134. Smith DJ, Zhu Y, Zhang J, Cheng JF, Rubin EM. Construction of a panel of transgenic mice containing a contiguous 2-Mb set of YAC/P1 clones from human chromosome 21q22.2. Genomics 1995; 27(3):425–434.

135. Smith DJ, Stevens ME, Sudanagunta SP, Bronson RT, Makhinson M, Watabe AM, O'Dell TJ, Fung J, Weier HU, Cheng JF, Rubin EM. Functional screening of 2 Mb of human chromosome 21q22.2 in transgenic mice implicates minibrain in learning defects associated with Down syndrome. Nat Genet 1997; 16(1):28–36.

136. Guimera J, Casas C, Pucharcos C, Solans A, Domenech A, Planas AM, Ashley J, Lovett M, Estivill X, Pritchard MA. A human homologue of Drosophila minibrain (MNB) is expressed in the neuronal regions affected in Down syndrome and maps to the critical region. Hum Mol Genet 1996; 5(9): 1305–1310.

137. Hernandez D, Mee PJ, Martin JE, Tybulewicz VL, Fisher EM. Transchromosomal mouse embryonic stem cell lines and chimeric mice that contain freely segregating segments of human chromosome 21. Hum Mol Genet 1999; 8(5):923–933.

138. Inoue T, Shinohara T, Takehara S, Inoue J, Kamino H, Kugoh H, Oshimura M. Specific impairment of cardiogenesis in mouse ES cells containing a human chromosome 21. Biochem Biophys Res Commun 2000; 273(1):219–224.

139. Shinohara T, Tomizuka K, Miyabara S, Takehara S, Kazuki Y, Inoue J, Katoh M, Nakane H, Iino A, Ohguma A, Ikegami S, Inokuchi K, Ishida I, Reeves RH, Oshimura M. Mice containing a human chromosome 21 model behavioral impairment and cardiac anomalies of Down's syndrome. Hum Mol Genet 2001; 10(11):1163–1175.

140. Smithies O, Kim H-S. Targeted gene duplication and disruption for analyzing quantitative genetic traits in mice. Proc Natl Acad Sci USA 26; 1994; 91(9):3612–3615.

141. Yu YE, Morishima M, Pao A, Qi Y, Rivera S, Baldini A, Bradley A. Engineering chromosomal rearrangements in mice to model del(17)(q21q23) and Down syndrome. Am J Med Genet 2002; 71(suppl 4):195.

142. Olsen LE, Reeves RH. Generation of segmental aneuploidy to create a mouse model of Down syndrome [abstr]. Molecular biology of chromosome 21 and Down syndrome. 19 Suppl, Sitges, Spain, Sep 26–29, 2002.

143. Ogawa S, Pfaff DW. Application of antisense DNA method for the study of molecular bases of brain function and behavior. Behav Genet 1996; 26(3):279–292.

144. Ogawa S, Pfaff DW. Current status of antisense DNA methods in behavioral studies. Chem Senses 1998; 23(2): 249–255.

145. Bourc'his D, Viegas-Pequignot E. Direct analysis of chromosome methylation. Methods Mol Biol 2001; 181:229–242.

146. Cassidy SB, Schwartz S. Prader–Willi and Angelman syndromes: disorders of genomic imprinting. Medicine (Baltimore) 1998; 77:140–151.

147. Nicholls RD, Saitoh S, Horsthemke B. Imprinting in Prader–Willi and Angelman syndromes. Trends Genet 1998; 14(5): 194–200.

148. Clayton-Smith J, Laan L. Angelman syndrome: a review of the clinical and genetic aspects. J Med Genet 2003; 40(2): 87–95.

149. Williams CA, Zori RT, Hendrickson J, Stalker H, Marum T, Whidden E, Driscoll DJ. Angelman syndrome. Curr Probl Pediatr 1995; 25:216–231.

150. Rougeulle C, Glatt H, Lalande M. The Angelman syndrome candidate gene, UBE3A/E6-AP, is imprinted in brain. Nat Genet 1997; 17(1):14–15.

151. Kishino T, Lalande M, Wagstaff J. Mutations cause Angelman syndrome UBE3A/E6-AP. Nat Genet 1997; 15(1): 70–73.

152. Vu TH, Hoffman AR. Imprinting of the Angelman syndrome gene, UBE3A, is restricted to brain. Nat Genet 1997; 17(1): 12–13.

153. Albrecht U, Sutcliffe JS, Cattanach BM, Beechey BV, Armstrong D, Eichele G, Beaudet AL. Imprinted expression of the murine Angelman syndrome gene, Ube3a, in hippocampal and Purkinje neurons. Nat Genet 1997; 17(1):75–78.

154. Nicholls RD, Knepper JL. Genome organization, function, and imprinting in Prader–Willi and Angelman syndromes. Annu Rev Genomics Hum Genet 2001; 2:153–175.

155. Buiting K, Lich C, Cottrell S, Barnicoat A, Horsthemke B. A 5-kb imprinting center deletion in a family with Angelman syndrome reduces the shortest region of deletion overlap to 880 bp. Hum Genet 1999; 105(6):665–666.

156. Jiang YH, Armstrong D, Albrecht U, Atkins CM, Noebels JL, Eichele G, Sweatt JD, Beaudet AL. Mutation of the Angelman ubiquitin ligase in mice causes increased cytoplasmic p53 and deficits of contextual learning and long-term potentiation. Neuron 1998; 21(4):799–811.

157. Miura K, Kishino T, Li E, Webber H, Dikkes P, Holmes GL, Wagstaff J. Neurobehavioral and electroencephalographic

abnormalities in Ube3a maternal-deficient mice. Neurobiol Dis 2002; 9(2):149–159.

158. Cassidy SB. Prader–Willi syndrome. J Med Genet 1997; 34: 917–923.

159. Ledbetter DH, Riccardi VM, Airhart SD, Strobel RJ, Keenen SB. Crawford JD. Deletions of chromosome 15 as a cause of the Prader–Willi syndrome. N Engl J Med 1981; 304:325–329.

160. Yang T, Adamson TE, Resnick JL, Leff S, Wevrick R, Francke U, Jenkins NA, Copeland NG, Brannan CI. A mouse model for Prader–Willi syndrome imprinting-centre mutations. Nat Genet 1998; 19(1):25–31.

161. Gabriel JM, Merchant M, Ohta T, Ji Y, Caldwell RG, Ramsey MJ, Tucker JD, Longnecker R, Nicholls RD. A transgene insertion creating a heritable chromosome deletion mouse model of Prader–Willi and Angelman syndromes. Proc Natl Acad Sci USA 1999; 96(16):9258–9563.

162. Muscatelli F, Abrous DN, Massacrier A, Boccaccio I, Le Moal M, Cau P, Cremer H. Disruption of the mouse necdin gene results in hypothalamic and behavioral alterations reminiscent of the human Prader–Willi syndrome. Hum Mol Genet 2000; 9(20):3101–3110.

163. Keverne EB, Fundele R, Narasimha M, Barton SC, Surani MA. Genomic imprinting and the differential roles of parental genomes in brain development. Brain Res Dev Brain Res 1996; 92(1):91–100.

164. Huppke P, Held M, Laccone F, Hanefeld F. The spectrum of phenotypes in females with Rett syndrome. Brain Dev 2003; 25(5):346–351.

165. Dunn HG, MacLeod PM. Rett syndrome: review of biological abnormalities. Can J Neurol Sci 2001; 28(1):16–29.

166. Takagi N. The role of X-chromosome inactivation in the manifestation of Rett syndrome. Brain Dev 2001; 23(suppl 1):S182–S185.

167. Moog U, Smeets EE, van Roozendaal KE, Schoenmakers S, Herbergs J, Schoonbrood-Lenssen AM, Schrander-Stumpel CT. Neurodevelopmental disorders in males related to the

gene causing Rett syndrome in females (MECP2). Eur J Paediatr Neurol 2003; 7(1):5–12.

168. Johnston MV, Jeon OH, Pevsner J, Blue ME, Naidu S. Neurobiology of Rett syndrome: a genetic disorder of synapse development. Brain Dev 2001; 23(suppl 1):S206–S213.

169. Percy AK. Rett syndrome. Current status and new vistas. Neurol Clin 2002; 20(4):1125–1141.

170. Chen RZ, Akbarian S, Tudor M, Jaenisch R. Deficiency of methyl-CpG binding protein-2 in CNS neurons results in a Rett-like phenotype in mice. Nat Genet 2001; 27: 322–326.

171. Guy J, Hendrich B, Holmes M, Martin JE, Bird A. A mouse Mecp2-null mutation causes neurological symptoms that mimic Rett syndrome. Nat Genet 2001; 27(3):322–326.

172. Shahbazian M, Young J, Yuva-Paylor L, Spencer C, Antalffy B, Noebels J, Armstrong D, Paylor R, Zoghbi H. Mice with truncated MeCP2 recapitulate many Rett syndrome features and display hyperacetylation of histone H3. Neuron 2002; 35:243–254.

173. Tudor M, Akbarian S, Chen RZ, Jaenisch R. Transcriptional profiling of a mouse model for Rett syndrome reveals subtle transcriptional changes in the brain. Proc Natl Acad Sci USA 2002; 99(24):15536–15541.

174. Pieretti M, Zhang FP, Fu YH, Warren ST, Oostra BA, Caskey CT, Nelson DL. Absence of expression of the FMR-1 gene in fragile X syndrome. Cell 1991; 66(4):817–822.

175. O'Donnell WT, Warren ST. A decade of molecular studies of fragile X syndrome. Annu Rev Neurosci 2002; 25:315–338.

176. Verheij C, Bakker CE, de Graaff E, Keulemans J, Willemsen R, Verkerk AJ, Galjaard H, Reuser AJ, Hoogeveen AT, Oostra BA. Characterization and localization of the FMR-1 gene product associated with fragile X syndrome. Nature 1993; 363(6431):722–724.

177. Bardoni B, Mandel JL, Fisch GS. FMR1 gene and fragile X syndrome. Am J Med Genet 2000; 97(2):153–163.

178. Khandjian EW. Biology of the fragile X mental retardation protein, an RNA-binding protein. Biochem Cell Biol 1999; 77(4):331–342.

179. The Dutch–Belgian Fragile X Consortium. Fmr1 knockout mice: a model to study fragile X mental retardation. Cell 1994; 78:23–33.

180. Peier AM, McIlwain KL, Kenneson A, Warren ST, Paylor R, Nelson DL. (Over)correction of FMR1 deficiency with YAC transgenics: behavioral physical features. Hum Mol Genet 2000; 9:1145–1159.

181. Hinton VJ, Brown WT, Wisniewski K, Rudelli RD. Analysis of neocortex in three males with the fragile X syndrome. Am J Med Genet 1991; 41:289–294.

182. Rudelli RD, Brown WT, Wisniewski K, Jenkins EC, Laure-Kamionowska M, Connell F, Wisniewski HM. Adult fragile X syndrome. Clinico-neuropathologic findings. Acta Neuropathol 1985; 67:289–295.

183. Comery TA, Harris JB, Willems PJ, Oostra BA, Irwin SA, Weiler IJ, Greenough WT. Abnormal dendritic spines in fragile X knockout mice: maturation and pruning deficits. Proc Natl Acad Sci USA 1997; 94(10):5401–5404.

184. Nimchinsky EA, Oberlander AM, Svoboda K. Abnormal development of dendritic spines in FMR1 knock-out mice. J Neurosci 2001; 21:5139–5146.

185. Brown WT. The FRAXE Syndrome: is it time for routine screening? Am J Hum Genet 1996; 58(5):903

186. Knight SJ, Flannery AV, Hirst MC, Campbell L, Christodoulou Z, Phelps SR, Pointon J, Middleton-Price HR, Barnicoat A, Pembrey ME, et al. Trinucleotide repeat amplification and hypermethylation of a CpG island in FRAXE mental retardation. Cell 1993; 74(1):127–134.

187. Gu Y, McIlwain KL, Weeber EJ, Yamagata T, Xu B, Antalffy BA, Reyes C, Yuva-Paylor L, Armstrong D, Zoghbi H, Sweatt JD, Paylor R, Nelson DL. Impaired conditioned fear and enhanced long-term potentiation in Fmr2 knock-out mice. J Neurosci 2002; 22(7):2753–2763.

188. Kim JJ, Fanselow MS. Modality-specific retrograde amnesia of fear. Science 1992; 256(5057):675–677.

189. Phillips RG, LeDoux JE. Differential contribution of amygdala and hippocampus to cued and contextual fear conditioning. Behav Neurosci 1992; 106(2):274–285.

190. Wright TJ, Ricke DO, Denison K, Abmayr S, Cotter PD, Hirschhorn K, Keinanen M, McDonald-McGinn D, Somer M, Spinner N, Yang-Feng T, Zackai E, Altherr MR. A transcript map of the newly defined 165 kb Wolf–Hirschhorn syndrome critical region. Hum Mol Genet 1997; 6(2):317–324.

191. Naf D, Wilson LA, Bergstrom RA, Smith RS, Goodwin NC, Verkerk A, van Ommen GJ, Ackerman SL, Frankel WL, Schimenti JC. Mouse models for the Wolf–Hirschhorn deletion syndrome. Hum Mol Genet 2001; 10:91–98.

192. Wassif CA, Zhu P, Kratz L, Krakowiak PA, Battaile KP, Weight FF, Grinberg A, Steiner RD, Nwokoro NA, Kelley RI, Stewart RR, Porter FD. Biochemical, phenotypic and neurophysiological characterization of a genetic mouse model of RSH/Smith–Lemli–Opitz syndrome. Hum Mol Genet 2001; 10(6):555–564.

193. Thomas DG, Jacques SM, Flore LA, Feldman B, Evans MI, Qureshi F. Prenatal diagnosis of Smith–Magenis syndrome (del 17p11.2). Fetal Diagn Ther 2000; 15(6):335–337.

194. Walz K, Caratini-Rivera S, Bi W, Fonseca P, Mansouri DL, Lynch J, Vogel H, Noebels JL, Bradley A, Lupski JR. Modeling del(17)(p11.2p11.2) and dup(17)(p11.2p11.2) contiguous gene syndromes by chromosome engineering in mice: phenotypic consequences of gene dosage imbalance. Mol Cell Biol 2003; 23(10):3646–3655.

195. Tarantino LM, Bucan M. Dissection of behavior and psychiatric disorders using the mouse as a model. Hum Mol Genet 2000; 9(6):953–965.

196. Bucan M, Abel T. The mouse: genetics meets behaviour. Nat Rev Genet 2002; 3(2):114–123.

7

Medical Care of the Child with Down Syndrome

WILLIAM I. COHEN

Children's Hospital of Pittsburgh, University of
Pittsburgh School of Medicine, Pittsburgh,
Pennsylvania, U.S.A.

I. INTRODUCTION

Down syndrome (DS) remains the most commonly occurring genetic disorder causing intellectual disability (mental retardation). Despite the widespread availability and promotion of prenatal screening and diagnosis to detect fetuses with DS, the incidence remains steady and estimated at 1 per 800–1000 live births.

Fortunately, an extensive body of literature exists to support the primary care physician in caring for children with DS (1). The Medical Home initiative of the American Academy of

Pediatrics, first disseminated in 1992 and recently updated in July 2002, beseeches primary care physicians to provide children with special health care needs a single place where their comprehensive medical and developmental needs can be met (2). Nevertheless, families frequently report a lack of standardized approaches to the diagnosis of DS and failure to consistently receive comprehensive information about this condition at the time of initial diagnosis, and, later in the life of the child (3).

Several factors explain this dilemma. First of all, it is estimated that the average pediatric practice has 2.5/children per 1000 patients with DS, and these individuals are likely to be of various ages. (Some practices, it should be noted, may concentrate individuals with DS if they develop a reputation for compassionate and/or knowledgeable care). These numbers may not provide enough opportunities to keep the clinician up to date.

The physician factors, which affect the success of delivery of care to individuals with DS, include the physician's *attitudes* re: individuals with intellectual disability (mental retardation) and the need for specific *knowledge* about medical issues, developmental trajectory, educational interventions, and social and emotional needs.

This chapter will provide an overview of these issues to support the primary care physician in delivering optimal care. Patient satisfaction at the time of diagnosis is felt to be related to both the attitudes and the knowledge of the clinician, and therefore, we will begin with a discussion of these factors in order to effectively support the family, not only at the time of diagnosis, but throughout the lifespan.

II. ATTITUDES

In spite of the high degree of medical vulnerability of children with DS, it seems that both parents and physicians are affected by the fact that these children are expected to have an intellectual disability (mental retardation). In the past, children with correctable problems (such as cardiac and gastrointestinal malformations) were left untreated, leading to the untimely death of the child. (In 1982, the Baby Doe case, in which a child with such a problem was allowed to die, is only the most notorious example). Note that parents often colluded with physicians in these decisions, although the physicians doubtless had a powerful influence on shaping the outcome. Parents continue to report that they are told about institutionalization for children with DS, even though virtually all such facilities have closed. Many physicians were trained to believe that raising a child with a condition such as DS would damage the family, siblings, and marriage. Unfortunately, those ideas have not fully disappeared. The same attitudes are reflected in the suggestion that families consider placing their child for adoption. While this is an option for those parents who do not believe they can raise their child with DS (and there are parents looking to adopt these babies), most parents are offended when this suggestion is made.

Many families come to appreciate the potential for satisfying and productive lives for individuals with intellectual disabilities. This often develops in spite of the initial negative discussion with respect to DS at the time of the informing interview. This is more likely to occur when, during residency, the physician has not had an opportunity to care for children with DS of various ages and abilities. Even in the absence of negative or disparaging comments, families may sense the physician's pessimistic attitude by the tone of voice, failure to provide specific information, or in some instances, lack of contact after the news is given. And while it is understandable that physicians often feel guilty about having to give this news, the parents frequently report that they feel abandoned. This is often the case when the family and physician have not had an opportunity to establish a relationship. These attitudes may also inhibit physicians from taking advantage of the abundant material designed to address the needs of the child and family, starting from the time of diagnosis through adulthood.

The current generation of physicians, especially those pediatricians who have trained in academic medical center, have had a greater opportunity over the last 10–15 years to participate in specialized DS clinics or centers, where they can meet children with DS from birth to adolescence (and in some instances, through adulthood) and thereby come to appreciate first hand the medical issues and needs, as well as the abilities of individuals with DS and the commitment, capabilities, and knowledge of their families (15).

III. HISTORICAL KNOWLEDGE

In 1866, J. Langdon Down, working in Surrey, England, described a group of children in an institution for retarded children who had a characteristic facial appearance (flat profile, upslanting palpebral fissures, and brachycephaly) together with hypotonia and intellectual disability. Reflecting the racial theory of intelligence, these individuals were described as "Mongoloid idiots." It was not until 1959 that Jerome LeJeune and colleagues discovered that the presence of a third copy of chromosome 21 was the genetic basis for this disorder. This was the first step on a path that, thanks to the Human Genome Project, has led to our current knowledge of the approximately 225 genes on chromosome 21 that exist in triplicate and thereby providing opportunities to look for specific therapeutic interventions.

IV. GENETICS

Most individuals (95%) with the DS phenotype have a 47 chromosome count with an extra chromosome 21 referred to as trisomy 21 (Fig. 1). This is a result of nondisjunction during meiosis I, when the paired 21st chromosomes fail to separate. The extra chromosome number 21 is of maternal origin in 95% of DS subjects. The only substantiated factor associated with nondisjunction is advanced parental age, particularly maternal age.

About 3% of individuals with DS are found to have a chromosome translocation, in which the extra chromosome 21 is attached to either a chromosome number 13, 14, 15, 21, or 22 (Fig. 2). Although 50% of chromosome translocations occur *de novo*, the other 50% are inherited from a parent who is a balanced carrier (i.e., the parent has one of their chromosome 21's attached to another chromosome). This parent (mother

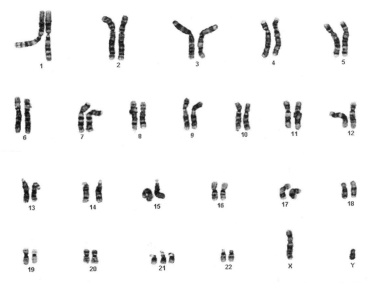

Figure 1 A 47,XY,+21 karyotype from a male with Down syndrome or trisomy 21.

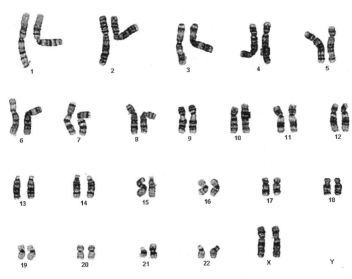

Figure 2 A 46,XX,der (21;21)(q10;q10),+21 karyotype in a female with Down syndrome due to an unbalanced translocation involving two chromosome 21s which appears as only one chromosome.

or father) can transmit the translocated chromosome to a subsequent child in an unbalanced fashion (and have another child with DS), or in a balanced fashion to the affected child's siblings, who would be at risk for having a child of their own with DS if the chromosome translocation is inherited in an unbalanced fashion. Table 1 shows the empiric recurrence risk for the parents depending on the chromosome translocation status and parent of origin. Consequently, it is necessary to obtain a karyotype of both parents of children with transloca- tion DS to determine the type of chromosome translocation, if present, which impacts on the recurrence risk.

The last genotype of DS to discuss is a mosaic form. This represents the smallest percentage of individuals with DS (about 2%) and is the one that is most confusing to predict outcome. Mosaicism represents the presence in the individual of two cell lines: one with an extra 21 and one with a normal 46 chromosome count. The effect on the individual of the mosaic cell lines varies with which tissues have been affected and the degree of mosaicism. In most instances, the tissues with "normal" cells began with the extra chromosome 21 or trisomy 21, but lost it during early development. In other cases, non- disjunction occurs in early development of the embryo. In either case, the time at which this occurs in embryogenesis determines the phenotype. Interestingly, medical problems of individuals with mosaic DS have been found to occur in the same frequency as in children with trisomy 21 (4). In addition, intellectual functioning is often similarly affected. Indeed, most of the ascertained cases of mosaic DS have the same physical and intellectual features as individuals with trisomy 21. We have seen children with a very low percentage of

Table 1 Empiric Risk for Unbalanced (Down Syndrome) Offspring from Balanced Chromosome Translocation Carriers

Translocation	Female Carrier (%)	Male Carrier (%)
14;21	10	2
21;22	10	5
21;21	100	100

mosaicism, who would not have been detected had not a karyotype been done for reasons other than ruling out DS. The confounding issue for clinicians is that DS, like all biological disorders, is a spectrum condition: there is a wide range of expression of the condition among individuals with trisomy 21. Parents frequently report that their primary care physician suggested that their baby had mosaic DS because muscle tone was close to normal, or because the facial features were subtle. This has not been found to be true.

V. PRENATAL SCREENING AND TESTING

Down syndrome was the first condition to be definitively diagnosed prenatally (via amniocentesis and culturing fetal cells). The recommended age for definitive prenatal diagnosis has been 35 years, reflecting the age at which the risk for fetal loss secondary to amniocentesis was equivalent to the risk of having a child with DS. In addition to amniocentesis, which is typically performed between 14 and 18 weeks gestation, chorionic villus sampling can be performed between 10 and 12 weeks gestation, although it has a higher risk of miscarriage than amniocentesis.

Serum screening protocols, using primarily maternal serum alpha-feto-protein (MSAFP) have been widely used. Maternal serum alpha-feto-protein is an excellent screen for neural tube defects, and a rather poor screen for DS. For this reason, human chorionic gonadotrophin and estradiol have been added (triple screen) and, in some centers, inhibin A (quad screen). More recently, the addition of ultrasound evaluation for nuchal translucency at 11–13 weeks appears to increase the sensitivity of serum screening. (Ultrasound evaluations alone are not recommended because of the high false negative rate.) Regarding serum screening, the 40% false negative rate causes as many problems as the 5–8% false positive. The false positives are distressing in the short run, but leads to more definitive testing which turns out to reveal a healthy fetus. Unfortunately, the false negatives cause parents to believe they have an unaffected child, only to discover their child has a condition that they had been lead to believe was ruled out. This reflects the frequent lapse of failing to distinguish between screening and definitive diagnostic testing.

VI. MAKING THE DIAGNOSIS IN THE NEWBORN PERIOD

Most physicians consider the diagnosis of DS in the newborn infant when they find a variety of physical characteristics in conjunction with low muscle tone (hypotonia). The facial appearance is often the first clue: flat profile, upslanted palpebral fissures, epicanthal folds, flat nasal bridge, small auricles (external ears), nuchal fat pad, and short head (brachycephaly) (Fig. 3). Many clinicians associate DS with one or two findings, such as a single palmar crease, even though this is found in only 50% of children with DS. Sometimes the absence of this finding has caused many physicians to doubt the clinical diagnosis.

In the newborn period, the common findings are listed in Table 2. It is important to confirm the diagnosis with a karyotype. This will, of course, necessitate a discussion of your concerns with the family, which is a challenging task. It is

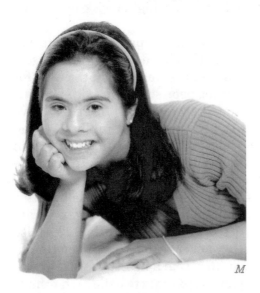

Figure 3 A photograph of an 18-year-old female with Down syndrome showing facial findings recognized in this condition.

Table 2 Common Diagnostic Findings for Down Syndrome in the Newborn Period

Features	Frequency
Flat nasal bridge	83%
Epicanthal folds	60%
Upslanting palpebral fissures	98%
Short head (brachycephaly)	75%
Loose skin on nape of neck	87%
Brushfield spots	75%
Single palmar crease	50–60%
Clinodactyly	51%
–curved fifth fingers unilaterally or bilaterally	
Gap between 1st and 2nd toes	96%
Low muscle tone	Majority of infants

possible to deliver this news sensitively and respectfully. Table 3 contains recommendations that can make this difficult task more manageable and tolerable for the family and the physician. If at all possible, speak to both parents together. In any event, if the mother is alone, make every effort to contact her husband, partner, or significant support

Table 3 Suggestions for the Informing Interview

Parents should be told:
  As soon as possible.
  By someone with sufficient knowledge to inspire credibility.
  With both parents present, if possible.
  With the baby present, if possible, and referred to by name.
  In a private, comfortable place, away from distractions.
  In a straightforward manner, using understandable language, with as much time needed for questions.
  With a balanced point of view, instead of list of problems.
  With a follow-up planned, and phone number to call for information.
  With additional information sources, including contact with other parents.
  With an opportunity to freely express all emotions,
  –Especially sadness, anger, guilt, and fear
  Followed by uninterrupted time for the parents and child to be alone together

Source: From Ref. 14.

person yourself, to tell that individual that you believe that the child may have DS and have ordered further investigations. (Although many pediatricians are confident in making this clinical diagnosis, a medical genetics consultation is always an appropriate step).

Families appreciate talking to other parents of children with DS, and you may be able to facilitate such parent-to-parent contact by identifying support groups in your area. Contact the local Association for Retarded Citizens (ARC) or check with an organization such as the National Down Syndrome Society (+1-800-221-4602) to learn if there is a local affiliate in your area. NDSS also provides information to new parents, and has a variety of educational resources available (Table 4).

VII. HEALTH CARE

Optimal health care for the child with DS includes the following components:

1. identification of congenital malformations;
2. adherence to standard well child protocols of the American Academy of Pediatrics or the American Academy of Family Practice;

Table 4   Resources for Parents

---

1. National Down Syndrome Society
    www.ndss.org
    Phone: +1-800-221-4602
2. National Down Syndrome Congress
    1370 Center Drive, Suite 102, Atlanta, GA, 30338
    www.ndsccenter.org
    Phone: +1-800-232-NDSC
3. ARC of the United States (Association for Retarded Citizens)
    To find a local chapter: http://www.thearc.org/chaptersearch/
    Phone: +1-301-565-3842
4. Down Syndrome Health Issues
    This site contains a wealth of information, including DS clinics, both
    nationally and internationally, links to DS growth charts and the
    Health Care Guidelines in both English and Spanish
    www.ds-health.com

---

3. recognition of the medical vulnerability of children and adults with DS to a variety of conditions which occur more frequently than in the population of typically developing individuals. It is possible to screen for these in order to minimize or prevent potential morbidity.

VIII.   CONGENITAL ABNORMALITIES

A.   Cardiovascular

Approximately 50% of children with DS have a congenital heart defect. The most commonly occurring condition is atrioventricular septal defect (AVSD) which is also known as endocardial cushion defect (see Table 5). In most of these conditions, the diagnosis of a serious disorder will be made by the presence of signs and symptoms, such as a murmur, cyanosis, or congestive heart failure. Children with DS are prone to develop high pulmonary vascular resistance. In children with AVSD, this would prevent the left to right intracardiac shunt, minimize the heart murmur, and prevent heart failure from occurring. This, in turn, has the potential to lead to significant pulmonary hypertension. The only way to detect this problem with a high degree of accuracy is to perform a cardiac evaluation, including an echocardiogram on every infant with DS. (Note that in some centers, asymptomatic children with DS may be able to get a screening echocardiogram).

Table 5   Frequency of Congenital Cardiovascular Malformations in Down Syndrome

Overall	*46–62%*
Atrioventricular septal defect	59%
Ventricular septal defect	19%
Atrial septal defect	9%
Tetralogy of fallot	6%
Patent ductus areterious	4%
Other	3%

B. Gastrointestinal

Gastrointestinal malformations occur in approximately 5% of children with DS (see Table 6). The most commonly occurring abnormality is duodenal atresia, which presents with vomiting and the inability to tolerate feedings in the first 12 hr of life. This diagnosis is frequently suspected prenatally via the ultrasound findings of a "double bubble" or in the presence of polyhydramnios. Hirschsprung disease is 25 times more likely to occur in individuals with DS than in the general population, and failure to pass meconium within the first 24 hr of life should raise the index of suspicion. New techniques in minimally invasive surgery have led to single stage repairs of such conditions as Hirschsprung disease and imperforate anus, avoiding the need for multiple procedures.

C. Cataracts

Dense congenital cataracts are an ophthalmologic emergency, because amblyopia can begin to develop within 7 days. In a recent retrospective study of cataracts in Metropolitan Atlanta, spanning 31 years, the incidence of cataracts was 2/10,000 children. Twenty-three of the 199 children had a syndrome diagnosis, and trisomy 21 was seen in 6 of the 23. This would translate to a rate of 0.6% of children with DS (5). The failure to detect a red reflex on ophthalmoscopic exam warrants immediate referral to a pediatric ophthalmologist for evaluation and surgical intervention, as indicated.

Table 6 Frequency of Gastrointestinal Malformations in Down Syndrome

Overall	*5%*
Duodenal stenosis/atresia	50%
Imperforate anus	20%
Hirschsprung disease	10%
Tracheoesophageal fistula	9%
Pyloric stenosis	6%
Malrotation	4%
Other	1%

D. Hearing Loss

In general, DS is associated with increased incidence of hearing loss, which may be conductive, sensorineural, or mixed. Roizen et al. (6) found that 66% of 47 unselected children had hearing loss. The loss was sensorineural in 16 ears, mixed in 14 ears, and conductive in 19 ears. This study led to the recommendation to objectively assess hearing in all children with DS by 6 months of age. While universal hearing screening has now superseded this recommendation, it is important to remember that DS is a disorder with a high risk for hearing loss.

E. Hypothyroidism

Congenital hypothyroidism has been reported to occur in as many as 3% of infants with DS depending on the series. This indicates the need for diligence in verifying the results of mandatory newborn screening and follow-up in the DS patient.

IX. MEDICAL VULNERABILITIES

In addition to the above abnormalities, which occur more frequently in the newborn with DS, individuals with DS in general are more likely to develop a variety of medical conditions over their lifetime, and the astute practitioner should be mindful of these conditions. The goal of this third component of health supervision is to prevent secondary disabilities, thus the need for disease specific health care guidelines. For example, children with DS have delayed acquisition of speech and language. The failure to recognize and treat significant hearing problems in these children can further hamper language development.

X. HEMATOLOGIC CONDITIONS

Polycythemia occurs in approximately 18% of newborns with DS and it may be necessary to check a complete blood count and hematocrit. If polycythemia is present, a partial exchange transfusion may be required. An unusual, severe, transient myelodysplastic syndrome is seen in children with DS. This disorder, also called transient leukemia or leukemoid reaction, is characterized by elevated peripheral leukocyte count and predominance of megakaryoblasts. In the majority of these cases, the condition resolves by 2–3 months without treatment. However, 20% of these children develop nonlymphocytic leukemia several years later.

Children with DS account for 2% of all leukemias. Most of the leukemias in children under 3 years of age are nonlymphocytic. After 3 years, only 20% are nonlymphocytic. Interestingly, the response to treatment of children with DS and acute myelocytic leukemia is better than expected and bone marrow transplantation has not been found to be necessary. However, the dose of chemotherapeutic agents, especially methotrexate, must be adjusted.

XI. ENDOCRINOLOGICAL DISORDERS

In addition to congenital hypothyroidism, 14–20% of individuals with DS develop hypothyroidism. Usually, this has an autoimmune origin. In addition, hyperthyroidism also occurs in this population, though less frequently. Juvenile diabetes mellitus has also been reported.

XII. IMMUNOLOGICAL/INFECTIOUS DISORDERS

As can be seen, autoimmune disorders are often seen in individuals with DS. In addition to hypo- and hyperthyroidism, and juvenile onset diabetes mellitus, there is an increased incidence in alopecia areata, celiac disease, and juvenile rheumatoid arthritis.

There are deficits in cellular and humoral immunity reported. Individuals with DS are likely to develop frequent otolaryngologic infections (nasopharyngitis/sinusitis and otitis), which are also based on the anatomic predisposition.

XIII. AUDIOLOGIC AND OTOLARYNGOLOGIC PROBLEMS

Individuals with DS are prone to conductive loss because of the anatomic abnormalities (eustachian tube position and dysfunction) which predispose them to recurrent otitis media, both acute and serous varieties (7). Stenotic external auditory canals may make otoscopy difficult, leading to the failure to detect serous otitis media (SOM). Vigorous assessment of hearing and diligent treatment of the conductive hearing loss associated with SOM via medical and surgical means can result in optimal hearing levels and minimize the impact on speech language development. Periodic hearing assessment is mandatory. The current recommendations suggest assessment every 6 months until 3 years, or whenever pure tone audiometry can be performed via headphones. Periodic screening is recommended yearly thereafter (7).

The midfacial hypoplasia, which provides the characteristic facial appearance of children with DS often, results in narrow airways and sinus ostia. As such, these children are frequently susceptible to chronic infections. Obstructive sleep apnea often occurs in the face of tonsillar and adenoidal tissue blocking the narrow airways. Hypotonia of the pharyngeal musculature and blockage of the hypopharynx by the tongue may also be contributing factors. Snoring and sleep apnea warrant an evaluation by an otolaryngologist and/or sleep center.

XIV. OPHTHALMOLOGIC DISORDERS

Nasolacrimal duct stenosis and nystagmus commonly occur in infants with DS. High-frequency low-amplitude nystagmus is usually benign. Detection of strabismus warrants referral in order to rule out those conditions that can lead to amlyopia. In general, there is a 50% incidence of refractive errors in children with DS. Children should be evaluated routinely by 6 months of age, and, in general, yearly thereafter.

XV. GASTROINTESTINAL DISORDERS

Gastroesophageal reflux is frequently encountered in children with DS, and can be particularly challenging for children with congenital heart disease being treated for congestive heart failure. Infants and children with DS frequently are constipated, and dietary management with fiber (fruit juices) or other osmotic agents (Karo Syrup, MiraLax) is usually sufficient. Intractable constipation will warrant an evaluation to rule out Hirschsprung disease. Celiac disease (gluten enteropathy) is reported to occur in between 7% and 16% of individuals with DS. Most individuals present with failure to thrive, diarrhea, and bloating, although some have constipation, while a few present solely with behavioral changes. Currently, it is recommended that children with DS get screened at 2 years of age by checking tissue transglutaminase antibody (as well as total IgA, to be certain the individual is not IgA deficient). Positive studies should then be followed up by duodenal biopsy, looking for characteristic villous atrophy. Treatment with gluten-free diet is the same as that used for typical individuals with this condition.

XVI. FEEDING ISSUES AND PHYSICAL GROWTH

Oral motor weaknesses in the newborn period may manifest itself by poor coordination of suck/swallow. This may make nursing a challenge, but with appropriate support, most infants with DS can be breast-fed. Towards the end of the first year, a group of children with DS have difficulty handling a variety of textures. Occupational therapists and/or speech language pathologists can assist in this area. Some children have sufficient difficulty to warrant a referral to a functional feeding team.

Individuals with DS are shorter than typically developing individuals. In general, they are microcephalic, although their heads are proportionate to the length/height. Children with DS have been shown to have a lower metabolic rate, which translates into an increased likelihood for their weight to plot at a higher percentile than height on typical growth charts. There are growth charts available for children with DS, and it is recommended they be used in conjunction with those for typical individuals (8). As is the case with typically developing individuals, body mass index (BMI) should be determined.

XVII. MUSCULOSKELETAL DISORDERS

Individuals with DS often have ligamentous laxity, which manifests itself in the unusual flexibility seen in these children. Interestingly, there is no increase in hip dislocation in infants, although adolescents may develop hip and knee problems.

The cervical spine has been an area of focus for some time. There are abnormalities found at the cervical/occipital junction, as well as the well-described atlanto-axial abnormalities at C_1 and C_2. There has been much concern that children with DS are at risk for spinal cord compression from excess movement of the transverse cervical ligament. This has led to the requirement that all children participating in Special Olympics need a radiological screening. Atlanto-axial instability is the term used to describe more than 5 mm of movement between the atlanto-dens interval when looking at the cervical spine in neutral, flexion, and extension. However, there is no compelling evidence that sports injuries have caused cord compression which is reported to occur in approximately 2% of individuals with DS. Most instances occur spontaneously, or in response to cervical manipulation. Measurement of the neural canal width provides a better indication of the possibility of cord compression (9).

XVIII. NEURODEVELOPMENTAL ISSUES

Unfortunately, DS does not protect a child from having attention deficit/hyperactivity disorder (ADHD), although some clinicians may misinterpret the child's activity level as normal for age. More problematic for families is the increased incidence of autism in children with DS (5–9%) as compared to the general population. As is the case with ADHD, diagnosis may be delayed, because of failure to recognize the defect in reciprocal social relationships, which is the core of this condition.

A. Alzheimer Disease

Many parents express fear of Alzheimer disease (AD) at the time of diagnosis of DS. While it is true that the gene for amyloid precursor protein seen in familial AD is on chromosome 21, much of the behavior change in the aging population of individuals with DS has been found to be related to other, treatable conditions, such as depression, hypothyroidism, and hearing loss (10).

B. Developmental and Educational Needs

All children with DS in the United States from birth to 3 years are eligible for federally funded developmental services which are known by a variety of names (e.g., early intervention, infant stimulation). These services are based on the child's developmental profile, and they often include physical, occupational, speech-language therapies, as well as developmental (cognitive) support. There is a well-described pattern of a relative weakness in expressive language skills when compared to cognitive and receptive language. This has led to the recommendation to teach sign language as part of a total communication approach to language. Note that learning sign language does not interfere with spoken language development.

When the child turns 3 years of age, local school districts become responsible for the child's education, under the mandate of IDEA, the federal Individuals with Disabilities Education Act. There has been much interest in educating children with both physical and cognitive disabilities along with their peers (inclusion). The value is seen as much from the positive modeling by the typical students as from the opportunities for the typical students to learn tolerance of individuals with disabilities.

XIX. COMPLEMENTARY AND ALTERNATIVE MEDICAL TREATMENTS

As is common for conditions associated with cognitive impairments, parents of children with DS, similar to those of children with autism, often search for treatments which offer hope of improving cognitive functioning, or, in the case of autism, decreasing the target symptoms. A variety of such treatments have been promoted for children with DS. Those involving nutritional supplements have been quite popular over the years. Physicians generally evaluate such treatments on the basis of plausibility of the theoretical basis (is there evidence, for instance, a vitamin or mineral deficiency) and the evidence of controlled trials, if available. Parents, on the other hand, usually make their decisions on an emotional basis, and consequently the decision to use these treatments represents the parents' hope for improvement in the face of a condition that seems to limit their child's future. Physicians are cautioned to respond to inquiries about these treatments in a way that respects the parents' hopefulness while at the same time being certain that the treatments are not harmful. Cooley describes this process with great sensitivity to the conflicts between the physician's biomedical model as it clashes with the family's fear of losing a potentially narrow window of opportunity to help their child. He offers respectful advice on how to continue the discussion without alienating the family and without putting the child at risk (11).

XX. HEALTH CARE GUIDELINES FOR INDIVIDUALS WITH DOWN SYNDROME

Health Care Guidelines for Individuals with DS provide a framework for screening from birth to adulthood. The 1999 revision closely matches the "Health Supervision for Down Syndrome" recommendations of the Committee on Genetics of the American Academy of Pediatrics (12,13). It is available on-line at http://www.denison.edu/dsq/. For example, in the newborn period, the recommendations include evaluation for congenital heart defects, hearing and vision problems, and referral to early intervention services (see Table 7 for a summary).

XXI. PRACTICAL SUGGESTIONS

The most commonly asked question by parents of children recently diagnosed is, "Can you tell me if this is a mild case?

Table 7 Summary of Health Care Guidelines for Down Syndrome from Birth to Adolescence

---

Birth
Cardiac evaluation (should include echocardiogram)
Objective hearing evaluation (auditory brainstem response test or
    evoked otoacoustic emissions test)
Ophthalmoscopic exam to detect dense congenital cataracts
Thyroid function testing (check state-mandated screening)
Refer for early intervention services
Discuss availability of family services support
Medical genetics consultation, as indicated, re: discussion of future
    risk in subsequent pregnancies

First year of life
Repeat hearing evaluation periodically (every 6 months) until pure
    tone audiograms can be performed. Then yearly
Eye examination by pediatric vision specialist by 6 months
Repeat thyroid function testing (TSH and Free T_4) at 6 and 12 months

Ages 1–12 years
Continue periodic hearing evaluations
Continue eye examinations
Yearly thyroid function testing
Screen for celiac disease (beginning at 2–3 years of age). Repeat
    every 2 years
Lateral cervical spine x-rays (flexion, neutral, and extension)
    between 3 and 5 years of age looking for atlanto-axial instability.
Measure neural canal width

Adolescence
Continue yearly thyroid function testing
Continue periodic vision and hearing assessment
Adolescent medicine consult re: sexual health concerns
Educational programming should focus on transition planning

---

or "How affected is my child?" It is impossible to answer that question with any degree of certainty in the newborn period, and still difficult to do when the child is 3 or 4 years of age. Physicians who are tempted to give an answer are likely to make an over- or under-estimation. On the other hand, pleading ignorance or the inability to accurately answer fails to acknowledge the parents' understandable fears and concerns about their child's well being. Many parents have appreciated this description:

"Your family is like a flower garden, and you know quite well what the flowers look like. The new plant in the garden is your baby, and we know that the flower that will grow on that plant will look like the other flowers in a number of ways. At the same time, we know that this flower will have some differences when it opens. It may be smaller, or have fewer petals. Perhaps the color will not exactly match the other flowers or the fragrance may be different. And we think that it will take longer for the flower to open. We are often impatient to see exactly what the flower will look like, and we do not like having to wait. We want to help assure that the flower is the most beautiful it can be. And that is why we put the plant in the best part of the garden, in that spot that has the right amount of sunlight, and shade, and moisture. We keep the plant healthy and free of anything that will weaken it. We give it the best nutrition, fertilizing it periodically. And after a while, we discover that we enjoy watching the flower open, at its own speed, discovery the magic of the unfolding. Sometimes, we find that we are able to be patient, appreciating the flower's unique beauty as it emerges."

This story seeks to capture the family's hopes for their child's future, and the wise physician discovers that he or she does not need to prognosticate since the process, as it unfolds, is self-revealing. What parents want and need is a trusted professional to walk with them down this path, without abandoning them to their worst fears and anxieties. Preserving hope and discovering possibilities are priceless gifts that are never forgotten (15).

REFERENCES

1. Cooley WC, Graham JM. Down syndrome—an update and review for the primary care physician. Clin Pediatr 1991; 30(4):233–253.

2. American Academy of Pediatrics "The Medical Home." Pediatrics 2002; 110(1):184–186.

3. Collins V, Williamson R. Providing services for families with a genetic condition: a contrast between cystic fibrosis and Down syndrome. Pediatrics. In press.

4. McClain A, Bodurtha J, Meyer J, Jackson-Cook C. Mosaic Down Syndrome. Richmond: Medical College of Virginia/ Virginia Commonwealth University, 1996:1–44.

5. Bhatti TR, Dott M, Yoon PW, Moore CA, Gambrell D, Rasmussen SA. Descriptive epidemiology of infantile cataracts in metropolitan Atlanta, GA, 1968–1998. Arch Pediatr Adol Med 2003; 157(4):341–347.

6. Roizen NJ, Walters C, Nicol T, Blondis T. Hearing loss in children with Down syndrome. J Pediatr 1993; 123(1):S9–S11.

7. Shott SR, Joseph A, Heithaus D. Hearing loss in children with Down syndrome. Int J Pediatr Otorhinolaryngol 2001; 61(3): 199–205.

8. Growth charts for children with Down syndrome. Available at: www.growthcharts.com. Accessed January 14, 2005.

9. Cohen WI. Atlanto-axial instability. What's next? Arch Pediatr Adolesc Medic 1998; 152(2):119–122

10. Chicoine B, McGuire D, Rubin S. Adults with Down syndrome: specialty clinic perspectives. In: Janicki MP, Dalton AJ, eds. Dementia, Aging, and Intellectual Disabilities: A Handbook. New York: Brunner/Mazel, 1998.

11. Cooley WC. Nonconventional therapies for Down syndrome: a review and framework for decision making. In: Cohen WI, Nadel L, Madnick ME, eds. Down Syndrome: Visions for the 21st Century. New York: Wiley–Liss, 2002.

12. WI Cohen, ed. Health Care Guidelines for individuals with Down syndrome—1999 revision. Down Syndrome Quarterly 1999; 4(1):1–19.

13. Committee on Genetics, American Academy of Pediatrics. Health supervision for children with Down syndrome. Pediatrics 2001; 107(2):442–449.

14. Holan JE, Cohen WI. Reflections on the informing process: why are these people angry with me? Down Syndrome Papers and Abstracts for Professionals 1992; 15(2):4–5

15. Skotko B. Mothers of children with Down syndrome reflect on their postnatal support. Pediatrics 2005; 115:64–77.

8

Fragile X and X-linked Mental Retardation

SEBASTIEN JACQUEMONT

M.I.N.D. Institute, UC Davis Medical
Center, Sacramento, California, U.S.A.

VINCENT DES PORTES

INSERM U129, Institut Cochin de
Génétique Moléculaire, Paris, France

RANDI HAGERMAN

Department of Pediatrics, University
of California, Davis; M.I.N.D. Institute,
UC Davis Medical Center,
Sacramento, California, U.S.A.

I. FRAGILE X SYNDROME

A. Introduction

The prevalence of X-linked mental retardation (XLMR) is approximately 1.8 males per 1000 (1). Approximately two-thirds of these patients have nonspecific (nonsyndromic) forms of XLMR in which the cognitive impairment is not associated with any recognizable physical features such as skeletal abnormalities or dysmorphic facial features.

The most common form of XLMR is fragile X syndrome (FXS), which is a syndromic form of XLMR. It has a prevalence of one in 4,000–6,000 males (2). In the past 5 years important progress was made in identifying nonspecific *XLMR* genes. However, routine genetic screening is not yet available for clinicians following patients with MR except for DNA testing for the FXS and high resolution cytogenetic testing.

The clinical syndrome delineated by Martin and Bell (3) led to the identification of the fragile site on the X chromosome (Xq27.3) for which the disorder was named. Geneticists subsequently used this syndrome in order to identify the fragile X mental retardation 1 gene (FMR1) and the CGG repeat expansion within the 5' untranslated region. Individuals with 55–200 repeats are carriers of the premutation and those with FXS have greater than 200 repeats (full mutation). The clinical and molecular research has revealed a broad spectrum of involvement in those with the full mutation. More recently, an effort to characterize patients with CGG repeats in the high premutation range has revealed that those patients present with a mild phenotype (4,5). Lower CGG expansions in the premutation range have also been associated with emotional symptoms and premature ovarian failure (POF) in women and recently to a new neurological syndrome in older males (6,7).

The mean age at diagnosis for the FXS is 35 months (8), however, Crawford et al. (9) reported that one-quarter to one-third of the children attending Atlanta public schools were not diagnosed before the age of 10 years. In the first year of life, delays are not usually detected but hypotonia, feeding problems, and vomiting are common. By 24 months, language delays are apparent followed by irritability and tantrums by age 3 years.

B. Physical Involvement in Males with Fragile X Syndrome

In males affected with the full mutation (with complete methylation), little or no FMR1 protein (FMRP) is produced.

The clinician can observe the classic association of facial and connective tissue anomalies, macroorchidism, cognitive delay, and behavioral anomalies (Fig. 1). The facial features include long wide and protruding ears in the prepubertal boy and later on a long face with a high arched palate and a prominent jaw in adolescents and adults. However, one-third of the boys with the FXS do not have any obvious dysmorphic features.

Macroorchidism is one of the most consistent findings (over 80% of the adult cases), but it is not usually seen in young children. By the age of 14 years old, 90% of the boys have testicular measurements above the 95th percentile (10). The endocrine function has been investigated in order to understand the mechanism underlying macroorchidism. Mild elevations of gonadotropin levels have been reported (11,12), suggesting a hypothalamo-pituitary dysfunction. A small subgroup of patients with FXS present with a Prader–Willi syndrome (PWS) phenotype including extreme obesity, short stature, small extremities, and hypogonadism (13–15). It is likely that this subgroup represents a more severe form of hypothalamic dysfunction. It is recommended to test for fragile X in patients presenting with obesity or other PWS features and developmental delay.

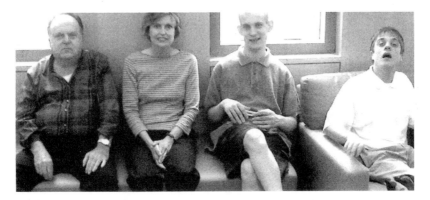

Figure 1 On the right are two brothers affected with FXS presenting with physical features such as prominent ears and slightly elongated face particularly in the brother identified second from the right. A carrier mother is second from the left, without physical features. Her father (on the left) has FXTAS.

The connective tissue anomalies include the orthopedic problems of flat feet and scoliosis. Joint laxity is also common, but joint dislocation occurs in only 3% (16). Mitral valve prolapse (MVP) is uncommon in childhood but is present in about one-half of the adult patients (17). This is another manifestation of the connective tissue dysplasia, but significant mitral regurgitation is rare. When a click or murmur is present during auscultation, an echocardiogram is recommended.

The growth in patients with FXS is often above the 50th percentile in prepubertal boys. However, adults tend to be shorter with as much as one-quarter of the patients below the 5th percentile (18). Studies indicate a mild increase in head circumference with 7% of the cases above the 97th percentile (19). Occasionally, children with FXS have been misdiagnosed with Sotos syndrome or cerebral gigantism.

Seizures occur in approximately 23% of the cases (20). They are generally complex partial and generalized tonic-clonic seizures. The EEG studies have shown certain recurrent patterns including temporal or central spikes typical of benign rolandic epilepsy. Seizures are usually well controlled with anticonvulsants such as carbamazepine or valproic acid and do not usually persist into adulthood (21). Neuroimaging studies have reported volumetric anomalies such as asymmetrical ventriculomegaly (40% of the cases) (22), hippocampal and caudate nucleus hypertrophy, and a small posterior vermis (23–25).

The physician must be vigilant about the high prevalence of otitis media in this patient population. Although this is certainly not specific of FXS, recurrent otitis media have been documented in 63% of boys with FXS as opposed to 38% in developmentally disabled children and 15% of age-matched controls (26). Recurrent otitis is associated with fluctuating conductive hearing loss which can be an additional factor leading to language delay and cognitive deficits. If there is a positive history of otitis media, it is imperative that the child be followed by an ENT physician to evaluate potential hearing loss and need for polyethylene (PE) tubes.

Schinzel and Largo (27), Maino et al. (28), and King et al. (29) described strabismus in 30–55% of males with FXS.

However, a more recent prospective study showed that 8% of a group of 48 males were diagnosed with strabismus and 17% with refractive errors (mainly hyperopia and astigmatism) (30). In order to prevent amblyopia, all children with FXS should be evaluated before 4 years of age by an ophthalmologist.

C. Behavioral Phenotype in Males with Fragile X Syndrome

The behavioral phenotype can be the most important clue leading to the diagnosis of FXS. The behavioral phenotype is marked by the association of four main features: hyperarousal, attention deficit hyperactivity disorder (ADHD), social anxiety, and autism.

Individuals with FXS are extrasensitive to sensory stimuli. These sensory difficulties have been studied using psychophysiological paradigms. Electrodermal reactivity (EDR) studies show that individuals with fragile X demonstrate an enhanced sweat response in a variety of stimuli including auditory, tactile, olfactory, and vestibular modalities (31). Heart rate studies also demonstrated that boys with FXS have a faster heart rate and a lower parasympathetic activity (32,33).

Hyperactivity is also a very prevalent symptom and has been documented in 70% of boys with FXS (16,34). In general, the hyperactivity improves in adolescence, however, the impulsiveness and poor attention span usually persist into adulthood.

Individuals with FXS display many of the clinical features found in patients diagnosed with autism including stereotypies (hand flapping), gaze avoidance, shyness, tactile defensiveness, and perseverative speech (35,36). However, only a subgroup (approximately 30%) of patients presents with the core social deficits required for the diagnosis of autism (37). This suggests that there may be additional genetic or environmental effects that predispose to autism (37,38). Clinically, patients with severe anxiety leading to social avoidance are more likely to meet DSM IV criteria for autism or pervasive developmental disorder, not otherwise specified (PDDNOS). Shyness and social anxiety are a consistent finding even in high functioning males who are not mentally retarded.

There is clinical overlap between FXS and Tourette syndrome such as tics, stereotypies, and obsessive–compulsive behaviors. Stereotypies and tics can be motor and vocal (coprolalia, repetitive burst of swearing) and are influenced and increased in stressful situations. Tics occur in approximately 20% of males with FXS (16).

As boys with FXS reach adolescence and adulthood, aggressive outbursts become a problem in approximately 50% of adult patients (16). The outburst is often triggered by excessive stimuli in the environment or anxiety secondary to misperception of social confrontation. These outbursts are also related to mood instability, which is addressed in the treatment section.

Other psychiatric symptoms such as psychosis have been inconsistently described in males. We have seen psychotic ideation in over 10% of males; however, the distinction between psychosis and fragile X behaviors such as self-talk, perseverations, extreme shyness, and odd mannerisms is difficult. Nevertheless, the clinician needs to recognize psychotic or disorganized thinking when it is present because antipsychotic medication can be helpful.

D. Neuropsychological Involvement in Males with Fragile X Syndrome

The cognitive function or IQ of males with FXS is correlated to the residual amount of FMRP produced by the affected allele (39,40). Adult males with a full mutation and little or no FMRP have a mean IQ of 41 whereas mosaic males have a mean IQ of 60. Partially unmethylated males with the highest FMRP levels have a mean IQ of 88 (41).

Although FXS is considered as a "nonprogressive disorder" (as opposed to a neurodegenerative disorder), several studies show consistent evidence of a decline in IQ of males in childhood through adolescent (42–44). Although the tiology of the IQ decline remains unknown, there is no evidence of neurodegeneration. Many studies of the neuropsychological profile of patients with FXS have attempted to delineate a specific pattern. There is evidence for specific deficits in short-term auditory memory, sequential motor planning, spatial skills, and arithmetic (42,45). Preliminary evidence suggests that males with FXS have specific deficits in certain areas of executive function, especially those requiring holding information or sequences on-line in working memory (42). Males with FXS also seem to have a distinct pattern of abilities including memory for meaningful information and preliminary evidence suggests that males with FXS can encode and use perceptual gestalt to improve performance on visuospatial tasks (42,45).

E. Physical and Behavioral Involvement in Females with Fragile X

Like many X-linked disorders in which females are heterozygous, clinical involvement in females is more discrete and can range from the classic presentation described in males to little or no symptoms. The degree of phenotypic involvement in females with the full mutation has been correlated to the X-inactivation ratio and to FMRP expression (40,46–48).

Females with FXS also suffer less behavioral difficulties than males. Shyness and social anxiety are the most prominent behavioral challenge in girls with FXS (49,50). This feature can lead in some severe cases to selective mutism in which the patient is mute in certain settings (46,51). Hyperactivity is less frequent in girls, while attention deficit and impulsivity can be a significant problem in approximately 30% of the females with the full mutation.

Females with a full mutation have mean IQs of 74.4–90.8 that fall in the low average range (46,47). However, a significant number of women with FXS are mentally retarded. Cronister et al. (52,53) reported a group of 43 females with FXS in which 23% had an IQ < 70. De Vries et al. (47) found that 70% of females with the full mutation have an IQ < 85 or lower. Of those with a normal IQ, most have executive function deficits (54). The IQ decline observed in males has been inconsistently reported in females. There seems to be certain specificities in the neuropsychological profile such as a relative strength in their verbal memory and pronounced weaknesses in executive functions (42).

II. PREMUTATION CARRIERS: COMPLEXITY OF AN EMERGING PHENOTYPE

The premutation allele was not initially associated to any particular phenotype. The first clinical feature confirmed by large studies was POF found in 16–21% of female carriers (55). More recently, we reported a distinctive form of clinical involvement in some older male carriers of the fragile X premutation (6,7,56–58). These carriers, in their 50s and older, develop progressive intention tremor and ataxia. These movement disorders are often accompanied by progressive cognitive and behavioral difficulties, including memory loss, anxiety, irritable or reclusive behavior, and executive function deficits. In some individuals, dementia develops. Additionally, patients may have features of Parkinsonism, peripheral neuropathy, lower limb proximal muscle weakness, and autonomic dysfunction (urinary/bowel incontinence and impotence). This disorder has been designated the fragile X-associated tremor/ataxia syndrome (FXTAS) (7) and its penetrance appears to be similar to POF for females, although the data are still preliminary. Brain MRIs of patients with FXTAS reveal approximately symmetric increases in T2-weighted signal intensity in the middle cerebellar peduncles (MCP) and adjacent cerebellar white matter (56). This unusual radiological finding, visible in the majority of published permutation carriers with FXTAS, is not seen in controls.

Genetic counseling is important in all patients and their families presenting with significant developmental delay, mental retardation (MR), or autism and FMR1 DNA testing for the FXS is essential. Once the diagnosis is confirmed, the family history should be reviewed carefully to identify potential, carriers, and other affected individuals. Siblings should systematically be tested, as early intervention is beneficial as discussed in the treatment section.

III. X-LINKED MENTAL RETARDATION (XLMR) NOT DUE TO FRAGILE X

During the last 5 years, fifteen new *XLMR* genes have been identified, and the pace of new gene discovery is dramatically increasing (Fig. 2). Nearly 100 genes are expected to be identified (59). These new *XLMR* genes led to the understanding of the etiology of some familial cases of MR. However, clinical diagnostic criteria associated with nonspecific *XLMR* genes are not available yet, especially for isolated MR, without distinctive somatic, metabolic, radiological, or neurological features. Inversely, syndromic *XLMR* genes are usually involved in well-defined clinical conditions characterized with recognizable clinical features. Only a few families share a

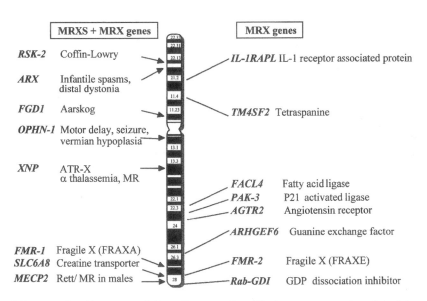

Figure 2 Genes and location on the X chromosome involved in syndromic (MRXS) and nonsyndromic XLMR (MRX).

mutation in each of the new nonspecific *XLMR* genes recently discovered, and little clinical data have been published. Genes associated with nonspecific MR can also be responsible for syndromic conditions, demonstrating a continuum between "syndromic" and "nonspecific" MR. Some of these clinical hallmarks will be detailed in this chapter. However, for some families affected with only MR, no striking clinical features are exhibited despite thorough clinical assessments.

IV. FROM NONSPECIFIC XLMR TO SYNDROMIC XLMR: A CONTINUUM

In order to illustrate the clinical diversity of the rapidly evolving XLMR field of research, syndromic *XLMR* genes will be described in this chapter. If needed, specific and updated information can be found on the international *XLMR* Genes Update Web Site (http://xlmr.interfree.it/home.htm).

A. *OPHN-1*: A Nonspecific *XLMR* Gene Involved in a Well-Defined Syndromic Condition

After the cloning of the fragile X (*FMR1* and *FMR2*) genes, *Oligophrenin-1* (*OPHN-1*) was the first new "MRX" gene to be identified in "nonspecific" MR (60). In order to identify specific clinical and radiological characteristics associated with the *OPHN-1* gene, affected subjects published by Billuart et al. (60) were revisited. Clinical and 3D brain MRI studies were performed in a female with an X;12-balanced translocations encompassing *OPHN-1*, and four affected males of family MRX 60 sharing a frameshift mutation in *OPHN-1*, leading to the description of a new distinctive phenotype (61). Clinical data shared by affected individuals were neonatal hypotonia with motor delay but no obvious ataxia in adults, marked strabismus, early onset complex partial seizures, and moderate to severe MR. Brain MRIs exhibited a specific vermian dysgenesis including an incomplete sulcation of the anterior and posterior vermis with the most prominent defect in lobules VI and VII. In addition, a nonspecific cerebral fronto-temporal atrophy was also observed with enlarged lateral ventricles. Concurrently, two independent groups published similar clinical and radiological features in three unrelated families (62,63). In Bergman et al. (62), myoclonic-astatic epilepsy, ataxia, and hypogenitalism were also observed. Philip et al. (63) also noticed in a large family macrocephaly in males and mildly affected obligate carriers. Interestingly, the partial vermian agenesis can be isolated (61) or associated with a large cisterna magna (63). This clinical presentation will be helpful for further targeted mutation screening of the *OPHN-1* gene.

B. Syndromic *XLMR* Genes Can Be Involved in Nonspecific Mental Retardation

In some cases syndromic *XLMR* genes were associated with nonsyndromic forms of XLMR. For instance, the gene RSK2 is usually mutated in the Coffin–Lowry syndrome, a condition with distinctive craniofacial and skeletal features (64). However, a missense mutation in exon 14 has been identified in a family with males presenting with nonspecific MR (65). Similarly, three brothers with nonsyndromic X-linked MR shared a mutation (P312L) in the *FGD1* gene (66), which is involved in the Aarskog syndrome (67). Although the brothers have short stature and small feet, they lack distinct craniofacial, skeletal, or genital findings suggestive of Aarskog syndrome. Inversely, their cognitive impairment (moderate to severe MR) is more severe than the cognitive deficit usually observed in Aarskog subjects.

In similar fashion, a missense mutation in the *XNP* gene, involved in alpha thalassemia/MR syndrome (ATR-X) (68), has been described in a family with borderline to moderate MR (69). This mutation has been found through a systematic mutation screening in nonspecific XLMR pedigrees. Only retrospective examination revealed childhood facial hypotonia and HbH inclusions in some of the affected males. Interestingly, a complete skewed X-inactivation was found in all carrier females in this family, which remains a consistent finding in XNP families. Authors have suggested that the

inactivation ratio may be used as screening criteria for XNP
in subjects with MR.

C. *ARX* and *MECP2*: Two *XLMR* Genes Involved in Both Syndromic and Nonspecific Mental Retardation

Two recently discovered *XLMR* genes have been shown to be
involved in several syndromic disorders and highly mutated
in nonspecific MR: the methyl-CpG-binding protein 2 (*MECP2*)
gene, and the Aristaless-related homeobox (*ARX*) gene. The
first gene, *MECP2*, is mutated in 80% of females affected with
Rett syndrome, a severe pervasive development disorder. In
addition, numerous mutations in males presenting with an
early onset encephalopathy or a mild mental deficiency have
been reported (70). As expected, missense mutations responsible for mild MR in males do not overlap with those involved in
Rett syndrome. Interestingly, a similar mutation in *MECP2*,
named "A140V", is involved in diverse syndromic disorders
including spastic paraplegia (71) and atypical schizophrenia
(72,73), and is also found in nonspecific MR (74). Another key
point about *MECP2* is a very high rate of polymorphism (75).
Therefore, cautious segregation studies within a family are
needed before suggesting the pathogenicity of the mutation
(69,76).

   The novel human *ARX* gene was recently identified as the
causative gene in X-linked infantile spasms (ISSX), severe lissencephaly with abnormal genitalia called XLAG (77), and in
some families with X-linked syndromic and nonsyndromic MR
(78). In addition, Frints et al. (79) found mild distal dystonia
after revisiting one of the latter nonspecific XLMR families.
Nevertheless, a thorough clinical examination performed in
some of these large families failed to exhibit any striking clinical feature despite a careful neurological assessment looking
for distal dystonia or epilepsy. For instance, a 35-year-old male
bearing a 24 bp duplication in exon 2 (the most common mutation in the *ARX* gene) was a very good drummer and recorded
two CDs and his affected brother worked as a skilled waiter in
a restaurant (des Portes, personal communication, 2003).

V. MANY *XLMR* GENES REMAIN WITHOUT RECOGNIZABLE PHENOTYPE

A. *XLMR* Genes Involved in Heterogeneous Clinical Presentations

In contrast to the *OPHN1* gene, the *Creatine transporter* (*SCL6A8/CT1*) gene illustrates the difficulty in defining a pattern of clinical features for a new syndrome diagnosed through a brain proton magnetic resonance spectroscopy revealing the absence of creatine signal (80). Loss of function of the Creatine transporter leads to motor delay and severe MR associated with epilepsy, dystonia, and autistic features (81,82). However, the clinical presentation is not specific enough to define practical guidelines for *SCL6A8/CT1* screening. In four families recently diagnosed, no specific clinical feature was described in addition to the MR and severe expressive language impairment (83). Moreover, some carrier females may exhibit a nonspecific mild cognitive impairment (82,83). Proton magnetic resonance spectroscopy remains the only reliable and sensitive way for the diagnosis of creatine deficiency syndromes, which include two autosomal-recessive disorders (GAMT and AGAT deficiencies) in addition to the X-linked Creatine transporter defect (84). Early diagnosis of these conditions can be helpful since GAMT and AGAT deficits are sensitive to exogenous creatine intake (84).

B. Nonspecific *XLMR* Genes Without Specific Clinical Features

At least eight nonspecific *XLMR* genes remain involved in "nonspecific" MR: *Rab-GDI* (85,86), *PAK3* (85,87,88) *AGTR2* (89), *TM4SF2* (90,91), FRAXE (*FMR2*) (92,93), *ARHGEF6/ αPIX* (94), and the *Fatty acid ligase* (*FACL4*) gene (95). It is still questionable whether MR is effectively the only hallmark in these families. Subtle consistent clinical features may be identified. It is worth noting that a complete skewed X-chromosome inactivation pattern is always observed in females carrying a mutation in the *ARHGEF6*, and the *FACL4* genes (94–96). For the latter disorder, a rapid enzymatic assay for screening MR patients could also be developed (96).

VI. CLINICAL INSIGHTS FOR MUTATION SCREENING IN NEW *XLMR* GENES: A PRACTICAL APPROACH

Genetic screening criteria remain unavailable, but several relevant clinical, imaging, and biological features have already been identified and may prove useful for the clinician: Hypotonia in infancy is usually associated with *OPHN-1* and *SLC6A8* (Creatine transporter) mutations. A short and transitory period of regression may be noticed in *MECP2* affected males. Mutations in most of the nonspecific *XLMR* genes lead to a moderate to severe MR in males, except for *MECP2* and FMR2, which are involved in mild MR. Psychiatric features may be prominent, such as atypical schizophrenia with *MECP2*. Autism has been described sporadically in many families and is not specific to any gene. Carrier females with a mutation in *RAB-GDI*, *FACL4*, or *SCL6A8* may show mild cognitive impairment. Neurological features are also helpful: spasticity has been described in patients with *MECP2* mutation; dystonia is observed in families with mutation in *ARX* and *SCL6A8*; infantile spasms, partial motor seizures, and undefined seizure may occur in children with a mutation in *ARX*, *OPHN-1*, and *SCL6A8*, respectively. Bilateral strabismus is a constant feature in *OPHN-1* patients. New imaging techniques are also powerful: (i) a striking vermian hypoplasia with cystic fossa magna or subtler partial agenesis may suggest *OPHN-1* mutations; (ii) creatine deficiency due to mutation in *SLC6A8* is exhibited on brain proton magnetic resonance spectroscopy. Finally, a complete skewed X-inactivation pattern in obligate carrier females is always associated with mutations in *ARHGEF6* and *FACL4*.

For the remaining core of "nonspecific" MR, it is likely that technological advances in mutation detection, such as HPLC or DNA chips, will allow implementation of large routine screening for dozens of genes. However, a wide molecular screening will never replace a good clinical assessment of the child and family, which remains the most powerful tool for an accurate and reliable approach to MR diagnosis.

VII. TREATMENT OF FRAGILE X AND X-LINKED MENTAL RETARDATION

There are no published controlled studies regarding treatment of XLMR with a few exceptions including FXS (35). However general information is available regarding behavioral interventions in those with MR and/or autism and medical treatment and follow-up are often applicable to those with a variety of forms of X-linked MR including FXS (61,97). Some of the highlights of treatment will be emphasized here.

A. Infants and Toddlers

A variety of medical problems occur in the first year of life and require medical intervention. Many infants with FXS or nonspecific *XLMR* present with hypotonia and motor delays either at birth or in the first year of life. A difficulty in organizing a suck is often the first clue and this may require motor therapy by either a feeding specialist, occupational, or physical therapist. Attention to normalizing vision and hearing problems in the first year is important for optimizing learning. Strabismus, which may be a problem for 8–30% of infants with FXS and for infants with an OPHN1 mutation, requires referral to the ophthalmologist within the first year. Recurrent otitis media occur in approximately 60% of children with FXS and it requires treatment with either prophylactic antibiotics or placement of PE tubes (97). Many young children with FXS may also have problems with gastrointestinal reflux and this can usually be treated with positioning and thickened feedings, although on occasion medications or surgery may be needed. There is a paucity of literature regarding infant early intervention protocols for any specific disorder, but stimulation of language, visual perception, play initiation, and social skills have been described for those with cognitive deficits and/or autism and should be utilized for FXS and nonspecific XLMR (98,99).

In FXS, there is a significant problem with hyperarousal to sensory stimuli leading to tactile defensiveness, particularly around the mouth and later social withdrawal and anxiety (31). In approximately 30% of those with FXS, autism is an additional clinical diagnosis (100), which may be related to the sensory integration problems and anxiety. These individuals would benefit from a structured discrete trials training program developed for autism intervention that has empirically demonstrated efficacy (98,99,101). The sensory hyperarousal problems in FXS can be treated by an occupational therapist with experience in sensory integration therapy (102). In the first year of life, this can include oral motor stimulation and desensitization. Work on oral motor mechanisms is also utilized in PROMPT therapy which has been shown to be helpful in children who have not developed language by 3 years of age related to oral motor dysphasia (103).

Seizures may be a problem for 20% of children with FXS. An EEG is required for the evaluation of any clinical signs of seizures including starring spells, repetitive movements not under voluntary control or unusual outbursts that do not have a precipitant. The documentation of spike wave discharges combined with a clinical history of seizures would lead to treatment with an anticonvulsant (104). In some cases, treatment with an anticonvulsant can lead to improvement in developmental domains such as language, particularly because the spike wave discharges can interfere with appropriate processing of information and coordination of responses in language and motor areas (105,106).

Psychotropic medications are typically not utilized in the toddler period; however, a few exceptions exist. Sleep disturbance after age 2 can be problematic for the child because it can cause sedation during the day when they should be learning from environmental stimulation and because sleep deprivation can cause behavioral problems including hyperactivity. In addition, sleep-deprived parents can be significantly stressed and seek treatment for their child. Behavioral routines to calm at bedtime include a hot bath and relaxing stories. If additional treatment is needed, melatonin can be helpful for approximately 60% of children with FXS and also for other causes of developmental disabilities (97,107,108). When the child is at least 3 years old, other sedating compounds such as diphenhydramine, clonidine, or guanfacine can be used although the later two medications should have an ECG in follow-up to identify any prolongation of cardiac conduction (97).

B. Parent Education

Genetic counseling is helpful in all X-linked MR syndromes. Explanation of the disorder, the genetics, and penetrance of the symptoms is essential for the family and their future reproductive decisions. For the trinucleotide repeat disorders, FXS and FRAXE, the genetics are more complicated and ongoing follow-up is often helpful (109).

Parents can make an important contribution to early intervention and treatment that has been empirically validated for infants and toddlers with MR (110,111). Training time should be spent with the parents to educate them regarding how to elicit, prompt, and shape the communication of their child on a daily basis. Teaching them the principles of responsivity to the child's interest areas, positive reinforcers for language, flexibility, and scaffolding and shaping responses can lead to multiple hours per day of parent-mediated therapy. Parents can also be taught how to structure discipline and behavioral interventions so that behavior can be molded and episodes of behavioral decomposition can be avoided (112).

C. School-Aged Interventions

By the time the child is 5 years old, problems such as ADHD, anxiety, episodic discontrol, mood instability, and aggression have typically declared themselves if they are going to be problematic for the child's development. Each of these problems can be treated by both therapy and medication and when the problems are severe a synergistic effect of both interventions is often utilized (97,102,112). These interventions have been utilized most consistently with FXS and have been described elsewhere (102,112), but controlled studies have not been carried out except regarding the use of medication as described below.

Stimulants have been studied in a controlled fashion in FXS and approximately two-thirds respond to them compared to placebo (113). Since stimulants are effective for a similar number of individuals with MR and ADHD or autism and ADHD (114), they should be utilized for the treatment of X-linked MR and ADHD. Although many previous studies have used short acting stimulants such as methylphenidate and dextroamphetamine, some of the newer long acting preparations such as Concerta®, Adderall XR®, and Ritalin LA® often help in avoiding withdrawal behavior, rebound, or mood swings related to fluctuating levels of medication. Other medications used to treat ADHD including atomoxetine, buproprion, and venlafaxine may also be helpful for mood and ADHD symptoms. Buproprion should be used cautiously in patients with a propensity for seizures.

Anxiety is a significant problem in FXS, and it is related to sensory hyperarousal. Medication intervention includes the use of selective serotonin reuptake inhibitors (SSRIs), although only survey information is available regarding efficacy (115). If a child also has autism, an SSRI, particularly fluoxetine may promote improvement in socialization and language and is worthy of a clinical trial (116,117). Open trials of fluoxetine in children with autism spectrum disorder have shown that the majority responds with improvements in language and socialization (116,117). Risperidone has also been documented to be efficacious in autism and behavioral problems including aggression (118). Patients with FXS were included in the Aman et al. (118) controlled trial but other forms of X-linked MR have not been studied. The atypical antipsychotics not only decrease aggression, but also have a positive effect in mood stabilization, which is often needed in those significantly affected by fragile X (97).

VIII. CONCLUSIONS

There are over 200 genes on the X chromosome associated with MR and FXS cause approximately 30% of all XLMR. FMR1 DNA testing should be routinely carried out in the evaluation of any child with MR. The mutations in several other genes are just beginning to be characterized and available for assessment clinically, such as *MECP2*, but the assessments are expensive and are not ordered unless phenotypic features are present suggesting the disorder. Recent research has demonstrated that many syndromic XLMR disorders can also cause nonsyndromic MR so routine screening for more causes of XLMR will hopefully be a reality in the future with advances in genetic diagnostic techniques.

ACKNOWLEDGMENTS

Grants form the French Foundation for Medical Research (FRM), and the Foundation "Jérôme Lejeune" supported Dr. des Portes. This work was also supported by the M.I.N.D. Institute (Dr. Jacquemont) and by NICHD grant # HD36071 (Dr. Hagerman). We thank Faraz Farzin for her expertise in the preparation of this manuscript.

REFERENCES

1. Herbst DS, Miller JR. Nonspecific X-linked mental retardation II: the frequency in British Columbia. Am J Med Genet 1980; 7(4):461–469.

2. Crawford DC, Acuna JM, Sherman SL. FMR1 and the fragile X syndrome: human genome epidemiology review. Genet Med 2001; 3(5):359–371.

3. Martin JP, Bell J. A pedigree of mental defect showing sex linkage. J Neur Psych 1943; 6:154–157.

4. Tassone F, Hagerman RJ, Taylor AK, Gane LW, Godfrey TE, Hagerman PJ. Elevated levels of *FMR1* mRNA in carrier

males: a new mechanism of involvement in fragile X syndrome. Am J Hum Genet 2000; 66:6–15.

5. Tassone F, Hagerman RJ, Taylor AK, Mills JB, Harris SW, Gane LW, Hagerman PJ. Clinical involvement and protein expression in individuals with the *FMR1* premutation. Am J Med Genet 2000; 91:144–152.

6. Hagerman RJ, Leehey M, Heinrichs W, Tassone F, Wilson R, Hills J, Grigsby J, Gage B, Hagerman PJ. Intention tremor, parkinsonism, and generalized brain atrophy in male carriers of fragile X. Neurology 2001; 57:127–130.

7. Jacquemont S, Hagerman RJ, Leehey M, Grigsby J, Zhang L, Brunberg JA, Greco C, des Portes V, Jardini T, Levine R, Berry-Kravis E, Brown WT, Schaeffer S, Kissel J, Tassone F, Hagerman PJ. Fragile X premutation tremor/ataxia syndrome: molecular, clinical and neuroimaging correlates. Am J Hum Genet 2003; 72:869–878.

8. Bailey DB, Skinner D, Hatton D, Roberts J. Family experiences and factors associated with the diagnosis of fragile X syndrome. J Dev Behav Pediatr 2000; 21(5):315–321.

9. Crawford DC, Meadows KL, Newman JL, Taft LF, Scott E, Leslie M, Shubek L, Holmgreen P, Yeargin-Allsopp M, Boyle C, Sherman SL. Prevalence of the fragile X syndrome in African–Americans. Am J Med Genet 2002; 110(3): 226–233.

10. Butler MG, Brunschwig A, Miller LK, Hagerman RJ. Standards for selected anthropometric measurements in males with the fragile X syndrome. Pediatr 1992; 89(6 Pt 1): 1059–1062.

11. Ruvalcaba RH, Myhre SA, Roosen-Runge EC, Beckwith JB. X-linked mental deficiency megalotestes syndrome. JAMA 1977; 238:1646–1650.

12. McDermott A, Walters R, Howell RT, Gardner A. Fragile X chromosome: clinical and cytogenetic studies on cases from seven families. J Med Genet 1983; 20(3):169–178.

13. de Vries BB, Fryns JP, Butler MG, Canziani F, Wesby-van Swaay E, van Hemel JO, Oostra BA, Halley DJJ, Niermeyer MF. Clinical and molecular studies in fragile X patients

with a Prader–Willi-like phenotype. J Med Genet 1993; 30: 761–766.

14. Schrander-Stumple C, Gerver WT, Meyer H, Engelen J, Mulder H, Fryns JP. Prader–Willi-like phenotype in fragile X syndrome. Clin Genet 1994; 45:175–180.

15. Fryns JP, Dereymaeker AM, Volcke P, Van den Berghe H. A peculiar subphenotype in the fra(X) syndrome: extreme obesity-short stature-stubby hands and feet-diffuse hyperpigmentation. Further evidence of disturbed hypothalamic function in the fra(X) syndrome? Clin Genet 1987; 32(6):388–392.

16. Hagerman RJ. The physical and behavioral phenotype. In: Hagerman RJ, Hagerman PJ, eds. Fragile X Syndrome: Diagnosis, Treatment, and Research. Baltimore: The Johns Hopkins University Press, 2002:3–110.

17. Loehr JP, Synhorst DP, Wolfe RR, Hagerman RJ. Aortic root dilatation and mitral valve prolapse in the fragile X syndrome. Am J Med Genet 1986; 23:189–194.

18. Loesch DZ, Huggins RM, Hoang NH. Growth in stature in fragile X families: a mixed longitudinal study. Am J Med Genet 1995; 58(3):249–256.

19. Sutherland GR, Hecht F. Fragile Sites on Human Chromosomes. New York: Oxford University Press, 1985.

20. Musumeci SA, Hagerman RJ, Ferri R, Bosco P, Dalla Bernardina K, Tassinari CA, DeSarro GB, Elia M. Epilepsy and EEG findings in males with fragile X syndrome. Epilepsia 1999; 40(8):1092–1099.

21. Wisniewski KE, Segan SM, Miezejeski CM, Sersen EA, Rudelli RD. The Fra(X) syndrome: neurological, electrophysiological and neuropathological abnormalities. Am J Med Genet 1991; 38(2–3):476–480.

22. Schapiro MB, Murphy DG, Hagerman RJ, Azari NP, Alexander GE, Miezejeski CM, Hinton VJ, Horwitz B, Haxby JV, Kumar A, White B, Grady CL. Adult fragile X syndrome: neuropsychology, brain anatomy, and metabolism. Am J Med Genet 1995; 60(6):480–493.

23. Mazzocco MMM, Freund LS, Baumgardner TL, Forman L, Reiss AL. The neurobehavioral and neuroanatomical effects

of the FMR1 full mutation: monozygotic twins dyscordant for fragile X syndrome. Neuropsychology 1995; 9:470–480.

24. Mostofsky SH, Mazzocco MMM, Aakalu G, Warsofsky IS, Denckla MB, Reiss AL. Decreased cerebellar posterior vermis size in fragile X syndrome. Am Acad Neurol 1998; 50:121–130.

25. Reiss AL, Aylward E, Freund LS, Joshi PK, Bryan RN. Neuroanatomy of fragile X syndrome: the posterior fossa. Ann Neurol 1991; 29(1):26–32.

26. Hagerman RJ, Altshul-Stark D, McBogg P. Recurrent otitis media in boys with the fragile X syndrome. Am J Dis Child 1987; 141:184–187.

27. Schinzel A, Largo RH. The fragile X syndrome (Martin–Bell syndrome). Clinical and cytogenetic findings in 16 prepubertal boys and in 4 of their 5 families. Helvetica Paediatr Acta 1985; 40(2–3):133–152.

28. Maino DM, Wesson M, Schlange D, Cibis G, Maino JH. Optometric findings in the fragile X syndrome. Optom Vis Sci 1991; 68(8):634–640.

29. King RA, Hagerman RJ, Houghton M. Ocular findings in fragile X syndrome. Develop Brain Dysfunct 1995; 8:223–229.

30. Hatton DD, Buckley EG, Lachiewicz A, Roberts J. Ocular status of young boys with fragile X syndrome: a prospective study. J Am Assoc Pediatr Ophthal Strabismus 1998; 2(5): 298–301.

31. Miller LJ, McIntosh DN, McGrath J, Shyu V, Lampe M, Taylor AK, Tassone F, Neitzel K, Stackhouse T, Hagerman RJ. Electrodermal responses to sensory stimuli in individuals with fragile X syndrome: a preliminary report. Am J Med Genet 1999; 83:268–279.

32. Roberts JE, Boccia ML, Bailey DB, Hatton D, Skinner M. Cardiovascular indices of physiological arousal in boys with fragile X syndrome. Develop Psychobiol 2001; 39(2): 107–123.

33. Roberts J, Mirrett P, Burchinal M. Receptive and expressive communication development of young males with fragile X syndrome. Am J Men Retard 2001; 106(3):216–230.

34. Baumgardner TL, Reiss AL, Freund LS, Abrams MT. Specification of the neurobehavioral phenotype in males with fragile X syndrome. Pediatr 1995; 95(5):744–752.

35. Hagerman RJ, Hagerman PJ. In: Hagerman RJ, Hagerman PJ, eds. Fragile X Syndrome: Diagnosis, Treatment and Research. 3rd ed. Baltimore: The Johns Hopkins University Press, 2002.

36. Turk J, Graham P. Fragile X syndrome, autism and autistic features. Autism 1997; 1(2):175–197.

37. Rogers SJ, Wehner EA, Hagerman RJ. The behavioral phenotype in fragile X: symptoms of autism in very young children with fragile X syndrome, idiopathic autism, and other developmental disorders. J Develop Behav Pediatr 2001; 22(6): 409–417.

38. Bailey DB Jr, Hatton DD, Skinner M, Mesibov GB. Autistic behavior, FMR1 protein, and developmental trajectories in young males with fragile X syndrome. J Autism Develop Disorders 2001; 31(2):165–174.

39. Kaufmann WE, Abrams MT, Chen W, Reiss AL. Genotype, molecular phenotype, and cognitive phenotype: correlations in fragile X syndrome. Am J Med Genet 1999; 83:286–295.

40. Tassone F, Hagerman RJ, Iklé DN, Dyer PN, Lampe M, Willemsen R, Oostra BA, Taylor AK. FMRP expression as a potential prognostic indicator in fragile X syndrome. Am J Med Genet 1999; 84(3):250–261.

41. Merenstein SA, Sobesky WE, Taylor AK, Riddle JE, Tran HX, Hagerman RJ. Molecular-clinical correlations in males with an expanded FMR1 mutation. Am J Med Genet 1996; 64(2): 388–394.

42. Bennetto L, Pennington BF. In: Hagerman RJ, Hagerman PJ, eds. Neuropsychology in Fragile X Syndrome: Deagnosis, Treatment, and Research. 3rd ed. Baltimore: Johns Hopkins University Press, 2002:206–248.

43. Hodapp RM, Dykens EM, Hagerman RJ, Schreiner R, Lachiewicz AM, Leckman JF. Developmental implications of changing trajectories of IQ in males with fragile X

syndrome. J Am Acad Child Adol Psych 1990; 29(2): 214–219.

44. Wright Talamante C, Cheema A, Riddle JE, Luckey DW, Taylor AK, Hagerman RJ. A controlled study of longitudinal IQ changes in females and males with fragile X syndrome. Am J Med Genet 1996; 64(2):350–355.

45. Cornish KM, Munir F, Cross G. Spatial cognition in males with fragile-X syndrome: evidence for a neuropsychological phenotype. Cortex 1999; 35(2):263–271.

46. Sobesky WE, Taylor AK, Pennington BF, Bennetto L, Porter D, Riddle J, Hagerman RJ. Molecular-clinical correlations in females with fragile X. Am J Med Genet 1996; 64(2):340–345.

47. de Vries BB, Wiegers AM, Smits AP, Mohkamsing S, Duivenvoorden HJ, Fryns JP, Curfs LM, Halley DJ, Oostra BA, van den Ouweland AM, Niermeijer MF. Mental status of females with an *FMR1* gene full mutation. Am J Med Genet 1996; 58(5):1025–1032.

48. Riddle JE, Cheema A, Sobesky WE, Gardner SC, Taylor AK, Pennington BF, Hagerman RJ. Phenotypic involvement in females with the *FMR1* gene mutation. Am J Men Retard 1998; 102(6):590–601.

49. Hagerman RJ, Jackson C, Amiri K, Silverman AC, O'Connor R, Sobesky W. Girls with fragile X syndrome: physical and neurocognitive status and outcome. Pediatr 1992; 89(3): 395–400.

50. Sobesky WE, Porter D, Pennington BF, Hagerman RJ. Dimensions of shyness in fragile X females. Devel Brain Dysfunc 1995; 8:280–292.

51. Hagerman RJ, Hills J, Scharfenaker S, Lewis H. Fragile X syndrome and selective mutism. Am J Med Genet 1999; 83: 313–317.

52. Cronister A, Hagerman RJ, Wittenberger M, Amiri K. Mental impairment in cytogenetically positive fragile X females. Am J Med Genet 1991; 38(2–3):503–504.

53. Cronister A, Schreiner R, Wittenberger M, Amiri K, Harris K, Hagerman RJ. Heterozygous fragile X female: historical,

physical, cognitive, and cytogenetic features. Am J Med Genet 1991; 38(2–3):269–274.

54. Mazzocco MM, Pennington BF, Hagerman RJ. The neurocognitive phenotype of female carriers of fragile X: additional evidence for specificity. J Develop Behav Pediatr 1993; 14(5):328–335.

55. Allingham-Hawkins DJ, Babul-Hirji R, Chitayat D, Holden JJA, Yang KT, Lee C, Hudson R, Nolin SL, Glicksman A, Jenkins EC, Brown WT, Howard-Peebles PN, Becchi C, Cummings E, Fallon L, Seitz S, Black SH, Vianna-Morgante AM, Costa SS, Otto PA, Mingroni-Netto RC, Murray A, Webb J, MacSwinney F, Dennis N, Jacobs PA, Syrrou M, Georgiou I, Patsalis PC, Giovannucci Uzielli ML, Guarducci S, Lapi E, Gecconi A, Ricci U, Ricotti G, Biondi C, Scarselli B, Vieri F. Fragile X premutation is a significant risk factor for premature ovarian failure: the international collaborative POF in fragile X study—preliminary data. Am J Med Genet 1999; 83:322–325.

56. Brunberg JA, Jacquemont S, Hagerman RJ, Berry-Kravis E, Grigsby J, Leehey M, Tassone F, Brown WT, Greco C, Hagerman PJ. Fragile X premutation carriers: characteristic MR imaging findings in adult males with progressive cerebellar and cognitive dysfunction. Am J Neuroradiol 2002; 23(10): 1757–1766.

57. Leehey MA, Munhoz RP, Lang AE, Brunberg JA, Grisby J, Greco C, Jacquemont S, Tassone F, Lozano AM, Hagerman PJ, Hagerman RJ. The fragile X premutation presenting as essential tremor. Arch Neurol 2003; 60:117–121.

58. Berry-Kravis E, Lewin F, Wuu J, Leehey M, Hagerman R, Hagerman P, Goetz CG. Tremor and ataxia in fragile X premutation carriers: blinded videotape study. Ann Neurol 2003; 53(5):616–623.

59. Chelly J, Mandel JL. Monogenic causes of X-linked mental retardation. Nat Rev Genet 2001; 2(9):669–680.

60. Billuart P, Bienvenu T, Ronce N, des Portes V, Vinet MC, Zemni R, Crollius HC, Carrie A, Fauchereau F, Cherry M, Briault S, Hamel B, Fryns JP, Beldjord C, Kahn A, Moraine C, Chelly J. Oligophrenin 1, a novel gene encoding a

rho-GAP protein involved in X-linked non-specific mental retardation. Nature 1998; 392:923–926.

61. des Portes V, Boddaert N, Sacco S, Briault S, Maincent K, Bahi N, Gomot M, Ronce N, Bursztyn J, Adamsbaum C, Zilbovicius M, Chelly J, Moraine C. Specific clinical and brain MRI features in mentally retarded patients with mutations in the *Oligonephrenin-1* gene. Am J Med Genet 2004; 124(4):364–371.

62. Bergman C, Zerres K, Senderek J, Rudnik-Schoneborn S, Eggermann T, Hausler M, Mull M, Ramaekers VT. Oligophrenin 1 (OPHN1) gene mutation causes syndromic X-linked mental retardation with epilepsy, rostral entricular enlargement and cerebellar hypoplasia. Brain 2003; 126:1537–1544.

63. Philip N, Chabrol B, Lossi AM, Cardoso C, Guerrini R, Dobyns WB, Raybaud C, Villard L. Mutations in the oligonephrin-1 gene (OPHN1) cause X-linked congenital cerebellar hypoplasia. J Med Genet 2003; 40(6):441–446.

64. Trivier E, De Cesare D, Jacuot S, Pannetier S, Zachai E, Young I, Mandel JL, Sassone-Corsi P, Hanauer A. Mutations in the kinase Rsk-2 associated with Coffin–Lowry syndrome. Nature 1996; 384:567–570.

65. Merienne K, Jaquot S, Pannetier S, Zeniou M, Bankier A, Gecz J, Mandell JL, Mulley J, Sassone-Corsi P, Hanauer A. A missense mutation in RPS6KA3 (RSK2) reponsible for non-specific mental retardation. Nat Genet 1999; 22(1): 13–14.

66. Lebel RR, May M, Pouls S, Lubs HA, Stevenson RE, Schwartz CE. Non-syndromic X-linked mental retardation associated with a missense mutation (P312L) in the FGD1 gene. Clin Genet 2002; 61(2):139–145.

67. Pasteris NG, Cadle A, Logie L, Porteous MEM, Schwatz CE, Stevenson RE, Glover TW, Wilroy RS, Gorski JL. Isolation and characterization of the faciogenital dysplasia (Aarskog–Scott syndrome) gene: a putative Rho/Rac guanine nucleotide exchange factor. Cell 1994; 79:669–678.

68. Gibbons R, Picketts DJ, Villard L, Higgs D. Mutations in a putative global transcriptional regulator cause X-linked

mental retardation with a-thalassemia (ATR-X syndrome). Cell 1995; 80:837–845.

69. Yntema HG, Kleefstra T, Oudakker AR, Romein T, de Vries BB, Nillesen W, Sistermans EA, Brunner HG, Hamel BC, van Bokhoven H. Low frequency of MECP2 mutations in mentally retarded males. Eur J Human Genet 2002; 10(8): 487–490.

70. Moog U, Smeets EE, van Roozendaal KE, Schoenmakers S, Herbergs J, Schoonbrood-Lenssen AM, Schrander-Stumpel CT. Neurodevelopmental disorders in males related to the gene causing Rett syndrome in females (MECP2). Eur J Pediatr Neurol 2003; 7(1):5–12.

71. Dotti MT, Orrico A, De Stefano N, Battisti C, Sicurelli F, Severi S, Lam CW, Galli L, Sorrentino V, Federico A. A Rett syndrome MECP2 mutation that causes mental retardation in men. Neurol 2002; 58(2):226–230.

72. Cohen D, Lazar G, Couvert P, des Portes V, Lippe D, Mazet P, Heron D. MECP2 mutation in a boy with language disorder and schizophrenia. Am J Psych 2002; 159:148–149.

73. Klauck SM, Lindsay S, Beyer KS, Splitt M, Burn J, Poustka A. A mutaiton hot spot for nonspecific X-linked mental retardation in the MECPR2 gene causes the PPM-X syndrome. Am J Hum Genet 2002; 70(4):1034–1037.

74. Couvert P, Bienvenu T, Aquaviva C, Poirier K, Moraine C, Gendrot C, Verloes A, Andrès C, Le Fevre AC, Souville I, Steffann J, des Portes V, Ropers HH, Yntema HG, Fryns JP, Briault S, Chelly J, Cherif B. *MECP2* gene is highly mutated in X-linked mental retardation. Hum Mol Genet 2001; 10(9):941–946.

75. Laccone F, Zoll B, Huppke P, Hanefeld F, Pepinski W, Trappe R. MECP2 gene nucleotide changes and their pathogenicity in males; proceed with caution. J Med Genet 2002; 39(8):586–588.

76. Moncla A, Jaquot S, Pannetier S, Zeniou M, Bankier A, Gecz J, Mandel JL, Mulley J, Sassone-Corsi P, Hanauer A. A missense mutation in RPS6KA3 (RSK2) responsible for non-specific mental retardation. Nat Genet 1999; 22(1):13–14.

77. Kitamura K, Yanazawa M, Sugiyama N, Miura H, Iizuka-Kogo A, Kusaka M, Omichi K, Suzuki R, Kato-Fukui Y, Kamiirisa K, Matsuo M, Kamijo S, Kasahara M, Yoshioka H, Ogata T, Fukuda T, Kondo I, Kato M, Dobyns WB, Yokoyama M, Morohashi K. Mutation of ARX causes abnormal development of forebrain and testes in mice and X-linked lissencephaly with abnormal genitalia in humans. Nat Genet 2002; 32(3): 359–369.

78. Stromme P, Mangelsdorf ME, Shaw MA, Lower KM, Lewis SM, Bruyere H, Lutcherath V, Gedeon AK, Wallace RH, Scheffer IE, Turner G, Partington M, Frints SG, Fryns JP, Sutherland GR, Mulley JC, Gecz J. Mutations in the human ortholog of Aristaless cause X-linked mental retardation and epilepsy. Nat Genet 2002; 30(4):441–445.

79. Frints SG, Froyen G, Marynen P, Willekens D, Legius E, Fryns JP. Re-evaluation of MRX36 family after discovery of an ARX gene mutation revelas mild neurological features of Partington syndrome. Am J Med Genet 2002; 112(4): 427–428.

80. Salomons GS, can Dooren SJ, Verhoeven NM, Cecil KM, Ball WS, Degrauw TJ, Jakobs C. X-linked creatine-transporter gene (SLC6A8) defect: a new creatine-deficiency syndrome. Am J Hum Genet 2001; 68(6):1497–1500.

81. Cecil KM, Salomons GS, Ball WS Jr, Wong B, Chuck G, Verhoeven NM, Jakobs C, DeGrauw TJ. Irreversible brain creatine deficiency with elevated serum and urie creatine: a creatine transporter defect? Ann Neurol 2001; 49(3):401–404.

82. Hahn KA, Salomons GS, Tackels-Horne D, Wood TC, Taylor HA, Schroer RJ, Lubs HA, Jakobs C, Olson RL, Holden KR, Stevenson RE, Schwartz CE. X-linked mental retardation with seizures and carrier manifestations is caused by a mutation in the creatine-transporter gene (SLC6A8) located in Xq28. Am J Hum Genet 2002; 70(5):1349–1356.

83. deGrauw TJ, Salomons GS, Cecil KM, Chuck G, Newmeyer A, Schapiro MB, Jakobs C. Congenital creatine transporter deficiency. Neuropediatr 2002; 33(5):232–238.

84. Schulze A. Creatine deficiency syndromes. Mol Cell Biochem 2003; 244(1–2):143–150.

85. Bienvenu T, des Portes V, de Saint Martin A, McDonnell N, Billuart P, Carrie A, Vinet MC, Couvert P, Toniolo O, Ropers H, Moraine C, van Bokhoven H, Fryns JP, Kahn A, Beldjord C, Chelly J. Non-specific X-inked semidominant mental retardation by mutations in Rab GDP-dissociation inhibitor. Hum Mol Genet 1998; 7:1311–1315.

86. d'Adamo P, Menegon A, Lo Nigro C, Grasso M, Gulisano M, Tamanini F, Bienvenu T, Gedeon A, Oostra B, Wu-S K, Tandon A, Valtorta F, Balch W, Chelly J, Toniolo D. Mutations in GDI1 are responsible for X-linked non-specific mental retardation. Nature Genet 1998; 19(2):134–139.

87. Allen K, Gleeson J, Bagrodia S, Partington M, MacMillan J, Cerione R, Mulley J, Walsh C. PAK3 mutation in nonsyndromic X-linked mental retardation. Nat Genet 1998; 20(1): 25–30.

88. Bienvenu T, des Portes V, McDonell N, Carrie A, Zemni R, Couvert P, Ropers HH, Moraine C, van Bokhoven H, Fryns JP, Allen K, Walsh CA, Boue J, Kahn A, Chelly J, Beldjord C. A missense mutation in PAK-3, R67C, causes X-linked non-specific mental retardation. Am J Med Genet 2000; 93(4): 294–298.

89. Vervoort VS, Beachem MA, Edwards PS, Ladd S, Miller KE, de Mollerat X, Clarkson K, DuPont B, Schwartz CE, Stevenson RE, Boyd E, Srivastava AK. AGTR2 mutations in X-linked mental retardation. Science 2002; 296(5577): 2401–2403.

90. Zemni R, Bienvenu T, Vinet MC, Sefiani A, Carrie A, Billuart P, McDonell N, Couvert P, Francis F, Chafey P, Fauchereau F, Friocourt G, des POrtes V, Cardona A, Frints S, Meindl A, Brandau O, Ronce N, Moraine C, van Bokhoven H, Ropers H, Sudbrak R, Kahn A, Fryns JP, Beldjord C, Chelly J. A new gene involved in X-linked mental retardation identified by analysis of an X; 2 balanced translocation. Nat Genet 2000; 24(2):167–170.

91. Carrie A, Jun L, Bienvenu T, Vinet MC, McDonell N, Couvert P, Zemni R, Cardona A, Van Buggenhout G, Frints S, Hamel B, Moraine C, Ropers HH, Strom T, Howell GR, Whittaker A, Ross MT, Kahn A, Fryns JP, Beldord C, Maynen P, Chelly J. A new member of the IL-1 receptor family highly expressed in

hippocampus and involved in X-linked mental retardation. Nat Genet 1999; 23(1):25–31.

92. Knight SJ, Flannery AV, Hirst MC, Campbell L, Christodoulou Z, Phelps SR, Pointon J, Middleton Price HR, Barnicoat A, Pembrey ME. Trinucleotide repeat amplification and hypermethylation of a CpG island in FRAXE mental retardation. Cell 1993; 74(1):127–134.

93. Gecz J. The FMR2 gene, FRAXE and non-specific X-linked mental retardation: clinical and molecular aspects. Ann Hum Genet 2000; 64(pt 2):95–106.

94. Kutsche K, Yntema H, Brandt A, Jantke I, Nothwang HG, Orthu U, Boavida MG, David D, Chelly J, Fryns JP, Moraine C, Ropers HH, Hamel BC, van Bokhoven H, Gal A. Mutations in ARHGEF6, encoding a guanine nucleotide exchange factor for RHo GTPases, in patients with X-linked metal retardation. Nat Genet 2000; 26(2):247–250.

95. Meloni I, Muscettola M, Raynaud M, Longo I, Bruttini M, Moizard MP, Gomot M, Chelly J, des Portes V, Fryns JP, Ropers HH, Magi B, Bellan C, Volpi N, Yntema HG, Lewis SE, Schaffer JE, Renieri A. FACL4, encoding fatty acid-CoA ligase 4, is mutated in nonspecific X-linked mental retardation. Nat Genet 2002; 30(3):436–440.

96. Longo I, Frints SG, Fryns JP, Meloni I, Pescucci C, Ariani F, Borghgraef M, Raynaud M, Marynen P, Schwartz C, Renieri A, Froyen G. A third MRX family (MRX68) is the result of mutation in the long chain fatty acid-CoA ligase 4 (FACL4) gene: proposal of a rapid enzymatic assay for screening mentally retarded patients. J Med Genet 2003; 40(1):11–17.

97. Hagerman RJ. Medical follow-up and pharmacotherapy. In: Hagerman RJ, Hagerman PJ, eds. Fragile X Syndrome: Diagnosis, Treatment, and Research. 3rd ed. Baltimore: The Johns Hopkins University Press, 2002:287–338.

98. Schreibman L. Intensive behavioral/psychoeducational treatments for autism: research needs and future directions. J Autism Develop Disord 2000; 30:373–378.

99. Mastergeorge AM, Rogers SJ, Corbett BA, Solomon M. Non-medical interventions for autism spectrum disorders. In: Ozonoff S, Rogers SJ, Hendren RL, eds. Autism Spectrum

Disorders: A Research Review for Practitioners. Arlington: American Psychiatric Publishing, Inc, 2003.

100. Rogers S, Stackhouse T, Hepburn S, Wehner E. Imitation performance in toddlers with autism and those with other developmental disorders. Poster presented at: The Developmental Psycholobiology Research Group, Estes Park, Colorado, May 15–17, 2002.

101. Lovaas OI. Behavioral treatment and normal educational and intellectual functioning in young autistic children. J Consult Clin Psych 1987; 55(1):3–9.

102. Scharfenaker S, O'Connor R, Stackhouse T, Noble L. An integrated approach to intervention. In: Hagerman RJ, Hagerman PJ,eds. Fragile X Syndrome: Diagnosis, Treatment, and Research. 3rd ed. Baltimore: The Johns Hopkins University Press, 2002:363–427.

103. Square-Storer P, Hayden D. Prompt treatment. In: Square-Storer P, ed. Acquired Apraxia of Speech in Aphasic Adults. New York: Taylor and Francis, 1987:190–219.

104. Tharp BR. Contributions of neurology. In: Ozonoff S, Rogers SJ, Hendren RL, eds. Autism Spectrum Disorders: A Research Review for Practitioners. Arlington: American Psychiatric Publication Inc, 2003:111–133.

105. Uvebrant P, Bauziene R. Intractable epilepsy in children. The efficacy of lamotrigine treatment, including non-seizure-related benefits. Neuropediatrics 1994; 25(6):284–289.

106. Di Martino A, Tuchman RF. Antiepileptic drugs: affective use in autism spectrum disorders. Pediatr Neurol 2001; 25:199–207.

107. Acalman S, Jacquemont S, Goodlin-Jones B. Melatonin and sleep problems in children with autism and fragile X. Paper presented at: The International Meeting for Autism Research (IMFAR), Orlando, FL, 2002.

108. Jan JE, Espezel H, Appleton RE. The treatment of sleep disorders with melatonin. Dev Med Child Neurol 1994; 36(2):97–107.

109. Gane L, Cronister A. Genetic counseling. In: Hagerman RJ, Hagerman PJ, eds. The Fragile X Syndrome: Diagnosis, Treatment, and Research. Baltimore: Johns Hopkins University Press, 2002:251–286.

110. Yoder PJ, Warren SF. Intentional communication elicits language-facilitating maternal responses in dyads with children who have developmental disabilities. Am J Ment Retard 2001; 106(4):327–335.

111. Yoder PJ, Warren SF. Effects of prelinguistic milieu teaching and parent responsivity education on dyads involving children with intellectual disabilities. J Speech Lang Hear Res 2002; 45(6):1158–1174.

112. Hills-Epstein J, Riley K, Sobesky W. The treatment of emotional and behavioral problems. In: Hagerman RJ, Hagerman PJ, ed. Fragile X Syndrome: Diagnosis, Treatment, and Research. 3rd ed. Baltimore: Johns Hopkins University Press, 2002:39–362.

113. Hagerman RJ, Murphy MA, Wittenberger MD. A controlled trial of stimulant medication in children with the fragile X syndrome. Am J Med Genet 1988; 30(1–2):377–392.

114. Handen BL, Johnson CR, Lubetsky M. Efficacy of methylphenidate among children with autism and symptoms of attention-deficit hyperactivity disorder. J Autism Dev Disord 2000; 30(3):245–255.

115. Hagerman RJ, Riddle JE, Roberts LS, Brease K, Fulton M. A survey of the efficacy of clonidine in fragile X syndrome. Dev Brain Dysfunct 1995; 8:336–344.

116. DeLong GR, Teague LA, McSwain Kamran M. Effects of fluoxetine treatment in young children with idiopathic autism [see comments]. Dev Med Child Neurol 1998; 40(8):551–62.

117. DeLong GR, Ritch CR, Burch S. Fluoxetine response in children with autistic spectrum disorders: correlation with familial major affective disorder and intellectual achievement. Dev Med Child Neurol 2002; 44(10):652–659.

118. Aman MG, De Smedt G, Derivan A, Lyons B, Findling RL, Hagerman RJ, Handen B, Hellings J, Lesem M, Pahl J, Pearson D, Rieser M, Singh N, Swanson J. Double-blind, placebo-controlled study of risperidone for the treatment of disruptive behaviors in children with subaverage intelligence. Am J Psych 2002; 159(8):1337–1346.

9

Prader–Willi Syndrome: An Example of Genomic Imprinting

MERLIN G. BUTLER

Section of Medical Genetics and Molecular
Medicine, Children's Mercy Hospitals and
Clinics, University of Missouri–Kansas City
School of Medicine, Kansas City
Missouri, U.S.A.

I. BACKGROUND AND HISTORICAL OVERVIEW

Prader–Willi syndrome (PWS) is a complex disorder with cardinal features of infantile hypotonia (94% of subjects), mental deficiency (average IQ of 65, range 20–90; 97%), hypogonadism (95%), early onset of childhood obesity (94%), small hands and feet (83%), short stature (76%), and a characteristic facial appearance (e.g., narrow bifrontal diameter, almond-shaped eyes, and a triangular mouth) (1). Prader–Willi syndrome is the most common genetic cause of marked obesity in humans (1). It is estimated that there are 350,000–400,000 people with this syndrome worldwide with more than 4000 persons with PWS known to the Prader–Willi Syndrome Association (U.S.A.) out of an approximate 17,000–22,000 (2). Prader–Willi syndrome has an incidence of 1 in 8000–25,000 individuals (1,3). The population prevalence is estimated at 1–50,000 (4). Prader–Willi syndrome and Angelman syndrome, an entirely different clinical condition, were the first examples in humans of genomic imprinting. Genomic imprinting or the differential expression of genetic information depending on the parent of origin plays a significant role in other conditions including malignancies (5,6).

Prader–Willi syndrome is thought to be one of the most common disorders seen for genetic services but yet sufficiently uncommon such that most pediatricians may encounter only a few patients during their lifelong clinical practice. Over 1500 reports on PWS have been published in the medical literature. Patients with this syndrome do present to developmental and behavioral specialists for assessment and treatment of their behavioral and learning problems, beginning in the early childhood. Prader–Willi syndrome is present in all races and ethnic groups but reported disproportionately more in Caucasians (7). Most cases are sporadic; however, at least 20 families have been reported in the literature with more than one affected member. The chance for recurrence is generally low, i.e., <1% (8).

Features of PWS were first described in an adolescent female by Down (9) in 1887. In 1956, Prader et al. (10) later reported nine individuals with similar findings, which now bears their name. In 1981, Ledbetter et al. (11) first reported an interstitial deletion of the proximal long arm of chromosome 15 at region q11–q13 in the majority of subjects studied using high resolution chromosome analysis (Fig. 1). In 1983, Butler and Palmer (12) were the first to report that the origin of the chromosome 15 deletion was de novo in origin and donated from the father as determined by chromosome 15 polymorphism studies (12). This puzzling observation of finding only a paternal deletion in PWS subjects and the reporting of a maternal deletion in patients with Angelman

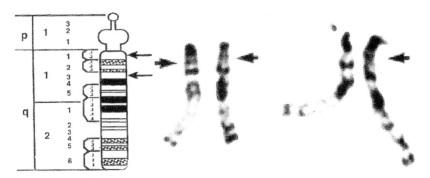

Figure 1 High resolution chromosome 15 ideogram on the (left) showing the pattern of bands and location of the breakpoints at 15q11 and 15q13 (arrows). A normal chromosome 15 pair (in the middle) with the 15q12 band designated by the arrows in each normal chromosome 15. The chromosome 15 pair (on the right) demonstrates the 15q11–q13 deletion from a PWS subject [deleted chromosome 15 on the left and normal chromosome 15 on the right (arrow shows the 15q12 band in the normal chromosome 15)].

syndrome was clarified by molecular genetic techniques in the late 1980s.

About 70% of PWS subjects are reported with a paternally derived de novo interstitial deletion of about 3–4 million DNA bases from the chromosome 15q11–q13 region. In addition, about 25% have maternal disomy of chromosome 15 (both 15s from the mother) and the remaining PWS subjects have either a mutation defect of the imprinting center controlling the activity or expression of selected genes in the 15q11–q13 region or translocations/other chromosome anomalies. In 1986, Butler et al. (13) reported clinical differences in those PWS subjects with or without the chromosome 15 deletion. Prader–Willi syndrome subjects with the deletion were more homogenous in their clinical presentation and were hypopigmented compared with their family members. This pigmentary change is due to loss of the P gene which is involved with skin pigment production and found in the 15q11–q13 region.

In 1989, molecular genetic methods and Southern hybridization of newly identified polymorphic DNA markers isolated from the 15q11–q13 chromosome region were reported by Nicholls et al. (14) in PWS individuals with normal appearing chromosomes and both chromosome 15s were from the mother. This phenomenon was termed maternal uniparental disomy 15 or UPD. Both members of the chromosome 15 pair were inherited from the mother as a result of nondisjunction or an error in the separation of the 15th chromosome pair in meiosis during egg production. One normal chromosome 15 was received from the father resulting in trisomy 15 (or three 15s) in the fetus. After fertilization, the father's chromosome 15 is lost in the fetal cells during early pregnancy. If the trisomic 15 condition would have continued, a spontaneous miscarriage would have resulted. The loss of the father's chromosome 15 in subsequent cells rescues the fetus. Chromosome abnormalities, specifically trisomy 15 and other trisomy and monosomy events, are common causes of spontaneous miscarriages. Approximately 50% of early miscarriages in the general population are due to chromosome problems.

II. GENETICS

Prader–Willi syndrome arises from loss of expression of paternally derived genes from the chromosome 15q11–q13 region. Nearly one dozen genes or transcripts have been mapped to the 15q11–q13 region and are paternally expressed (or maternally imprinted) including *SNURF–SNRPN, NDN, snoRNAs, MKRN3* (formerly called *ZNF127*), and *MAGEL2* (5). The location of genes and genetic markers on chromosome 15q11–q13 region is shown in Fig. 2. Candidate genes for PWS are imprinted (silenced on the maternally inherited chromosome 15), located within the 15q11–q13 region and are involved with brain function leading to the condition recognized as PWS. The best-characterized paternally expressed gene studied to date is *SNRPN* (small nuclear ribonucleoprotein N) (15) in which exons 4–10 encode a core spliceosomal and protein (SmN) involved with mRNA splicing in the brain. A second DNA sequence of *SNRPN* is termed *SNURF (SNRPN upstream reading frame)*. The promotor and first exon of

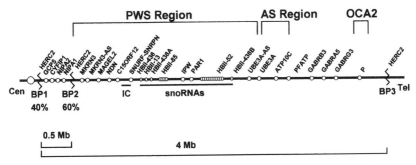

Figure 2 Illustration of the 15q11–q13 region showing the location and position of genes identified in the region. The PWS and AS regions and candidate genes involved with the two syndromes are designated. The P gene that causes oculocutaneous albinism type II (OCA2) is also shown. BP1, BP2, and BP3 represent common breakpoints (type I deletion results from a break at BP1 and BP3 in about 40% of PWS deletion subjects and type II deletion results from a break at BP2 and BP3 in about 60% of PWS deletion subjects). Type I deletion is about 4 Mb of DNA in size, whereas type II deletion is smaller at about 3.5 Mb in size.

SNURF–SNRPN are an integral part of the imprinting center or genetic locus that controls the regulation of imprinting or gene activity throughout the chromosome 15q11–q13 region (16). A disruption of this locus, as evidenced by small microdeletions generally found in PWS patients with imprinting mutations or in those with balanced chromosome 15 translocations having a classical PWS phenotype, will cause loss of function of paternally expressed genes in this chromosome region. Recent studies have shown that the *SNURF–SNRPN* gene is an exceedingly complex locus spanning over 450 kb of DNA with nearly 150 possible exons or segments of the gene undergoing alternative splicing (16,17). This locus also encodes novel small nucleolar RNAs (*snoRNAs*), prefixed as HBII, which do not code for proteins and found at the 3' end of the gene locus (17). How the two independent proteins from *SNURF–SNRPN* and the snoRNAs play a role in the causation of PWS or regulation of gene expression is unknown. The imprint signal generated by the imprinting center which is transmitted bidirectionally over 0.5–1 million DNA bases in either direction, and the impact on chromatin structure and spreading (or stopping) of the imprint is also not clearly understood.

Genomic imprinting appears important for growth in humans and other mammals. Many conditions are now thought to be due to imprinting (e.g., Beckwith–Weidemann, Silver–Russell syndromes) and present with either overgrowth or growth retardation (5,6). Many imprinted genes identified to date are involved with regulation of cell proliferation or differentiation and may play a role in tumorigenesis. Other imprinted genes are known to represent fetal growth factors. Maternal genes generally tend to suppress growth of the developing fetus, whereas paternal genes enhance growth. The competition for expression of maternal and paternal genes has evolved to control fetal growth, and fine tuning of expression of genes depends on the parent of origin and a complex balance of maternal and paternal genes. Hence, a disruption of the genetic balance results in growth anomalies in the fetus or found postnatally.

The *UBE3A* gene found in the 15q11–q13 region is maternally expressed (or paternally imprinted) and associated with Angelman syndrome (5,18). This syndrome is characterized by severe mental retardation, seizures, lack of speech, ataxia, and inappropriate laughter (8). Further description of Angelman syndrome will be presented in Chapter 10. Both *SNURF–SNRPN* and *UBE3A* are imprinted genes expressed in brain tissue and play a significant role in the causation of the phenotypic findings seen in PWS and Angelman syndrome, respectively.

Among other imprinted candidate genes for PWS is *NDN* (19) that encodes the MAGE family NECDIN protein and has received attention. In mice, the highest level for this gene expression is in the hypothalamus but is found in other regions of the brain particularly during late embryonic and early postnatal development (5). A second imprinted MAGE member is *MAGEL2* that is located adjacent to *NDN* in human and mouse but with the highest expression in the late developmental stages in the hypothalamus and other brain regions. These genes may play a role in neural differentiation and cell survival suggesting potential roles for several PWS features such as growth retardation, hypotonia, behavioral problems, appetite control, and abnormal genital development.

The chromosome 15q11–q13 region consists of about 4 million base pairs (Mb) of DNA including a large cluster of imprinted genes (2–3 Mb) that cause PWS and a nonimprinted domain (1–2 Mb). Novel DNA sequences have been identified with low copy repeats clustered at or near the two major proximal and distal 15q11–q13 chromosome breakpoint regions in individuals with PWS. Two breakpoint clusters (BP1 and BP2) have been reported at the proximal end of the 15q11–q13 region (20,21). The deletion occurring at the third breakpoint (BP3) occurs at the distal end of the 15q11–q13 region but on the telomere side of the P gene locus involved in hypopigmentation in nearly all PWS subjects with the typical deletion. The deletion (type I) that occurs at breakpoints BP1 and BP3 is about 4 Mb in size, whereas the second smaller deletion (type II) that occurs at breakpoints BP2 and BP3 is about 3.5 Mb in size. The source of the chromosome breaks may be attributed to repeated DNA sequences in these areas leading to genetic instability. These DNA sequence repeats are derived from a large duplication of a novel gene (*HERC2*) (22). Recently, clinical differences have been reported in PWS subjects with type I or type II deletions particularly in adaptive and maladaptive behavior (23) and will be discussed later.

Besides imprinted genes in the 15q11–q13 region, three gamma amino butyric acid receptor genes (*GABRB3, GABRA5,* and *GABRG3*) and the P gene for pigment production are located toward the telomere end of the 15q11–q13 region (5). The expression status of the GABA receptor genes has recently been studied with microarray technology and reported to have a paternal bias of expression (more expression from the paternal allele than from the maternal allele) that may impact on the phenotype (24). Mouse models for PWS, whereby the human chromosome equivalent (15q11–q13) located on mouse chromosome 7 is deleted, have also been produced and their phenotypes have also been described

(25). By studying the phenotype of these mice with equivalent genetic anomalies seen in humans, a better understanding of the role of specific genes causing PWS will be gained. In addition, studies with animal models (e.g., transgenic knockout mice) involving single genes, such as SNRPN, have shown that loss of a single specific candidate gene does not necessarily correlate with the PWS phenotype. Therefore, PWS is termed a contiguous gene syndrome with several genes involved.

There are five molecular genetic subclasses for PWS. Approximately 70% of subjects have a *de novo* paternally derived deletion from the proximal 15q11–q13 region, 25% have maternal disomy 15, and a third class of subjects (<3%) have very small microdeletions in the imprinted-controlling center termed imprinting mutations or defects. The smallest region of deletion overlap is reported to be 4 kb in size and localized in the imprinting center (26). Most deletions in PWS subjects are detected with fluorescence *in situ* hybridization (FISH) (Fig. 3) using 15q11–q13 DNA probes (e.g., *SNRPN*), whereas other subjects with atypical or small microdeletions or with maternal disomy 15 will require additional specialized testing using DNA microsatellites and sequencing (Fig. 4), but all will have abnormal DNA methylation testing (Fig. 5). A fourth class of subjects with features of PWS are those with a balanced reciprocal chromosome translocation involving the 15q11–q13 region, which disrupts a gene in the region. This rare class probably accounts for <0.1% of PWS subjects. The fifth class of PWS subjects is hypothesized to be those with structural gene mutations within the chromosome 15q11–q13 region. They have not been reported to date. Targeting unusual PWS subjects (those with imprinting mutations, reciprocal translocations, or possibly structural gene mutations of chromosome 15) may allow for a better understanding of the genetic impact on the clinical phenotype and identification and location of candidate genes that cause specific clinical features.

Genetic testing available for PWS includes the following: (**1**) Chromosome analysis to rule out translocations. (**2**) FISH with DNA probes from chromosome 15q11–q13 to detect

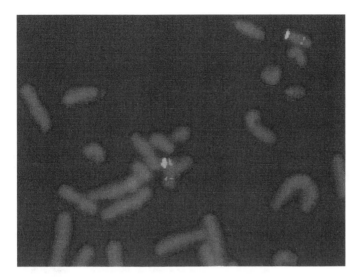

Figure 3 Fluorescence in situ hybridization using the *SNRPN* probe (red color) from the proximal 15q11–q13 region, a centromeric probe (green color) from chromosome 15, and a distal control probe (red color) from the distal end of the long arm of chromosome 15. The lack of the red *SNRPN* signal close to the centromere on the deleted chromosome 15 (shown at the top) is demonstrated from a PWS subject with the 15q11–q13 deletion. (*See color insert.*)

deletions. (**3**) DNA Methylation testing of the *SNURF–SNRPN* gene with polymerase chain reaction (PCR) to identify the male (unmethylated) and female (methylated) chromosome 15, which is 99% accurate for diagnosing PWS. However, it will not distinguish deletions from maternal disomy 15 or identify those PWS patients with chromosome 15 translocations. (**4**) Polymorphic DNA microsatellite analysis using PCR, which will confirm a paternal 15q11–q13 deletion in subjects with PWS or identify maternal disomy 15. A DNA sample from the patient and each parent will be required to identify the parental source of the chromosome 15 and determine the genetic finding (e.g., deletion or maternal disomy). (**5**) Gene expression studies for imprinted genes (e.g., paternally expressed *SNRPN* gene) from the 15q11–q13 region. The lack of paternally expressed genes will confirm the diagnosis of PWS but will

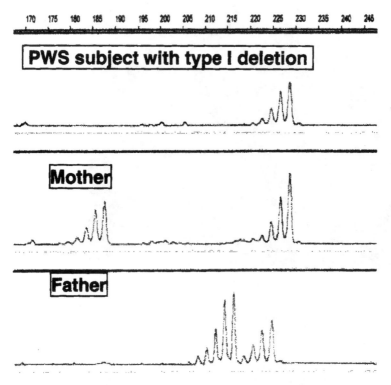

Figure 4 Microsatellite DNA pattern generated using an automated DNA sequencer for the 1035 locus isolated from the chromosome 15q11–q13 region from a PWS subject and parental DNA isolated from peripheral blood. Only one DNA signal is seen in the PWS subject that matches one of the mother's chromosome 15 signals. No DNA signal was seen from the father indicating a paternal deletion of the chromosome 15q11–q13 region consistent with the diagnosis of PWS.

not determine the genetic subtype (e.g., deletion or maternal disomy). (**6**) DNA replication patterns using specialized techniques showing variations in the parental source of the chromosome 15. Tests **1–3** are generally performed in subjects presenting with features of PWS and available in most genetic laboratories. Tests **4–6** are generally research based and available in only selected laboratories.

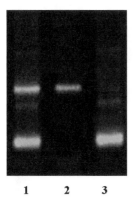

1   2   3

Figure 5 Representative methylation testing for chromosome 15 from DNA isolated from three individuals (normal, Prader–Willi Syndrome, Angelman syndrome) using the *SNPRN* probe and PCR. Two DNA bands (upper band from the mother's chromosome 15q11–q13 region and the lower band from the father's chromosome 15q11–q13) are seen in the normal individual (lane1), whereas an individual with PWS shows only the upper band from the mother (lane 2), and an individual with Angelman syndrome shows only the lower band from the father (lane 3).

III. CLINICAL DESCRIPTION

Many clinical features in PWS may be subtle or nonspecific, whereas other features are more characteristic. The primary features of PWS include infantile hypotonia, feeding difficulties, mental deficiency, hypogonadism, behavior problems (temper tantrums, stubbornness, obsessive–compulsive disorder), hyperphagia and early onset of childhood obesity, small hands and feet, endocrine disturbances including growth hormone deficiency, and a characteristic facial appearance (small upturned nose, narrow bifrontal diameter, dolichocephaly, downturned corners of the mouth, sticky saliva, almond-shaped eyes, and strabismus) (Fig. 6). Table 1 lists the clinical findings and time period when they occur.

Subtle physical characteristics may be recognized by only clinical geneticists trained in dysmorphology; however, a greater awareness by pediatricians, other physicians, and

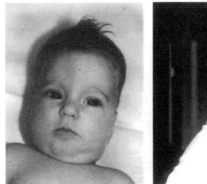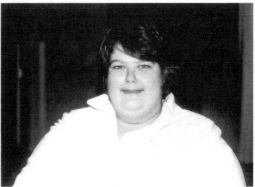

Figure 6 Frontal facial views of two subjects (6-month-old female and 23-year-old female) with PWS showing the typical facial features (short upturned nose, downturned corners of the mouth, narrow bifrontal diameter, almond-shaped eyes) and obesity in the older female.

health care providers now exists. Because of better recognition and awareness of PWS by the medical community during the past 10 years and of more accurate and reliable genetic testing, the diagnosis is made earlier than in the past and extensive diagnostic procedures are generally avoided. Many children with PWS were not diagnosed in the past until rapid weight gain was evident leading to obesity and until the presence of specific learning/behavioral problems. For example, the average age of diagnosis for patients with PWS was >6 years of age reported in the mid 1980s (13).

Prader–Willi syndrome can be divided into two distinct stages on the basis of clinical course and natural history. The first stage is characterized by neonatal hypotonia, a weak cry, hypogenitalism, and feeding difficulties, whereas the second stage, which usually occurs between 1 and 2 years of age, is characterized by psychomotor retardation, speech articulation problems, and early onset of childhood obesity (1–3). Food foraging and physical inactivity are found during this stage. The average onset for crawling, walking, and talking (>10 words) is 16, 28, and 39 months, respectively (13). Although 60% of individuals with PWS have IQs in the normal

Table 1 Clinical Findings in the Majority of Subjects with
Prader–Willi Syndrome and Time Period in which They Appear

Pregnancy and delivery	Neonatal and early infancy	Childhood	Adolescence and adulthood
Reduced fetal activity	Hypotonia	Almond-shaped eyes	Short stature
Breech delivery	Absent or poor suck	Strabismus	Lack of puberty
Pre-term or post-term delivery	Weak or febile cry	Myopia	Diabetes mellitus
	Temperature instability	Enamel hypoplasia (dental caries)	Depression
	Feeding problems	Hypopigmentation	Osteoporosis
	Cryptorchidism	Short stature	Scoliosis
	Hypogenitalism	Small hands and feet	Obesity complications
	Narrow frontal diameter	Onset of obesity	
	Thick, viscous saliva	Excessive appetite and eating	
	Developmental delay	Decreased intellectual functioning	
		Temper tantrums	
		Stubbornness	
		Obsessive–compulsive symptoms	
		Skin picking	

or borderline range, cognitive dysfunction is nearly always present.

Early in the second stage, infants and toddlers are usually easy going and affectionate, but in about 50% of PWS individuals, personality problems develop between 2 and 5 years of age. These problems include temper tantrums, depression, intolerance of changes in routine, obsessive compulsivity, and sudden acts of violence. These behavioral changes may be initiated by withholding of food particularly during adolescence and young adulthood. Poor peer interactions, immaturity, and inappropriate social behavior may also occur during this time. Other recognized findings seen in PWS individuals during the second stage include speech articulation problems, foraging for food, rumination, unmotivated sleepiness, physical inactivity, decreased pain sensitivity, skin picking, strabismus, prolonged periods of low body temperature, pale pigmentation, dental problems, and scoliosis.

Obesity is the most significant health problem in PWS and an increasingly common trait found in about one-half of the US adult population. It is on the rise in children. Obesity is a risk factor in 5 of the top 10 causes of death (heart disease, stroke, diabetes, atherosclerosis, and malignancies) in this country (27). Weight control and diet restrictions are constant key management issues in PWS. Because growth hormone deficiency is a common finding in PWS children, many of them are placed on growth hormone treatment which decreases obesity (fat mass), increases muscle mass and stature, and improves physical activity (28,29). Caloric restriction of 6–8 calories/cm of height beginning in early childhood should allow for weight loss, and 10–12 calories/cm of height may be required to maintain weight in PWS subjects. This caloric requirement to maintain weight is about 60% of normal. To be successful, a diet plan should include close consultation with a dietitian and an exercise program designed specifically for the individual to meet the growth needs and ensure overall good health and development.

The onset of obesity usually occurs during the second stage but may occur as early as 6 months of age (30). About one-third of nongrowth hormone treated subjects with PWS weigh more than 200% of ideal body weight, and without intervention significant morbidity, mortality may occur from complications of obesity (e.g., cardiopulmonary compromise, hypertension, diabetes mellitus). Individuals with PWS may have 40–50% body fat which is two to three times more than in the general population (31). In addition, the fatness pattern appears to be sex reversed with males having more fat than females. The heaviest deposition of subcutaneous fat in PWS individuals is on the trunk and limb regions. A different peripheral–visceral fat storage pattern in PWS subjects may be present compared to obese controls and could account for abnormal pathways of fat storage and lipolysis in PWS (32).

Obesity in PWS results from overeating, decreased metabolic rate, decreased physical activity, and impaired vomiting (1). Stomach rupturing has been reported as a cause of death in this syndrome. Diet medications have met with little success in PWS individuals, and surgical intervention is not helpful. Adolescents with PWS may weigh 250–300 lb by their late teens. The average adult male with PWS without growth hormone therapy is 155 cm (61 in.) and the adult female is 147 cm (58 in.) (33). Additional classical findings of this syndrome, including small hands and feet, are particularly evident during adolescence and adulthood. This eating disorder and its complications including obesity can reduce life expectancy. The oldest described person with PWS reported to date was 71 years of age (34).

Recently, ghrelin, an endogenous ligand of the growth hormone secretagogue receptor which is G-protein coupled and located in the hypothalamus, is produced by the stomach (35). It is involved with energy balance and appetite stimulation. Adults and children (including infants during stage one or failure to thrive period) have been reported with fasting ghrelin levels three to five times higher than obese or nonobese control subjects (36–38). Additional testing of this peptide and others (e.g., peptide YY) involved in eating behavior in PWS subjects will be needed to understand their role in the hyperphagia and insatiable appetite seen as cardinal features of PWS.

In 1993, Holm et al. (39) developed consensual diagnostic criteria to assist in the diagnosis of PWS using major and minor findings and established a scoring system for patients presenting with features seen in this syndrome. The scoring system consisted of three categories (major, minor, and supportive criteria) and scoring was based on a point system. The major criteria included infantile hypotonia, feeding problems, excessive or rapid weight gain, characteristic facial appearance (narrow face, dolichocephaly, almond-shaped eyes, small appearing mouth with thin upper lip), hypogonadism, global developmental delay, hyperphagia, and a 15q11–q13 deletion or maternal disomy 15 were weighed at one point each. Minor criteria such as decreased fetal movement or a weak cry, typical behavioral problems (temper tantrums, violent outbursts, stubbornness, manipulative, stealing), sleep disturbances, short stature for family background, hypopigmentation, small hands and feet, narrow hands with straight ulnar border, esotropia or myopia, thick, viscous saliva, speech articulation defects, and skin picking were weighed at one-half point each. Supportive criteria such as high pain threshold, reduced vomiting, temperature instability, scoliosis and/or kyphosis, early adrenarche, osteoporosis, unusual skills with jigsaw puzzles, and normal neuromuscular findings (EMG, NCV) received no points but may be helpful to confirm the diagnosis. Children of age ≤3 years required five points for diagnosis and four of the points should come from the major group. Children of age 3 years to adulthood required a total score of eight points necessary for the diagnosis. Major criteria comprised five or more points of the total score of eight.

IV. NATURAL HISTORY

A. Pregnancy and Delivery

In nearly all PWS pregnancies, the mothers note decreased fetal movement. About one-fourth of all babies with PWS were delivered in breech presentation. Approximately, one-half of babies with PWS are born pre- or post-term (i.e., 2 weeks early or later than the anticipated delivery date). Mild parental growth retardation is noted with an average birth weight of 2.8 kg. Low birth weight is seen in about 30% of deliveries.

B. Infancy

Neonates with PWS are profoundly floppy due to generalized hypotonia. Their presentation can be mistaken for neuromuscular disorders such as Werdnig–Hoffman or trisomy 18. The infants are frequently evaluated for a brain anomaly, a metabolic disturbance, or an environmental insult. The central hypotonia may lead to asphyxia, and extensive medical evaluations which in the past have included muscle biopsies and brain imaging studies. However, most of the brain imaging studies and muscle biopsies have been reported as normal or not diagnostic for a specific syndrome.

Most infants with PWS have a weak or absent cry with little spontaneous movement. Hyporeflexia, excessive sleepiness, and poor feeding due to diminished swallowing and sucking reflexes may necessitate gavage feedings that may last for several months. However, feeding difficulties generally improve by 6 months of age. Owing to failure to thrive, feeding difficulties, and hormone deficiencies, the growth of the PWS infant may fall below the third centile. Temperature instability may be present during early infancy. Hyperthermia may trigger medical investigations to pursue an infectious agent which is generally not found. Infants with PWS may also have significant respiratory abnormalities including sleep related central and obstructive apnea and a reduced response to changes in oxygen and carbon dioxide levels (40) and should be monitored closely during this stage of development.

The hands and feet may be small at birth and become remarkably smaller relative to age. Cryptorchidism, a hypoplastic penis and scrotum, in males and hypogenitalism in females are commonly noted. Cryptorchidism may require treatment (hormone and/or surgery). Prader–Willi syndrome subjects tend to have a high pain threshold as evidenced by skin picking and self-injurious behavior as they become older. Developmental milestones are typically delayed in PWS infants that continue into childhood.

Mild dysmorphic features are recognized during the infancy period. A narrow forehead, mild upward slanting of the palpebral fissures, a long, narrow-appearing head (dolichocephaly), a small upturned nose, and downturned corners of the mouth with a thin upper lip and sticky saliva are noted. Prader–Willi syndrome subjects may have diminished facial mimic activity due to the muscular hypotonia, as they grow older. Hypopigmentation for family background with fair skin and light hair color may also be recognized during the infancy period. Depigmentation relative to family background is a feature in about three-fourths of PWS subjects and correlates with the 15q11–q13 deletion and loss of the P gene (causes OCA2) (41).

C. Childhood

Although infants with PWS may be tube fed during infancy, by 18 months to 2 years of age, their feeding behavior changes radically and an insatiable appetite develops. This leads to major somatic and psychological problems in early childhood. Along with global developmental delays, temper tantrums, difficulty in changing routines, stubbornness, controlling or manipulative behavior, and obsessive–compulsive characteristics become more apparent during childhood. Lying, stealing, and aggressive behavior are common during the childhood years and continue into adolescence and adulthood. Frequently, medical and/or behavior management advice is sought to treat the behavioral problems, although no specific medication has been of great benefit. However, specific serotonin reuptake inhibitors have been helpful in controlling behavior and psychiatric disturbances in some PWS children particularly as they become older (3,8,42).

On average, toddlers with PWS learn to walk at about 28 months of age (13). By the time they enter kindergarten, they are nearly always overweight and are short for their age. Recently, growth hormone has been approved for treating the short stature in children with PWS. Growth hormone also significantly improves body composition (decreased fat mass, increased muscle mass) and improves energy level and metabolism in PWS children. Other endocrine abnormalities such as hypothyroidism and diabetes mellitus should also be ruled out in these children. Generally, their lipid levels are within normal range but their insulin levels are low (2,28). Therefore, a consultation with an endocrinologist experienced with growth hormone treatment is advised for the PWS child and their family. Additional findings including orthopedic problems such as scoliosis, particularly if the child is being treated with growth hormone, may occur. Enamel hypoplasia, malocclusion, and dental caries are frequently seen during childhood in PWS. During early childhood, PWS children may develop nystagmus or strabismus. The most common recognized eye finding is myopia, followed by decreased visual acuity and impaired stereoscopic vision, the later finding is more common in PWS subjects with maternal disomy 15 (43). The hypopigmentation becomes more pronounced during childhood, but pigment appears to increase as they enter adulthood. Obstruction sleep apnea and respiratory problems relating to PWS may be recognized at this time or earlier. Sleep assessments may be warranted, particularly if the child is to undergo treatment with growth hormone.

The small hands and feet may not be apparent at birth but become more recognized during mid-childhood. The foot appears smaller than the hand. Almond-shaped eyes may be more noticeable during childhood due to periorbital tissue shape. A characteristic body habitus, including sloping shoulders, heavy mid-section and genu valgus with straight lower leg borders and sparing of distal extremities from fat deposition, is usually present in toddlerhood.

Decreased intellectual functioning was among the four original defining characteristics of PWS. The IQ is typically in the mild range (55–70) with an average of 65 and a range of 20–100. About one-half of children with PWS will have borderline retardation or low normal intelligence and about 20% have moderate retardation. Early reports suggested IQ values in PWS declined with age; however, more recent studies failed to reveal that IQ decreases over time. However, body composition and chromosome factors may correlate with IQ in PWS subjects. Individuals with PWS who were never obese had significantly higher IQs (mean = 80.2) compared with PWS subjects who were currently obese (mean = 57.3) or had been obese and lost weight, although participating in a comprehensive weight management program (mean = 59.9) (44). Academic achievement is generally poor for cognitive ability. During the first 6 years of life, children with PWS often do not achieve normal levels of cognition, motor, or language development. There are reported differences in behavior, academic and intelligence testing between the PWS subjects with deletion vs. maternal disomy and will be discussed later.

Many children with PWS begin school in mainstream settings. By elementary school age, children with PWS may steal or hide food at home or during school to be eaten later. About 5% of PWS children attend normal school until secondary level, but the intellectual impairment and behavioral problems present in the vast majority of PWS children require special education and support services. It is common for PWS subjects to have relatively strong reading, visual, spatial, and long memory skills but relatively weak math, sequential processing, and short-term memory skills (45), although few studies on learning and memory have been reported in PWS subjects. Verbal skills are relative strengths particularly in those PWS subjects with maternal disomy, although speech articulation is often poor with nasal or slurred characteristics. An unusual skill with jigsaw puzzles and motor skills are particularly common in those PWS children with the 15q11–q13 deletion (46), as well as visual perception and organization skills. Recent studies have shown genotype/phenotype correlations between genetic sub-types (deletion vs. maternal disomy) which may impact on these skills and will be discussed later.

D. Adolescence and Adulthood

Puberty is absent or delayed in both males and females with PWS during adolescence. They do not mature sexually as rapidly as their peers. Gonadotropin hormone production is low (28). As a result, adolescents and young adults with PWS look young for their chronologic age. The occurrence of reduced growth hormone secretion and hypogonadotropic hypogonadism in the majority of children and adolescents with PWS, along with an insatiable appetite and high pain threshold, suggests a hypothalamic pituitary dysfunction that has been supported by recent brain imaging studies (PET and MRI scans) (47,48). Studies by Swaab (49) also showed a 30% reduction in the growth hormone releasing hormone neurons in the arcuate nucleus in the brain, and a key nucleus in the release of neuropeptides involved in eating behavior. Gabreels et al. (50) studied for the presence of 7B2 peptide in the supraoptic and paraventricular nucleus of the hypotha-lamus in PWS subjects by the use of antibody analysis. 7B2 is a neuroendocrine chaperone protein, which interacts with prohormone conversion PC2 and involved with the regulation of secretory pathways in the brain. Thus, a disturbance of 7B2 may interfere with the release of hormones in this brain region. Antibodies against the 7B2 precursor polypeptide showed no reaction in three of five PWS subjects, but a positive reaction was seen in the brains of 30 control subjects. Similarly, no antibody reaction was found in the brain nuclei against vasopressin (51). In addition, plasma GABA levels were reported to be high in PWS subjects compared with control individuals (52). GABA is a major inhibitory neurotransmitter in the brain and involved with brain function and in controlling behavior. Thus, evidence exists whereby regulatory genes/proteins (e.g., 7B2) and their derangements may interfere with several neurological functions through transcription errors affecting regulatory proteins and impacting on neurotransmitters or release of neurohormones. Prader–Willi syndrome may be an example of such a syndrome due to these derangements. There is a high probability that the hypothalamus/pituitary axis deficiency seen in children with PWS is also present in adults. Therefore, adults may also benefit from growth hormone therapy, but a paucity of data exists regarding the use of growth hormone in PWS adults.

Hypogonadism and hypogenitalism occur in the vast majority of males or females with PWS and become more evident during adolescence. Cryptorchidism occurs with a hypoplastic penis and scrotum in males and can be identified in early infancy, but the hypoplastic labia minora and clitoris in females may not be as easily recognized. Sertoli cells and a variable number of Leydig and germinal cells are usually present in the testicles, although no reports of fertility in males have been reported. The tubules are usually small and atrophic. The hypogonadism is due to hypothalamic hypogonadotrophism, as it is often associated with low gonadotropin and gonadal steroid levels (28). Penile size increases modestly in many males during the third or fourth decade of life, but testicular size remains small. Treatment of the small penis with topical or parenteral testosterone has achieved penile growth in PWS males (3). However, mature genital development in males is rarely seen. Gonadotropin treatment may also be helpful in treating PWS males with cryptorchidism. Cryptorchid testes may descend spontaneously in some patients during childhood and puberty. Precocious developmental of pubic and axillary hair occurs frequently as a consequence of premature adrenarche. The degree of hypogonadism is variable from patient to patient but more marked in males. In males with palpable testes, the size is small and seldom >6 mL. Beard and body hair are variable occurring later than normal, if at all. Beard growth is absent in about 50% of men.

Menarche is often late or does not occur in PWS females. In 98 appropriately aged females reported in the literature, 38 developed spontaneous menstruation (1). In a study of mostly adult PWS females, breast development was normal in about 50% with onset between 9 and 13 years of age. Primary amenorrhea occurred in about 70% of females and oligomenorrhea in the remaining. Age of menarche is variable with a range from $7\frac{1}{2}$ to 38 years. In a series of 106 females between the ages of 15 and 63, 13 were given hormones to induce menses. Very few of the women who had spontaneous menarche had regular menses, most were scant and infrequent (53). Pubic hair is normal in about 40% of females with PWS (54).

Two women with presumed PWS were reported in the 1970s with established pregnancies (one woman was pregnant on two separate occasions) (55). However, the diagnosis of PWS was not confirmed with genetic testing in the two females. More recently, two women with documented PWS confirmed by cytogenetic and molecular genetic methods were reported with established pregnancies. One woman with PWS was 33 years of age and had suspected maternal disomy (i.e., abnormal methylation testing and normal chromosome study with FISH). She gave birth to a healthy girl by C-section delivery after an estimated 41-week gestation. The other adult female with a reported 15q deletion gave birth, not surprisingly, to a child with Angelman syndrome. The mother with PWS and suspected maternal disomy had low cerebrospinal fluid concentration of 5-hydroxyindoleacetic acid, a serotonin metabolite (56). These findings were similar to those of other cases of PWS possibly reflecting low serotonin synaptic transmission. Owing to behavioral problems before pregnancy, she was medically treated with serotonergic drugs which may have influenced gonadotropin release to induce hormonal conditions required for pregnancy. Therefore, fertility in women with PWS is exceedingly rare, but fertility issues should be addressed in reproductive age females.

Typical behavior problems include rigidity of personality, perseveration in conversation, tantrums, obsessive–compulsive symptoms and noncompliance. Typical adolescent rebelliousness is often exaggerated by a constant struggle with parents and teachers over access to food. Occasionally, behavior worsens during adulthood and symptoms of psychosis may be seen. Psychotropic agents can be helpful in controlling abnormal behavior, but no specific medication has been effective in controlling abnormal behavior or food seeking. When an adult with PWS is surrounded by caregivers who have been trained in the management of PWS, behaviors are usually manageable. Many persons become happy members of their community. When the environment is one in which caregivers are not aware of the specific needs of adults with PWS, behavioral deterioration can be expected.

Approximately 90% of subjects with PWS without growth hormone treatment will have short stature by adulthood. Growth standards for Caucasian PWS males and females aged 2–22 years, without a history of growth hormone therapy, have been developed by Butler and Meaney (33) in 1991 and used in the clinical setting to monitor growth parameters of PWS and to compare with healthy and normal subjects. For example, the 50th centile for height in the PWS group fell below the normal 5th centile by the age of 12–14 years, whereas the 50th centile for weight in the PWS group approximated the 95th centile in the healthy control group. Height may follow the 10th centile or below until the age of 10 years for females and 12 years for males at which time the height velocity often declines relative to normal due to the lack of a growth spurt. Growth hormone therapy will increase the growth spurt and impact positively on the ultimate height and body composition in the PWS subject.

Small hands with thin tapering fingers and small feet (acromicria) are seen during infancy and childhood and become more pronounced during adolescence and adulthood but less frequently in African-Americans (57). There is a relative sparing of the hands and feet from obesity with fat distribution often appearing to end abruptly at the ankle and wrist. There is a straight ulnar border of the hands. Foot length tends to be smaller than hand length when compared with normative standards. The average adult shoe size in males in size 5 and size 3 in females. Scoliosis may also become more pronounced during the adolescent period and kyphosis may be present by early adulthood. Inverse correlations have been reported with linear measurements (e.g., height, hand and foot length) and age indicating a deceleration of linear growth with increasing age relative to normal individuals (58).

By late adolescence, some with PWS begin stealing food from stores and rummaging through discarded lunch bags or trash cans to find partially eaten left-over food or inedible food items (e.g., frozen food). Some parents find it necessary to lock the refrigerator and cabinets containing food to prevent excessive eating. Overeating can lead to immediate life-threatening events such as stomach rupturing as a cause of death. Despite these precautions, some with PWS pry open locked cabinets to gain access to food. The eating behavior, complications of obesity which can reduce the life expectancy of a PWS person, and cognitive impairments will preclude normal adult independent living. Behavioral and psychiatric problems interfere with the quality of life in adulthood and may require medical treatment and behavioral management. However, if weight is adequately controlled and in view of the lack of internal organ problems in PWS individuals, life expectancy should be similar to that of other mildly retarded individuals. Hence, caloric diet restriction is life long and important to control the obesity and its complications. Continued consultation with a dietitian is required.

Many persons with PWS live into their seventh decade of life. A person who died at age 71 was described in 1994 (34), and a second individual at 68 years of age was described in 2000 (59). A review of causes of death in 25 persons with PWS in 1994 indicated that obesity and related complications caused the death in 14 subjects (60). The average age of death was 23 years.

Sleep disorders and respiratory dysfunctions, such as hypoventilation and oxygen desaturation, are common from childhood to adulthood for the PWS subject. Sleep apnea and sleep assessments to check for obstructive airway problems should be considered in all PWS subjects. The PWS adolescents have a tendency to fall asleep during the day particularly when they are inactive. They do not sleep soundly and may awaken often during the night and forage for food.

Adults with PWS have generalized mild hypotonia and decreased muscle bulk and tone, poor coordination, and often decreased muscle strength. However, muscle electrophysiological and biopsy studies are generally normal or nonspecific. The decreased muscle tone and muscle mass contributes to the lower metabolic rate contributing to physical inactivity and obesity (61,62), although thyroid function tests have generally been within the normal range (28).

Behavioral and learning problems may become more prominent, particularly temper tantrums and obsessions during the teenage years. An analysis of 232 individuals with PWS conducted by Greenswag (54) showed that 75% had received special education services. They typically performed at the sixth grade level in reading and the third grade level or lower in mathematics. Acute psychosis can be seen in young adulthood in about 10% of PWS patients and recently reported to correlate with maternal disomy (63).

The adult with PWS has goals for himself or herself similar to those of any other person entering adulthood: establishing vocational goals, deciding where to live, and desiring to become independent in decision making. Daily living skills in PWS become more of strength with increasing age (45). Living goals sometimes lead to conflict and frequently causes an exacerbation of health and behavior problems. For most persons with PWS, formal education ends between ages 18 and 21. If vocational training has been successfully introduced before, then a smooth transition to the world can occur. Unfortunately, many individuals do not have access to training and a gap exists between completion of school and entrance into a job setting. This loss of daytime structured activities usually results in behavioral deterioration, and health problems may occur or increase. The challenge to family and caregivers is establishing an appropriate environment for the adult, which includes a supervised living arrangement (with food restrictions), a vocational setting appropriate for the skills and behavior of the young adult, and professional sources knowledgeable about PWS. As in childhood, limiting access to food is essential, as it is skill in management of typical behavior problems. If this does not happen, deterioration in health occurs.

Assignment of legal guardianship to another adult is frequently helpful and necessary to assure a safe environment for adults with PWS. Decisions regarding living arrangements and availability of food are usually made unwisely by persons with the syndrome, and therefore, it is in the best interest of the person to have guardianship legally assigned to a parent or other adult.

V. CLINICAL DIFFERENCES IN PRADER–WILLI SYNDROME GENETIC SUBTYPES

Clinical differences in individuals with PWS with the different genetic subtypes (deletion, maternal disomy, or imprinting defects) are important to identify and to learn more about the role of specific genes and their clinical consequences. The correlation of specific clinical manifestations and genetic findings will enhance our understanding of genetic imprinting and genotype/phenotype correlations in PWS. However, the rarity of individuals with imprinting defects has limited their comparison to those PWS individuals with deletions or maternal disomy for genetic and clinical correlation studies.

Previous studies have shown that individuals with PWS and the chromosome 15 deletion were more homogeneous in their clinical presentation, including anthropometric and physical characteristics such as hand bone measurements and dermatoglyphic findings (64,65). Molecular genetic studies also associated the hypopigmentation status of deletion patients with the P gene for pigment formation (41,66). In addition, Gillessen-Kaesbach et al. (67) reported lower birth weights in PWS individuals with deletions, whereas individuals with maternal disomy had increased maternal age. Mitchell et al. (68) also reported a shorter birth length in PWS males with maternal disomy compared with PWS males with the deletion and a shorter course of gavage feeding with a later onset of hyperphagia in PWS females with maternal disomy. In 1997, Cassidy et al. (42) observed that people with PWS and maternal disomy were less likely to have the typical facial appearance and less likely to show certain behavioral features of PWS, including skin picking, skill with jigsaw puzzles, a high pain threshold, and articulation problems. No significant differences were found between the groups (deletion or maternal disomy) in most other clinical findings, including neonatal hypotonia, need for gavage feeding, cryptorchidism, genital hypoplasia, small hands and feet, scoliosis, dental anomalies, sticky saliva, behavioral disturbances, hyperphagia, and decreased vomiting or sleeping disorder. Gunay-Aygun et al. (69) also reported that the diagnosis of PWS was made later in individuals with maternal disomy compared with those with the deletion, possibly reflecting a milder phenotype in maternal disomy subjects.

Subjects with PWS are known to have behavioral problems including obsessive compulsivity and self-injurious behavior. Self-injurious behavior in persons with intellectual impairment, autism, and related developmental disabilities ranges from 5% to 60%, depending on the methods used and populations studied (70). Serious health problems can occur relating to this behavior. Investigators have previously reported that self-injurious behavior is a prevalent behavioral problem for 69% of adolescents with PWS (71) and in 81% of adults (72). A study reported by Symons et al. (73) characterized self-injurious behavior in 62 PWS subjects via a questionnaire survey and found skin picking to be the most common form of self injury. Prader–Willi syndrome individuals with the 15q11–q13 deletion injured at significantly more body sites than did individuals with maternal disomy.

Subjects with PWS hoard, arrange and clean repetitively and excessively. Dykens et al. (74) found compulsive symptoms in up to 60% of persons with PWS. In 1999, Dykens et al. (75) also described differences in genetic subtypes in PWS subjects such that the deletion group had higher scores using the Child Behavior Checklist, indicating more compulsive symptoms and more symptom-related distress than in maternal disomy subjects. Dykens (46) further studied children with PWS in order to characterize their presumed ability at jigsaw puzzles. She reported relative strengths on standardized visual–spatial tasks such as object assembly, and the scores were significantly higher in PWS subjects compared with age and IQ matched control subjects with mixed mental retardation, but lower scores were found than in age-matched normal children with average IQs. In contrast, children with PWS scored similar to normal peers on word searches and outperformed them on jigsaw puzzles placing more than twice as many pieces as the typically developing group. Within the PWS group, puzzle proficiency was not predicted by age, IQ, gender, degree of obesity, or obsessive–compulsive symptoms but by the genetic status (higher in the deletion subgroup).

Thompson and Butler (76) collected clinical, genetic, cognitive, academic, and behavioral data from 49 individuals with PWS (22 males, 27 females; 27 with 15q deletions; 21 with maternal disomy 15, and 1 with an imprinting defect) ranging in age from 10 to 50 years and 27 control participants in order to examine for genotype–phenotype relationships. Prader–Willi syndrome participants in the study obtained significantly lower scores in performance IQ ($p < 0.05$), visual-motor skills ($p < 0.01$) and adaptive functioning as assessed by the broad independence ($p < 0.01$), community independence ($p < 0.01$), and motor skill ($p < 0.001$) dimensions of the Scales of Independent Behavior. No significant differences were found for measures of academic achievement. With respect to maladaptive behaviors, PWS participants demonstrated significantly higher levels of self-injury on the Reiss ($p < 0.05$) and scores on the general maladaptive index ($p < 0.05$) of the Scales of Independent Behavior indicating worse behavior. On the Yale-Brown Obsessive–Compulsive Scale (Y-BOCS), group differences between PWS and control participants were found for the total ($p < 0.05$) and compulsion ($p < 0.01$) scores, as well as for specific aspects of severity of compulsions: time spent performing compulsions ($p < 0.01$), length of compulsion-free intervals ($p < 0.01$), interference with daily activities ($p < 0.01$), and degree of control over compulsions ($p < 0.01$). In contrast, significant group differences were not obtained for any of the Y-BOCS obsession scores or for internal aspects of compulsive behaviors, such as the individual's effort to resist against compulsions.

Prader–Willi syndrome subjects with deletions exhibited significantly greater self-injury than both the control group and the maternal disomy subgroup ($p < 0.01$). The deletion subgroup displayed higher compulsivity scores ($p < 0.05$) than the control group and spent more time engaging in compulsive behavior. Their compulsive rituals interfered with their daily living. They were also less able to control their compulsive behavior. Both PWS subgroups (deletion and maternal disomy) showed significantly greater global severity of compulsive behaviors ($p < 0.01$) than the control group. The deletion group consistently showed the most severe symptoms of OCD, with subjects with maternal disomy having intermediate level OCD symptoms. In addition, Vogels et al. (63) recently reported that psychosis in PWS subjects occurs more often in those adults with maternal disomy 15 compared with those with the deletion.

Subgroup comparisons revealed additional differences between PWS deletion and maternal disomy participants (77). In this study, measures of intelligence and academic achievement were administered to 38 (16 males and 22 females) individuals with PWS (24 with deletion and 14 with maternal disomy). Prader–Willi syndrome subjects with maternal disomy 15 had significantly higher verbal IQ scores than those with the deletion ($p < 0.01$). The magnitude of difference in verbal IQ was 9.1 points (69.9 vs. 60.8 for maternal disomy and deletion PWS subjects). Only 17% of the subjects with the 15q11–q13 deletion had a verbal IQ ≥ 70, whereas 50% of those with maternal disomy had a verbal IQ ≥ 70. However, performance IQ scores did not differ between the two PWS genetic subtypes (62.2 vs. 64.7 for maternal disomy and deletion PWS subjects). The full scale IQ did not differ between the two groups (64.1 vs. 61.0 for maternal disomy and deletion).

Specific subtest differences were noted in numeric calculation skill, attention, word meanings, factual knowledge, and social reasoning with the maternal disomy PWS subgroup scoring higher than the deletion subgroup. Deletion PWS subgroup subjects scored higher than the maternal disomy subgroup on the object assembly subtest which further supports specific visual perceptual skills being a relative strength for the deletion subgroup. This may explain anecdotal accounts of subjects with PWS having an uncanny ability to assemble jigsaw puzzles and the study reported by Dykens (46).

The mechanisms whereby certain skills appear to be preserved in the maternal disomy subgroup have yet to be identified. Whether this phenomenon is caused by genetic imprinting against the nonimprinting status of genes in the 15q11–q13 region is not known. The presence of more active or expressed genes in maternal disomy individuals may be due to possible dosage mechanisms whereby only one allele or member of a gene pair is normally functional or expressed. If a gene is paternally imprinted (inactive) and if two functional (active) maternal alleles are now present in maternal disomy PWS individuals in contrast to those with a deletion and no expression (a normal individual would have only one gene member or allele expressed), then there may be a relative strength for the PWS individual with maternal disomy to have over expression of a gene and its product. Evidence to date further documents the difference between verbal and performance IQ score patterns among subjects with PWS and the deletion vs. the maternal disomy subtype.

A. Visual Perception and Visual Memory

Discrimination of shape of motion testing was previously reported by Fox et al. (43), and forms were generated by random dot elements that vary in element density and temporal correlation. This testing was done in four participant groups

(PWS deletion, PWS maternal disomy, comparison subjects, and normal controls). The array produced for the participant to visualize on the computer screen generated a letter "E" that varied in element density and degree of correlation with the blinking dots. Performances of normal controls exceeded that of all other groups (78% correct, $p < 0.009$). The PWS deletion (66%) and equivalent controls (59%) did not differ significantly. However, performance of the maternal disomy group was significantly worse (38%) than any of the other groups ($p < 0.04$). The inferior performance of the maternal disomy group may be attributed to receiving two active alleles of maternally expressed genes influencing development of the visual system. Other possibilities include requirements of paternally expressed genes, residual mosaic trisomy in brain tissue, or complex interactions including specific ratios of differentially spliced gene products (43). Alternatively, as we know people with PWS have elevated plasma GABA, and it has been shown from other studies that excessive GABA levels have deleterious effects on retinal functioning, it is possible that visual signal strengths could be compromised at the level of initial input, which would manifest itself as a perceptual deficit.

Joseph et al. (78) also studied 17 individuals with PWS, 7 with deletions, 10 with maternal disomy and 9 with matched controls (78). Each participant performed a visual recognition task. A series of color digital photographs were presented; most were presented twice, the remainder appeared only once. Photographs presented twice were separated by 0, 10, 30, 50, or 100 intervening photographs. After viewing each photograph, participants indicated whether or not the photograph had been presented previously. This procedure was conducted twice, once using photographs of foods and the second time using nonfood items. As the number of intervening photographs increased between the first and the second presentation, participants were less likely to remember having seen the photograph previously. Performance by the maternal disomy participants was less affected by increasing the number of intervening photographs relative to the other two groups (deletion or controls) suggesting superior visual recognition memory.

B. Clinical Findings Associated with Longer vs. Shorter Typical Deletions

The majority of people with PWS have a paternally derived interstitial deletion of the 15q11–q13 chromosome region including 3.5–4 Mb of DNA. There are two types of this typical interstitial deletion depending on size. Type I deletions are larger than type II deletions by about 500 kb of DNA (79). We recently analyzed clinical, anthropometric, and behavioral data in 12 PWS subjects (5 males, 7 females; mean age 25.9 ± 8.8 years) with type I deletion and 14 PWS subjects (6 males, 8 females; mean age 19.6 ± 6.5 years) with type II deletion determined by the presence or absence of DNA markers between breakpoints BP1 and BP2. Prader–Willi syndrome subjects with longer deletions scored significantly higher in self-injurious behavior and maladaptive behavior tests compared with PWS subjects with shorter deletions. In addition, obsessive–compulsive behavior was more evident in PWS subjects with longer deletions (23). Apparently, loss of genetic material between breakpoints BP1 and BP2 significantly increases the severity of behavioral and psychological problems in this syndrome. Recently, four genes including NIPA-1, which is expressed in brain tissue, have been identified and located between BP1 and BP2 (80). They may play a role in brain development or function accounting for our observed clinical differences.

In summary, PWS is a classical contiguous gene disorder with several genes in the 15q11–q13 region contributing to the phenotype. Prader–Willi syndrome and Angelman syndrome were the first examples in humans of genomic imprinting or due to difference in gene expression depending on the parent of origin. Significant behavioral differences distinguish the two major genotypes (deletion vs. maternal disomy). Generally, those with deletions have the most severe behavioral phenotype with more skin picking, lower verbal IQ scores, and hypopigmentation. Those with maternal disomy are more impaired in visual perception but have superior visual recognition memory. Recently, those with typical deletions were categorized into two deletion subtypes, a longer and a shorter deletion. The phenotypes of individuals with the longer deletion were more severe in their clinical presentation with more maladaptive behavior including self-injurious behavior than those with shorter deletions. Within the region between the long and the short deletion breakpoints are four genes including the NIPA-1 gene which is expressed in brain tissue. These genes may be implicated in the observed clinical differences. Additional research is needed to clarify these observations.

ACKNOWLEDGMENTS

The author thanks Linda A. Heim and Deborah Moore for their expert preparation of the manuscript. Partial funding support was received from the NICHD (PO1HD30329 and RO1HD41672), The Hall Foundation (GL01.3905), and the Physician Scientist Award from Children's Mercy Hospitals and Clinics (GL01.4871).

REFERENCES

1. Butler MG. Prader–Willi syndrome: current understanding of cause and diagnosis. Am J Med Genet 1990; 35(3):319–332.

2. Butler MG, Thompson T. Prader–Willi syndrome: clinical and genetic findings. Endocrinology 2000; 10:3S–16S.

3. Cassidy SB. Prader–Willi syndrome. J Med Genet 1997; 34(11): 917–923.

4. Whittington JE, Holland AJ, Webb T, Butler J, Clarke D, Boer H. Population prevalence and estimated birth incidence and mortality rate for people with Prader–Willi syndrome in one UK Health Region. J Med Genet 2001; 38(11):792–798.

5. Nicholls RD, Knepper JL. Genome organizations, function and imprinting in Prader–Willi and Angelman syndromes. Ann Rev Genom Hum Genet 2001; 2:153–175.

6. Butler MG. Imprinting disorders: non-Mendelian mechanisms affecting growth. J Ped Endocrinol Metab 2002; 5:1279–1288.

7. Butler MG, Weaver DD, Meaney FJ. Prader–Willi syndrome: are there population differences? Clin Genet 1982; 22(5): 292–294.

8. Cassidy SB, Dykens E, Williams CA. Prader–Willi syndromes: sister imprinted disorders. Am J Med Genet 2000; 97(2): 136–146.

9. Down JL. Mental Affections of Childhood and Youth. London, England: Churchill Publisher, 1887:172.

10. Prader A, Labhart A, Willi H. Ein syndrome von adipositas, kleinwuchs, kryptochismus and oligophrenie nach myatonieartigem zustand in neugeborenenalter. Schweiz Med Wochenschr 1956; 86:1260–1261.

11. Ledbetter DH, Riccardi VM, Airhart SD. Deletions of chromosome 15 as a cause of the Prader–Willi syndrome. New Eng J Med 1981; 304(6):325–329.

12. Butler MG, Palmer CG. Parental origin of chromosome 15 deletion in Prader–Willi syndrome. Lancet 1983; 1:1285–1286.

13. Butler MG, Meaney FJ, Palmer CG. Clinical and cytogenetic survey of 39 individuals with Prader–Labhart–Willi syndrome. Am J Med Genet 1986; 23(3):793–809.

14. Nicholls RD, Knoll HM, Butler MG, Karum S, Lalande M. Genetic imprinting suggested by maternal heterodisomy in nondeletion Prader–Willi syndrome. Nature 1989; 342:281–285.

15. Ozcelik T, Leff S, Robinson W, Donlon T, Lalande M, Sanjines E, Schinzel A, Francke U. Small nuclear ribonucleoprotein polypeptide N (SNRPN), an expressed gene in the Prader–Willi syndrome critical region. Nat Genet 1992; 2(4):265–269.

16. Runte M, Huttenhofer A, Gross S, Kiefmann M, Horsthemke B, Buiting K. The IC–SNURF–SNRPN transcript serves as a host for multiple small nucleolar RNA species and as an antisense RNA for UBE3A. Hum Mol Genet 2001; 10(23):2687–2700.

17. Gallagher RC, Pils B, Albalwi M, Francke U. Evidence for the role of PWCR1/HB11-85 C/D box small nucleolar RNAs in Prader–Willi syndrome. Am J Hum Genet 2002; 71(3): 669–678.

18. Malzac P, Webber H, Moncla A, Graham JM, Kukolich M, Williams C, Pagon RA, Ramsdell LA, Kishino T, Wagstaff J. Mutation analysis of UBE3A in Angelman syndrome patients. Am J Hum Genet 1998; 62(6):1353–1360.

19. Sutcliffe JS, Han M, Christian SL, Ledbetter DH. Neuronally-expressed necdin gene: an imprinted candidate gene in Prader–Willi syndrome. Lancet 1997; 350(9090):1520–1521.

20. Christian SL, Fantes JA, Mewborn SK, Huang B, Ledbetter DH. Large genomic duplicons map to sites of instability in the Prader–Willi/Angelman syndrome chromosome region (15q11–q13). Hum Mol Genet 1999; 8(6):1025–1037.

21. Amos-Landgraff JM, Ji Y, Gottlieb W, Depinet T, Wandstrat AE, Cassidy SB, Driscoll DJ, Rogan PK, Schwartz S, Nicholls RD. Chromosome breakage in Prader–Willi and Angelman syndromes involves recombination between large, transcribed repeats at proximal and distal breakpoints. Am J Hum Genet 1999; 65(2):370–386.

22. Ji Y, Walkowicz MJ, Buiting K, Johnson DK, Tarvin RE, Rinchik EM, Horsthemke B, Stubbs L, Nicholls RD. The ancestral gene for transcribed, low-copy repeats in the Prader–Willi/Angelman region encodes a large protein implicated in protein trafficking, which is deficient in mice with neuromuscular and spermiogenic abnormalities. Hum Mol Genet 1999; 8(3):533–542.

23. Butler MG, Bittel DC, Kibiryeva N, Talebizadeh Z, Thompson T. Behavioral differences among subjects with Prader–Willi syndrome and type I or type II deletion and maternal disomy. Pediatrics 2004; 113 (3pt 1):565–573.

24. Bittel DC, Kibiryeva N, Talebizadeh Z, Butler MG. Microarray analysis of gene/transcript expression in Prader–Willi syndrome: deletion versus UPD. J Med Genet 2003; 40(8): 558–574.

25. Gabriel JM, Merchant M, Ohta T, Ji Y, Caldwell RG, Ramsey MJ, Tucker TD, Longnecker R, Nicholls RD. A transgene insertion creating a heritable chromosome deletion mouse model of Prader–Willi and Angelman syndromes. Proc Natl Acad Sci USA 1999; 96(16):9258–9263.

26. Ohta T, Gray TA, Rogan PK, Buiting K, Gabriel JM, Saitoh S, Muralidhar B, Bilienska B, Krajewska-Walasek M, Driscoll DJ, Horsthemke B, Butler MG, Nicholls RD. Imprinting-mutation mechanisms in Prader–Willi syndrome. Am J Hum Genet 1999; 64(2):397–413.

27. Flegal KM, Carroll MD, Kucamarski RJ. Overweight and obesity in the United States: Prevalence and trends. Int J Obes Rel Metab Dis 1998; 22:39–47.

28. Burman P, Ritzén EM, Lindgren AC. Endocrine dysfunction in Prader–Willi syndrome: a review with special reference to GH. Endocrinol Rev 2001; 22(6):787–799.

29. Carrel AL, Myers SE, Whitman BY, Allen DB. Benefits of long-term GH therapy in Prader–Willi syndrome: a 4-year study. J Clin Endocrinol Metab 2002; 87(4):1581–1585.

30. Butler MG, Butler RI, Meaney FJ. The use of skinfold measurements to judge obesity during the early phase of Prader–Labhart–Willi syndrome. Int J Obes 1988; 12: 417–422.

31. Meaney FJ, Butler MG. Characterization of obesity in the Prader–Labhardt–Willi syndrome: fatness patterning. Med Anthropol Quart 1989; 3:294–305.

32. Goldstone AP, Thomas EL, Brynes AE, Bell JD, Frost G, Saeed N, Hajnal JV, Howard JK, Holland A, Bloom SR. Visceral adipose tissue and metabolic complications of obesity are reduced in Prader–Willi syndrome female adults: evidence for novel influences on body fat distribution. J Clin Endocrinol Metab 2001; 86(9):4430–4338.

33. Butler MG, Meaney FJ. Standards for selected anthropometric measurements in Prader–Willi syndrome. Pediatrics 1991; 88: 853–860.

34. Carpenter PK. Prader–Willi syndrome in old age. J Intellect Disabil Res 1994; 38:529–531.

35. Tschop M, Devanarayan V, Weyer C, Tataranni P, Ravussin E. Circulating ghrelin levels are decreased in human obesity. Diabetes 2001; 50:707–709.

36. Cummings DE, Clement K, Purnell JQ, Vaisse C, Foster KE, Frayo RS, Schwartz MW, Basdevant A, Weigle DS. Elevated plasma ghrelin levels in Prader–Willi syndrome. Nat Med 2002; 8(7):643–644.

37. Haqq AM, Farooqi IS, O'Rahilly S, Stadler DD, Rosenfeld RG, Pratt KL, LaFranchi SH, Purnell JQ. Serum ghrelin levels is inversely correlated with body mass index, age, and insulin

concentrations in normal children and are markedly increased in Prader–Willi syndrome. J Clin Endocrinol Metab 2003; 88(1):174–178.

38. Butler MG, Bittel DC, Talebizadeh Z. Plasma ghrelin and peptide YY levels in infants and children with Prader–Willi syndrome. J Pediatr Endocrinol Metab 2004; 17(9):1177–1184.

39. Holm VA, Cassidy SB, Butler MG, Hanchett JM, Greenberg F. Prader–Willi syndrome: consensus diagnostic criteria. Pediatrics 1993; 91:398–402.

40. Arens R, Gozal D, Omlin KL, Livingston FR, Liu J, Keens TG, Ward SL. Hypoxic and hypercapnic ventilatory responses in Prader–Willi syndrome. J Appl Physiol 1994; 77:2224–2230.

41. Butler MG. Hypopigmentation: a common feature of Prader–Labhart–Willi syndrome. Am J Hum Genet 1989; 45:140–146.

42. Cassidy SB, Forsythe M, Heeger S, Nicholls RD, Schork N, Benn P, Schwartz S. Comparison of phenotype between patients with Prader–Willi syndrome due to deletion 15q and uniparental disomy 15. Am J Med Genet 1997; 68:433–440.

43. Fox R, Yang GS, Feurer ID, Butler MG, Thomspon T. Kinetic form discrimination in Prader–Willi syndrome. J Intellect Dis Res 2001; 45:317–325.

44. Crnic KA, Sulzbacher S, Snow J, Holm VA. Preventing mental retardation associated with gross obesity in the Prader–Willi syndrome. Pediatrics 1980; 66(5):787–789.

45. Dykens EM, Hodapp EM, Walsh K, Nash LJ. Profiles, correlates, and trajectories of intelligence in Prader–Willi syndrome. J Am Acad Child Adolesc Psych 1992; 31(6):1125–1130.

46. Dykens EM. Are jigsaw puzzle skills 'spared' in persons with Prader–Willi syndrome? J Child Psychol Psychiatry 2002; 43(3): 343–352.

47. Butler MG, Kessler RM. Positron emission tomography of three adult patients with Prader–Willi syndrome. Dysmorphol Clin Genet 1992; 6:30–31.

48. Yoshii A, Krishnamoorthy KS, Grant PE. Abnormal cortical development shown by 3D MRI in Prader–Willi syndrome. Neurology 2002; 59(4):644–645.

49. Swaab DF. Prader–Willi syndrome and the hypothalamus. Acta Paediatr Suppl 1997; 423:50–54.

50. Gabreels BA, Swabb DF, Seidah NG, van Duijnhoven HL, Martens GJ, van Leeuwen FW. Differential expression of the neuroendocrine polypeptide 7B2 in hypothalamus of Prader–(Labhart)–Willi syndrome patients. Brain Res 1994; 657(1–2): 281–293.

51. Gabreels BA, Swaab DF, de Kleijn DP, Seidah NG, Van de Loo JW, Van de Ven WJ, Martens GJ, van Leeuwen FW. Attenuation of the polypeptide 7B2, prohormone convertase PC2, and vasopressin in the hypothalamus of some Prader–Willi patients: indications for a processing defect. J Clin Endocrinol Metab 1998; 83(2):591–599.

52. Ebert MH, Schmidt DE, Thompson T, Butler MG. Elevated plasma gamma-aminobutyric acid (GABA) levels in individuals with either Prader–Willi syndrome or Angelman syndrome. J Neuropsych Clin Neurosci 1997; 9(1):75–80.

53. Hanchett JM. Menstrual periods in Prader–Willi syndrome women. Am J Med Genet 1996; 64:577.

54. Greenswag LR. Adults with Prader–Willi syndrome: a survey of 232 cases. Devel Med Child Neurol 1987; 29(2):145–152.

55. Laxova R, Gilderdale S, Ridler MAC. An aetiological study of 53 female patients from subnormality hospital and of their offspring. J Mental Defic Res 1973; 17:193–225.

56. Akefeldt A, Tornhage CJ, Gillberg C. A woman with Prader–Willi syndrome gives birth to a healthy baby girl. Develop Med Child Neurol 1999; 41(11):789–790.

57. Hudgins L, Geer JS, Cassidy SB. Phenotypic differences in African-Americans with Prader–Willi syndrome. Genet Med 1998; 1(1):49–51.

58. Butler MG, Meaney FJ. An anthropometric study of 38 individuals with Prader–Labhart–Willi syndrome. Am J Med Genet 1987; 26:445–455.

59. Butler MG. A 68-year-old white female with Prader–Willi syndrome. Clin Dysmorphol 2000; 9(1):65-67.

60. Hanchett JM, Butler M, Cassidy SB, Holm V, Parker KR, Wharton R, Zipf W. Age and causes of death in Prader–Willi syndrome patients. Am J Med Genet 1996; 62:211.

61. Hill JO, Kaler M, Spetalnick B, Reed G, Butler MG. Resting metabolic rate in Prader–Willi syndrome. Dysmorphol Clin Genet 1990; 4:27–32.

62. Chen KY, Ming S, Butler MG, Thompson T, Carlson MG. Development and validation of a measurement system for assessment of energy expenditure and physical activity in Prader–Willi syndrome. Obesity Res 1999; 7(4):387–394.

63. Vogels A, Matthijs G, Legius E, Devriendt K, Fryns JP. Chromosome 15 maternal uniparental disomy and psychosis in Prader–Willi syndrome. J Med Genet 2003; 40(1):72–73.

64. Butler MG, Kaler SG, Meaney FJ. Metacarpophalangeal pattern profile analysis in Prader–Willi syndrome. Clin Genet 1982b; 22:315–320.

65. Reed T, Butler MG. Dermatologic features in Prader–Willi syndrome with respect to chromosomal findings. Clin Genet 1984; 25:341–346.

66. Spritz RA, Bailin T, Nicholls RD, Lee ST, Park SK, Mascari MJ, Butler MG. Hypopigmentation in Prader–Willi syndrome correlates with P gene deletion but not with haplotype of the hemizygous P allelle. Am J Med Genet 1997; 71:57–62.

67. Gillessen-Kaesbach G, Gross S, Kaya-Westerloh S, Passarge E, Horsthemke B. DNA methylation based testing of 450 patients suspected of having Prader–Willi syndrome. J Med Genet 1995; 32(2):88–92.

68. Mitchell J, Schinzel A, Langlois S, Gillessen-Kaebach G, Schuffenhauer S, Michaelis R, Abeliovich D, Lerer I, Christian S, Guitart M, McFadden DE, Robinson WP. Comparison of phenotype in uniparental disomy and deletion Prader–Willi syndrome: sex specific differences. Am J Med Genet 1996; 65(2):133–136.

69. Gunay-Aygun M, Heeger S, Schwartz S, Cassidy SB. Delayed diagnosis in patients with Prader–Willi syndrome due to maternal uniparental disomy 15. Am J Med Genet 1997; 71(1): 106–110.

70. Thompson T, Gray DB. Destructive behavior in developmental disabilities: diagnosis and treatment. In: Thompson T, Gray DB, eds. Behavior in Developmental Disabilities. Thousand Oaks, CA: Sage Publishers, 1994.

71. Whitman BY, Accardo P. Emotional symptoms in Prader–Willi syndrome adolescents. Am J Med Genet 1987; 28(4):897–905.

72. Thornton L, Dawson KP. Prader–Willi syndrome in New Zealand: A survey of 36 affected people. NZ Med J 1990; 103(885):97–98.

73. Symons FJ, Butler MG, Sanders MD, Feurer ID, In: Thompson T. Self-injurious behavior and Prader–Willi syndrome: behavioral forms and body locations. Am J Mental Retard 1999; 104:260–269.

74. Dykens EM, Leckman JF, Cassidy SB. Obsessions and compulsions in Prader–Willi syndrome. J Child Psychol Psych 1996; 37:995–1002.

75. Dykens EM, Cassidy SB, King BH. Maladaptive behavior differences in Prader–Willi syndrome due to paternal deletion versus maternal uniparental disomy. Am J Mental Retard 1999; 104:67–77.

76. Thompson T, Butler MG. Prader–Willi syndrome: Clinical, behavioral and genetic findings. In: Wolraich ML, ed. Disorders of Development and Learning. 3rd ed. Hamilton: B.C. Decker, Inc, 2003.

77. Roof E, Stone W, MacLean W, Feurer ID, Thompson T, Butler MG. Intellectual characteristics of Prader–Willi syndrome: comparison of genetic subtypes. J Intellect Disabil Res2000; 44:1–6.

78. Joseph B, Egli M, Sutcliffe JS, Thompson T. Possible dosage effect of maternally expressed genes on visual recognition memory in Prader–Willi syndrome. Am J Med Genet 2001; 105(1):71–75.

79. Ungaro P, Christian SL, Fantes JA, Mutirangura A, Black S, Reynolds J, Malcolm S, Dobyns WB, Ledbetter DH. Molecular characterization of four cases of intrachromosomal triplication of chromosome 15q11-q14. J Med Genet 2001; 38(1):26–34.

80. Chai JH, Locke DP, Eichler EE, Nicholls RD. Evolutionary transposition of 4 unique genes mediated by flanking duplicons in the Prader–Willi/Angelman syndrome deletion region. Am J Hum Genet 2002; 71:A395.

10

Angelman Syndrome

CHARLES A. WILLIAMS

Department of Pediatrics, Division of Genetics,
Raymond C. Philips Research and
Education Unit, University of Florida,
Gainesville, Florida, U.S.A.

I. INTRODUCTION

In 1965, Dr. Harry Angelman, an English physician, first described three children with characteristics now known as the Angelman syndrome (AS) (1). All these children had a stiff, jerky gait, absent speech, excessive laughter, and seizures. During the next 20 years, additional cases were noted but the condition was considered to be extremely rare and many doubted its existence. The first reports from North America appeared in the early 1980s, but during the last two decades several hundred cases have been reported and several thousand individuals are known worldwide to be affected. Angelman syndrome is now familiar to most clinical geneticists and child neurologists as a recognizable syndrome associated with mental retardation and infantile seizures. However, the AS clinical features are not yet widely appreciated among most general pediatricians or family practitioners. Several general reviews have recently appeared in the genetic literature (2–4) and this chapter reviews the salient neurological and diagnostic aspects of the condition.

II. INCIDENCE

It appears that AS occurs worldwide without geographic clustering. Studies on school age children, age 6–13 years, show a minimum prevalence of AS of 1/12,000 in Sweden (5) and 1/10,000 in Denmark (6). Several reports address the prevalence among individuals with established developmental delay, showing rates of 0% (7), 1.3% (8), 1.4% (9), and 4.8% (10). The latter study extrapolated data in order to compare it to the population of the state of Washington (using 1997 U.S. Census Bureau figures) and obtained an estimate of 1/20,000. It seems that AS has prevalence among children and young adults at between 1/10,000 and 1/20,000.

III. CLINICAL PRESENTATION

Clinical consensus criteria for the diagnosis have been published as is illustrated in Table 1 (11). Severe speech deficit (usually absent speech), severe mental retardation, behavioral abnormalities, and movement problems are ubiquitous in AS. Other features, such as microcephaly or seizures may be absent. The AS clinical gestalt is heavily dependent on the combination of behaviors, including excessive laughter and apparent happiness combined with tremulous movements and gait ataxia.

The physician often first encounters AS while consulting on an infant with developmental delay, microcephaly, or seizures (12). The normal prenatal and birth history typically provides no clues that AS is the diagnosis. However, feeding problems and muscle hypotonia are often reported. Brain MRI or CT scans are normal, but may show nonspecific

Table 1   Clinical Diagnostic Criteria for Angelman Syndrome

(A) Consistent (100%)
Developmental delay, functionally severe
Speech impairment, none or minimal use of words; receptive and
  nonverbal communication skills higher than verbal ones
Movement or balance disorder, usually ataxia of gait and/or tremulous
  movement of limbs
Behavioral uniqueness: any combination of frequent laughter/smiling;
  apparent happy demeanor; easily excitable personality, often with
  hand flapping movements; hypermotoric behavior; short attention span
(B) Frequent (more than 80%)
Delayed, disproportionate growth in head circumference, usually
    resulting in microcephaly (absolute or relative) by age 2
Seizures, onset usually < 3 years of age
Abnormal EEG, characteristic pattern with large amplitude slow-spike
  waves (usually 2–3 s^{-1}), facilitated by eye closure
(C) Associated (20–80%)
Flat occiput
Occipital groove
Protruding tongue
Tongue thrusting; suck/swallowing disorders
Feeding problems during infancy
Prognathia
Wide mouth, wide-spaced teeth
Frequent drooling
Excessive chewing/mouthing behaviors
Strabismus
Hypopigmented skin, light hair, and eye color (compared to family),
  seen only in deletion cases
Hyperactive lower extremity deep tendon reflexes
Uplifted, flexed arm position especially during ambulation
Increased sensitivity to heat
Sleep disturbance
Attraction to/fascination with water

Source: Ref. 11.

changes such as mild cortical atrophy or delay in myelination. Laboratory tests of blood and urine are also normal including metabolic screening. If the child is less than 12 months of age, tremulous movements, ataxia, or severe lack of speech may not be apparent. Likewise, seizures may not have occurred at this time. The facial features and general physical exami-

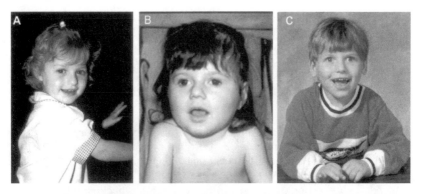

Figure 1   Children with genetically proven diagnosis of Angelman syndrome. The common 15q11.2–15q13 deletion was present in A and C. An UBE3A mutation was detected in B. (Author photos.)

nation are generally normal (Fig. 1), although protruding tongue, strabismus, brisk deep tendon reflexes, and an apparent happy demeanor may be present. For infants with AS due to a chromosome deletion, absolute or relative skin hypopigmentation may be present in infancy due to deletion of a pigment gene (the P gene) that resides within the deletion area (13). This hypopigmentation is usually overlooked unless the physician is specifically thinking about the possibility of AS.

As the child with AS develops, the correct diagnosis may become evident during follow-up neurology visits, especially when it becomes apparent that speech is essentially absent and attempts at walking are compromised because of severe jerkiness and ataxia. Additionally, onset of seizures, more common after 1 year of age, usually forces reassessment of the working diagnosis of such entities as cerebral palsy, static encephalopathy, or idiopathic mental retardation. The EEG in AS is usually very abnormal and more abnormal than clinically expected. It usually has symmetrical high-voltage slow-wave activity (4–6 c/s) persisting for most of the record and unrelated to drowsiness; and very large amplitude slow activity at 2–3 c/s occurring in runs and more prominent anteriorly. In addition, spikes or sharp waves, mixed with large amplitude 3–4 c/s components, are seen posteriorly and usually provoked by passive eye closure (4,14,15). The

EEG findings alone can point strongly to the AS diagnosis, but it can be normal at times in individuals genetically proven to have AS.

It is more likely to consider the clinical diagnosis of AS when the child is older than 3 years. Here, the behavioral and movement characteristics predominate, often in the setting of microcephaly and an established seizure disorder. In these children, there is no evidence of neurodeterioration as they are socially outgoing, quite hypermotoric, and are moving forward developmentally. They may be hyperexcitable with excessive laughing, grabbing, and pulling so as to engage others, often constantly putting objects in their mouth. Drooling is frequent. However, mild expression can be present in cases where there is no microcephaly, seizures, and only mild ataxia or tremulousness. In these cases, the EEG may be the first suggestion that AS is the correct diagnosis. Often the parents may be the first to suggest the possibility of AS.

IV. GENETIC ETIOLOGY

It was not until the 1980s that chromosome 15 was implicated in its causation. The first clue was the discovery that the majority of individuals with AS had microdeletion of 15q11.2–15q13. Initially confusing was the observation that Prader–Willi syndrome (PWS) could also be caused by the same microdeletion. It soon became evident that deletions on the paternally derived 15 caused PWS and ones on the maternally derived 15 caused AS. The two syndromes are, however, caused by different genes that lie in close proximity to one another.

The last decade led to the identification of UBE3A (encoding for a ubiquitin ligase enzyme) as the AS gene (16,17). In certain regions of the normal brain, UBE3A is expressed only from the maternal chromosome and its expression in the AS brain with 15q11.2–15q13 deletion is only about 10% of normal (18). This phenomenon of monoallelic or single chromosome regional expression is termed "genomic imprinting," one of the hallmarks of AS. Mice lacking the maternal UBE3A gene have very low level of mRNA in the hippocampus, cerebellar Purkinje cells, and olfactory bulb (19).

Imprinted genes like UBE3A often have novel as well as complex control mechanisms. This is illustrated in Fig. 2, where the current gene map of the 15q11.2–q13 region illustrates how a distant imprinting control (IC) area can affect the transcription of the UBE3A gene even though the IC is spatially located several hundred thousand base pairs from the UBE3A gene. It appears that the IC accomplishes this control through regulation of another gene, SNRPN, that indirectly affects whether UBE3A (and other genes in the region) are turned on or off. The general aspects of this control are nicely summarized in the related chapter on Prader–Willi syndrome (refer to text). The molecular details of this imprinting control are being rapidly dissected and are beyond the scope of this review (20–22). However, knowledge that UBE3A is an imprinted gene is fundamental to understanding the genetic defects that cause AS.

Figure 3 illustrates the four genetic mechanisms known to cause AS. Chromosome microdeletions are clearly the most common type and almost always involve consistent

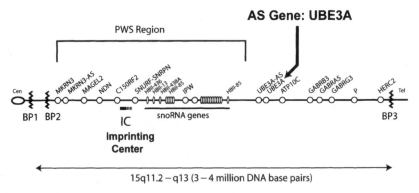

Figure 2 Illustration of the complexity of the genetic map in the 15q11.2–15q13 region. BP1, BP2, and BP3 represent common breakpoints related to the presence of repetitive genes (duplicons). The Imprinting center (IC) is depicted in the promoter region of the SNRPN gene. See text for details of regulation of UBE3A.

Deletion   UBE3A Mutation

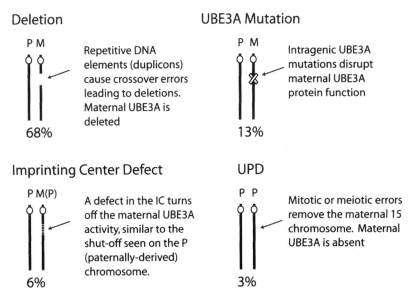

Figure 3 Summary of the four known genetic mechanisms that cause Angelman syndrome. Percentages below each mechanism indicate the proportion of all clinically diagnosed individuals in whom that mechanism is detected. About 10% of all clinically diagnosed individuals will have normal genetic testing. Percentages are approximated and may vary in reported surveys.

breakpoints in flanking cassettes of repetitive genes (sometimes called duplicons) (22–24). Unequal or misaligned crossing over between these chromosome 15 repetitive elements causes the AS deletion. These repetitive gene cassettes have accumulated from ancestral duplication events. Accordingly, there are similar sites for the proximal (centromeric) and distal (telomeric) break points: BP1 and BP2 occur proximally and BP3 distally (25,26) (refer to the PWS section also for discussion of BP breakpoints). A recent study indicated that normal mothers, in some families having an AS deletion children, had rearrangements or inversions related to these duplicated gene cassettes (27). It is unclear what the significance of this finding may prove to be.

Failure of the zygote to incorporate the normal maternal and paternal chromosome 15s can lead to only two paternal

15s, a term called paternal uniparental disomy (UPD). In such cases, UBE3A is not expressed in critical brain areas due to the presence of only two paternal chromosome 15s (with inactive UBE3As). The mechanism leading to the uniparental disomy appears to be mainly postzygotic, i.e., after fertilization, perhaps representing a mitotic "correction" event in response to normal fertilization of an abnormal egg that is nullisomic for chromosome 15 (28). This mechanism for paternal UPD in AS is somewhat different than that of the maternal UPD seen in PWS. In PWS, the maternal UPD is usually the result of trisomy "rescue" in that a trisomic 15 conceptus (e.g., early embryo) eventually loses the paternal 15 chromosome and thus corrects to a disomic status with two maternal 15 chromosomes (refer to text on PWS for further discussion). Imprinting center defects can involve small molecular deletions that can be detected by molecular or cytomolecular FISH methods. More likely however, no actual DNA deletion is found but DNA methylation abnormalities are present in the IC region interfering with the activity of the genes in the region (29). Intragenic UBE3A mutations can also cause AS by creating an abnormal protein that is either degraded or functions abnormally. Finally, about 10–15% of individuals with the appropriate clinical diagnosis of AS have negative testing for all four of the above mechanisms. For them, the diagnosis could be incorrect or they could still have AS due to, yet-to-be identified, genetic mechanisms.

There is some correlation between the clinical severity of AS and its type of genetic mechanism (4,30). Individuals with large chromosome deletions are more likely to have seizures and microcephaly and are more likely to have skin, eye, and hair hypopigmentation. These features are probably due to additional deleted genes in the 3–4 Mb deleted region. Those with uniparental disomy may be milder in their clinical presentation and are more likely to have no seizures, normal head circumferences, and better cognitive functioning although severe to profound impairment. Those with UBE3A and IC defects are more likely to have clinical severity between that seen with the large deletion or UPD. The presence of somatic mosaicism can result in milder clinical features in those with

IC defects (29) and has been noted in a case of 15q11.2–15q13 deletion (31). Overall, however, regardless of the mechanism, individuals with AS are more alike in their clinical features than they are different.

V. GENETIC DIAGNOSTIC TESTING

DNA methylation testing of blood is a sensitive and specific screening for three of the four known genetic mechanisms in AS. This methylation testing, using the SNRPN gene, is the same to detect PWS cases (refer to text for diagnostic testing for PWS). There are several methods available for testing and all rely on the observation that the DNA methylation pattern for AS in the IC control region is easily distinguishable from normal when AS is caused by chromosome deletions, UPD or IC defects. The diagnosis of AS is thus confirmed if the methylation result is abnormal but will not distinguish which of the above three mechanisms is operative. To determine the genetic subtype, the next step is to perform chromosome 15 FISH analysis (to detect 15q11.2–15q13 deletions that will be present in the majority of cases). If this FISH test is normal, additional specialized molecular genetic testing is necessary to determine if either UPD or IC defects are present.

If the initial DNA methylation test is normal, the child with AS could still have an intragenic UBE3A mutation since these mutations have no effect on the DNA methylation pattern in the 15q11.2–15q13 region. If UBE3A mutation testing is normal, these patients may still have AS and be one of the 10–15% in whom genetic test confirmation is not possible. It is also possible that this latter group is incorrectly diagnosed, as mimicking conditions, including other chromosome defects, have been reported (32). The disorders most commonly considered in the differential diagnosis of AS are cerebral palsy of undetermined etiology, Rett syndrome (particularly in infant girls), and idiopathic static encephalopathy. Accordingly, all children with AS-like features not diagnosed by the above genetic tests should have at least a routine chromosome study performed.

Families with AS should be offered genetic counseling since UBE3A mutations and IC defects can carry up to a 50% recurrence risk. However, the common deletion cases typically have less than 1% recurrence risk but exceptions to this can occur (33).

VI. UBE3A AND BRAIN DEVELOPMENT IN ANGELMAN SYNDROME

The UBE3A gene has at least 16 exons that span about 100 kb and produces an mRNA of 5–8 kb size, spliced into five different mRNA types (34,35). UBE3A produces a protein called the E6-associated protein (E6AP), which acts as a cellular ubiquitin ligase enzyme. It is termed "E6-associated," because it was first discovered as the protein able to associate with p53 in the presence of the E6 oncoprotein of the human papilloma virus, type 16 (36). The E6AP enzyme functions to create a covalent linkage (e.g., the "ligase" function) between the small ~76 amino acid ubiquitin molecule and its target protein (37). After initial ubiquitin attachment, for example, onto p53, E6AP can then add ubiquitins onto the first ubiquitin to create a polyubiquitylated substrate. Proteins modified in this way can then be targeted for degradation though the 26S proteasome complex (38,39). The E6AP is the prototype of what is termed the E3 component of the ubiquitin cycle; E1 and E2 proteins respectively activate and transfer the ubiquitin molecule to E3. The E3 is then able to bind to a target protein and transfer and ligate ubiquitin to the target (see Fig. 4). This ligation reaction occurs mainly in a catalytic region of the E3 enzyme, called the homologous to E6AP C terminus (HECT) domain (40). Most Angelman UBE3A mutations disrupt function of this region of the protein (41). Many E3 proteins (and their specific genes) have now been discovered and have distinct ways of mono- or polyubiquitylation. These proteins play a role in diverse cellular events such as DNA repair, cell cycle control, antigen presentation, chromosome organization, intracellular translocation of proteins, intracellular signaling, and apoptosis (42). Unfortunately, no clearly pathogenic target protein for UBE3A has yet been identified.

Ubiquitin Pathway

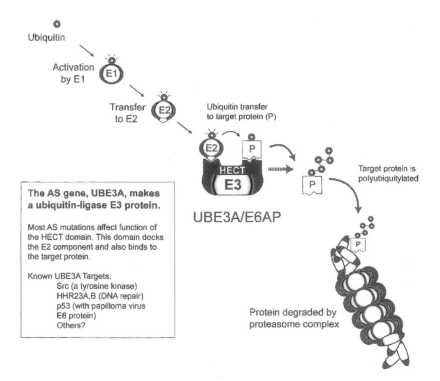

The AS gene, UBE3A, makes
a ubiquitin-ligase E3 protein.

Most AS mutations affect function of
the HECT domain. This domain docks
the E2 component and also binds to
the target protein.

Known UBE3A Targets:
   Src (a tyrosine kinase)
   HHR23A,B (DNA repair)
   p53 (with papilloma virus
   E6 protein)
   Others?

Figure 4 Illustration of the ubiquitin pathway and the role of the UBE3A (E6-AP) protein. It functions as a ubiquitin E3 ligase and transfers activated ubiquitin to target proteins resulting in their degradation by the 26S proteasome. Many types of E3 ligase proteins function to regulate the complex process of cellular protein homeostasis. Refer to text for details.

The cell cycle control protein p53, a target in the presence of the E6 protein, was first to be identified but its role in AS is unclear (43). The activated form of the Src family tyrosine kinase Blk, and HHR23A and HHR23B (homologues of RAD23, an excision repair protein in yeast) appear to be targets (44,45). However, these targets do not yet give insight into the neuronal pathophysiology of AS.

The UBE3A deficient mouse model provides some insight into regional brain dysfunction with recent work focused on the well-studied phenomenon of long-term potentiation (LTP). Learning in the context of LTP is abnormal in the AS mouse (43,46). In recent LTP studies involving mouse hippocampus, abnormal ratios of phospho-calcium/calmodulin-dependent protein kinase II (CaMKII) have been found. Other downstream effectors of the LPT process such as protein kinase C (PKC) and cAMP-dependent protein kinase A (PKA) appeared to function normally. It appears however that CaMKII is not an actual target for ubiquitylation by UBE3A. Presumably, there is some indirect connection to this protein's phosphorylation status (43).

Theoretically, UBE3A disruption could cause mental retardation and seizures of AS at many cellular sites. Ubiquitin processes have been implicated in axonal guidance (47) and synapse development (48) although UBE3A per se has not yet been implicated in such events.

ACKNOWLEDGMENTS

Funding for this work was supported in part by the Raymond C. Philips Research and Education Unit, Department of Children and Family Services, State of Florida.

REFERENCES

1. Angelman H. "Puppet" children: a report on three cases. Dev Med Child Neurol 1965; 7:681–688.

2. Jiang Y, Lev-Lehman E, Bressler J, Tsai TF, Beaudet AL. Genetics of Angelman syndrome. Am J Hum Genet 1999; 65(1):1–6.

3. Mann MR, Bartolomei MS. Towards a molecular understanding of Prader–Willi and Angelman syndromes. Hum Mol Genet 1999; 8(10):1867–1873.

4. Clayton-Smith J, Laan L. Angelman syndrome: a review of the clinical and genetic aspects. J Med Genet 2003; 40(2):87–95.

5. Steffenburg S, Gillberg CL, Steffenburg U, Kyllerman M. Autism in Angelman syndrome: a population-based study. Pediatr Neurol 1996; 14(2):131–136.

6. Petersen MB, Brondum-Nielsen K, Hansen LK, Wulff K. Clinical, cytogenetic, and molecular diagnosis of Angelman syndrome: estimated prevalence rate in a Danish county. Am J Med Genet 1995; 60(3):261–262.

7. Vercesi AM, Carvalho MR, Aguiar MJ, Pena SD. Prevalence of Prader–Willi and Angelman syndromes among mentally retarded boys in Brazil. J Med Genet 1999; 36(6):498.

8. Aquino NH, Bastos E, Fonseca LC, Llerena JC Jr. Angelman syndrome methylation screening of 15q11–q13 in institutionalized individuals with severe mental retardation. Genet Test 2002; 6(2):129–131.

9. Jacobsen J, King BH, Leventhal BL, Christian SL, Ledbetter DH, Cook EH Jr. Molecular screening for proximal 15q abnormalities in a mentally retarded population. J Med Genet 1998; 35(7): 534–538.

10. Buckley RH, Dinno N, Weber P. Angelman syndrome: are the estimates too low? Am J Med Genet 1998; 80(4):385–390.

11. Williams CA, Angelman H, Clayton-Smith J, Driscoll DJ, Hendrickson JE, Knoll JH, Magenis RE, Schinzel A, Wagstaff J, Whidden EM, et al. Angelman syndrome: consensus for diagnostic criteria. Angelman Syndrome Foundation. Am J Med Genet 1995; 56(2):237–238.

12. Fryburg JS, Breg WR, Lindgren V. Diagnosis of Angelman syndrome in infants. Am J Med Genet 1991; 38(1):58–64.

13. King RA, Wiesner GL, Townsend D, White JG. Hypopigmentation in Angelman syndrome. Am J Med Genet 1993; 46(1):40–44.

14. Boyd SG, Harden A, Patton MA. The EEG in early diagnosis of the Angelman (happy puppet) syndrome. Eur J Pediatr 1988; 147(5):508–513.

15. Laan LA, Renier WO, Arts WF, Buntinx IM, vd Burgt IJ, Stroink H, Beuten J, Zwinderman KH, van Dijk JG, Brouwer OF. Evolution of epilepsy and EEG findings in Angelman syndrome. Epilepsia 1997; 38(2):195–199.

16. Kishino T, Lalande M, Wagstaff J. UBE3A/E6-AP mutations cause Angelman syndrome [published erratum appears in Nat Genet 1997; 15(4):411]. Nat Genet 1997; 15(1):70–73.

17. Matsuura T, Sutcliffe JS, Fang P, Galjaard RJ, Jiang YH, Benton CS, Rommens JM, Beaudet AL. De novo truncating mutations in E6-AP ubiquitin-protein ligase gene (UBE3A) in Angelman syndrome. Nat Genet 1997; 15(1):74–77.

18. Rougeulle C, Glatt H, Lalande M. The Angelman syndrome candidate gene, UBE3A/E6-AP, is imprinted in brain [letter]. Nat Genet 1997; 17(1):14–15.

19. Albrecht U, Sutcliffe JS, Cattanach BM, Beechey CV, Armstrong D, Eichele G, Beaudet AL. Imprinted expression of the murine Angelman syndrome gene, UBE3A, in hippocampal and Purkinje neurons. Nat Genet 1997; 17(1):75–78.

20. Runte M, Huttenhofer A, Gross S, Kiefmann M, Horsthemke B, Buiting K. The IC–SNURF–SNRPN transcript serves as a host for multiple small nucleolar RNA species and as an antisense RNA for UBE3A. Hum Mol Genet 2001; 10(23):2687–2700.

21. Perk J, Makedonski K, Lande L, Cedar H, Razin A, Shemer R. The imprinting mechanism of the Prader–Willi/Angelman regional control center. EMBO J 2002; 21(21):5807–5814.

22. Nicholls RD, Knepper JL. Genome organization, function, and imprinting in Prader–Willi and Angelman syndromes. Annu Rev Genomics Hum Genet 2001; 2:153–175.

23. Pujana MA, Nadal M, Guitart M, Armengol L, Gratacos M, Estivill X. Human chromosome 15q11–q14 regions of rearrangements contain clusters of LCR15 duplicons. Eur J Hum Genet 2002; 10(1):26–35.

24. Pujana MA, Nadal M, Gratacos M, Peral B, Csiszar K, Gonzalez-Sarmiento R, Sumoy L, Estivill X. Additional complexity on human chromosome 15q: identification of a set of newly recognized duplicons (LCR15) on 15q11–q13, 15q24, and 15q26. Genome Res 2001; 11(1):98–111.

25. Amos-Landgraf JM, Ji Y, Gottlieb W, Depinet T, Wandstrat AE, Cassidy SB, Driscoll DJ, Rogan PK, Schwartz S, Nicholls RD. Chromosome breakage in the Prader–Willi and Angelman syndromes involves recombination between large, transcribed

repeats at proximal and distal breakpoints. Am J Hum Genet 1999; 65(2):370–386.

26. Christian SL, Fantes JA, Mewborn SK, Huang B, Ledbetter DH. Large genomic duplicons map to sites of instability in the Prader–Willi/Angelman syndrome chromosome region (15q11–q13). Hum Mol Genet 1999; 8(6):1025–1037.

27. Gimelli G, Pujana MA, Patricelli MG, Russo S, Giardino D, Larizza L, Cheung J, Armengol L, Schinzel A, Estivill X, Zuffardi O. Genomic inversions of human chromosome 15q11–q13 in mothers of Angelman syndrome patients with class II (BP2/3) deletions. Hum Mol Genet 2003; 12(8):849–858.

28. Robinson WP, Christian SL, Kuchinka BD, Penaherrera MS, Das S, Schuffenhauer S, Malcolm S, Schinzel AA, Hassold TJ, Ledbetter DH. Somatic segregation errors predominantly contribute to the gain or loss of a paternal chromosome leading to uniparental disomy for chromosome 15. Clin Genet 2000; 57(5):349–358.

29. Buiting K, Gross S, Lich C, Gillessen-Kaesbach G, El-Maarri O, Horsthemke B. Epimutations in Prader–Willi and Angelman syndromes: a molecular study of 136 patients with an imprinting defect. Am J Hum Genet 2003; 72(3):571–577.

30. Lossie AC, Whitney MM, Amidon D, Dong HJ, Chen P, Theriaque D, Hutson A, Nicholls RD, Zori RT, Williams CA, Driscoll DJ. Distinct phenotypes distinguish the molecular classes of Angelman syndrome. J Med Genet 2001; 38(12): 834–845.

31. Tekin M, Jackson-Cook C, Buller A, Ferreira-Gonzalez A, Pandya A, Garrett CT, Bodurtha J. Fluorescence in situ hybridization detectable mosaicism for Angelman syndrome with biparental methylation. Am J Med Genet 2000; 95(2):145–149.

32. Williams CA, Lossie A, Driscoll D. Angelman syndrome: mimicking conditions and phenotypes. Am J Med Genet 2001; 101(1):59–64.

33. Stalker HJ, Williams CA. Genetic counseling in Angelman syndrome: the challenges of multiple causes [see comments]. Am J Med Genet 1998; 77(1):54–59.

34. Yamamoto Y, Huibregtse JM, Howley PM. The human E6-AP gene (UBE3A) encodes three potential protein isoforms generated by differential splicing. Genomics 1997; 41(2):263–266.

35. Kishino T, Wagstaff J. Genomic organization of the UBE3A/E6-AP gene and related pseudogenes. Genomics 1998; 47(1):101–107.

36. Scheffner M, Huibregtse JM, Vierstra RD, Howley PM. The HPV-16 E6 and E6-AP complex functions as a ubiquitin-protein ligase in the ubiquitination of p53. Cell 1993; 75(3):495–505.

37. Huibregtse JM, Scheffner M, Beaudenon S, Howley PM. A family of proteins structurally and functionally related to the E6-AP ubiquitin-protein ligase. Proc Natl Acad Sci USA 1995; 92(7):2563–2567.

38. Scheffner M, Nuber U, Huibregtse JM. Protein ubiquitination involving an E1–E2–E3 enzyme ubiquitin thioester cascade. Nature 1995; 373(6509):81–83.

39. Ciechanover A. The ubiquitin–proteasome proteolytic pathway. Cell 1994; 79(1):13–21.

40. Verdecia MA, Joazeiro CA, Wells NJ, Ferrer JL, Bowman ME, Hunter T, Noel JP. Conformational flexibility underlies ubiquitin ligation mediated by the WWP1 HECT domain E3 ligase. Mol Cell 2003; 11(1):249–259.

41. Malzac P, Webber H, Moncla A, Graham JM, Kukolich M, Williams C, Pagon RA, Ramsdell LA, Kishino T, Wagstaff J. Mutation analysis of UBE3A in Angelman syndrome patients. Am J Hum Genet 1998; 62(6):1353–1360.

42. Conaway RC, Brower CS, Conaway JW. Emerging roles of ubiquitin in transcription regulation. Science 2002; 296(5571):1254–1258.

43. Miura K, Kishino T, Li E, Webber H, Dikkes P, Holmes GL, Wagstaff J. Neurobehavioral and electroencephalographic abnormalities in UBE3A maternal-deficient mice. Neurobiol Dis 2002; 9(2):149–159.

44. Oda H, Kumar S, Howley PM. Regulation of the Src family tyrosine kinase Blk through E6AP-mediated ubiquitination. Proc Natl Acad Sci USA 1999; 96(17):9557–9562.

45. Kumar S, Talis AL, Howley PM. Identification of HHR23A as a substrate for E6-associated protein-mediated ubiquitination. J Biol Chem 1999; 274(26):18785–18792.

46. Jiang YH, Armstrong D, Albrecht U, Atkins CM, Noebels JL, Eichele G, Sweatt JD, Beaudet AL. Mutation of the Angelman ubiquitin ligase in mice causes increased cytoplasmic p53 and deficits of contextual learning and long-term potentiation [see comments]. Neuron 1998; 21(4):799–811.

47. Murphey RK, Godenschwege TA. New roles for ubiquitin in the assembly and function of neuronal circuits. Neuron 2002; 36(1):5–8.

48. Hegde AN, DiAntonio A. Ubiquitin and the synapse. Nat Rev Neurosci 2002; 3(11):854–861.

11

Williams–Beuren Syndrome

HUI ZHANG

Department of Genetics, Yale University
School of Medicine, New Haven,
Connecticut, U.S.A.

BARBARA POBER

Department of Pediatrics,
MassGeneral Hospital for Children,
and Department of Surgery, Division
of Genetics, Children's Hospital,
Boston, Massachusetts, U.S.A.

**CHERYL KLAIMAN and
ROBERT SCHULTZ**

Child Study Center, Yale University
School of Medicine, New Haven,
Connecticut, U.S.A.

I. INTRODUCTION

In 1961, Williams et al. (1) recognized that individuals with supravalvular aortic stenosis (SVAS), unusual facial features, growth retardation and mental "subnormality" constituted a distinct clinical entity. Shortly, thereafter, Beuren et al. (2) independently described this condition expanding the phenotype to include other vascular stenoses, dental anomalies, and

---

Drs. Zhang and Klaiman contributed equally in the preparation of this Chapter.

a friendly personality. It has now been recognized that this condition, Williams syndrome, or Williams–Beuren syndrome (WBS), is caused by a microdeletion of chromosome 7 surrounding the elastin gene (3), which results in a characteristic developmental disability associated with a distinct facies and a constellation of medical problems. A clinical diagnosis of WBS can be confirmed by a laboratory test, fluorescent in situ hybridization (FISH), which reveals a submicroscopic deletion on the long arm of chromosome 7.

The reported incidence of WBS is between 1/10,000 and 20,000 (4,5), but this number may increase now that an accurate diagnostic tool is available. Although relatively rare, WBS has become increasingly well known in both professional and lay circles for its distinctive cognitive, personality, and behavior profiles. Williams–Beuren syndrome may present during infancy with characteristic physical features, cardiovascular problems, hypercalcemia, and/or failure to thrive. Diagnosis of WBS in older children is most often made during a workup for developmental delay. Recognition of WBS in adults frequently results from caregiver-referral following increased public awareness of this condition.

This chapter begins with a review of the medical and cognitive profiles of WBS, is followed by a discussion of the genetic etiology of WBS, and ends with some practical recommendations for medical monitoring, educational, and vocational support.

II. MEDICAL PROFILE

Patients with WBS can have many distinctive physical features and medical problems; fortunately, no single patient will have all the potential problems listed below. The frequency of certain problems is well known whereas the frequency of other problems is less clear, either due to inadequate study or under ascertainment. Listed below are the most important medical problems found in WBS.

Characteristic facial features are an invariant component of WBS, though the degree of dysmorphology varies among individuals, as well as over time in the same individual (6,7).

The key features of the WBS facial "gestalt" among infants and children include periorbital fullness, stellate or starburst irides among blue-eyed individuals, short up-turned nose, long philtrum, macrostomia, flat facial profile, full lower cheeks, and a small chin. Over time some coarsening of facial features occurs (Fig. 1).

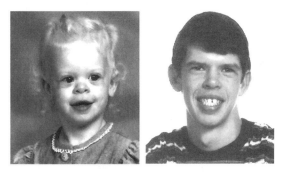

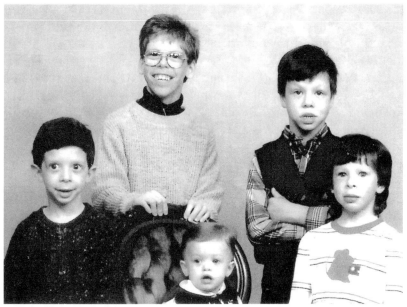

Figure 1 Frontal views of several individuals (2-year-old-female, 18-year-old-male, group picture at different ages) with Williams–Beuren syndrome.

Intrauterine growth retardation occurs in a significant proportion of WBS individuals (8). Mean growth rates of WBS children are below normal by 1–2 cm/year in the first few years of life (9). Syndrome-specific growth rate curves for WBS reveal a premature and abbreviated pubertal growth spurt in both sexes (9). These factors contribute to a final adult height in WBS that typically falls in the low range of normal adult height (7,8).

Cardiovascular disease occurs in 75–80% of WBS individuals (6,7). A recent study detected cardiovascular disease in only 53% of the 75 WBS individuals studied (10); this decreased prevalence may reflect ascertainment of WBS individuals with milder phenotypes due to more accurate diagnostic testing. The hallmark of WBS vascular disease is a generalized arteriopathy that can lead to discrete and/or diffuse arterial stenoses (11); this pathology often suggests the diagnosis of WBS. The single most common lesion is SVAS, which can be found in isolation or in conjunction with other vascular stenoses. Central or peripheral pulmonary artery stenoses are the second most common type of cardiovascular involvement (10,12,13). Stenoses of other vessels such as thoracic and abdominal aorta (14), renal, mesenteric, and/or coronary arteries are observed though the true frequency of such stenoses is unknown. Pulmonary stenoses are likely to improve spontaneously with time (15), but as many as 39% of all cardiovascular lesions require surgical intervention (10). This generalized arteriopathy significantly increases the risk of hypertension in WBS individuals, which is life long, and may be progressive. Hypertension is noted in 40–60% of the WBS individuals (16,17), some of whom require treatment with antihypertensive medications.

Arteriopathy of the coronary arteries and severe biventricular outflow tract obstruction in WBS individuals may result in sudden death by causing myocardial ischemia, decreased cardiac output, and/or arrhythmia (18–20). Most of the reported sudden death cases occurred perioperatively, while a few cases occurred unprecipitated in ambulatory settings. Though the true risk of sudden death in WBS is unknown, exposure to anesthetic agents seems to increase this risk (18–20). Ischemic stroke is another serious complication of the arteriopathy if it involves intracranial arteries (21).

A highly characteristic constellation of oral and dental problems is present in WBS. This includes small, widely spaced teeth, malocclusions, persistent tongue thrust, and absence of one or more teeth (22). One recent study finds 40.5% of the WBS individuals had agenesis of one or more permanent teeth and 11.9% had agenesis of six permanent teeth or more (23).

Virtually all WBS children suffer from hyperacusis (heightened sensitivity to certain sounds). This can be very disruptive and anxiety provoking especially in younger children. The common offending sounds include firecrackers, motorcycles, thunder, vacuum cleaners, and sirens (24). Recurrent otitis media occurs more frequently among WBS children than normal controls (7,24). More recently, hearing loss, specifically, high frequency sensorineural hearing loss has been noted as a common problem in WBS adults (25,26).

Aside from the stellate irides, the main ophthalmologic finding in WBS is strabismus, typically esotropia, which occurs in more than half of the individuals (27,28). Vision disturbance is generally limited to hyperopia and presbyopia in adults. Development of cataract at a young age has also been reported (28,29).

Musculoskeletal problems are extremely common in WBS and may evolve with time. During infancy and childhood, hypotonia and joint laxity are more prominent, whereas contractures of the large and small joints, as well as spinal abnormalities can develop in adolescence and adulthood (16,30,31). Kyphosis, scoliosis, and lordosis have all been observed, and may worsen with time if untreated. However, severe spinal abnormalities necessitating surgery are uncommon. Radioulnar synostosis is found in 5–25% of the WBS individuals (32,33).

Gastrointestinal problems are common in both children and adults with WBS. Young infants are frequently colicky and have feeding difficulties (71%); these may contribute to failure to thrive in some of the WBS infants (7). Gastroesophageal reflux and constipation occur in almost half of the infants (7) and many WBS infants and young children experience textured food intolerance. Constipation can continue to be a problem throughout childhood while in the adult WBS population, the most frequent gastrointestinal problems are constipation, abdominal pain, and diverticular diseases (16). Chronic constipation can be complicated by rectal prolapse, hemorrhoids, and increases the risk of diverticulosis and diverticulitis; therefore, it requires aggressive ongoing medical management. Celiac disease may be another contributing factor to gastrointestinal problems in WBS. Biopsy-proven celiac disease has been reported in 6 of 63 WBS children all of whom were treated successfully with a gluten free diet (34).

Among the endocrine problems WBS individuals may experience, hypercalcemia is the most frequently discussed. The true incidence of hypercalcemia is not known, as hypercalcemia is most often asymptomatic. The highest risk period for hypercalcemia appears to be during infancy and when present, it may cause irritability, poor feeding, vomiting, constipation, and failure to thrive (35). However, the risk of hypercalcemia persists throughout childhood into adult life, though of a lesser magnitude. Hypercalciuria can be present in the absence of hypercalcemia, and increases the risk of nephrocalcinosis (7). The etiology of abnormal calcium metabolism in WBS continues to evade our knowledge (36).

Other endocrine problems that may manifest in WBS individuals include early puberty, hypothyroidism, and glucose intolerance/diabetes mellitus. One study found that puberty in WBS occurred 2 years earlier than in published population controls (37). A more recent study confirms that the average menarcheal age in WBS girls is 11.5, one and a half years younger than that of the contemporary normal controls (38). This is consistent with the early onset growth spurt observed in both sexes (9). In the same study, central precocious puberty (defined as thelarche before the 8th birthday and/or menarche before the 9th birthday) was found in 17 (18.3%) of the 86 WBS girls; 5 of them received treatment with a gonadotropin-releasing hormone agonist. Hypothyroidism has been reported in children with WBS (39). We have observed clinical or subclinical hypothyroidism in ~20% of our WBS population which indicates that periodic monitoring of thyroid function is required (40). Case reports mentioning diabetes mellitus in adults with WBS exist (7,31,41–43). In our experience, in addition to the small percent of WBS adults with clinical diabetes, the majority have abnormal glucose tolerance on standard oral glucose tolerance testing, which may progress to diabetes (26,44).

Structural abnormalities of the kidney such as solitary, duplicated, hypoplasic, or scarred kidney have been identified on ultrasonography in 15–20% of the WBS individuals (45,46). Nephrocalcinosis is identified in a small percent of the WBS individuals, presumably secondary to hypercalcemia. Structural abnormalities of the kidneys and/or ureters may contribute to recurrent urinary tract infections occasionally seen in WBS adults (16,31). Renal failure has been reported in a few cases possibly as a result of nephrocalcinosis, renal dysplasia, recurrent infections, and/or renal artery stenosis (47–50). Voiding frequency and urinary incontinence are the most common genitourinary problems in WBS, present in half of the individuals (7). One study documented bladder diverticuli and abnormal detrusor contraction in more than one-third of the individuals with such symptoms (51).

Neurological findings in infants and young children are generally normal save for hypotonia. Hypertonia, hyperreflexia, gait and fine motor disturbances have been noted in a high percentage of older children and adults with WBS (52,53). We have also found signs of cerebellar dysfunction such as impairment of oculomotor control, dysmetria, dysdiadokinesis, limb and gait ataxia in WBS adults (54). Chiari malformation type I has been reported in both children and adults with WBS (30,55,56).

WBS individuals are often described as having "soft" skin and concerns have been raised whether their skin prematurely ages (3). The majority of the WBS adults have premature graying of the hair (16), which can occur as early as 16 years (BP personal observation). These findings and the earlier than expected onset of other medical findings (such as early puberty, high frequency sensorineural hearing loss, diabetes, and cataracts) raise the question whether mild premature aging is a component of the natural clinical course for WBS.

III. COGNITIVE AND BEHAVIORAL FEATURES

A. Cognitive Profiles

Most individuals with WBS function in the mild-to-moderate ranges of mental retardation, with a mean IQ in the 50–60 range. However, the FSIQ range is broad with a subgroup of individuals who score in the borderline to low average ranges of intelligence (IQ scores 70–90). Individuals with WBS tend to do better on tests of vocabulary and verbal abstract reasoning, but poorer on tests of general knowledge, memory for digits, numeracy, and visual sequencing (57). Studies of IQ stability over time have resulted in contradictory results, with studies finding both increases and decreases over time (58–60). Dykens et al. (61) suggest that conflicting IQ findings may be a result of the different aspects of cognition in WBS with variable developmental trajectories.

Individuals with WBS have uneven cognitive profiles such that overall IQ scores may be misleading. Typically, individuals with WBS show slightly better developed verbal than nonverbal reasoning abilities (57); when averaged out to provide an overall IQ score, such discrepancies are masked. An area of strength typically includes auditory short-term memory. Compared with chronological (CA) and mental-aged (MA)-matched individuals with Down syndrome, individuals with WBS can recall significantly longer strings of digits (62,63) as well as verbal items (63). In fact, in one study (62), 65% of children with WBS scored in the typical range on the digit recall subtest of the Differential Abilities Scale (DAS).

Areas of weakness in individuals with WBS include visual–spatial functioning, perceptual planning, and fine motor control. With regard to visual–spatial functioning, individuals with WBS show profound impairments in visual–spatial tasks such as long-term visual–spatial memory tasks (64), and construction and puzzle tests. Individuals with WBS are less able than CA and MA-matched individuals to copy two- to four-piece block designs, suggesting poor motor planning, spatial orientation, and eye-hand coordination (61,65). With regard to perceptual planning and fine motor control, individuals with WBS show weaknesses on standardized drawing tests, such as the Developmental Test of Visual-Motor Integration (VMI) (66); as well as freeform drawing tasks, typically scoring lower than MA- or CA-matched comparison groups (62,67–69). Many individuals with WBS draw disorganized, disjointed depictions of objects, such as a bicycle or an elephant (67–70), though improvements are found with practice and age (71). In addition, individuals with WBS also have difficulty in the basic academic areas of reading, spelling, and mathematics. Often persons with WBS reach only about the 7–8 age year level in these areas (57).

B. Language Profiles

Most young children with WBS have delays in the acquisition of language and in early speech (72). The median age for first words is about 2 years, and for first sentences, is about 3 years (73). Despite the slow start, over time, gains are made in some areas. One area of relative strength for individuals with WBS is in their basic vocabulary skills or lexicon. Early studies showed that relative to others as well as to their own abilities, individuals with WBS excel in the extent of their word knowledge (74,75); however, more recent research on a large cohort of children and adolescents with WBS studied with the Peabody Picture Vocabulary Test-Revised (PPVT-R) (76) found an average score of 66, indicating overall mild levels of delay for the group.

With regard to syntax and grammar, some research suggests strengths whereas other work indicates these skills are impaired. For instance, specific difficulties have been found in gender assignment, past tense, and agreement among people and number (77,78). Semantics, the meaning and organization of words, also show conflicting results. Bellugi et al. (70), on a word fluency test, found that adolescents and adults with WBS produced more unusual words than MA-matched controls. They concluded that high rates of low-frequency words suggest an unusual or atypical semantic organization in WBS. However, Volterra et al. (79) and Scott et al. (80) found no differences in word fluency test performance among children with WBS and MA-matched controls.

A consistent area of strength is in linguistic affect. The language of individuals with WBS is permeated with affect, both in prosody and narrative enrichment techniques (70,75). Linguistic affect and a hyperverbal conversational style (81) may contribute to the positive social interactions observed in individuals with WBS.

C. Additional Strengths

Facial recognition and a fascination with faces are considered defining features of individuals with WBS (70,82). Even in infancy, individuals with WBS seem extremely attentive to the faces of others (83). People with WBS perform significantly better on the Benton Test of Facial Recognition (84) than do MA-matched controls, in which people must match a stimulus face to several choices presented under different light and angle conditions (85,86). In addition, on Theory of Mind tasks, specifically inferring the intentions and goals of others using the direction of eye-gaze, individuals with WBS do better than those with Prader–Willi syndrome, befitting their socially oriented, empathic personalities (87–89).

Another area of reported strength is in musical talents, including singing, playing instruments, and recognizing songs. It is unclear, however, how representative these findings are. In a study comparing 36 children with WBS to those with Down syndrome, Dykens et al. (61) found that both groups enjoyed listening to music or singing, but that people with WBS were more likely to play an instrument. The musical abilities in individuals with WBS do not seem to be related to IQ, nor does it have a savant quality (90). Musical rhythm was assessed in an echo clapping task on a small selected WBS and control group, and the two groups performed similarly, with the same low rate of errors. However, when children with WBS made errors, they produced creative embellishments or extensions of the reference rhythm; hence individuals with WBS were more likely to improvise. One recent study suggested that persons with WBS may have different neural organization with regard to processing music (91). While listening to music, individuals with WBS showed less activation on fMRI scanning in specific areas of the temporal lobe compared to age-matched controls; however, they activated a wider set of neural structures, recruiting portions of the amygdala, cerebellum, and brain stem.

D. Adaptive Profiles

Adaptive behavior is defined on the basis of day-to-day activities necessary to take care of oneself and to get along with others. It is measured in terms of typical performance rather than the potential ability of the individual—what a person actually does as opposed to what a person is capable of doing. Children with WBS show relative strengths in adaptive behavior around communication and socialization and relative weaknesses in daily living skills (92). On average, adaptive behavior scores fall slightly below IQ scores indicating moderate levels of adaptive delay for the group as a whole (92). Adults with WBS show conflicting patterns of adaptive skills. Some studies indicate relative strengths in communication and relative weakness in personal self-care (41), others show significantly higher socialization skills and significantly lower communication skills. Overall, adaptive behavior age-equivalents in this adult sample were around a 6-year age level, indicating impaired ability to use their intellectual aptitudes within a general social context. Other data suggest that about 75–80% of adults live at home with their parents (31,93) and most are enrolled in supervised vocational, recreational, or continuing educational programs.

E. Behavioral and Personality Profiles

Beuren et al. (2) first described that individuals with WBS "all have the same kind of friendly nature, they love everyone, are loved by everyone, and are very charming" (see Ref. 2, p. 472). This friendly and charming image has persisted through the literature; however, these labels can be misleading at times. These basic attributes simplify a more complicated personality and behavioral picture. Many individuals with WBS experience significant externalizing and internalizing difficulties that impede their day-to-day functioning.

1. Externalizing Behaviors

The most common behavioral difficulty exhibited by individuals with WBS seems to be attentional, as most children with WBS have hyperactivity and attention problems (82, 94–96). The attentional problems tend to peak in childhood and are less common among adults (93,97). Gosch and Pankau (97) reported difficulties sitting still in 64% of 48 children younger than 10 years of age and in only 19% of 27 adults ages 20 years and older. Unlike this manifestation of hyperactivity, difficulties sustaining attention seem to persist in the adult years, with 90% of 70 adults showing distractibility (98). High rates of other externalizing behaviors have been shown in several studies (87,93,95–100). These behaviors include attention-seeking, disobedience, and temper tantrums. Severe aggression, fighting, or destroying property are uncommon. Compared with typically developing children, children with WBS show higher activity, more negative moods, less persistence, lower adaptability, and greater impulsivity in their approach to others (101).

Additional maladaptive behaviors observed in individuals with WBS also prevent them from achieving better functional outcomes. Checklist data suggest increased difficulties regulating bodily states, increased frequency of socially uninhibited behaviors (97), and vulnerability to exploitation (61). Davies et al. (98) found that 59% of adults in their sample were physically over-demonstrative, including touching, hugging, and kissing others. Further, 10% of the sample reported to the police that they had been sexually assaulted, and an additional 10% made allegations of assault that were not reported to the police. Clearly, the personalities of individuals with WBS place them at increased risk for being taken advantage of by others.

2. Internalizing Behaviors

Most older children and adults with WBS experience significant problems with anxiety (102), greater than those with other developmental disabilities (59,87,99,103). They typically show a high baseline of generalized anxiety as well as specific phobias (104). The baseline level of anxiety differs between persons but can also wax and wane over time in a single individual. Anxiety can be sufficiently intense and negatively impact quality of life requiring treatment with counseling and/or medication.

An increased frequency of other psychiatric disorders such as depression, obsessive compulsive symptoms, phobias, panic attacks, and post-traumatic stress disorder have been observed in our cohort of adult WBS patients (Pober, personal communication, 2003). Sensory-based stimuli, such as sensitivity to sounds, seem to trigger considerable anxiety in individuals with WBS. Unanticipated environmental changes can also be a cause of extreme anxiety. Our pilot work using the startle response paradigm (L. Mayes, personal communication, 2003) is showing an extreme increase in startle responses in persons with WBS compared to individuals with typical development as well as mental-aged-matched controls. In addition to anxiety, many persons with WBS, especially as they age into adolescence and adulthood, have unsatisfactory peer relations resulting in loneliness (105). A majority of individuals with WBS are very socially isolated from others their own age (93).

3. Other Behaviors

As mentioned earlier, almost all individuals with WBS show hypersensitivity to certain sounds (24,106). A small portion of individuals with WBS seem to outgrow auditory hyperacusis (24), but most continue to be sensitive enough to be able to detect a specific sound in a noisy environment (106).

F. Neurological Profiles

Using magnetic resonance imaging techniques, several studies have shown global cerebral tissue reduction in individuals with WBS (by about 15% compared to typical controls), as well as reductions in specific brain regions (50), such as the right occipital lobe and brainstem (107). Other brain areas, however, such as the amygdala and hippocampus (108,109), the cerebellum (70), the superior temporal gyrus (107), and the volume of the frontal cortex are similar to typically developing controls. It is hypothesized that the relative sparing of the frontal cortex and neocerebellar structures may be associated with the linguistic competencies seen in individuals with WBS while the sparing of the limbic system and amygdala may underlie strengths in facial processing and affect recognition (110,111). Functional MRI studies are beginning to show that brain regions supporting face recognition demonstrate normal patterns of activation among persons with WBS (111). Finally, there are now two reports (112,113) finding that the dorsal extension of the central sulcus, in both hemispheres, is significantly less developed, not reaching the interhemispheric fissure in WBS as compared to low and normal IQ controls. The clinical significance of this finding is not known.

Event-related potentials (ERPs) allow the examination of electrical brain activity that is time locked to stimulus events or higher cognitive events. ERP studies of WBS have shown unique markers for certain aspects of language functioning and face perception processes (114,115). The patterns of electrical activity distinguish people with WBS from typical controls, suggesting that distinct neural systems underlie different cognitive processes in persons with WBS.

IV. GENETICS

The cause of WBS remained unknown until the early 1990s when unequivocal evidence of monozygotic twin concordance for WBS and parent-to-child transmission of WBS were presented (116–118). These findings indicated that although WBS occurs sporadically in most instances, it is genetically caused, and can be transmitted in an autosomal dominant manner. One of the characteristic features of WBS, SVAS, is by itself an autosomal dominant trait and is referred to as familial SVAS (119–121). Identical vascular pathology showing abnormal elastic fiber architecture is seen in familial SVAS and WBS (122). Molecular genetic techniques demonstrated that familial SVAS is caused by disruption of the elastin gene located on chromosome 7 (123–125). This finding was the springboard for the discovery that one copy of the elastin gene is deleted in individuals with WBS (3). Deletion of the elastin gene occurs in greater than 95% of the individuals with a clinical diagnosis of typical WBS (126–128). Further physical and genetic mapping revealed that WBS actually is a "contiguous gene deletion" or "microdeletion" syndrome on the long arm of chromosome 7 (7q11.23). Specifically, WBS is caused by a common deletion of 1.5 million base pairs of DNA extending far beyond the elastin gene and involving loss of as many as 17 nearby genes (Fig. 2) (129–132). This commonly deleted region is referred to as the WBS critical region. Since the common deletion is below the threshold detectable by conventional cytogenetic banding techniques, it requires the specialized technique, FISH, to

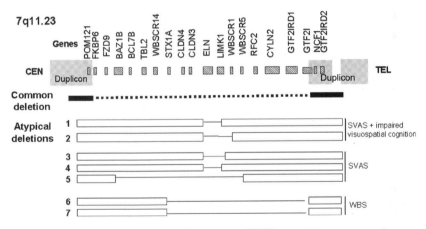

Figure 2 A map of the Williams or Williams–Beuren syndrome (WBS) critical region on human chromosome 7q11.23 adapted from Osborne in 1999 (136). The orientations of the map are indicated by CEN for centromeric, and TEL for telomeric. The hatched boxes indicate the locations of the genes in the regions (not drawn to scale), and the names of the genes are illustrated above the boxes. The large gray boxes symbolize the duplicons, the thick dotted line indicates the size of the common deletion, and the thin straight lines indicate the atypical deletions. The references of the atypical deletions can be found in the text. (From Ref. 136.)

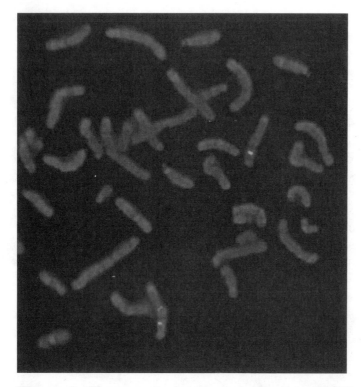

Figure 3 Fluorescence in situ hybridization (FISH) using the elastin probe (red color) from the 7q11.23 chromosome band and a control probe from 7q31 (green color) showing the absence of the elastin signal in the deleted chromosome 7 (at upper right) from an individual with Williams–Beuren syndrome. (*See color insert.*)

confirm its presence (Fig. 3). This deletion occurs with equal frequency on the maternally or paternally inherited chromosome 7 (129,133,134). As seen in other microdeletion syndromes, susceptibility to the WBS deletion is caused by DNA duplications (duplicons) that are flanking the deleted region with the duplicons containing highly homologous DNA sequences of genes and pseudogenes (135–137). Specifically, these homologous sequences predispose the intervening WBS region to misalignment and unequal crossing-over during DNA replication, which in turn can result in the common deletion responsible for WBS. These duplicons also predispose to a much rarer genetic phenomenon, inversion of the WBS critical region; this has been observed in individuals with a subset of the WBS phenotypes, as well as in phenotypically normal parents of children with the typical WBS deletion (138). Finally, a few cases with "atypical" deletions (e.g., smaller than the 1.5 million base pair common deletion) have been reported (139–141). The genetic mechanism predisposing to these atypical deletions is not known.

Loss of one copy of the elastin gene (ELN) has been unequivocally linked to the WBS cardiovascular phenotype. It is far less clear how many other deleted genes are important in WBS pathogenesis. Table 1 lists currently identified genes and their recognized functions in the WBS critical region; and though a comprehensive description of all known deleted genes (135,136) is beyond the scope of this chapter, several of the genes that have already been implicated in the WBS phenotype will be briefly discussed. The putative role of genes in the pathogenesis of the WBS phenotype has been gleaned from individuals and families with "atypical" deletions involving the WBS critical region and/or experimental animal studies.

The elastin gene encodes the protein tropoelastin that assembles on a scaffold of microfibrils into elastic fibers. These fibers are the major component of elastic tissues such as the lung, the arterial vessels, the epiglottis, and the skin. Multiple lines of evidence indicate that loss of normal elastin protein production is responsible for the cardiovascular phenotypes of WBS. Analysis of mice that have both copies of the elastin gene disrupted (so called homozygous knockout) has subendothelial smooth muscle cell accumulation, which eventually leads to obliteration of the vascular lumen (178,179). Heterozygous knockout mice (with only one copy of the elastin gene disrupted) have increased number of elastic lamellae and smooth muscle rings similar to findings in the aorta of human SVAS and WBS patients. Several authors speculate that inadequate elastin may also contribute to other connective tissue abnormalities seen in WBS including premature sagging of skin, hoarse voice, hernia, and diverticuli of the colon and bladder.

Table 1 Genes in the Williams–Beuren Syndrome Critical Region

Gene	Protein product	Function/putative function	Reference
POM121	Pore membrane protein of the nuclear envelope	Nuclear pore complex assembly	(142)
FKBP6	FK506 binding protein 6	FK506 binding protein class of immunophillins, essential for homologous chromosome pairing during male meiosis and male fertility	(143,144)
FZD9	Frizzled 9	Member of the seven-transmembrane-receptor family for WNT proteins. Upon binding to Wnt2 and Wnt8 ligand, activates β-catenin pathway	(145–147)
BAZ1B/WBSCR9/WSTF	Bromodomain adjacent zinc finger 1B/WBS critical region 9/Williams syndrome transcription factor	Contains PHD (Plant homeodomain) finger and bromodomain, participates in ATP-dependent chromatin-remodeling. Overexpression of WSTF restores the impaired recruitment of vitamin D receptor to vitamin D regulated promoters in fibroblasts from WBS patients	(148–151)
BCL7B	B-cell lymphoma 7B	Member of a protein family involved in translocation in Burkitt's lymphoma. Also found as atopy-related IgE autoantigen	(131,152,153)
TBL2/WS-βTRP	Transducin β-like 2/Williams syndrome β transducin repeat protein	Contains putative transducin (WD40) repeats. Unknown function	(131,154)

WBSCR14/WS-bHLH	WBS critical region 14/Williams syndrome basic helix–loop–helix protein	Basic helix–loop–helix leucine zipper transcription factor of the Myc/Max/Mad superfamily. Heterodimerizes with Mlx to cause transcription repression	(131,155)
STX1A	Syntaxin 1A	Part of a trimeric complex at the presynaptic membrane which mediates exocytosis of neurotransmitter-containing vesicles	(130)
CLDN4 and CLDN3	*Clostridium perfringens* enterotoxin receptors 1 and 2	Members of the claudin family of transmembrane proteins, essential components of intercellular tight junction structures that regulate paracellular ion flux	(156,157)
ELN	Elastin	Main component of the elastic tissue, crucial role in arterial development	(3)
LIMK1	LIM kinase 1	LIM domain containing protein that regulates actin filament dynamics, important for neuronal synaptic function	(139,158–160)
EIF4H/WBSCR1	Eukaryotic initiation factor 4H/WBS critical region 1	Part of the eukaryotic translation initiation complex, facilitates the function of eIF4A, an RNA helicase	(159,161)
WBSCR5/NTAL	WBS critical region 5/Non-T-cell activation linker	A transmembrane adaptor protein involved in immunoreceptor signaling	(162,163)

(Continued)

Table 1   Genes in the Williams–Beuren Syndrome Critical Region (*Continued*)

Gene	Protein product	Function/putative function	Reference
RFC2	Replication factor C subunit 2	Third-largest subunit of the replication factor C (RF-C) complex, an auxiliary factor for DNA polymerases delta and Epsilon. RFC2 is important for both DNA replication and checkpoint function	(159,164–166)
CYLN2	Cytoplasmic linker protein, CLIP-115	Mediates interaction between cell organelles and microtubules, important for organelle shape, localization, and translocation	(159,167)
GTF2IRD1 /WBSCR11/ CREAM1/ MusTRD/BEN	GTF2I-related domain 1/WBS critical region 11	Member of the transcription factor TFII-I family	(168–172)
GTF2I	TFII-I, transcription factor II, subunit I	Functions in both basal and inducible transcription, also involved in chromatin structure remodeling	(173–175)
NCF1	Neutrophilic cytosolic factor 1, p47-phox	Component of phagocyte NADPH oxidase. Homozygous mutation causes autosomal recessive chronic granulomatous disease (CGD)	(176)

Adapted from review by Osborne (136). Several other novel genes have been identified in the WBS critical region which are not included in this table (177).

Impaired visuospatial constructive cognition similar to that seen in WBS was observed in patients who had only SVAS and normal intelligence. These patients carried a very small deletion in the WBS critical region involving loss of only ELN and its immediate neighboring gene LIMK1 (139). The authors proposed that loss of one copy of LIMK1 results in the impaired visuospatial construction found in WBS. The LIMK1 gene encodes LIM-kinase1 protein which is highly expressed in neurons and accumulates at high levels at mature synapses; the protein regulates actin filament dynamics and is a key component of a network that connects extracellular stimuli to changes in cytoskeletal structure. Mice with homozygous knockout of LIMK1 had abnormal synaptic function and altered fear responses and spatial learning (180) providing additional tantalizing evidence for the role of LMK1 in visuospatial construction. However, in another report, three other SVAS patients whose deletion included LIMK1 in addition to ELN did not have visuospatial impairment (141). One of these three patients had a deletion that included all but the three most telomeric genes in the WBS region, CYLN2, GTF2IRD1, and GTF2-I, but had none of the WBS phenotype except for SVAS. This suggests that these three telomeric genes may be responsible for most of the WBS phenotype. This assumption is further supported by the report of two WBS individuals with typical or classical WBS features who harbored smaller deletions that included all the telomeric genes but not STX1A and the genes centromeric to it (140).

The CYLN2 gene encodes CLIP-115, a cytoplasmic linker protein (CLIP), that mediates interaction between cell organelles and microtubules which are important for cell organelle shape, intracellular localization, and translocation (181). CLIP-115 is most abundantly expressed in the brain. Disruption of the Cyln2 gene in mice results in mild growth deficiency, increased brain ventricle volume, and decreased corpus callosum size, hippocampal dysfunction, and impaired motor coordination (167). These findings strongly implicate deletion of CYLN2 in the cognitive and neurological phenotypes of WBS.

Another gene that is highly expressed in the central nervous system, Syntaxin 1A (STX1A), codes for a protein that is one member of a multicomponent complex responsible for neurotransmitter release (182,183). Loss of another component of this complex results in hyperactivity in mice. Whether loss of one copy of STX1A has a similar effect thus contributing to attention deficit/hyperactivity seen in WBS individuals remains to be determined.

GTF2I is the most telomeric gene in the WBS critical region and codes for TFII-I, which functions as part of the basal transcription machinery, as well as an inducible transcription factor that regulates the expression of other genes (174). TFII-I is involved in histone deacetylation and chromatin structure remodeling (175,185,186). Although TFII-I is expressed ubiquitously (186), its function may be dosage sensitive only in certain tissues such as the brain. The multifaceted ability of TFII-I with effects on multiple down-steam target genes makes it a likely candidate responsible for some aspects of the WBS phenotype.

Immediately adjacent to GTF2I resides a structurally and functionally related gene GTF2IRD1 (WBSCR11, CREAM1, MusTRD1, BEN) which encodes a transcription factor in the TFII-I family (169–172). The role of loss of one copy of GTF2IRD1 in the pathogenesis of the WBS phenotype is unclear as a transgenic mouse model with homozygous disruption of this gene has a normal life span without any striking morphological or behavioral abnormalities despite greatly reduced expression of Gtf2ird1 mRNA (187). However, a combined deletion of both GTF2IRD1 and GTF2I may affect the regulation of developmental programs differently than loss of only one of these genes at a time (175).

V. PRACTICAL IMPLICATIONS

The diagnosis of WBS, based on clinical criteria, can be confirmed by FISH testing using a probe for the elastin gene. More than 95% of the WBS individuals have a submicroscopic deletion detectable by this FISH test. Individuals with clinical features of WBS and a negative FISH test should be referred to a clinical geneticist for further evaluation (either for consideration of other diagnoses or for research genetic testing to determine if an atypically sized deletion is present).

Comprehensive medical monitoring guidelines for WBS individuals have recently been published (Table 2) by the American Academy of Pediatrics (188). Upon confirmation of a diagnosis of WBS, the patient should receive baseline evaluation of all systems that may be affected including cardiovascular, renal, hearing, vision, endocrine, and neurological. The family should receive counseling regarding the medical, developmental, and genetic aspects of the condition. Addressing growth and feeding issues plays a prominent part of management during infancy. Multivitamin preparations containing vitamin D should not be prescribed as this may potentiate hypercalcemia. Lifelong cardiovascular monitoring including blood pressure determinations is indicated in WBS individuals even if the initial evaluation is normal. Any procedure requiring anesthesia should be preceded by a careful evaluation of the anesthesia risk particular to WBS individuals. Hearing, vision, and dental problems require appropriate referrals and follow up. Musculoskeltal problems should be addressed with early intervention programs and routine physical therapies. Aggressive management of constipation is necessary for quality of life and prevention of more complicated gastrointestinal problems. Calcium metabolism should be monitored by periodically evaluating serum and urine calcium levels; any abnormality should prompt further evaluation of calcium regulatory hormones. The issue of early menarche may need to be addressed in very delayed young girls with WBS; in selected cases, pharmacologic intervention to defer menses should be discussed with an endocrinologist. Thyroid function and glucose metabolism are other endocrine issues that require continued monitoring, the latter especially in adulthood. Sufficiently frequent findings of genitourinary structural and functional abnormalities necessitate baseline assessment and regular monitoring of this organ system. Likewise, the high prevalence of abnormal neurological findings and the risk of stroke and symptomatic Chiari malformation

Table 2 Medical Problems in Williams–Beuren Syndrome[a]—by Organ System and Age

Gene	Incidence (%)[a]	Infancy	Childhood	Adult
Oscular and visual				
Esotropia	50	X		
Hyperopia	50		X	X
Auditory				
Chronic otitis media	50	X	X	
Hypersensitivity to sound	90	X	X	X
Dental				
Malocclusion	85		X	X
Microdontia	95		X	X
Cardiovascular				
Any abnormality	80	X	X	X
SVAS	75	X	X	X
SVPS	25	X	X	X
PPS	50	X		
Renal artery stenosis	45	X	X	X
Other arterial stenosis	20		X	X
VSD	10	X		
Hypertension	50		X	X
Genitourinary				
Structural anomaly	20	X	X	X
Enuresis	50		X	
Nephrocalcinosis	<5	X	X	X
Recurrent urinary tract infections	30			X
Gastrointestinal				
Feeding difficulties	70	X	X	
Constipation	40	X	X	X
Colon diverticula	30		X	X
Rectal prolapse	15	X	X	
Integument				
Soft lax skin	90	X	X	X
Inguinal hernia	40	X		
Umbilical hernia	50	X		
Premature gray hair	90			X
Musculoskeletal				
Joint hypermobility	90	X	X	
Joint contractures	50	X	X	X

(Continued)

Table 2 *(Continued)*

Gene	Incidence (%)[a]	Infancy	Childhood	Adult
Radioulnar synostosis	20	X	X	X
Kyphosis	20			X
Lordosis	40		X	X
Awkward gait	60		X	X
Calcium				
Hypercalcemia	15	X		X
Hypercalciuria	30	X	X	X
Endocrine				
Hypothyroidism	2	X	X	X
Early puberty (but rarely true precocious puberty)	50		X	
Diabetes mellitus	15			X
Obesity	30			X
Neurologic				
Hyperactive deep tendon reflexes	75		X	X
Chiari I malformation	10	X	X	X
Hypotonia (central)	80	X	X	
Hypertonia (peripheral)	50		X	X
Cognitive				
Developmental delay	95	X	X	
Mental retardation	75		X	X
Borderline intellectual functioning	20		X	X
Normal intelligence	5		X	X
Impaired visuospatial constructive cognition	95		X	X
Behavioral				
Attention-deficit hyperactivity disorder	70		X	
Generalized anxiety disorder	80		X	X

[a]Percentages based on the following: (1) review of rates of complications in several reports of series of patients with Williams syndrome, and (2) database of 315 children and adults with Williams syndrome evaluated by Colleen A. Morris, MD. SVAS indicates supravalvular aortic stenosis; SVPS, supravalvular pulmonic stenosis; PPS, peripheral pulmonary artery stenosis; and VSD, ventricular septal defect.
Source: Ref. 188.

warrant that the primary caregiver performs ongoing neurological examinations and makes prompt referral for further evaluation for any acute changes in neurological status.

VI. EDUCATIONAL AND VOCATIONAL INTERVENTIONS

Specific therapeutic interventions should target language difficulties, visual-motor difficulties and maladaptive behaviors to enable individuals with WBS to live up to their potentials. Most individuals with WBS require special educational services throughout their schooling. These interventions can run the spectrum from resource room pull-out services to a fully segregated special educational setting. Regardless of the setting, additional services should include speech and language therapy, occupational therapy, physical therapy, and counseling services. Speech and language therapy is recommended for essentially all children with WBS (7,189,190) due to language delays and other language difficulties. Further, speech therapists can use language strengths as a means to increase performance in other areas, such as with some of the visual–spatial difficulties. Occupational therapy services can help remediate some of the visual-motor difficulties, as well as some of the hypersensitivities. However, it is the maladaptive behaviors, including anxieties and fears, distractibility, impulsivity, resistance to change and vulnerabilities that create unstable and stressful conditions in the families of individuals with WBS that are the most important to receive services for. Counseling as well as psychopharmacologic treatments are useful therapeutic modalities.

REFERENCES

1. Williams JC, Barratt-Boyes BG, Lowe JB. Supravalvular aortic stenosis. Circulation 1961; 24:1311–1318.

2. Beuren AJ, Apitz J, Harmjanz D. Supravalvular aortic stenosis in association with mental retardation and certain facial appearance. Circulation 1962; 26:1235–1240.

3. Ewart AK, Morris CA, Atkinson D, Jin W, Sternes K, Spallone P, Stock AD, Leppert M, Keating MT. Hemizygosity at the elastin locus in a developmental disorder, Williams syndrome. Nat Genet 1993; 5(1):11–16.

4. Greenberg F. Williams syndrome professional symposium. Am J Med Genet 1990; 6(suppl):89–96.

5. Grimm T, Wesselhoeft H. Zur Genetik des Williams–Beuren-Syndroms und der Ioslierten Form der Supravalvularen Aortenstenose Untensuchungenvon 128 Familien. Z Kardiol 1980; 69:168–172.

6. Burn J. Williams syndrome. J Med Genet 1986; 23(5):389–395.

7. Morris CA, Demsey SA, Leonard CO, Dilts C, Blackburn BL. Natural history of Williams syndrome: physical characteristics. J Pediatr 1988; 113(2):318–326.

8. Pankau R, Partsch CJ, Gosch A, Oppermann HC, Wessel A. Statural growth in Williams–Beuren syndrome. Eur J Pediatr 1992; 151(10):751–755.

9. Partsch CJ, Dreyer G, Gosch A, Winter M, Schneppenheim R, Wessel A, Pankau R. Longitudinal evaluation of growth, puberty, and bone maturation in children with Williams syndrome. J Pediatr 1999; 134(1):82–89.

10. Eronen M, Peippo M, Hiippala A, Raatikka M, Arivo M, Johansson R, Kahkonen M. Cardiovascular manifestations in 75 patients with Williams syndrome. J Med Genet 2002; 39(8):554–558.

11. Rein AJ, Preminger TJ, Perry SB, Lock JE, Sanders SP. Generalized arteriopathy in Williams syndrome: an intravascular ultrasound study. J Am Coll Cardiol 1993; 21(7): 1727–1730.

12. Hallidie-Smith KA, Karas S. Cardiac anomalies in Williams–Beuren syndrome. Arch Dis Child 1988; 63(7):809–813.

13. Zalzstein E, Moes CA, Musewe NN, Freedom RM. Spectrum of cardiovascular anomalies in Williams–Beuren syndrome. Pediatr Cardiol 1991; 12(4):219–223.

14. Rose C, Wessel A, Pankau R, Partsch CJ, Bursch J. Anomalies of the abdominal aorta in Williams–Beuren syndrome-another

cause of arterial hypertension. Eur J Pediatr 2001; 160(11): 655–658.

15. Giddins NG, Finley JP, Nanton MA, Roy DL. The natural course of supravalvular aortic stenosis and peripheral pulmonary artery stenosis in Williams's syndrome. Br Heart J 1989; 62(4):315–319.

16. Morris CÅ, Leonard CO, Dilts C, Demsey SA. Adults with Williams syndrome. Am J Med Genet 1990; 6:102–107.

17. Broder K, Reinhardt E, Ahern J, Lifton R, Tamborlane W, Pober BR. Elevated ambulatory blood pressure in 20 subjects with Williams syndrome. Am J Med Genet 1999; 83(5): 356–360.

18. Kececioglu D, Kotthoff S, Vogt J. Williams–Beuren syndrome: a 30–year follow-up of natural and postoperative course. Eur Heart J 1993; 14(11):1458–1464.

19. Bird LM, Billman GF, Lacro RV, Spicer RL, Jariwala LK, Hoyme HE, Zamora-Salinas R, Morris C, Viskochil D, Frikke MJ, Jones MC. Sudden death in Williams syndrome: report of ten cases. J Pediatr 1996; 129(6):926–931.

20. Horowitz PE, Akhtar S, Wulff JA, Fadley F, Halees Z. Coronary artery disease and anesthesia-related death in children with Williams syndrome. J Cardiothorac Vasc Anesth 2002; 16(6):739–741.

21. Soper R, Chaloupka JC, Fayad PB, Greally JM, Shaywitz BA, Awad IA, Pober BR. Ischemic stroke and intracranial multifocal cerebral arteriopathy in Williams syndrome. J Pediatr 1995; 126(6):945–948.

22. Hertzberg J, Nakisbendi L, Needleman HL, Pober BR. Williams syndrome—oral presentation of 45 cases. Pediatr Dent 1994; 16(4):262–267.

23. Axelsson S, Bjornland T, Kjaer I, Heiberg A, Storhaug K. Dental characteristics in Williams syndrome: a clinical and radiographic evaluation. Acta Odontol Scand 2003; 61(3): 129–136.

24. Klein AJ, Armstrong BL, Greer MK, Brown FR III. Hyperacusis and otitis media in individuals with Williams syndrome. J Speech Hear Disord 1990; 55(2):339–344.

25. Johnson LB, Comeau M, Clarke KD. Hyperacusis in Williams syndrome. J Otolaryngol 2001; 30(2):90–92.

26. Pober BR, Wang E, Morgan T. Abnormal glucose tolerance and sensorineural hearing loss in adults with William syndrome. Long Beach, CA: Ninth International Professional Conference on Williams Syndrome, 2002.

27. Greenberg F, Lewis RA. The Williams syndrome. Spectrum and significance of ocular features. Ophthalmology 1988; 95(12):1608–1612.

28. Winter M, Pankau R, Amm M, Gosch A, Wessel A. The spectrum of ocular features in the Williams–Beuren syndrome. Clin Genet 1996; 49(1):28–31.

29. Knudtzon J, Aksnes L, Akslen LA, Aarskog D. Elevated 1,25-dihydroxyvitamin D and normocalcaemia in presumed familial Williams syndrome. Clin Genet 1987; 32(6):369–374.

30. Kaplan P, Kirschner M, Watters G, Costa MT. Contractures in patients with Williams syndrome. Pediatrics 1989; 84(5): 895–899.

31. Lopez-Rangel E, Maurice M, McGillivray B, Friedman JM. Williams syndrome in adults. Am J Med Genet 1992; 44(6): 720–729.

32. Charvat KA, Hornstein L, Oestreich AE. Radio-ulnar synostosis in Williams syndrome. A frequently associated anomaly. Pediatr Radiol 1991; 21(7):508–510.

33. Bzduch V. Radioulnar synostosis in Williams syndrome: a historical overview. Am J Med Genet 1994; 50(4):386.

34. Giannotti A, Tiberio G, Castro M, Virgilii F, Colistro F, Ferretti F, Digilio MC, Gambarara M, Dallapiccola B. Coeliac disease in Williams syndrome. J Med Genet 2001; 38(11): 767–768.

35. Martin MD, Snodgrass GJ, Cohen RD. Idiopathic infantile hypercalcaemia—a continuing enigma. Arch Dis Child 1984; 59(7):605–613.

36. Kruse K, Pankau R, Gosch A, Wohlfahrt K. Calcium metabolism in Williams–Beuren syndrome. J Pediatr 1992; 121(6): 902–907.

37. Cherniske EM, Sadler LS, Schwartz D, Carpenter TO, Pober BR. Early puberty in Williams syndrome. Clin Dysmorphol 1999; 8(2):117–121.

38. Partsch CJ, Japing I, Siebert R, Gosch A, Wessel A, Sippell WG, Pankau R. Central precocious puberty in girls with Williams syndrome. J Pediatr 2002; 141(3):441–444.

39. Cammareri V, Vignati G, Nocera G, Beck-Peccoz P, Persani L. Thyroid hemiagenesis and elevated thyrotropin levels in a child with Williams syndrome. Am J Med Genet 1999; 85(5): 491–494.

40. Pober BR, Carpenter TO, Breault D. Prevalence of hypothyroidism and compensated hypothyroidism in Williams syndrome. In: Twenty First David W. Smith Workshop on Malformation and Morphogenesis, La Jolla, CA, 2000.

41. Plissart L, Borghgraef M, Volcke P, Van den Berghe H, Fryns JP. Adults with Williams–Beuren syndrome: evaluation of the medical, psychological and behavioral aspects. Clin Genet 1994; 46(2):161–167.

42. Imashuku S, Hayashi S, Kuriyama K, Hibi S, Tabata Y, Todo S. Sudden death of a 21-year-old female with Williams syndrome showing rare complications. Pediatr Int 2000; 42(3):322–324.

43. Nakaji A, Kawame Y, Nagai C, Iwata M. [Clinical features of a senior patient with Williams syndrome]. Rinsho Shinkeigaku 2001; 41(9):592–598.

44. Pober BR, Wang E, Petersen K, Osborne LR, Caprio S. Impaired glucose tolerance in Williams syndrome. Am J Hum Genet 2001; 69(4):302A.

45. Pober BR, Lacro RV, Rice C, Mandell V, Teele RL. Renal findings in 40 individuals with Williams syndrome. Am J Med Genet 1993; 46(3):271–274.

46. Pankau R, Partsch CJ, Winter M, Gosch A, Wessel A. Incidence and spectrum of renal abnormalities in Williams–Beuren syndrome. Am J Med Genet 1996; 63(1):301–304.

47. Biesecker LG, Laxova R, Friedman A. Renal insufficiency in Williams syndrome. Am J Med Genet 1987; 28(1):131–135.

48. Steiger MJ, Rowe PA, Innes A, Burden RP. Williams syndrome and renal failure. Lancet 1988; 2(8614):804.

49. Ichinose M, Tojo K, Nakamura K, Matsuda H, Tokudome G, Ohta M, Sakai S, Sakai O. Williams syndrome associated with chronic renal failure and various endocrinological abnormalities. Intern Med 1996; 35(6):482–488.

50. Davies M, Howlin P, Udwin O. Independence and adaptive behavior in adults with Williams syndrome. Am J Med Genet 1997; 70(2):188–195.

51. Schulman SL, Zderic S, Kaplan P. Increased prevalence of urinary symptoms and voiding dysfunction in Williams syndrome. J Pediatr 1996; 129(3):466–469.

52. Chapman CA, du Plessis A, Pober BR. Neurologic findings in children and adults with Williams syndrome. J Child Neurol 1996; 11(1):63–65.

53. Trauner DA, Bellugi U, Chase C. Neurologic features of Williams and Down syndromes. Pediatr Neurol 1989; 5(3): 166–168.

54. Pober BR, Szekely A. Distinct neurological profile in Williams syndrome. Am J Hum Genet 1999; 65(4):367A.

55. Pober BR, Filiano JJ. Association of Chiari I malformation and Williams syndrome. Pediatr Neurol 1995; 12(1):84–88.

56. Wang PP, Hesselink JR, Jernigan TL, Doherty S, Bellugi U. Specific neurobehavioral profile of Williams' syndrome is associated with neocerebellar hemispheric preservation. Neurology 1992; 42(10):1999–2002.

57. Howlin P, Davies M, Udwin O. Cognitive functioning in adults with Williams syndrome. J Child Psychol Psych Allied Discipl 1998; 39:183–189.

58. Crisco JJ. Rate of cognitive development in young children with Williams syndrome. Clin Res 1990; 38:536A.

59. Gosch A, Pankau R. Longitudinal study of the cognitive development in children with Williams–Beuren syndrome. Am J Med Genet 1996; 61:26–29.

60. Udwin O, Davies M, Howlin P. A longitudinal study of cognitive abilities and educational attainment in Williams syndrome. Dev Med Child Neurol 1996; 38:1020–1029.

61. Dykens E, Hodapp RM, Finucane BM. Genetics and Mental Retardation Syndromes: a New Look at Behavior and Interventions. Baltimore, MD: Paul H. Brookes, 2000.

62. Mervis CB, Robinson BF, Pani JR. Visuospatial construction. Am J Hum Genet 1999; 65:1222–1229.

63. Wang PP, Bellugi U. Evidence from two genetic syndromes for a dissociation between verbal and visual–spatial short-term memory. J Clin Exp Neuropsychol 1994; 16:317–322.

64. Vicari S, Brizzolara D, Carlesimo GA, Pezzini G, Volterra V. Memory abilities in children with Williams syndrome. Cortex 1996; 32:503–514.

65. Farran EK, Jarrold C, Gathercole SE. Block design performance in the Williams syndrome phenotype: a problem with mental imagery? J Child Psychol Psych Allied Discipl 2001; 42:719–728.

66. Berry KE. Revised Administration, Scoring, and Teaching Manual for the Developmental Test of Visual-Motor Integration. Cleveland, OH: Modern Curriculum Press, 1982.

67. Bellugi U, Sabo H, Vaid V. Spatial defects in children with Williams syndrome. In: Bellugi U, ed. Spatial Cognition: Brain Bases and Development. Hillsdale, NJ: Lawrence Erlbaum Associates, 1988:273–298.

68. Bertrand J, Mervis CB, Eisenberg JD. Drawing by children with Williams syndrome: a developmental perspective. Dev Neuropsychol 1997; 13:41–67.

69. Wang PP, Doherty S, Rourke SB, Bellugi U. Unique profile of visuo-perceptual skills in a genetic syndrome. Brain Cognition 1995; 29:54–65.

70. Bellugi U, Wang PP, Jernigan TL. Williams syndrome: an unusual neuropsychological profile. In: Grafman J, ed. Atypical Cognitive Deficits in Developmental Disorders: Implications for Brain Function. Hillsdale, NJ: Erlbaum, 1994:23–56.

71. Bertrand J, Mervis CB. Longitudinal analysis of drawings by children with Williams syndrome: preliminary results. Visual Arts Res 1996; 22:19–34.

72. Jarrold C, Baddeley AD, Hewes AK. Verbal and nonverbal abilities in the Williams syndrome phenotype: evidence for diverging developmental trajectories. J Child Psychol Psych Allied Discipl 1998; 39:511–523.

73. Semel E, Rosner SR. The behavioral characteristics of children with Williams syndrome: analysis of the Utah survey. Report Presented to a Meeting of the Laboratory for Language and Cognition. La Jolla, CA: Salk Institute, 1991.

74. Bellugi U, Marks S, Bihrle A, Sabo H. Dissociation between language and cognitive functions in Williams syndrome. In: Mogford K, ed. Language Development in Exceptional Circumstances. London: Churchill Livingstone, 1988:171–189.

75. Reilly J, Klima ES, Bellugi U. Once more with feeling: affect and language in atypical populations. Dev Psychopathol 1990; 2:367–391.

76. Dunn LM, Dunn LM. Peabody Picture Vocabulary Test—Revised. Circle Pines, MN: American Guidance Service, 1981.

77. Karmiloff-Smith A, Grant J, Berthoud I, Davies M, Howlin P, Udwin O. Language and Williams syndrome: how intact is "intact"? Child Dev 1997; 68:246–262.

78. Kataria S, Goldstein DJ, Kushnick T. Developmental delays in Williams ("elfin facies") syndrome. Appl Res Ment Retard 1981; 5:419–423.

79. Volterra V, Capirci O, Pezzini G, Sabbadini L, Vicari S. Linguistic abilities in Italian children with Williams syndrome. Cortex 1996; 32:663–677.

80. Scott P, Mervis CB, Bertrand J, Klein BP, Armstrong SC, Ford AJ. Semantic organization and word fluency in 9- and 10-year-old children with Williams syndrome. Genet Counsel 1995; 6:172–173.

81. Udwin O, Yule W. Expressive language of children with Williams syndrome. Am J Med Genet Suppl 1990; 6:108–114.

82. Udwin O, Yule W. A cognitive and behavioural phenotype in Williams syndrome. J Clin Exp Neuropsychol 1991; 13: 232–244.

83. Mervis CB, Bertrand J. Developmental relations between cognition and language: evidence from Williams syndrome. In: Romski MA, ed. Research on Communication and Language Disorders: Contributions to Theories of Language Development. Baltimore, MA: Brookes, 1997:75–106.

84. Benton AL, Hamsher KS, Varney NR, Spreen O. Contributions to Neuropsychological Assessment. New York: Oxford University Press, 1983.

85. Gagliardi C, Frigerio E, Burt DM, Cazzaniga I, Perrett DI, Borgatti R. Facial expression recognition in Williams syndrome. Neuropsychologia 2003; 41:733–738.

86. Pezzini G, Vicari S, Volterra V, Milani L, Ossella MT. Children with Williams syndrome: is there a single neuropsychological profile? Dev Neuropsychol 1999; 15:141–155.

87. Dykens EM, Rosner BA. Refining behavioral phenotypes: personality-motivation in Williams and Prader–Willi syndromes. Am J Ment Retard 1999; 104:158–169.

88. Karmiloff-Smith A, Klima ES, Bellugi U, Grant J, Baron-Cohen S. Is there a social module? Language, face processing, and theory of mind in individuals with Williams syndrome. J Cognitive Neurosci 1998; 7:196–208.

89. Tager-Flusberg H, Boshart J, Baron-Cohen S. Reading the windows to the soul: evidence of domain-specific sparing in Williams syndrome. J Cognitive Neurosci 1998; 10:631–639.

90. Lenhoff HM, Perales O, Hickok G. Absolute pitch in Williams syndrome. Music Perception 2001; 18:491–503.

91. Levitin DJ, Menon V, Schmitt JE, Eliez S, White CD, Glover GH, Kadis J, Korenberg JR, Bellugi U, Reiss AL. Neural correlates of auditory perception in Williams syndrome: an fMRI study. Neuroimage 2003; 18:74–82.

92. Greer MK, Brown FR III, Pai GS, Choudry SH, Klein AJ. Cognitive, adaptive, and behavioral characteristics of Williams syndrome [comment]. Am J Med Genet 1997; 74: 521–525.

93. Udwin O. A survey of adults with Williams syndrome and idiopathic infantile hypercalcaemia. Dev Med Child Neurol 1990; 32:129–141.

94. Pagon RA, Bennett FC, LaVeck B, Stewart KB, Johnson J. Williams syndrome: features in late childhood and adolescence. Pediatrics 1987; 80:85–91.

95. Dilts CV, Morris C, Leonard CO. Hypothesis for development of a behavioral phenotype in Williams syndrome. Am J Med Genet 1990; 6:126–131.

96. Gosch A, Pankau R. Social—emotional and behavioral adjustment in children with Williams—Beuren syndrome. Am J Med Genet 1994; 53.

97. Gosch A, Pankau R. Personality characteristics and behaviour problems in individuals of different ages with Williams syndrome. Dev Med Child Neurol 1997; 39:527–533.

98. Davies M, Udwin O, Howlin P. Adults with Williams syndrome. Preliminary study of social, emotional and behavioural difficulties [comment]. Brit J Psychiat 1998; 172:273–276.

99. Einfeld SL, Tonge BJ, Florio T. Behavioral and emotional disturbance in individuals with Williams syndrome. Am J Ment Retard 1997; 102:45–53.

100. Udwin O, Yule W, Martin N. Cognitive abilities and behavioural characteristics of children with idiopathic infantile hypercalcaemia. J Child Psychol Psychiat 1987; 28:297–309.

101. Tomc SA, Williamson NK, Pauli RA. Temperament in Williams syndrome. Am J Med Genet 1990; 36:345–352.

102. Bregman J. Social, affective, and behavioral impairments in Williams syndrome. Paper Presented at the Seventh International Professional Conference on Williams Syndrome. King of Prussia, PA, 1996.

103. Sarimski K. Behavioural phenotypes and family stress in three mental retardation syndromes. Euro Child Adol Psychiat 1997; 6:26–31.

104. Levine K, Wharton R. Williams syndrome and happiness. Am J Ment Retard 2002; 105:363–371.

105. Udwin O, Howlin P, Davies M, Mannion E. Community care for adults with Williams syndrome: how families cope and the availability of support networks. J Intellect Disability Res 1992; 42:238–245.

106. Van Borsel J, Curfs L, Fryns JP. Hyperacusis in Williams syndrome: a sample survey study. Genet Counsel 1997; 8: 121–126.

107. Reiss AL, Eliez S, Schmitt JE, Straus E, Lai Z, Jones W, Bellugi U. IV. Neuroanatomy of Williams syndrome: a high-resolution MRI study. J Cognitive Neurosci 2000; 12(suppl 1): 65–73.

108. Galaburda A, Wang PP, Bellugi U, Rosen M. Cytoarchitectronic findings in a genetically-based disorder: Williams syndrome Neuroreport 5, 1994.

109. Jernigan TL, Bellugi U, Sowell E, Doherty S, Hesselink J. Cerebral morphologic distinctions between Williams and Down syndromes. Arch Neurol 1993; 50:186–191.

110. Baron-Cohen S, Ring H. A model of the mindreading system: neuropsychological and neurobiological perspectives. In: Lewis C, ed. Origins of an Understanding of Mind. Hillsdale, NJ: Erlbaum, 1994.

111. Schultz RT, Grelotti DJ, Pober BR. Genetics of childhood disorders: XXVI. Williams syndrome and brain–behavior relationships. J Am Acad Child Adolesc Psychiat 2001; 40: 606–609.

112. Jackowski AP, Schultz RT. Foreshortened dorsal extension of the central sulcus in Williams syndrome. Cortex. In press.

113. Galaburda AM, Schmitt JE, Atlas SW, Eliez S, Bellugi U, Reiss AL. Dorsal forebrain anomaly in Williams syndrome. Arch Neurol 2001; 58:1865–1869.

114. Mills DL, Alvarez TD, St George M, Appelbaum LG, Bellugi U, Neville H III. Electrophysiological studies of face processing in Williams syndrome. J Cognitive Neurosci 2000; 12(suppl 1): 47–64.

115. Neville HJ, Mills DL, Bellugi U. Effects of altered auditory sensitivity and age of language acquisition on the development of language-relevant neural systems: preliminary

studies of Williams syndrome. In: Grafman J, ed. Atypical Cognitive Deficits in Developmental Disorders: Implications for Brain Function. Hillsdale, NJ: Erlbaum, 1994:67–83.

116. Murphy MB, Greenberg F, Wilson G, Hughes M, DiLiberti J. Williams syndrome in twins. Am J Med Genet Suppl 1990; 6: 97–99.

117. Morris CA, Thomas IT, Greenberg F. Williams syndrome: autosomal dominant inheritance. Am J Med Genet 1993; 47(4):478–481.

118. Sadler LS, Robinson LK, Verdaasdonk KR, Gingell R. The Williams syndrome: evidence for possible autosomal dominant inheritance. Am J Med Genet 1993; 47(4):468–470.

119. Schmidt MA, Ensing GJ, Michels VV, Carter GA, Hagler DJ, Feldt RH. Autosomal dominant supravalvular aortic stenosis: large three-generation family. Am J Med Genet 1989; 32(3): 384–389.

120. Eisenberg R, Young D, Jacobson B, Boito A. Familial supravalvular aortic stenosis. Am J Dis Children 1964; 108: 341–347.

121. Merritt DA, Palmar CG, Lurie PR, Petry EL. Supravalvular aortic stenosis: genetic and clinical studies. J Lab Clin Med 1963; 62:995.

122. O'Connor WN, Davis JB Jr, Geissler R, Cottrill CM, Noonan JA, Todd EP. Supravalvular aortic stenosis. Clinical and pathologic observations in six patients. Arch Pathol Lab Med 1985; 109(2):179–185.

123. Ewart AK, Morris CA, Ensing GJ, Loker J, Moore C, Leppert M, Keating M. A human vascular disorder, supravalvular aortic stenosis, maps to chromosome 7. Proc Natl Acad Sci USA 1993; 90(8):3226–3230.

124. Olson TM, Michels VV, Lindor NM, Pastores GM, Weber JL, Schaid DJ, Driscoll DJ, Feldt RH, Thibodeau SN. Autosomal dominant supravalvular aortic stenosis: localization to chromosome 7. Hum Mol Genet 1993; 2(7):869–873.

125. Curran ME, Atkinson DL, Ewart AK, Morris CA, Leppert MF, Keating MT. The elastin gene is disrupted by a translocation

associated with supravalvular aortic stenosis. Cell 1993; 73(1):
159–168.

126. Nickerson E, Greenberg F, Keating MT, McCaskill C, Shaffer LG.
     Deletions of the elastin gene at 7q11.23 occur in approximately
     90% of patients with Williams syndrome. Am J Hum Genet
     1995; 56(5):1156–1161.

127. Lowery MC, Morris CA, Ewart A, Brothman LJ, Zhu XL,
     Leonard CO, Carey JC, Keating M, Brothman AR. Strong
     correlation of elastin deletions, detected by FISH, with
     Williams syndrome: evaluation of 235 patients. Am J Hum
     Genet 1995; 57(1):49–53.

128. Mari A, Amati F, Mingarelli R, Giannotti A, Sebastio G,
     Colloridi V, Novelli G, Dallapiccola B. Analysis of the elastin
     gene in 60 patients with clinical diagnosis of Williams
     syndrome. Hum Genet 1995; 96(4):444–448.

129. Perez Jurado LA, Peoples R, Kaplan P, Hamel BC, Francke
     U. Molecular definition of the chromosome 7 deletion in Wil-
     liams syndrome and parent-of-origin effects on growth. Am J
     Hum Genet 1996; 59(4):781–792.

130. Osborne LR, Soder S, Shi XM, Pober BR, Costa T, Scherer
     SW, Tsui LC. Hemizygous deletion of the syntaxin 1A gene
     in individuals with Williams syndrome. Am J Hum Genet
     1997; 61(2):449–452.

131. Meng X, Lu X, Li Z, Green ED, Massa H, Trask BJ, Morris
     CA, Keating MT. Complete physical map of the common
     deletion region in Williams syndrome and identification and
     characterization of three novel genes. Hum Genet 1998;
     103(5):590–599.

132. Wu YQ, Sutton VR, Nickerson E, Lupski JR, Potocki L,
     Korenberg JR, Greenberg F, Tassabehji M, Shaffer LG. Deli-
     neation of the common critical region in Williams syndrome
     and clinical correlation of growth, heart defects, ethnicity,
     and parental origin. Am J Med Genet 1998; 78(1):82–89.

133. Dutly F, Schinzel A. Unequal interchromosomal rearrange-
     ments may result in elastin gene deletions causing the
     Williams–Beuren syndrome. Hum Mol Genet 1996; 5(12):
     1893–1898.

134. Urban Z, Helms C, Fekete G, Csiszar K, Bonnet D, Munnich A, Donis-Keller H, Boyd CD. 7q11.23 deletions in Williams syndrome arise as a consequence of unequal meiotic crossover. Am J Hum Genet 1996; 59(4):958–962.

135. Francke U. Williams–Beuren syndrome: genes and mechanisms. Hum Mol Genet 1999; 8(10):1947–1954.

136. Osborne LR. Williams–Beuren syndrome: unraveling the mysteries of a microdeletion disorder. Mol Genet Metab 1999; 67(1):1–10.

137. Peoples R, Franke Y, Wang YK, Perez-Jurado L, Paperna T, Cisco M, Francke U. A physical map, including a BAC/PAC clone contig, of the Williams–Beuren syndrome—deletion region at 7q11.23. Am J Hum Genet 2000; 66(1):47–68.

138. Osborne LR, Li M, Pober BR, Chitayat D, Bodurtha J, Mandel A, Costa T, Grebe T, Cox S, Tsui LC, Scherer SW. A 1.5 million-base pair inversion polymorphism in families with Williams–Beuren syndrome. Nat Genet 2001; 29(3): 321–325.

139. Frangiskakis JM, Ewart AK, Morris CA, Mervis CB, Bertrand J, Robinson BF, Klein BP, Ensing GJ, Everett LA, Green ED, Proschel C, Gutowski NJ, Noble M, Atkinson DL, Odelberg SJ, Keating MT. LIM-kinase1 hemizygosity implicated in impaired visuospatial constructive cognition. Cell 1996; 86(1):59–69.

140. Botta A, Novelli G, Mari A, Novelli A, Sabani M, Korenberg J, Osbourne LR, Digilio MC, Giannotti A, Dallapiccola B. Detection of an atypical 7q11.23 deletion in Williams syndrome patients which does not include the STX1A and FZD3 genes. J Med Genet 1999; 36(6):478–480.

141. Tassabehji M, Metcalfe K, Karmiloff-Smith A, Carette MJ, Grant J, Dennis N, Reardon W, Splitt M, Read AP, Donnai D. Williams syndrome: use of chromosomal microdeletions as a tool to dissect cognitive and physical phenotypes. Am J Hum Genet 1999; 64(1):118–125.

142. Bodoor K, Shaikh S, Enarson P, Chowdhury S, Salina D, Raharjo WH, Burke B. Function and assembly of nuclear pore complex proteins. Biochem Cell Biol 1999; 77(4):321–329.

143. Crackower MA, Kolas NK, Noguchi J, Sarao R, Kikuchi K, Kaneko H, Kobayashi E, Kawai Y, Kozieradzki I, Landers R, Mo R, Hui CC, Nieves E, Cohen PE, Osbourne LR, Wada T, Kunieda T, Moens PB, Penninger JM. Essential role of Fkbp6 in male fertility and homologous chromosome pairing in meiosis. Science 2003; 300(5623):1291–1295.

144. Meng X, Lu X, Morris CA, Keating MT. A novel human gene FKBP6 is deleted in Williams syndrome. Genomics 1998; 52(2):130–137.

145. Momoi A, Yoda H, Steinbeisser H, Fagotto F, Kondoh H, Kudo A, Driever W, Furutani-Seiki M. Analysis of Wnt8 for neural posteriorizing factor by identifying Frizzled 8c and Frizzled 9 as functional receptors for Wnt8. Mech Dev 2003; 120(4):477–489.

146. Karasawa T, Yokokura H, Kitajewski J, Lombroso PJ. Frizzled-9 is activated by Wnt-2 and functions in Wnt/beta-catenin signaling. J Biol Chem 2002; 277(40):37479–37486.

147. Wang YK, Samos CH, Peoples R, Perez-Jurado LA, Nusse R, Francke U. A novel human homologue of the Drosophila frizzled wnt receptor gene binds wingless protein and is in the Williams syndrome deletion at 7q11.23. Hum Mol Genet 1997; 6(3):465–472.

148. Jones MH, Hamana N, Nezu J, Shimane M. A novel family of bromodomain genes. Genomics 2000; 63(1):40–45.

149. Kitagawa H, Fujiki R, Yoshimura K, Mezaki Y, Uematsu U, Matsui D, Ogawa S, Unno K, Okubo M, Tokita A, Nakagawa T, Ito T, Ishimi Y, Nagasawa H, Matsumoto T, Yanagisawa J, Kato S. The chromatin-remodeling complex WINAC targets a nuclear receptor to promoters and is impaired in Williams syndrome. Cell 2003; 113(7):905–917.

150. Lu X, Meng X, Morris CA, Keating MT. A novel human gene, WSTF, is deleted in Williams syndrome. Genomics 1998; 54(2):241–249.

151. Peoples RJ, Cisco MJ, Kaplan P, Francke U. Identification of the WBSCR9 gene, encoding a novel transcriptional

regulator, in the Williams–Beuren syndrome deletion at 7q11.23. Cytogenet Cell Genet 1998; 82(3–4):238–246.

152. Jadayel DM, Osborne LR, Coignet LJ, Zani VJ, Tsui LC, Scherer SW, Dyer MJ. The BCL7 gene family: deletion of BCL7B in Williams syndrome. Gene 1998; 224(1–2):35–44.

153. Natter S, Seiberler S, Hufnagl P, Binder BR, Hirschl AM, Ring J, Abeck D, Schmidt T, Valent P, Valenta R. Isolation of cDNA clones coding for IgE autoantigens with serum IgE from atopic dermatitis patients. FASEB J 1998; 12(14): 1559–1569.

154. Perez Jurado LA, Wang YK, Francke U, Cruces J. TBL2, a novel transducin family member in the WBS deletion: characterization of the complete sequence, genomic structure, transcriptional variants and the mouse ortholog. Cytogenet Cell Genet 1999; 86(3–4):277–284.

155. Cairo S, Merla G, Urbinati F, Ballabio A, Reymond A. WBSCR14, a gene mapping to the Williams–Beuren syndrome deleted region, is a new member of the Mlx transcription factor network. Hum Mol Genet 2001; 10(6):617–627.

156. Paperna T, Peoples R, Wang YK, Kaplan P, Francke U. Genes for the CPE receptor (CPETR1) and the human homolog of RVP1 (CPETR2) are localized within the Williams–Beuren syndrome deletion. Genomics 1998; 54(3):453–459.

157. Morita K, Furuse M, Fujimoto K, Tsukita S. Claudin multigene family encoding four-transmembrane domain protein components of tight junction strands. Proc Natl Acad Sci USA 1999; 96(2):511–516.

158. Tassabehji M, Metcalfe K, Fergusson WD, Carette MJ, Dore JK, Donnai D, Read AP, Proschel C, Gutowski NJ, Mao X, Sheer D. LIM-kinase deleted in Williams syndrome. Nat Genet 1996; 13(3):272–273.

159. Osborne LR, Martindale D, Scherer SW, Shi XM, Huizenga J, Heng HH, Costa T, Pober BR, Lew L, Brinkman J, Rommens J, Koop B, Tsui LC. Identification of genes from a 500-kb region at 7q11.23 that is commonly deleted in Williams syndrome patients. Genomics 1996; 36(2):328–336.

160. Khurana T, Khurana B, Noegel AA. LIM proteins: association with the actin cytoskeleton. Protoplasma 2002; 219(1–2): 1–12.

161. Rogers GW Jr, Richter NJ, Lima NJ, Merrick WC. Modulation of the helicase activity of eIF4A by eIF4B, eIF4H, and eIF4F. J Biol Chem 2001; 276(33):30914–30922.

162. Brdicka T, Imrich M, Angelisova P, Brdickova N, Horvath O, Spicka J, Hilgert I, Luskova P, Draber P, Novak P, Engels N, Wienands J, Simeoni L, Osterreicher J, Aguado E, Malissen M, Schraven B, Horejsi V. Non-T cell activation linker (NTAL): a transmembrane adaptor protein involved in immunoreceptor signaling. J Exp Med 2002; 196(12):1617–1626.

163. Martindale DW, Wilson MD, Wang D, Burke RD, Chen X, Duronio V, Koop BF. Comparative genomic sequence analysis of the Williams syndrome region (LIMK1-RFC2) of human chromosome 7q11.23. Mamm Genome 2000; 11(10):890–898.

164. Peoples R, Perez-Jurado L, Wang YK, Kaplan P, Francke U. The gene for replication factor C subunit 2 (RFC2) is within the 7q11.23 Williams syndrome deletion. Am J Hum Genet 1996; 58(6):1370–1373.

165. Noskov VN, Araki H, Sugino A. The RFC2 gene, encoding the third-largest subunit of the replication factor C complex, is required for an S-phase checkpoint in *Saccharomyces cerevisiae*. Mol Cell Biol 1998; 18(8):4914–4923.

166. Schmidt SL, Pautz AL, Burgers PM. ATP utilization by yeast replication factor C. IV. RFC ATP-binding mutants show defects in DNA replication, DNA repair, and checkpoint regulation. J Biol Chem 2001; 276(37):34792–34800.

167. Hoogenraad CC, Koekkoek B, Akhmanova A, Krugers H, Dortland B, Miedema M, van Alphen A, Kister WM, Jaegle M, Koutsourakis M, Van Camp N, Verhoye M, van der Linden A, Kaverina I, Grosveld F, De Zeeuw CI, Galjart N. Targeted mutation of Cyln2 in the Williams syndrome critical region links CLIP-115 haploinsufficiency to neurodevelopmental abnormalities in mice. Nat Genet 2002; 32(1):116–127.

168. Franke Y, Peoples RJ, Francke U. Identification of GTF2IRD1, a putative transcription factor within the Williams–Beuren

syndrome deletion at 7q11.23. Cytogenet Cell Genet 1999; 86(3–4):296–304.

169. O'Mahoney JV, Guven KL, Lin J, Joya JE, Robinson CS, Wade RP, Hardeman EC. Identification of a novel slow-muscle-fiber enhancer binding protein, MusTRD1. Mol Cell Biol 1998; 18(11):6641–6652.

170. Osborne LR, Campbell T, Daradich A, Scherer SW, Tsui LC. Identification of a putative transcription factor gene (WBSCR11) that is commonly deleted in Williams–Beuren syndrome. Genomics 1999; 57(2):279–284.

171. Bayarsaihan D, Ruddle FH. Isolation and characterization of BEN, a member of the TFII-I family of DNA-binding proteins containing distinct helix–loop–helix domains. Proc Natl Acad Sci USA 2000; 97(13):7342–7347.

172. Yan X, Zhao X, Qian M, Guo N, Gong X, Zhu X. Characterization and gene structure of a novel retinoblastoma-protein-associated protein similar to the transcription regulator TFII-I. Biochem J 2000; 345 Pt 3:749–757.

173. Perez Jurado LA, Wang YK, Peoples R, Coloma A, Cruces J, Francke U. A duplicated gene in the breakpoint regions of the 7q11.23 Williams–Beuren syndrome deletion encodes the initiator binding protein TFII-I and BAP-135, a phosphorylation target of BTK. Hum Mol Genet 1998; 7(3):325–334.

174. Roy AL. Biochemistry and biology of the inducible multifunctional transcription factor TFII-I. Gene 2001; 274(1–2):1–13.

175. Tussie-Luna MI, Bayarsaihan D, Seto E, Ruddle FH, Roy AL. Physical and functional interactions of histone deacetylase 3 with TFII-I family proteins and PIASxbeta. Proc Natl Acad Sci USA 2002; 99(20):12807–12812.

176. Nauseef WM. The NADPH-dependent oxidase of phagocytes. Proc Assoc Am Phys 1999; 111(5):373–382.

177. Merla G, Ucla C, Guipponi M, Reymond A. Identification of additional transcripts in the Williams–Beuren syndrome critical region. Hum Genet 2002; 110(5):429–438.

178. Li DY, Faury G, Taylor DG, Davis EC, Boyle WA, Mecham RP, Stenzel P, Boak B, Keating MY. Novel arterial pathology in

mice and humans hemizygous for elastin. J Clin Invest 1998; 102(10):1783–1787.

179. Li DY, Brooke B, Davis EC, Mecham RP, Sorensen LK, Boak BB, Eichwald E, Keating MY. Elastin is an essential determinant of arterial morphogenesis. Nature 1998; 393(6682):276–280.

180. Meng Y, Zhang Y, Tregoubov V, Janus C, Cruz L, Jackson M, Lu WY, MacDonald JF, Wang JY, Falls DL, Jia Z. Abnormal spine morphology and enhanced LTP in LIMK-1 knockout mice. Neuron 2002; 35(1):121–133.

181. Hoogenraad CC, Eussen BH, Langeveld A, van Haperen R, Winterberg S, Wouters CH, Grosveld F, De Zeeuw CI, Galjart N. The murine CYLN2 gene: genomic organization, chromosome localization, and comparison to the human gene that is located within the 7q11.23 Williams syndrome critical region. Genomics 1998; 53(3):348–358.

182. Zhang R, Maksymowych AB, Simpson LL. Cloning and sequence analysis of a cDNA encoding human syntaxin 1A, a polypeptide essential for exocytosis. Gene 1995; 159(2): 293–294.

183. Rettig J, Sheng ZH, Kim DK, Hodson CD, Snutch TP, Catterall WA. Isoform-specific interaction of the alpha1A subunits of brain Ca2+ channels with the presynaptic proteins syntaxin and SNAP-25. Proc Natl Acad Sci USA 1996; 93(14):7363–7368.

184. Wen YD, Cress WD, Roy AL, Seto E. Histone deacetylase 3 binds to and regulates the multifunctional transcription factor TFII-I. J Biol Chem 2003; 278(3):1841–1847.

185. Hakimi MA, Dong Y, Lane WS, Speicher DW, Shiekhattar R. A candidate X-linked mental retardation gene is a component of a new family of histone deacetylase-containing complexes. J Biol Chem 2003; 278(9):7234–7239.

186. Wang YK, Perez-Jurado LA, Francke U. A mouse single-copy gene, Gtf2i, the homolog of human GTF2I, that is duplicated in the Williams–Beuren syndrome deletion region. Genomics 1998; 48(2):163–170.

187. Durkin ME, Keck-Waggoner CL, Popescu NC, Thorgeirsson SS. Integration of a c-myc transgene results in disruption of the

mouse Gtf2ird1 gene, the homologue of the human GTF2IRD1 gene hemizygously deleted in Williams–Beuren syndrome. Genomics 2001; 73(1):20–27.

188. Committee on Genetics, American Academy of Pediatrics Health care supervision for children with Williams syndrome. Pediatrics 2001; 107(5):1192–1204.

189. Levine K. Information for teachers. Williams Syndrome Association National Newsletter. 10th ed. 1993:3–9.

190. Scheiber B. Fulfilling Dreams—Book 1. A Handbook for Parents of Williams Syndrome Children. Clawson, MI: Williams Syndrome Association, 2000.

12

Velo-Cardio-Facial Syndrome

**WENDY R. KATES, KEVIN ANTSHEL,
and WANDA FREMONT**

Department of Psychiatry and
Behavioral Sciences, State University of
New York Upstate Medical University,
Syracuse, New York, U.S.A.

NANCY ROIZEN

Department of Pediatrics, State
University of New York Upstate
Medical University, Syracuse,
New York, U.S.A.

ROBERT J. SHPRINTZEN

Departments of Pediatrics and
Otolaryngology and Communication
Sciences, State University of New York
Upstate Medical University,
Syracuse, New York, U.S.A.

I. INTRODUCTION

Velo-cardio-facial syndrome (VCFS) is a relatively common
genetic disorder that affects about 1 in 2000 individuals (1).
Caused by a microdeletion on chromosome 22q.11 (2,3), the
syndrome is associated with multiple congenital anomalies

383

and learning disabilities (4–8). The phenotypic spectrum of VCFS may be the most pleiotropic of any genetic syndrome. Over 180 clinical features have been reported in individuals with VCFS (1,9) with none being obligatory findings. Individuals with VCFS may have as few as four or five anomalies or over 50 depending on the severity of expression of the syndrome. Arguably, the most frequently described features of VCFS are behavioral, cognitive, and developmental problems (9).

Although the syndrome is often initially recognized by the presence of heart malformations or palatal anomalies, neither of these problems occurs in more than approximately three-quarters of affected individuals (9,10). However, behavioral disorders including developmental delay and learning disabilities occur in nearly 100% of cases and other behavioral manifestations such as language impairment, social immaturity, disinhibition, impulsivity, anxiety, and mood disorders (11,12) occur more commonly than the most common structural malformations. By adulthood, between 10% and 30% of individuals with VCFS are identified with severe psychiatric disorder (13).

The most common structural anomalies associated with the syndrome are probably vascular including anomalous internal carotid arteries, small caliber vessels, aberrant or absent major arteries, and abnormal perfusion (10). Other common structural anomalies found in VCFS include conotruncal heart malformations, palatal anomalies, minor external ear abnormalities including overfolding of the helices, slender digits with short nails, hypotonia and lax joints, characteristic facial appearance, prominent nasal root, and suborbital congestion. Also common but less frequent are facial asymmetry, renal anomalies, hernias, genitourinary tract anomalies, minor eye anomalies, and spine anomalies.

Although the clinical features of VCFS were described over 30 years ago, the mechanism for a genetic diagnosis was not known until 1993 (14). This factor coupled with the variable and complex phenotype in individuals with VCFS has slowed efforts to identify genotype–phenotype associations in this disorder. During the last decade, however, the functions of the genes with the 22q11 region have been the focus of increased attention. In this chapter, we will describe the genetic mechanism that underlies the syndrome, review its neuroanatomic, social/developmental, neuropsychological, and psychiatric phenotypes, and discuss the implications for continued research efforts to specify the genetic contribution to the complex phenotype that characterizes VCFS.

A. The History of the Delineation of VCFS

The diagnostic term *velo-cardio-facial syndrome* (often abbreviated as VCFS) was coined in a paper in 1978 delineating the features of this multiple anomaly disorder in 12 patients who had the association of cleft palate, hypernasal speech, learning disabilities, and a characteristic facial appearance (4). The 1978 paper described approximately a dozen clinical features in these cases and one familial case was included in the sample, a female-to-female transmission. Autosomal dominant inheritance was hypothesized and confirmed in follow-up reports (15,16). Although the 1978 paper is widely regarded as the initial description of the syndrome, an earlier paper by Strong (17) delineated the same syndrome in a single family with multiple affected members. Review of the photographs confirms that the family described by Strong (17) expressed dominant transmission of VCFS that was inherited from the mother. A case of male-to-male transmission described by Williams et al. (16) later confirmed autosomal dominant inheritance and ruled out X-linked dominant mode of inheritance.

A number of earlier reports described individuals with VCFS although the purpose of those reports was to discuss specific speech disorders, heart anomalies, or immune deficiencies (18–20). Sedlačková (21) reported a large series of cases that had the association of hypernasal speech with facial innervation anomalies. Cayler (22) described asymmetric crying facies and heart anomalies, a common association in VCFS. Kretschmer et al. (19) described three cases with absent thymus and showed photographs of a single case with "DiGeorge's syndrome" that clearly had the clinical features of VCFS. Kaplan (20) described the palatal anomalies

commonly found in VCFS and showed photographs of four
cases, of which three had VCFS and one clearly did not.
Kinouchi et al. (23) and Takao et al. (24) and Momma et al.
(25) also described the same syndrome in the Japanese literature. All of these early reports described the same syndrome
and because the authors who approached these clinical cases
often did so from different perspectives, we have the unfortunate circumstance of one condition having more than one
name. This nosologic dilemma has caused some confusion in
both the clinical and research approaches to children with
this common genetic syndrome. The disorder has been labeled
VCFS, DiGeorge syndrome, Cayler syndrome, conotruncal
anomalies face syndrome, Takao syndrome, Sedlačková syndrome, Shprintzen syndrome, 22q11 deletion syndrome, and
CATCH 22 (a regrettable acronym meant to invoke humor)
therefore leading some researchers and clinicians to conclude
that these are all separate disorders. However, let there be no
mistake that all of these conditions are one in the same.

B. Phenotype and Genotype

It is now well established that VCFS is a contiguous gene
syndrome and, in fact, is the most common contiguous gene
syndrome in humans (10). A contiguous gene syndrome is
typically referred to as a disorder that is caused by a deletion
of a submicroscopic segment of DNA from one of the nuclear
chromosomes with that deletion encompassing a region that
normally contains more than one gene. In the case of VCFS,
one copy of chromosome 22 has the deletion of the long arm
at the q11.2 band (Fig. 1). Approximately 90% of affected
individuals have a deletion that spans 3 million base pairs
of DNA and another 7% have a smaller deletion spanning
1.5 million base pairs so that 25–30 genes are deleted in the
large majority of cases. The remaining cases have unique,
smaller deletions.

Although familial cases have been reported as early as
the first delineation of the syndrome (4), the large majority
of people with VCFS represent new mutations often referred
to as *de novo* cases. This means that the DNA rearrangement

Chromosome 22

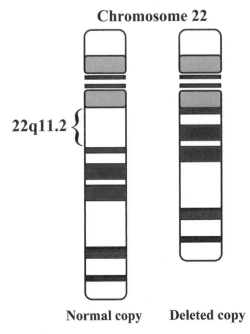

22q11.2 {

Normal copy **Deleted copy**

Figure 1 Graphic representation of chromosome 22 pair in an individual with velo-cardio-facial syndrome. The deleted copy is missing a segment of DNA just below the centromere.

that caused the deletion usually has happened during gametogenesis of the mother's egg or father's sperm. Our experience is that approximately 90% of cases of VCFS are not familial, but rather new occurrences with nearly all of the remaining 10% of cases being inherited from an affected parent. A very small number of cases are the result of unbalanced translocations and there have been reports of rare cases of somatic mutations, germ-line mutations, and inversions.

The anomalies associated with VCFS encompass nearly every organ system and are structural, behavioral, and metabolic including the central nervous system, cardiovascular system, endocrine system, integument, skeletal muscles, ocular system, auditory system, and skeletal system. Table 1 shows a list of the most common anomalies associated with VCFS with the frequency in the syndrome based on a sample of 815 cases from multiple ascertainment sources. These data

Table 1 A List of Anomalies and Their
Frequency in VCFS Based on Data Derived
from Examinations of 815 Individuals with the
Syndrome

Developmental delay	98%
Learning disorders	98%
Vascular anomalies	98%
Hypotonia	76%
Heart anomalies	76%
Palatal anomalies or dysfunction	75%
Behavioral disorders	68%
Chronic respiratory illness	65%
Severe speech disorders	62%
Minor structural ear anomalies	59%
Asymmetric crying facies	40%
Immune deficiency	31%
Scoliosis	30%
Seizures	28%
Hypocalcemia	25%
Raynaud's phenomenon	25%
Unilateral vocal cord paresis	22%
Renal anomalies	21%
Thrombocytopenia	21%
Hernias	17%
Hypospadias	14%
Anal anomalies	13%
Sprengel shoulder deformity	13%
Sensori-neural hearing loss	10%
Psychosis	10%
Laryngeal web	8%

were collected in a collaborative study supported by the
members of The Velo-Cardio-Facial Syndrome Educational
Foundation and is based on data from examinations at all
ages rather than birth records. The outcome of that study
showed that no anomaly occurred with 100% frequency and
the most common anomalies were behavioral and vascular.

The facial features of VCFS are usually minor in nature
and rather than describing the facies as dysmorphic it is more
appropriate to refer to it as characteristic of the syndrome
(Fig. 2). Vertical lengthening of the face, a long pear-shaped

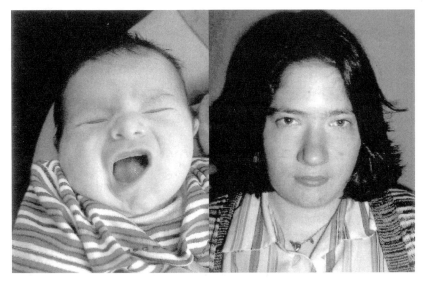

Figure 2 Characteristic appearance of a baby with VCFS and asymmetric crying facies (left) and a teenager with VCFS (right).

nose, eyes that seem vertically narrow, small ears with overfolded helices and attached lobules (often protuberant), and reduced facial animation are common. Facial asymmetry during smiling or crying is common, particularly in infants and young children, often leading to the diagnosis of "asymmetric crying facies." Even with these findings, children and adults with VCFS do not usually stand out from the general population based on appearance alone which may lead to underdetection of the syndrome.

The natural history of VCFS is marked by initial hypotonia with mild developmental delay in infancy and early childhood. Growth both in terms of linear growth velocity and weight gain often lags behind in the first two years of life followed by more rapid growth acceleration after the third birthday so that by school age nearly all children with VCFS are within normal limits. Developmental milestones are similar with early motor milestones slightly delayed but with more significant delay of speech and language milestones. The average age of onset of first word is 19 months with a similar delay in first independent steps. There is also a spurt of developmental milestones near the third birthday and with proper treatment, speech and language milestones are often close to normal by school age. Behavior is typically immature resulting in frequent social isolation. Learning disabilities become evident in early primary school years typically by second grade and educational difficulties tend to become more noticeable as learning involves more problem solving and abstraction. The onset of significant psychiatric disorders often precedes the 20th birthday (12) and can progress rapidly although it is a relatively small percentage of individuals with VCFS who develop psychosis, probably about 10%.

Because the phenotype of VCFS is so expansive, it is likely that many of the features will be shared by other syndromes. In addition, many of the anomalies found in VCFS are minor anomalies (such as umbilical hernia), variants of normal (such as widely spaced eyes and overfolded helices), or commonly occurring major anomalies (such as heart malformations and cleft palate) and as such are not syndrome specific nor uncommon in the general population. As a result, the phenotype of VCFS has been misidentified as Opitz syndrome (also known as the G/BBB syndrome) in a number of publications (26). Conversely, patients with other disorders such as del(10p) have been reported to have VCFS (27) but critical review of these cases shows that they are phenotypically different. To date, there is no evidence that VCFS has any cause other than 22q11.2 deletion.

As described above, the anomalies associated with VCFS encompass nearly every organ system. With these seemingly diverse regions of the body affected and because the syndrome is found in the presence of a deletion of 25–30 genes, it is natural to assume that the diverse features seen in VCFS are contributed to by at least several, if not many, genes. Therefore, research over the past decade has focused on trying to determine the specific causation of the many anomalies in VCFS based on knowledge of the deletion, the genes that are present in only a single copy, and any polymorphisms that might be present in the genes within the 22q11.2 region on the normal chromosome. The major focus has been on attempting to isolate the specific contributors to psychiatric illness and congenital heart disease. This research has been conducted in both humans and animal models (mice). Researchers have pondered if the majority of the phenotype is related to a single gene in the deleted region with minor modifications from the rest of the deletion, or major contributions from many genes. It has also been suggested that genes in the deleted region may interact with genes elsewhere in the genome to cause many anomalies. To date, there is not a definitive answer to these research questions but there is little doubt that the process of phenotype to genotype matching will be completed within the next decade.

The cytogenetic laboratory test used universally at this time to detect the deletion from 22q11.2 is *f*luorescent *in s*itu *h*ybridization (FISH). This relatively inexpensive and readily available procedure uses DNA probes found in the 22q11.2 region to detect the presence or absence of known sequences within the locus known to be deleted in cases of VCFS (Fig. 3). The test does not show the size of the deletion or the specific genes that are deleted but it does determine if DNA from a specific region that has been found to be deleted in all cases of VCFS is present or not. The test is easily performed from a small amount of peripheral blood that can be obtained by venipuncture. Because the DNA probes used are specific to 22q11.2, the test will not detect other genetic abnormalities. Therefore, when FISH is ordered for VCFS, it must be specified that the purpose of the procedure is to detect a deletion at 22q11.2.

Two previous studies have suggested that there are individuals with VCFS who do not have detectable deletions of DNA within the 22q11.2 locus (14,28). Both of these investigations accepted blood samples from multiple clinicians in order to determine if deletions from 22q11.2 were present. There was no control over the clinical diagnostic process so that errors in clinical diagnosis of VCFS were listed as "nondeleted" cases of VCFS. Some of the clinicians who submitted samples were more experienced than others with the diagnosis and no effort was made to control for individual clinician's rates of false negatives. Indeed, our own experience

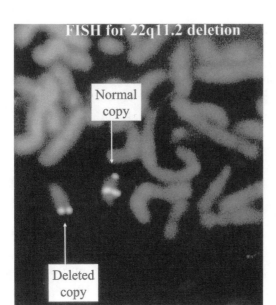

Figure 3 FISH (*fl*uorescent *in situ h*ybridization) of chromosome 22q11.2 in an individual with VCFS. Note that the normal copy of chromosome 22 had two bright signals (the double signal is a control probe) and the deleted copy has only the control probe signal.

has shown that over time the number of positive detections of deletions has risen to essentially 100% as the VCFS phenotype becomes more familiar. To date, there has been no single report of a "nondeleted" case with a point mutation or detection of a mutation outside of the 22q11.2 locus. Therefore, it is likely that the diagnostic test for deletions displays a high degree of sensitivity and specificity.

1. Candidate Genes

A number of studies have proposed candidate genes within the deleted region in relation to specific anomalies or groups of anomalies (29–32). At this time, it seems likely that at least two genes can be linked to some of the VCFS phenotype. Because the 22q11.2 genome is well preserved across species, its homolog has been isolated to mouse chromosome 16. Using animal models, investigators have determined that haploinsufficiency of the gene *TBX1* results in the same conotruncal heart anomalies commonly found in VCFS (31). The gene *COMT* (catechol-*O*-methyltransferase) has been linked to psychiatric disorders in relation to the metabolism and degradation of synaptic dopamine levels (30,33). *COMT* is responsible for the degradation of dopamines and therefore has been hypothesized to have an effect on neural transmission. *COMT* has been found to have a polymorphism, two alleles that have different activity levels with regard to their ability to degrade dopamines: a low secreting heat labile version, and a high secreting stable version (30). Hemizygosity for the low secreting version has been linked to a higher frequency of psychiatric disorders in individuals with VCFS (30). Both of these genes reside within the commonly deleted region for VCFS and all individuals who are FISH positive for the deletion will be missing single copies of *TBX1* and *COMT*.

2. The Mechanism for the Deletion

The loss of DNA that causes VCFS is an interstitial deletion from the long arm of chromosome 22 that resides within a region of the genome that is highly susceptible to mutation. This region of chromosome 22 seems to be one of the most mutable regions in the entire human genome, thus accounting for the high rate of spontaneous mutation and the large number of nonfamilial cases. The mechanism for the deletion has been determined to occur during gametogenesis (34). The rearrangement happens as a result of a recombinant event in the first meiotic prophase (Prophase I) during synapsis. There is an unusual arrangement of chromosome 22 in the region that marks the normal breakpoint for the proximal end of the deletion and the region at the distal end. In both of these regions, there occurs a series of low copy repeats (LCRs) of DNA that are largely homologous (Fig. 4).

As a result, these regions of homologous DNA on sister chromatids may misalign so that the proximal set of LCRs on one copy of chromosome 22 aligns with the distal series of LCRs on the other chromosome 22. When crossing over (recombination) occurs between the two copies of chromosome

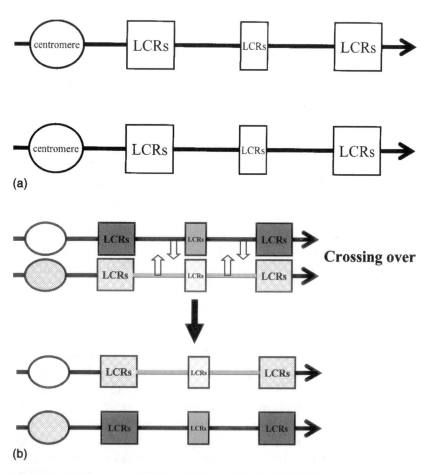

Figure 4 Cartoon of chromosome 22q11.2 (a) showing arrangement of a series of low copy repeats (LCRs). The first set of LCRs is located at the most common proximal breakpoint for VCFS. An identical series occurs at the most common distal breakpoint, and in between these two sets of identical LCR regions is a smaller set of LCRs which is the site of the distal breakpoint in approximately 7% of all cases of VCFS. The alignment of the LCRs during crossing over with the resulting recombinant 22q11.2 region (b).

22, the exchange of genetic material is not the same with one copy of chromosome 22 getting an extra segment of 22q11.2 and the other losing a segment of 22q11.2 (Fig. 5).

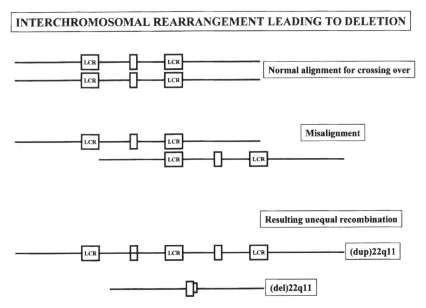

Figure 5 Cartoon of misalignment of 22q11.2 during crossing over with resulting chromosomes, one copy deleted (VCFS) and the other copy having a partial trisomy for 22q11.2. This type of recombinant event results in an interchromosomal mechanism for the deletion.

This type of interchromosomal recombination event resulting in a loss of 22q11.2 in the resulting sperm or egg is by far the most common mechanism for the deletion. In a smaller number of cases, perhaps 10% or less, the loss of material occurs in an intrachromosomal manner with a splicing out of 22q11.2 (Fig. 6).

In these intrachromosomal rearrangements, the proximal series of LCRs "reads" the distal series of repeats so that the region loops over on itself and splices out the segment between the breakpoints. These recombinant events represent true random genetic errors that are a part of the normal recombination process during gametogenesis but with the unusual arrangement of 22q11.2, the region becomes prone to these misreading errors and deletions. One might wonder why 22q11.2 deletions are encountered frequently but duplications of 22q11.2 are rare. Possible explanations include

INTRACHROMOSOMAL REARRANGEMENT LEADING TO DELETION

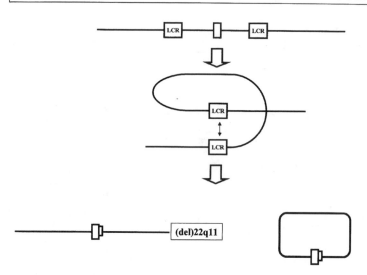

Figure 6 Cartoon of intrachromosomal deletion of 22q11.2 caused by the proximal set of LCRs aligning with the distal set of LCRs resulting in a splicing out of 22q11.2.

failure to diagnose a (dup) 22q11.2 syndrome. However, considering that in interchromosomal rearrangements one would expect an essentially equal number of cases of duplications as deletions it seems likely that fewer embryos with duplications reach term and survive.

II. NEUROANATOMIC PHENOTYPE

Parallel to the increased focus on the genetics of VCFS, the advent of high-resolution brain imaging (e.g., MRI) has permitted an upsurge of information about the developing and adult brain in VCFS. Initially, qualitative MRI studies (35,36) identified white matter hyperintensities, periventricular cysts, and reduced cerebellar vermi in the brains of individuals with VCFS. More recently, quantitative imaging studies have identified volumetric alterations in several brain regions of children and adults with this disorder. Although studies vary in sample composition and in methodology thus diluting the generalizability of anatomic imaging results, several consistent findings have emerged.

Relative to typically developing children, patients with VCFS exhibit reductions of approximately 11% in total brain volume (37,38). Although volumetric studies of the posterior fossa (39), cerebellum (37,40), and caudate nucleus (41,42) indicate that patients with VCFS exhibit alterations in these brain regions, the studies that have the greatest implications for understanding the neuropsychological and psychiatric correlates of VCFS have explored the morphology of the cerebral cortex and the lobar regions of which it consists. Volumetric studies of the morphology of the cerebral cortex in children with VCFS have revealed reductions in frontal (43) and parietal (37) gray matter volumes and in frontal (43), parietal and temporal white matter (38) volumes. Whereas gray matter reductions are not disproportionate to the 11% reduction in whole brain volume, the white matter volumes of the frontal, parietal, and temporal lobes is reduced between 15% and 23% in VCFS subjects relative to controls. Studies of cerebral cortical morphology in adults with VCFS have also found widespread differences in white matter volumes between patients and controls (38) and gray matter alterations in the frontal and temporal lobes (40,42,44). (Insofar as VCFS patients in adult studies are comorbid for schizophrenia, however, these findings may not be fully comparable to the studies of children.) All of these studies suggest that in patients with VCFS much of cortical white matter development is significantly compromised against a background of milder cortical gray matter deficits (43). Significant alterations in the cortical white matter in VCFS may be due to delays in myelin development, disturbances in the organization or density of axons within the cerebral cortex, or disturbances in the cellular structure of white matter. The application of imaging modalities that permit more specific analysis of white matter integrity in the brain (such as diffusion tensor imaging and magnetic resonance spectroscopy) are required to clarify this question.

Moreover, the functional consequences of the cortical white matter and gray matter reductions found in this disorder are poorly understood. The frontal, parietal, and temporal lobes mediate executive function, visual spatial perception, spatial working memory, and expressive language, all of which are neuropsychological deficits that have been observed in children with VCFS (as is described later in this chapter). In addition, frontal and temporal gray matter reductions have been identified in adults with schizophrenia for which individuals with VCFS are at significant risk.

Our understanding of the functional consequences of aberrant brain morphology in VCFS depends on identifying higher-order networks that may be anomalous in the brain. At least two functional networks are hypothesized to be anomalous in VCFS. Dysfunction of prefrontal–striatal networks (45–47) has been associated with impairments in attention, executive function, mood stability, and task inhibition (48), all features of the cognitive and behavioral phenotype in children with VCFS. Dysfunction of the orbitalfrontal–subcortical circuit, for example, is associated with mood lability, irritability, and impulsivity. These features have been described in children with ADHD and bipolar disorder both of which are observed consistently in children with VCFS (12,49–51). Dysfunction of the dorsolateral prefrontal–subcortical circuit is associated with deficits in executive function and ability to shift set, features that have also been described in children with VCFS.

A second network that may be anomalous in VCFS is the heteromodal association cortical network. The heteromodal association cortex has been described as a network of parallel, interconnected cortical regions that mediate higher-order cognitive functioning (52). Major components (53) include the dorsolateral prefrontal cortex, Broca's motor speech region, the inferior parietal lobule, and auditory association portions of the superior temporal gyrus. These regions mediate multimodal cognitive tasks such as executive function, working memory, focused attention, and auditory processing (54), all tasks which pose significant difficulties for patients with VCFS. Several neuroanatomic abnormalities that have been identified in studies of children with VCFS are included within this network of regions. Moreover, it has been hypothesized that dysfunction of this network may be associated with cognitive and behavioral features of schizo-phrenia, for which individuals with VCFS appear to be at risk. Additional studies are needed to test the extent to which either of these networks are, in fact, anomalous in VCFS.

To gain a fuller understanding of the networks of cortical deficits in VCFS, the implementation of functional magnetic resonance imaging (fMRI) studies is also essential. Published functional MRI studies of individuals with VCFS are limited. In an exploration of the neural correlates of mathematics performance, Eliez et al. (55) observed that in contrast to the control group activation of the left supramarginal gyrus in the VCFS group increased with the difficulty of the task pre-sented. These findings suggest that aberrant activation of the left supramarginal gyrus (which is part of the parietal lobe) may underlie the deficits in mathematics performance that is described frequently in children with this syndrome. Addi-tional functional imaging studies of VCFS patients that explore the precise neural correlates of cognitive skills thought to be mediated by the frontal and temporal lobes (such as executive function, verbal fluency, response inhibition, and auditory processing) are also critically needed.

In addition, we do not have a comprehensive understand-ing of the trajectory of brain development in VCFS. There is preliminary evidence that temporal lobe gray volume decreases with age during adolescence (56). This is consistent with the findings of absolute reductions of temporal gray matter volumes in adults with VCFS (40,44) but not children with VCFS (although as noted above, the sample composition of adult and child studies was different). Comprehensive longi-tudinal studies of children with VCFS are essential to our understanding of the effect of brain development on neuro-psychological function and risk for psychiatric disorder in individuals with this developmental disorder.

III. DEVELOPMENTAL PROFILE

Although precise brain–behavior associations in this disorder remain to be established, it is evident that dysfunction of the central nervous system derails key developmental achievements in a child with VCFS. If cardiac anomalies or a lack of clarity of speech have not stimulated the initiation of an evaluation for VCFS, then the associated developmental delays will often be the initiating concern (7). As noted above, the spectrum of severity of the major findings in VCFS is wide (57) but developmental and behavioral issues are present in most of the children, with learning difficulties reported in 82–100% (58). These may not be recognized in infancy as many of the children spend much time receiving medical and surgical treatment for their cardiac anomalies, cleft palates, low T-lymphocyte count, hypocalcemia, infections, or other less frequent findings. Any early delays may be attributed to their health problems. Alternatively, with the wide variability in function, the developmental delays may not be present or may be mild in infancy. Interestingly, the children with VCFS exhibit similar intelligence whether or not they have congenital heart defects (58). However, children with a familial deletion have a higher incidence of intellectual disability than those with a de novo deletion (58). This observation may reflect the dynamics of mate selection when one parent is cognitively impaired because they have VCFS. To the extent that intellectual levels between spouses are correlated (59), the increased incidence of intellectual disability in these families are most likely related to a confluence of inherited intellectual factors.

Scherer et al. (60) compared the performance on the Bayley Scales of Infant Development at 6, 18, and 30 months of age in four children with VCFS with normal children ($n = 8$), children with cleft lip and palate ($n = 8$), and children with isolate cleft palate ($n = 7$). At 6 months, there were no significant differences between the children with VCFS and the other three groups. In mental development by 18 months of age and continuing at 30 months of age, the children with VCFS were significantly behind both the normals and the children with cleft lip and palate. Mental Developmental Indexes decreased from 89.2 at 6 months of age to 82.5 at 30 months of age.

Mean age of walking has been reported to be 17 months of age with only 27% walking before age 15 months (5).

Hypotonia, which is more severe in infancy, is reported in 76–85% of children with VCFS (61) and problems with coordination and balance are also reported (57). In the Scherer et al. (60) study described in the previous paragraph, the Psychomotor Developmental Indexes (PDI) also decreased from 91.0 at 6 months of age to 82.5 at 30 months of age.

Most parents report delayed speech onset (5). In the study group described above, similar patterns of decreasing function in expressive and receptive language function were found. Impairments in language function were apparent from the onset of language and persisted with an increasing discrepancy between the VCFS group and the comparison groups from 6 to 30 months. Particularly striking was the lack of increase in the number of different words and consonants used by the VCFS group by 30 months. In a study of 28 toddlers using the Preschool Language Scale-Revised, the mean total language scores were 73.2 with expressive language being 71.2 and receptive language being 78.2. In the same study using the same scale in 12 preschoolers, the scores were unchanged (62).

IV. NEUROPSYCHOLOGICAL PROFILE

Individuals with VCFS often present with a tremendous range of neuropsychological abilities and it is very difficult to make broad generalizations about cognitive functioning in this population. Nevertheless, several distinctive neuropsychological features have been empirically demonstrated to exist at elevated levels.

A. General Intellectual Ability

A wide range of general cognitive abilities (mild mental retardation to average IQ) has been observed in VCFS with mean IQs in the borderline range of intellect (7). One of the more consistent findings in the literature is that verbal IQ scores are generally higher than performance (nonverbal) IQ scores (7,8). Difficulties in abstract reasoning, visuospatial abilities, and nonverbal reasoning have been proposed as possible reasons for this discrepancy. Our own clinical experience, however, suggests that this verbal/performance IQ divergence is by no means consistent across individuals with VCFS; it is not uncommon to find individuals who do not demonstrate this pattern or conversely exhibit the opposite pattern (nonverbal abilities stronger than verbal).

B. Academic Attainment

Consistent with less well-developed nonverbal abilities, children with VCFS generally have more pronounced difficulty in mathematics (63) and our experience suggests that difficulties in mathematics are often central features of the academic profile in children with VCFS. Long division misalignment of columns, fractions, decimals, and geometry are typically more difficult for these children in our experience. In addition, "survival math" concepts involving time, money, and measurement concepts are also sometimes poorly developed. Additional tutoring and physical models/manipulative aids may prove necessary to teach these basic mathematics concepts.

In the language domain, reading and spelling abilities are relatively stronger in children with VCFS although usually still behind their same-aged peers (63). Despite these areas of relative strength in the language domain, written language abilities are often significantly less well developed to some degree attributable to hypotonia and concomitant graphomotor difficulties that are common in this population (9,58). Reading comprehension abilities also often lag behind reading decoding and phonological processing abilities (63). In other words, these children are able to learn to read but frequently have trouble in reading to learn.

In general, children with VCFS frequently make adequate academic progress early in elementary school and may not begin to experience pronounced difficulty until near the end elementary school (e.g., 3rd or 4th grade) (9). At this time, school expectations shift from acquisition of basic skills and emphasis on concrete, discrete activities to more abstract, integrated learning. Children with VCFS frequently have more difficulty with abstract thinking (5) and often become more easily overwhelmed at this point in their schooling.

These intensified academic difficulties also coincide with heightening of social concerns. Often during the late elementary and early middle school years, children may become less tolerant of other children who are "different"; often as a result of their speech difficulties, children with VCFS may begin to experience amplified social difficulties including peer rejection.

C. Language/Verbal Abilities

In addition to the hypernasal resonance (associated with cleft palate), monotonous tone, limited range of affect, and poor articulation that typifies speech output (5,6), there are several other language features commonly found in VCFS. For example, although there is some evidence to suggest otherwise (64), receptive language abilities are generally stronger than expressive language abilities in children with VCFS (8).

D. Visuospatial/Perceptual Abilities

Diminished visuospatial and perceptual abilities are consistently cited as a primary area of neuropsychological deficit in VCFS (6,58). Furthermore, VCFS shares other features of a nonverbal learning disability (NLD) (65) and has been highlighted as prototypical of this learning disability and best suited to NLD remediation models (58). Visuospatial and visual–spatial memory deficits, possibly due to differences in the function of the right parietal lobe (66), are also often cited as the primary reasons for mathematics difficulties in VCFS (67).

Difficulties in navigating perceptual materials also raise the risk for motor difficulties including clumsiness and poor coordination. In our experience, it is not uncommon for parents to describe their child as frequently bumping into other people and objects and generally being unaware of the position in space that her/his body encompasses.

E. Memory Abilities

Also consistent with the population of children who are diagnosed with NLD, children with VCFS frequently have better developed rote memory skills particularly for auditory/verbal information. Research on the specific processes involved in memory have not been well defined in VCFS yet some evidence exists to suggest that memory abilities, particularly for rote information, may represent an area of relative strength when considering the neuropsychological phenotype of VCFS. It is our belief that children with VCFS frequently rely exclusively on a rote task approach and fail at integrating various pieces of information together. In other words, these children may "lose sight of the forest for the trees." Furthermore, this strategy quickly breaks down whenever these children encounter novel or complex situations and may only serve to exacerbate preexisting anxiety.

F. Attention/Executive Function Abilities

Despite the fact that very few empirical studies have explicitly addressed attention and/or executive function abilities in children with VCFS, there is an extant literature (12,68) that documents higher prevalence of attention deficit hyperactivity disorder (ADHD) than is seen in typically developing children. It is difficulty to discern, however, what is truly attention deficits due to the fact that these behaviors are typically elevated in children, like children with VCFS, who have developmental disabilities. Executive function deficits have also been described in VCFS including difficulties in shifting attention and less well-developed working memory abilities (70).

Our own clinical experience suggests that perseveration and difficulties in shifting attention can exact great social impairment and are frequently elevated in this population. For example, it is not uncommon for children to present in our office with one or two topics that they are interested in discussing and to have significant difficulty in moving past these topics. It is not hard to imagine how this relatively rigid social style may interfere with peer relations.

V. PSYCHIATRIC PHENOTYPE

A. Childhood Presentation

Behavioral and psychiatric complications are common in VCFS and attention, anxiety and mood disorders are most frequently observed (49). There is some evidence, however, to suggest that the psychiatric prevalence rates of these disorders in VCFS do not differ significantly from cognitively matched samples (49). The behavioral presentation can be quite variable; children with VCFS are often described in a wide range of terms including overactive, impulsive, emotionally labile, shy/withdrawn, or disinhibited (5,11,68). Many children with VCFS have been described as having a bland affect (9). It is our experience that children with VCFS also have difficulties with time perception; however, empirical data are needed to substantiate this observation. Social problems are also common, most often involving peer difficulties (7,11). A cross-sectional study of children with VCFS (11) reported a trend that increased with age of more internalizing problem behavior (withdrawn, somatic complaints, and anxious/depressed) than externalizing problem behavior (delinquent and aggressive). However, social problems, withdrawal, attention problems, and thought problems were consistently reported across the different ages.

Children with VCFS have been reported to have a higher prevalence than controls of night terrors, separation anxiety, obsessive compulsive disorder, mood swings, and ultrarapid cycling bipolar disorder with affective lability, anxiety, perseverative thoughts, and hallucinations (6,12,71–73). Some of the behaviors observed in children with VCSF are not uncommon in children with developmental delays. They include overreactivity, attentional problems, impulsivity, low frustration tolerance, perseveration, learning disabilities, and poor planning abilities and organizational skills. Like patients with VCFS, children with developmental delays and learning disabilities have been reported to have a higher rate of psychiatric disorders (69,74–76). Therefore, studies are needed to differentiate behaviors that are primary psychiatric conditions from behaviors that are due to other risk factors associated with developmental and cognitive deficits.

B. Later-Onset Conditions

It is possible that the behaviors observed in childhood are pro-dromal features of more severe psychiatric illnesses; there is some evidence to suggest that later-onset conditions may be causally connected with VCFS including schizophrenia (70,75,76), bipolar disorder (12), and major depressive disorder (13). In fact, there is some data to suggest that the risk of schizophrenia for an individual with VCFS approaches 25 times the risk in the general population (77). Furthermore, descriptions of psychosocial dysfunction that characterize children and adolescents at high risk for developing schizophrenia are consistent with descriptions of children with VCFS and include prominent anxiety and social withdrawal (78). Taken as a whole, the literature suggests that VCFS may be a genetic cause of schizophrenia although further work is needed.

As noted above, an association has been postulated between the role of the *COMT* gene and neuropsychiatric manifestations of VCFS (30,33). Functional polymorphisms of the *COMT* gene which codes for an enzyme involved in the breakdown of catecholamine neurotransmitters (dopamine, epinephrine, and norepinephrine), have been linked to neuropsychiatric disorders in the general population. Homozygosity for the COMT 108-met allele has been shown to be associated with obsessive compulsive disorder and ultra-rapid cycling bipolar disorder (30,81,82), whereas homozygosity for COMT 108-val is associated with poor performance on cognitive tasks of executive function (83) and possible risk for schizophrenia (84). It has been proposed that in patients with VCFS, deletion of the *COMT* gene from one chromosome 22 combined with the low-activity COMT allele (COMT 108-met) on the nondeleted chromosome results in an increase in cate-cholamine neurotransmission and consequent neuropsychiatric features in this disorder (85). However, this association has not yet been established (13) empirically; accordingly, future studies will need to determine the presence and nature of an association between allelic variation on COMT and the incidence of psychiatric disorder in VCFS.

Potentially, the establishment of a robust association between allelic variation on COMT and neuropsychiatric disorders in patients with VCFS would raise intriguing questions about treatment intervention. In order to improve the quality of life of patients with VCFS, innovative research studies (33) would need to examine the relationship between pharmacologic interventions targeted at the COMT enzyme and the resultant effects on neuropsychiatric symptoms in VCFS.

VI. CONCLUSIONS

Although investigations of the genetics and the phenotypic features of VCFS have mushroomed during the decade that has followed the identification of the 22q11.2 deletion in 1992, many questions remain unanswered. It is critical that we continue to specify candidate genes that contribute to the physical, neurocognitive, and psychiatric phenotypes in this disorder. Although recent interest has focused on the *TBX1* and *COMT* genes, additional genes of potential interest include the *UFDL-1*, *GSCL*, and *PROD-H* genes. Continuing to identify genotype–phenotype associations for likely candidate genes is also essential. The knowledge that is gained from studies of genotype–phenotype associations will ultimately inform treatment interventions. Insofar as 30 genes comprise the deleted region and appear to be associated with multiple phenotypic manifestations of the disorder, the study of gene–brain–behavior associations in VCFS will no doubt continue to fascinate scientists for many years to come.

One caveat, however, is that investigations of genotype–phenotype associations, particularly as they relate to the cognitive and behavioral manifestations of the disorder, assume that the phenotype is syndrome specific. Establishing, as one report has suggested, that the behavioral phenotype associated with VCFS is not significantly different from that of other developmental disabilities would have significant implications for genotype–phenotype association studies. If we learn that the overall dysfunction of the central nervous system accounts for the cognitive and behavioral features of

VCFS to a greater extent than the contribution of specific genes that regulate neurochemistry, for example our investigations of candidate genes might shift to an emphasis on genes that play a role in neuronal migration and neurodevelopment.

Our ability to establish whether the phenotype is syndrome specific will depend on the ascertainment of thoughtfully matched control samples. Many extant studies of cognitive, behavioral, and neuroanatomic features of VCFS (particularly in children) are based on comparisons with a control sample that is significantly discrepant in IQ. The recruitment of IQ-matched control samples as well as sibling samples (to control for family environment factors) is essential to determining the specificity of the VCFS phenotype.

Moreover, both scientists and practitioners must keep in mind that the phenotype itself is developmental: it changes over time. During infancy and early childhood, the child's medical status is predominant. Surgical interventions and hospitalizations often take precedence over the early developmental interventions that are also essential during this time. As children move into preschool and the early years of elementary school, many medical issues resolve only to give way to a focus on residual speech and language delays as well as academic difficulties. In the later elementary school years and in middle school, children with VCFS often experience emotional and behavioral problems as well as face significant peer difficulties and social problems.

Finally, as they move through high school and beyond, young adults with VCFS continue to be challenged by the demands of daily living and by the risk of severe psychiatric disorder. Accordingly, it is essential that medical and developmental professionals adopt the perspective of a "developmental phenotype" both to conceptualize the challenges that the patient with VCFS faces and to formulate appropriate interventions. Patients with VCFS require the expertise of a multidisciplinary team and families require ongoing community support and respite. To ensure that patients with VCFS achieve an adaptation to adulthood in which they can utilize their many strengths, appropriate interventions must be available to them throughout life.

REFERENCES

1. Shprintzen RJ. Velo-cardio-facial syndrome. In: Cassidy SB, Allanson J, eds. Management of Genetic Syndromes. New York: John Wiley & Sons, 2001:495–517.

2. Driscoll DA, Spinner NB, Budarf ML, McDonald-McGinn DM, Zackai EH, Goldberg RB, Shprintzen RJ, Saal HM, Zonana J, Jones MC, Mascarello JT, Emanuel BS. Deletions and microdeletions of 22q11.2 in velo-cardio-facial syndrome. Am J Med Genet 1992; 44:261–268.

3. Scambler PJ, Kelly D, Lindsay E, Williamson R, Goldberg R, Shprintzen R, Wilson DI, Goodship JA, Cross IE, Burn J. Velo-cardio-facial syndrome associated with chromosome 22 deletions encompassing the DiGeorge locus. Lancet 1992; 339:1138–1139.

4. Shprintzen RJ, Goldberg RB, Lewin ML, Sidoti EJ, Berkman MD, Argamaso RV, Young DA. A new syndrome involving cleft palate, cardiac, anomalies, typical facies, and learning disabilities: velo-cardio-facial syndrome. Cleft Palate 1978; 15:56–62.

5. Golding-Kushner KJ, Weller G, Shprintzen RJ. Velo-cardio-facial syndrome: language and psychological profiles. J Craniofac Genet Dev Biol 1985; 5:259–266.

6. Goldberg R, Motzkin B, Marion R, Scambler PJ, Shprintzen RJ. Velo-cardio-facial syndrome: a review of 120 patients. Am J Med Genet 1993; 45:313–319.

7. Swillen A, Devriendt K, Legius E, Eyskens B, Dumoulin M, Gewillig M, Fryns JP. Intelligence and psychosocial adjustment in velo-cardio-facial syndrome: a study of 37 children and adolescents with VCFS. J Med Genet 1997; 34:453–458.

8. Moss E, Batshaw M, Solot C, Gerdes M, McDonald-McGinn D, Driscoll D, Emanuel B, Zackai E, Wang P. Psychoeducational profile of the 22q11.2 microdeletion: a complex pattern. J Pediatr 1999; 134:193–198.

9. Shprintzen RJ. Velocardiofacial syndrome: a distinctive behavioral phenotype. Ment Retard Dev Disabil Res Rev 2000; 6:142–147.

10. Shprintzen R. Velo-cardio-facial syndrome. Otolaryngol Clin North Am 2000; 33:1217–1240.

11. Swillen A, Devriendt K, Legius E, Prinzie P, Vogels A, Ghesquiere P, Fryns JP. The behavioural phenotype in velo-cardio-facial syndrome (VCFS): from infancy to adolescence. Genet Couns 1999; 10:79–88.

12. Papolos DF, Faedda GL, Veit S, Goldberg R, Morrow B, Kucherlapati R, Shprintzen RJ. Bipolar spectrum disorders in patients diagnosed with velo-cardio-facial syndrome: does a hemizygous deletion of chromosome 22q11 result in bipolar affective disorder?Am J Psychiatry 1996; 153:1541–1547.

13. Murphy KC, Jones LA, Owen MJ. High rates of schizophrenia in adults with velo-cardio-facial syndrome. Arch Gen Psychiatry 1999; 56:940–945.

14. Driscoll DA, Salvin J, Sellinger B, Budarf ML, McDonald-McGinn DM, Zackai EH, Emanuel BS. Prevalence of 22q11 microdeletions in DiGeorge and velocardiofacial syndromes: Implications for genetic counselling and prenatal diagnosis. J Med Genet 1993; 30:813–817.

15. Shprintzen RJ, Goldberg RB, Young D, Wolford L. The velo-cardio-facial syndrome: a clinical and genetic analysis. Pediatrics 1981; 67:167–172.

16. Williams M, Shprintzen RJ, Goldberg RB. Male-to-male transmission of the velo-cardio-facial syndrome: a case report and review of 60 cases. J Craniofac Genet Dev Biol 1985; 5: 175–180.

17. Strong WB. Familial syndrome of right-sided aortic arch, mental deficiency, and facial dysmorphism. J Pediatr 1968; 73:882–888.

18. Sedlačková E. The syndrome of the congenitally shortening of the soft palate. Cas Lek Ces 1955; 94:1304–1307.

19. Kretschmer R, Say B, Brown D, Rosen FS. Congenital aplasia of the thymus gland (DiGeorge's syndrome). N Engl J Med 1968; 279:1295–1301.

20. Kaplan EN. The occult submucous cleft palate. Cleft Palate J 1975; 12:356–368.

21. Sedlačková E. The syndrome of the congenitally shortened velum. The dual innervation of the soft palate. Folia Phoniatr 1967; 19:441–450.

22. Cayler GG. Cardiofacial syndrome. Congenital heart disease and facial weakness, a hitherto unrecognized association. Arch Dis Child 1969; 44:69–75.

23. Kinouchi A, Mori K, Ando M, Takao A. Facial appearance of patients with conotruncal anomalies. Pediatr Jpn 1976; 17:84–87.

24. Takao A, Ando M, Cho K. Etiologic categorization of common congenital heart disease. In: Van Praagh R, Takao A, eds. Etiology and Morphogenesis of Congenital Heart Disease. Mount Kisco, NY: Futura, 1980:253–369.

25. Momma K, Kondo C, Matsuoka A, Takao A. Cardiac anomalies associated with a chromosome 22q11 deletion in patients with conotruncal anomaly face syndrome. Am J Cardiol 1996; 78: 591–594.

26. Fryburg JS, Lin YK, Golden WL. Chromosome 22q11.2 deletion in a boy with Opitz (G/BBB) syndrome. Am J Med Genet 1996; 62:274–275.

27. Daw SCM, Taylor C, Kraman M, Call K, Mao J, Schuffenhauer S, Meitinger T, Lipson T, Goodship J, Scambler P. A common region of 10p deleted in DiGeorge and velocardiofacial syndromes. Nat Genet 1996; 13:458–461.

28. Morrow B, Goldberg R, Carlson C, Das Gupta R, Sirotkin H, Collins J, Dunham I, O'Donnell H, Scambler P, Shprintzen R. Molecular definition of the 22q11 deletions in velo-cardio-facial syndrome. Am J Hum Genet 1995; 56:1391–1403.

29. Funke B, Saint-Jore B, Puech A, Sirotkin H, Edelmann L, Carlson C, Raft S, Pandita RK, Kucherlapati R, Skoultchi A, Morrow BE. Characterization and mutation analysis of goosecoid-like (GSCL), a homeodomain-containing gene that maps to the critical region for VCFS/DGS on 22q11. Genomics 1997; 46:364–372.

30. Lachman HM, Morrow B, Shprintzen R, Veit S, Parsia SS, Faedda G, Goldberg R, Kucherlapati R, Papolos DF. Association of codon 108/158 catechol-*O*-methyltransferase gene

polymorphism with the psychiatric manifestations of velo-cardio-facial syndrome. Am J Med Genet 1996; 67:468–472.

31. Merscher S, Funke B, Epstein JA, Heyer J, Puech A, Lu MM, Xavier RJ, Demay MB, Russell RG, Factor S, Tokooya K, Jore BS, Lopez M, Pandita RK, Lia M, Carrion D, Xu H, Schorle H, Kobler JB, Scambler P. TBX1 is responsible for cardiovascular defects in velo-cardio-facial/DiGeorge syndrome. Cell 2001; 104:619–629.

32. Yamagishi H, Garg V, Matsuoka R, Thomas T, Srivastava D. A molecular pathway revealing a genetic basis for human cardiac and craniofacial defects. Science 1999; 283:1158–1161.

33. Graf WD, Unis AS, Yates CM, Sulzbacher S, Dinulos MB, Jack RM, Dugaw KA, Paddock MN, Parson WW. Catecholamines in patients with 22q11.2 deletion syndrome and the low-activity COMT polymorphism. Neurology 2001; 57:410–416.

34. Edelmann L, Pandita RK, Spiteri E, Funke B, Goldberg R, Palanisamy N, Chaganti RS, Magenis E, Shprintzen RJ, Morrow BE. A common molecular basis for rearrangement disorders on chromosome 22q11. Hum Mol Genet 1999; 8: 1157–1167.

35. Mitnick R, Bello J, Shprintzen R. Brain anomalies in velo-cardio-facial syndrome. Am J Med Genet 1994; 54:100–106.

36. Chow EW, Mikulis DJ, Zipursky RB, Scutt LE, Weksberg R, Bassett AS. Qualitative MRI findings in adults with 22q11 deletion syndrome and schizophrenia. Biol Psychiatry 1999; 46:1436–1442.

37. Eliez S, Schmitt JE, White CD, Reiss AL. Children and adolescents with velocardiofacial syndrome: a volumetric MRI study. Am J Psychiatry 2000; 157:409–415.

38. Kates W, Burnette C, Jabs E, Rutberg J, Murphy A, Grados M, Geraghty M, Kaufmann W, Pearlson G. Regional cortical white matter reductions in velocardiofacial syndrome: a volumetric MRI analysis. Biol Psychiatry 2001; 49:677–685.

39. Eliez S, Schmitt J, White C, Wellis V, Reiss AL. A quantitative MRI study of posterior fossa development in velocardiofacial syndrome. Biol Psychiatry 2001; 49:540–546.

40. Van Amelsvoort T, Daly E, Robertson D, Suckling J, Ng V, Critchley H, Owen MJ, Henry J, Murphy KC, Murphy DGM. Structural brain abnormalities associated with deletion at chromosome 22q11: quantitative neuroimaging study of adults with velo-cardio-facial syndrome. Br J Psychiatry 2001; 178:412–419.

41. Eliez S, Barnea-Goraly N, Schmitt JE, Liu Y, Reiss AL. Increased basal ganglia volumes in velo-cardio-facial syndrome (deletion 22q11.2). Biol Psychiatry 2002; 52:68–70.

42. Sugama S, Bingham PM, Wang PP, Moss EM, Kobayashi H, Eto Y. Morphometry of the head of the caudate nucleus in patients with velocardiofacial syndrome (del 22q11.2). Acta Paediatr 2000; 89:546–549.

43. Kates WR, Burnette CP, Bessette BA, Folley BS, Strunge L, Jabs EW, Pearlson GD. Frontal and caudate alterations in velocardiofacial syndrome (deletion at chromosome 22q11.2). J Child Neurol 2004; 19(5):337–342.

44. Chow EW, Zipursky RB, Mikulis DJ, Bassett AS. Structural brain abnormalities in patients with schizophrenia and 22q11 deletion syndrome. Biol Psychiatry 2002; 51:208–215.

45. Mega MS, Cummings JL. Frontal–subcortical circuits and neuropsychiatric disorders. J Neuropsychiatry Clin Neurosci 1994; 6:358–370.

46. Alexander GE, DeLong MR, Strick PL. Parallel organization of functionally segregated circuits linking basal ganglia and cortex. Ann Rev Neurosci 1986; 9:357–381.

47. Middleton FA, Strick PL. Basal ganglia and cerebellar loops: motor and cognitive circuits. Brain Res Rev 2000; 31:236–250.

48. Cummings JL. Frontal–subcortical circuits and human behavior. Arch Neurol 1993; 50:873–880.

49. Feinstein C, Eliez S, Blasey C, Reiss AL. Psychiatric disorders and behavioral problems in children with velocardiofacial syndrome: usefulness as phenotypic indicators of schizophrenia risk. Biol Psychiatry 2002; 15:312–318.

50. Arnold PD, Siegel-Bartelt J, Cytrynbaum C, Teshima I, Schachar R. Velo-cardio-facial syndrome: implications of

microdeletion 22q11 for schizophrenia and mood disorders. Am J Med Genet (Neuropsychiatr Genet) 2001; 105:354–362.

51. Vogels A, Verhoeven WMA, Tuinier S, DeVriendt K, Swillen A, Curfs LMG, Frijns JP. The psychopathological phenotype of velo-cardio-facial syndrome. Annal de Genet 2002; 45:89–95.

52. Pearlson G, Petty R, Ross C, Tien A. Schizophrenia: a disease of heteromodal association cortex? Neuropsychopharmacology 1996; 14:1–17.

53. Mesulam M. A cortical network for directed attention and unilateral neglect. Arch Neurol 1981; 10:304–325.

54. Goldman-Rakic P. Higher functions of the brain. In: Plum F, Mountcastle V, eds. The Handbook of Physiology. Vol. V. Bethesda, MD: American Physiological Society, 1987:373–417.

55. Eliez S, Blasey CM, Menon V, White CD, Schmitt JE, Reiss AL. Functional brain imaging study of mathematical reasoning abilities in velocardiofacial syndrome (del22q11.2). Genet Med 2001; 3:49–55.

56. Eliez S, Blasey C, Schmitt E, White C, Hu D, Reiss A. Velocar-dio-facial syndrome: are structural changes in the temporal and mesial temporal regions related to schizophrenia? Am J Psychiatry. 2001; 158:447–453.

57. Ryan AK, Goodship JA, Wilson DI, Philip N, Levy A, Seidel H, Schuffenhauer S, Oechsler H, Belohradsky B, Prieur M, Aurias A, Raymond FL, Clayton-Smith J, Hatchwell E, McKeown C, Beemer FA, Dallapiccola B, Novelli G, Hurst JA, Ignatius J. Spectrum of clinical features associated with interstitial chromosome 22q11 deletions: a European colla-borative study. J Med Genet 1997; 34:798–804.

58. Swillen A, Vandeputte L, Cracco J, Maes B, Ghesquiere P, Devriendt K, Fryns J. Neuropsychological, learning and psy-chosocial profile of primary school aged children with the velo-cardio-facial syndrome (22q11 deletion): evidence for a nonverbal learning disability? Neuropsychol Dev Cogn Sect C Child Neuropsychol 1999; 5:230–241.

59. Gilger J. Differential assortative mating found for academic and demographic variables as a function of time of assessment. Behav Genet 1991; 21:131–150.

60. Scherer NJ, D'Antonio LL, Kalbfleisch JE. Early speech and language development in children with velocardiofacial syndrome. Am J Med Genet 1999; 88:714–723.

61. Lipson AH, Yuille D, Angel M, Thompson PG, Vandervoord JG, Beckenham EJ. Velo-cardio-facial (Shprintzen) syndrome: an important syndrome for the dysmorphologist to recognise. J Med Genet 1991; 28:596–604.

62. McDonald-McGinn DM, Kirschner R, Goldmuntz E, Sullivan K, Eicher P, Gerdes M, Moss E, Solot C, Wang P, Jacobs I, Handler S, Knightly C, Heher K, Wilson M, Ming JE, Grace K, Driscoll D, Pasquariello P, Randall P, Larossa D. The Philadelphia story: the 22q11.2 deletion: report on 250 patients. Genet Couns 1999; 10:11–24.

63. Simon TJ, Bearden CE, Moss EM, McDonald-McGinn D, Kackai E, Wang PP. Cognitive development in VCFS. Prog Ped Cardiol 2002; 15:109–117.

64. Glaser B, Mumme DL, Blasey C, Morris MA, Dahoun SP, Antonarakis SE, Reiss AL, Eliez S. Language skills in children with velocardiofacial syndrome (deletion 22q11.2). J Pediatr 2002; 140:753–758.

65. Rourke BP. Nonverbal Learning Disabilities: The Syndrome and the Model. New York: Guilford Press, 1989.

66. Warrington EK, James M. Visual apperceptive agnosia: a clinico-anatomical study of three cases. Cortex 1988; 24:13–32.

67. Wang PP, Woodin MF, Kreps-Falk R, Moss EM. Research on behavioral phenotypes: velocardiofacial syndrome (deletion 22q11.2). Dev Med Child Neurol 2000; 42:422–427.

68. Gerdes M, Solot C, Wang PP, Moss E, LaRossa D, Randall P, Goldmuntz E, Clark BJ III, Driscoll DA, Jawad A, Emanuel BS, McDonald-McGinn DM, Batshaw ML, Zackai EH. Cognitive and behavior profile of preschool children with chromosome 22q11.2 deletion. Am J Med Genet 1999; 85:127–133.

69. Einfeld SL, Tonge BJ. Population prevalence of psychopathology in children and adolescents with intellectual disability: II. Epidemiological findings. J Intellect Disabil Res 1996; 40:99–109.

70. Woodin M, Wang P, Bearden C, McDonald-McGinn D, Zakai E, Emanuel B. Attention, working memory and executive functions in children and adolescents with velocardiofacial syndrome: patterns, profiles, and presentation. Neuropsych Soc 2000; 6:160.

71. McCandless S, Scott J, Robin N. Deletion 22q11: a newly recognized cause of behavioral and psychiatric disorders. Arch Pediatr Adolesc Med 1998; 152:481–484.

72. Pulver AE, Nestadt G, Goldberg R, Shprintzen RJ, Lamacz M, Wolyniec PS, Morrow B, Karayiorgou M, Antonarakis SE, Housman D. Psychotic illness in patients diagnosed with velo-cardio-facial syndrome and their relatives. J Nerv Ment Dis 1994; 182:476–478.

73. Karayiorgou M, Morris M, Morrow B, Shprintzen R, Goldberg R, Borrow J, Gos A, Nestadt G, Wolyniec P, Lasseter V. Schizophrenia susceptibility associated with interstitial deletions of chromosome 22q11. Proc Natl Acad Sci USA 1995; 92:7612–7616.

74. Beitchman J, Nair R, Clegg M, Ferguson B, Patel P. Prevalence of psychiatric disorders in children with speech and language disorders. J Am Acad Child Psychiatry 1986; 25: 528–535.

75. Beitchman J, Young A. Learning disorders with a special emphasis on reading disorders: a review of the past 10 years. J Am Acad Child Adolesc Psychiatry 1997; 36:1020–1032.

76. Feinstein C, Reiss A. Psychiatric disorders in mentally retarded children and adolescents. Child Adolesc Psychiatr Clin N Am 1996; 5:827–852.

77. Carlson C, Papolos D, Pandita RK, Faedda GL, Veit S, Goldberg R, Shprintzen R, Kucherlapati R, Morrow B. Molecular analysis of velo-cardio-facial syndrome patients with psychiatric disorders. Am J Hum Genet 1997; 60:851–859.

78. Shprintzen RJ, Goldberg R, Golding-Kushner KJ, Marion RW. Late-onset psychosis in the velo-cardio-facial syndrome. Am J Med Genet 1992; 42:141–142.

79. Bassett AS, Chow EW. 22q11 deletion syndrome: a genetic subtype of schizophrenia. Biol Psychiatry 1999; 46:882–891.

80. Hans SL, Marcus J, Nuechterlein KH, Asarnow RF, Styr B, Auerbach JG. Neurobehavioral deficits at adolescence in children at risk for schizophrenia: the Jerusalem Infant Development Study. Arch Gen Psychiatry 1999; 56:741–748.

81. Karayiorgou M, Altemus M, Galke B, Goldman D, Murphy D, Ott J, Gogos J. Genotype determining low catechol-*O*-methyltransferase activity as a risk factor for obsessive–compulsive disorder. Proc Natl Acad Sci USA 1997; 94:4572–4575.

82. Papolos D, Veit S, Faedda G, Saito T, Lachman H. Ultra–ultra rapid cycling bipolar disorder is associated with the low activity atecholamine-*O*-methyltransferase allele. Mol Psychiatry 1998; 3:346–349.

83. Egan M, Goldberg T, Gscheidle T, Weirich M, Rawlings R, Hyde T, Bigelow L, Weinberger D. Relative risk for cognitive impairments in siblings of patients with schizophrenia. Biol Psychiatry 2001; 50:98–107.

84. Akil M, Kolachana B, Rothmond D, Hyde T, Weinberger D, Kleinman J. Catechol-*O*-methyltransferase genotype and dopamine regulation in the human brain. J Neurosci 2003; 23: 2008–2013.

85. Dunham I, Collins J, Wadey R, Scambler P. Possible role for COMT in psychosis associated with velo-cardio-facial syndrome. Lancet 1992; 340:1361–1362.

13

Smith–Magenis Syndrome—A Developmental Disorder with Circadian Dysfunction

ANN C. M. SMITH

National Human Genome Research
Institute, National Institutes of Health,
HHS, Bethesda, Maryland, U.S.A.
and
Department of Oncology, Institute of
Molecular and Human Genetics,
Georgetown University School of
Medicine, Washington, D.C., U.S.A.

WALLACE C. DUNCAN

Mood and Anxiety Disorders
Program, National Institute of Mental
Health, National Institutes of Health,
HHS, Bethesda, Maryland, U.S.A.

I. BACKGROUND AND HISTORICAL OVERVIEW

Smith–Magenis syndrome (SMS) is a rare complex developmental disorder with multisystem involvement that is the result of a heterozygous interstitial deletion of the p11.2

419

band of chromosome 17. The deletion was first identified cytogenetically in the early 1980s in two males with multiple congenital anomalies (MCA) (1). This report was followed by a clinical series of 15 patients ranging in age from 3 months to 65 years that more fully delineated the clinical aspects of this MCA/mental retardation (MR) syndrome (2,3). Comprehensive clinical reviews published in the 1990s further expanded the phenotypic spectrum and variability of features that distinguish the physical, developmental, and neurobehavioral aspects of the syndrome (4–14).

The phenotype of SMS is characterized by a distinct pattern of features that include infantile hypotonia, minor craniofacial and skeletal anomalies, middle ear/laryngeal anomalies and ocular abnormalities, marked early expressive speech/language delays, psychomotor and growth retardation, and, to a lesser extent, genitourinary and cardiac anomalies. In all cases, developmental delays and variable levels of mental retardation are found (5,13). A striking neurobehavioral SMS phenotype occurs that includes a specific pattern of stereotypies, hyperactivity, and self-injurious, aggressive and maladaptive behaviors (7,10,11,13,15,16). Chronic sleep disturbance is present that is likely aggravated by high daytime and low nighttime levels of melatonin (17,18). Hyper-cholesterolemia, low immunoglobulins, specifically IgA, and hypothyroidism are also noted (5,19).

Despite increased clinical recognition of the SMS phenotype, the diagnosis is frequently not made until school age or older when the neurobehavioral aspects of the syndrome often prompt clinical and diagnostic referral. Interestingly, the oldest individual (Case 8) (2) with SMS, now in her 80s, was originally diagnosed with Down syndrome (DS) in early childhood. She carried this diagnosis until cytogenetic tests in mid-1980s confirmed an interstitial deletion of 17p11.2 at age 65. This early case epitomizes the unfortunate fact that misdiagnosis occurs too frequently despite the abundance of diagnostic and genetic tools available to identify SMS. Early diagnosis requires an awareness of the often subtle clinical and neurobehavioral features that typify the early infant phenotype. The discovery of SMS rests on the technological advances made in the field of human cytogenetics and the observation by a skilled technologist in 1981 of the small interstitial deletion within the 17p11.2 band of one of the two chromosome 17 pairs (1). Most individuals with SMS have been identified in the last decade due to improved molecular cytogenetic techniques and an increased clinical awareness of the syndrome. In most cases, confirmation of the SMS diagnosis is accomplished cytogenetically and/or by fluorescence in situ hybridization (FISH). Approximately 75% of cases are associated with a common deletion interval spanning ~4 Mb, resulting in hemizygosity of multiple, functionally regulated genes located within the 17p11.2 interval (20,21). About 25% of reported cases represent a second subgroup of atypical, i.e., smaller or larger, deletions (20,21). A wide range of clinical variability is seen among those with the common deletion without a strong correlation between deletion size and clinical presentation (21). However, the frequency of EEG abnormalities and visceral anomalies tends to be more common in atypical deletion cases (21). These two major subgroups of deletions (common and atypical) account for over 95% of diagnosed cases. However, the recent report of mutations in a single gene, *RAI1* (retinoic acid-induced 1), identified in a third subgroup of patients with the SMS phenotype has implications for diagnosis in selected cases (22).

This chapter seeks to increase clinical awareness about SMS and assists the clinician in recognizing the salient and sometimes subtle constellation of features in SMS at different ages (Table 1). Many clues that go beyond physical appearance are present to alert the clinician and raise diagnostic suspicion in early childhood. Experience demonstrates the importance of listening to parents who tell stories about their child's first year of life. Embedded in these stories are key characteristics (archetypal findings) that resonate with an SMS diagnosis. For the parents and clinicians involved in the care of the undiagnosed SMS child, the road to diagnosis is usually paved by frequent pediatric office visits for upper respiratory infections, middle ear problems and/or growth delays, and numerous specialist and medical referrals for what may appear to be disparate symptoms. Individually,

Table 1 Characteristic Features of Smith–Magenis Syndrome by Age Group

	Infancy ≤1 year	Toddler/early childhood 1–5 years	School age 5–12 years	Adolescence/ adulthood >12 years
Very common (>75%)[a]				
Craniofacial/skeletal				
Brachycephaly	+	+	+	+
Midface hypoplasia	+	+	+	+
Micrognathia	+	±	0	0
Relative prognathism (prominent jaw)	0	0	+	+
Broad, square-shaped face	+	±	+	+
Down's-like appearance	+	+	+	0
Deep-set eyes	(+)	+	+	+
Closely set eyes	?	+	+	+
Upslanting palpebral fissures	+	+	±	(+)
Synophrys	(+)	(+)	+	+
Everted "tented" upper lip	+	+	+	+
Rosy cheeks	(+)	(+)	0	0
Short broad hands	+	+	+	+
Small feet	+	+	+	(+)
Dorsal edema feet/hands	(+)	±	(+)	(+)
Short stature (<5th percentile for age)	(+)	+	+	(+)
Otolaryngologic				
Middle ear and laryngeal anomalies	+	+	+	+
Hoarse, deep voice	NA	+	+	+

Diminished/weak cry	(+)	NA	NA	NA
Broad-based gait	NA	+	+	+
Neuro/behavioral				
Developmental delay/cognitive impairment	+	+	+	+
Generalized complacency/lethargy	+	0	0	0
Mild to moderate hypotonia	+	+	±	±
Hyporeflexia (decreased/absent DTRs)	+	+	+	(+)
Signs of peripheral neuropathy	+	+	+	+
Oral–sensory–motor dysfunction	+	+	+	(+)
Feeding/swallowing difficulties	+	+	(+)	?
Open mouth posture	+	+	±	?
Decreased lingual strength and movement	+	+	(+)	?
Speech/Language delay	+	NA	+	?
Articulation difficulties	NA	NA	+	+
Sleep disturbance	+	+	+	+
Inverted circadian rhythm of melatonin	?	+	+	+
Maladaptive behaviors	0	+	+	+
Attention seeking	?	+	+	+
Temper tantrums/sudden mood shifts	0	+	+	+
Impulsivity/hyperactivity	0	+	+	+
Self-injurious behaviors	0	+	+	+
Hitting/slapping self	0	+	+	+
Hand/wrist biting	0	+	+	+
Head-banging	(+)	+	+	+

(Continued)

Table 1 Characteristic Features of Smith–Magenis Syndrome by Age Group (*Continued*)

	Infancy ≤1 year	Toddler/early childhood 1–5 years	School age 5–12 years	Adolescence/ adulthood >12 years
Stereotypic behaviors (one or more)	0	+	+	+
Self-hug	0	(+)	+	+
Lick and page flipping	0	(+)	+	+
Hands in mouth	+++	+	(+)	?
Common (50–75%)				
REM sleep abnormalities	?	+	+	+
Hearing loss				
Conductive	+	+	+	+
Sensorineural	0ᵇ	0	+	+
Mild ventriculomegaly of brain	+	+	+	?
Ocular abnormalities	(+)	+	+	+
Strabismus	+	+	+	+ vs. (+)
Iris anomalies	+	+	+	+
Microcornea	?	(+)	+	+
Myopia	+	+	+	+
Wolfflin–Kruckmann and/or Brushfield spots				
Tracheobronchial problems	+	(+)	+	+
Velopharyngeal insufficiency (VPI)	NA	(+)	?	?
History GI reflux	(+)	(+)	?	?
Short stature(<5th percentage for age)	(+)	+	+	(+)

Feature	Infancy	Toddler/early childhood	School age	Adolescence/adulthood
Scoliosis	±	+	+	+
Hypercholesterolemia	+	+	+	(+)
History of constipation	+	+	+	+
Less common (25–50%)[a]				
Cardiac defects	+	+	+	+
Vertebral anomalies	+	+	+	+
Renal/urinary tract abnormalities	0	0	+	+
Thyroid function abnormalities	?	?	+	?
Immune function abnormalities	?	?	+	?
Obesity and/or increased BMI	?	+	+	+
Seizures ± EEG abnormality	?	(+)	+	?
Mild/diffuse atrophy of brain (CT scan)	+	+	?	?
Palatal dimpling	+	+	+	+
Exaggerated lingual papillae	?	?	+	(+)
Prominent fingertip pads	+	+	+	+
Onychotillomania (nail yanking)	0	±	+	+
Polyembolokoilamania (excluding mouth)	0	±	+	+
Occasional (under 25%)				
Forearm abnormalities	+	+	+	+
Cleft lip/palate	+	+	+	+
Retinal detachment	0	(+)	+	+

[a]Percentages are based on the overall frequency of features that define the syndrome, regardless of age. Since the presence/absence of certain features may be age dependent, additional codes (see below) are used to reflect whether the feature is present at the observed or different frequency level for a specific age group:

KEY: +, Documented presence at this age; (+), Reported or observed, but frequency unknown for age; ±, Low frequency at this age; 0, Absent at this age; ?, Insufficient data at this age; NA, Not applicable.

Source: Data derived from individual case reports, published reviews with age data, and/or personal observations as follows: Infancy: (1,2,19,26,39,46,54,66); Toddler/early childhood: (2,12,18,19,53,61,81,103,104); School age: (2,3,6,12,26,53,103–107; Adolescence/adulthood: (2,3,6,12,19,52,53,58,81).

these findings might not raise concern, but collectively they should alert one to the possibility of SMS. Once diagnosed, an interdisciplinary management approach that builds on practical and published experience is beneficial to persons with SMS, their families, and care providers.

Smith–Magenis syndrome has been identified worldwide among diverse ethnic groups. The prevalence is estimated to be 1/25,000 births (4), a likely underestimate since the syndrome remains vastly under diagnosed. Since initial description, more than 100 individuals with SMS have been described in the literature (23), and approximately 600 are registered with the international parent support group, parents and researchers interested in Smith–Magenis syndrome (PRISMS) (www.smithmagenis.org). Among individuals with mental retardation, the frequency of SMS (del 17p11.2) is estimated at approximately 1/600 (24–26).

II. GENETICS

As mentioned earlier, the diagnosis of SMS is usually confirmed by identification of an interstitial deletion of 17p11.2 (cytogenetically and/or by FISH with DNA-specific probes). Standard cytogenetic studies at a 500–600 band level of resolution are generally adequate to detect the SMS deletion in 90–95% of cases, especially in experienced hands (27). However, even with improved cytogenetic techniques, the deletion has gone undetected in the laboratory, especially when the indication for cytogenetic study fails to include SMS in the differential diagnosis.

In cases where results are equivocal and/or a visible deletion is not found, cytogenetic testing with FISH-specific probes for the SMS critical region (SMSCR) (e.g., *RAI1* or D17S258) is indicated. The specific FISH probe(s) used for diagnostic confirmation is important (22) and, if not used, retesting may be necessary (Fig. 1) (20). Specifically, FISH probes that do not contain *RAI1* may produce false negative results in some SMS patients (22). As discussed later, the newly recognized third subgroup of SMS includes at least three adults with SMS confirmed to have frameshift mutations of

RAI1 (28). Since *RAI1* sequencing is expensive, pursuing mutation analysis is still restricted to a case-by-case basis (20,22). In these special cases where the diagnosis of SMS is strongly suspected, but the SMS deletion has yet to be documented, thorough clinical re-evaluation by genetic clinicians experienced with the SMS phenotype is recommended before costly retesting is undertaken.

A. Contiguous Gene Syndrome

Smith–Magenis syndrome is classified as a contiguous gene deletion syndrome in which the phenotype results from physically linked, unrelated dosage-sensitive genes. Molecular advances arising from the Human Genome Project have helped define the SMSCR to approximately 1 Mb within 17p11.2, likely containing 13 known genes, 12 predicted genes and 3 expressed sequence tags (ESTs) (20).

Until recently, the specific gene(s) causing SMS was unknown, though several were speculated to play a role (8,19,28–32). As mentioned earlier, one of these, *RAI1*, exhibited individual frameshift mutations in three adults with clinically suspected SMS (28). In these cases, prior cytogenetic study including FISH failed to confirm a deletion. However, *RAI1* sequencing confirmed individual dominant mutations that led to protein truncation of *RAI1*. Although the role of *RAI1* in cellular function is not fully understood, haploinsufficiency of *RAI1* may be responsible for some of the core features of the syndrome (20,28). Additional cases are required to explore the role of *RAI1*, since at least two major SMS features (short stature, hypotonia) and other less common visceral anomalies (cardiac and renal anomalies) were not present in these three adult individuals. The possibility exists that haploinsufficiency of other genes mapping within the SMS critical interval is also likely to be involved with structural anomalies and variable features.

Deletions associated with the SMS phenotype range from <1.5 to >9 Mb (33). For the majority, a common de novo deletion interval spanning ~4 Mb can be documented by FISH analysis or by the presence of a junction fragment on pulse

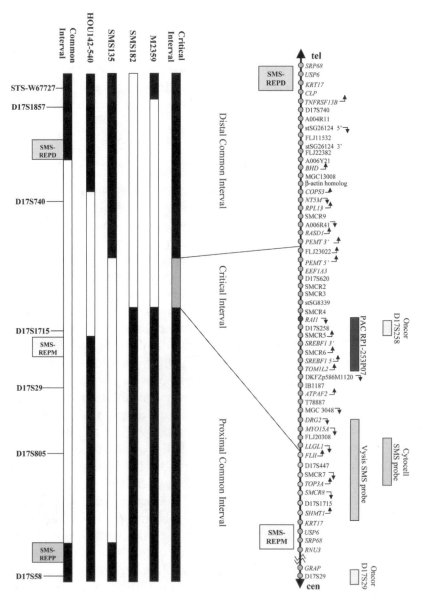

Figure 1 *(Caption on facing page)*

field gel electrophoresis (23). While early reports suggested the presence of the common deletion in over 90% of cases (23), more recent review of SMS patients with molecularly characterized deletions identified the common SMS deletion in approximately 74% of cases (20,21), a finding that has since been corroborated by others (21). Increased ascertainment of new cases has led to the identification of smaller or larger deletions involving 17p11.2 in the remaining 25% of cases (20,21). Identification of these atypical deletions remains critical to further refining the SMSCR. The SMS phenotype occurs in all cases where the deletion is identified cytogenetically and/or by FISH. The range and severity of features are variable even among individuals with SMS with the same sized common deletion (20,21).

No correlation exists between the deletion size and the variability of *cardinal* features of the syndrome (20,21,33). Less common features (Table 1), however, may be related to atypical deletions. Clinical correlations are hampered by the small number of atypical deletion cases that are molecularly

---

Figure 1 *(Facing page)* Smith–Magenis syndrome critical chromosome region. Refinement of the SMS critical chromosome interval, transcription map, and unusual 17p deletions. The SMS deletions important to the refinement of the SMS critical interval are indicated by the open/closed bars. Deleted DNA is represented by the open portion of the bars, while the closed portion represents nondeleted DNA. The common SMS deletion is labeled and represented by the largest openbar (bottom) includes the locations of the three SMS-REPs in relation to genomic markers mapped to this region of 17p. The SMS critical deletion region is represented by the pink bar. The current SMS transcription map (modified from Ref. 29 using the GenomeBrowser at UCSC and Unigene at NCBI information) is shown; genes, ESTs, and markers mapping to the critical interval are represented by pink circles. The *RAI1* gene is indicated by a blue circle. The green bars above the transcription map represent the currently available FISH probes from Vysis and Cytocell, the blue bar represents the PAC RP1-253P07 used in our FISH experiments, and the previously available FISH probes from Oncor are indicated by yellow bars. This figure is not to scale. (From Sarah Elsea, Ph.D., Virginia Commonwealth University, Richmond, Virginia.) *(See color insert.)*

and clinically characterized. For example, cardiac defects were identified in each of the four large deletion cases evaluated among 16 atypical published deletions (20,21,33). Interestingly, the two original cases reported by Smith in 1982 (1) both had large deletions and cardiac defects. Case 1 had multiple structural anomalies (cardiac defect, cleft palate, and a bilateral ureterovesicular obstruction with enlarged kidneys) and studied before the advent of FISH. Case 2 (2), currently in his 20s, has a large deletion that extends distally and includes PMP22 (4). While recent studies failed to identify renal anomalies among the large deletion cases, 50–60% of small deletion cases had renal anomalies compared to 15% of common deletion cases (20,21). The presence of renal anomalies in the original Case 1 illustrates the importance of identifying additional atypical deletion cases as they may help discern the role of specific genes in phenotypic expression.

B. Mechanism

The mechanism of the 17p11.2 microdeletion was first described in SMS by Chen et al. (23) and later shown to be a common feature of genomic disorders, including other contiguous gene syndromes (34,35). The mechanism involves nonallelic homologous recombination (NAHR) of large, highly homologous flanking low-copy repeat (LCR) gene clusters. Three LCR gene clusters are present, a proximal, middle, and distal referred to as SMS-REPs (Fig. 1). The clusters (SMS-REPs) are prone to deletion, duplication, and inversion (23). The ∼4-Mb genomic segment that is commonly deleted in individuals with SMS is flanked by two large complex LCRs, the proximal and distal SMS-REPs (23). The NAHR, using the proximal and distal SMS-REP as substrates, leads to the common interstitial deletion of chromosome 17p11.2 that occurs in 75% of cases (20,21). Newly described LCR elements flanking the SMS-REP sequences are thought to mediate recombination in the atypical deletions (36) at a much higher rate than previously thought (20,21). Although reciprocal duplication of the same segment, dup(17)(p11.2p11.2), is predicted to occur at the same frequency as deletions (34), it has been identified in only a few patients. Among the seven described cases (ages 3–41 years), clinical features differ phenotypically and behaviorally from those seen in SMS (37).

The genomic structure and evolutionary origin of SMS-REPs were determined by Park et al. (36) who elegantly showed that the proximal SMS-REP ($\sim$256 kb) and distal copy ($\sim$176 kb) are located in the same orientation and derive from a progenitor copy. In contrast, the middle SMS-REP ($\sim$241 kb) was found to be inverted and appears to be derived from the proximal SMS-REP (31,36).

C. Genetic Counseling

1. Risk Assessment

Smith–Magenis syndrome occurs de novo with few exceptions, suggesting a low recurrence risk. Only two reported cases of maternal vertical transmission from parent to child are described in the literature. The first case is a phenotypically normal mother of a child with SMS who had a structurally abnormal karyotype showing 47 chromosomes including a normal 17, deleted 17 (p11.2), and a supernumerary small marker presumed to be the missing portion derived from 17p (38). The second case involved maternal somatic mosaicism leading to the birth of a daughter with confirmed SMS (39). The mother of the second case had several mild features of SMS, including brachycephaly, brachydactyly, pes planus/cavus, and conductive hearing loss. Given these rare cases, parental chromosome analysis should be pursued for all newly diagnosed cases to permit accurate genetic counseling. In the presence of normal parental karyotypes, the recurrence risk for future affected offspring is low ($<$1%) (27). Random parental origin of the deletion is seen, arguing against an imprinting effect for expression of SMS phenotype (4). There is no evidence to suggest an obvious parental age effect (4) and/or an unusual gender distribution (40).

Originally identified in SMS, the genomic mechanism of NAHR or unequal crossing over leads to other contiguous gene syndromes (35), including Prader–Willi syndrome (PWS), Angelman syndrome, Williams syndrome, and

DiGeorge/Velocardiofacial syndrome. Recent data suggests that infants conceived via assisted reproductive technology (ART), specifically intracytoplasmic sperm injection or in vitro fertilization techniques, are at two-fold risk of major birth defects and chromosome abnormalities compared to naturally conceived infants (41). An association between ART and human imprinting disorders has been reported for at least two different conditions, Angelman syndrome (15q11.2-q13; 1/15,000 births) (42) and Beckwith–Wiedemann syndrome (BWS) (11p15.5; 1/13,700 births) (43). DeBaun et al. (44) argue that ART might affect the epigenetics of early embryogenesis leading to birth defects. This group found an increased prevalence of BWS (4.6%) in pregnancies conceived by ART. The observed prevalence of BWS births associated with ART was 4% over a 5 year period, significantly higher ($p = 0.009$) than the expected general population rate of 1.2% (45). While a relationship between ART and SMS remains unproven and requires further study, the authors are aware of at least two cases of dizygous twins discordant for SMS that resulted from pregnancies conceived by ART.

2. Counseling and Psychological Support

Public and professional awareness about SMS and its implications for families is not widespread, despite the syndrome's discovery over 2 decades ago. For the parent(s) of a child newly diagnosed with SMS, learning the diagnosis often generates mixed emotions and raises compelling needs for information. Currently, the best resources of this information are parent support advocacy group(s) and peer reviewed published literature. Unfortunately much information (sometimes erroneous) is exchanged word-of-mouth or via the internet. PRISMS, established in 1993 as a support advocacy organization focused on SMS (www.smithmagenis.org), currently serves as the international clearinghouse for disseminating reliable information about SMS. Other international groups also provide a network of regional support for families of persons with SMS worldwide. Information disseminated by the PRISMS Professional Advisory Board (PAB) is derived from the most recent clinical and research findings and is therefore often a good starting point for planning future treatment and management strategies. For example, some of the most current directions include findings from the intramural National Institutes of Health (NIH) "Natural History Study of SMS," as well as several other extramural NIH-funded research protocols.

While the information disseminated by PRISMS and other organizations can be helpful to the parent and clinician's planning for a patient's needs, it should be emphasized that management of persons with SMS requires an interdisciplinary approach to effectively assist the family and address the needs of the patient with SMS. Ideally, the interdisciplinary health care team includes a range of health care specialists (i.e., primary care physician, physical and occupational therapists, speech/language pathologists, audiologists, neurologists, behavioral specialists, and geneticists) as well as special educators. Development and implementation of a plan of care for the newly diagnosed individual should incorporate the published guidelines for evaluation and treatment adopted by the PRISMS PAB (27), as well as information from published reviews. The interdisciplinary team may also play a significant role in assisting in other areas including, genetic and cytogenetic referrals, ongoing education, managing behavior and sleep, assisting with the Individualized Educational Plan (IEP) and identifying community resources for respite care and emotional support.

D. Differential Diagnosis

Smith–Magenis syndrome is more easily recognized at later ages, but often under diagnosed in infants and toddlers. The average age of diagnosis is between 4–5 years of age (46,47) when the neurobehavioral aspects are highly prevalent and the characteristic facial appearance is more obvious. Frequently, initial pursuit of cytogenetic studies is for clinical indications other than suspected SMS. Fortuitous detection of the interstitial deletion [del(17)(p11.2p11.2)] may occur, but several cases have gone undetected until repeat cytogenetic analysis with FISH.

Clinically, several features of SMS overlap with other conditions. During the newborn period, a presumptive diagnosis of DS is the most common reason for initial cytogenetic workup, due to the striking degree of phenotypic overlap (2,47,48). Both conditions share hypotonia, feeding difficulties, delayed growth (short stature), small hands/feet, brachycephaly, round face with flattened midface, upslanting palpebral fissures, iris hamartomas (Brushfield spots in DS; Wolfflin–Kruckmann spots in SMS), and open mouth posture. Comparative craniofacial pattern analysis between DS (49) and SMS (12) shows strikingly similar patterns for facial width, nose, mouth, and eye measurements. It is not surprising that 3 of 9 cases originally described in 1986 (2) were presumed to have DS for many years (and decades) before confirmation of the SMS deletion (17p11.2). The presence of infantile hypotonia, generalized lethargy, and developmental delays has led to a diagnostic workup for other microdeletion syndromes, usually without consideration for SMS. Two neonatal infants presenting with tetralogy of Fallot, initially studied cytogenetically to exclude a diagnosis of DiGeorge syndrome (del 22q), were subsequently documented to have SMS (50). In some cases, the coarse facial appearance that occurs with age has actually led to a comprehensive workup for suspected metabolic storage disease. One reported male, initially felt to have facial dysmorphia consistent with fetal alcohol syndrome, was later suspected to have Coffin–Lowry syndrome due to coarse appearance. He was subsequently diagnosed with SMS after workup for fragile X syndrome (26). Thus, in the absence of cytogenetic confirmation of a clinically suspected diagnosis of DS or other microdeletion syndromes, SMS remains a strong possibility. Pursuit of multi-FISH analysis to assess for these microdeletions in different syndromes may actually prove cost effective given the overlap of features in early infancy.

As discussed later in this chapter, any clinical presentation associated with a behavioral phenotype including global developmental delays (cognitive, motor, and speech/language) in association with specific neurobehavioral findings (sleep disturbance, specific stereotypies, and self-injurious behaviors (SIB)) should raise diagnostic suspicion of SMS. If SMS has not been previously confirmed by school age, many children with SMS may carry a functional psychiatric diagnosis based on DSM-IV criteria, including attention deficit hyperactivity disorder (ADHD), attention deficit disorder, obsessive–compulsive disorder, and/or autistic spectrum disorder with MR/DD (dual diagnosis). Differential diagnosis and laboratory referrals for fragile X syndrome prior to confirmation of the SMS diagnosis have been reported in numerous cases (2,26). Developmental delay, speech delay, and behavioral problems including impulsivity, attention deficit, hyperactivity, and autistic-like features are common to both fragile X syndrome and SMS. Among referrals for fragile X testing, one center found del 17p11.2 to be the most common chromosomal abnormality detected outside of fra(X)(q27.3), representing 25% (4/16) of the unbalanced chromosome abnormalities identified (26). Today, these cases may have been missed, since DNA analysis for associated trinucleotide expansion (CGG repeat) in the *FMR1* is the current method of choice in testing specifically for fragile X syndrome (51). Thus, persons suspected to have fragile X syndrome, but for whom current DNA-based testing fails to confirm a diagnosis, warrant evaluation for SMS, both clinically and cytogenetically.

Observing distinct features (Fig. 2) and/or eliciting certain medical history can reveal salient clues to prompt diagnostic suspicion of SMS. The lingual papillae (Fig. 3) appear to be specific to the syndrome, although the implications of these are not yet understood. The digital anomalies are also useful clues, specifically the small broad hands and small feet (brachydactyly), dorsal edema of hands/feet in infancy, persistent fetal fingertip pads, and/or dorsiflexed great toes (hammer toes) (Fig. 3). Evidence of self-injury such as skin picking and nail or hand biting (47,52,53) may also serve as important behavioral markers. Hypercholesterolemia and low immunoglobulins can also serve as biochemical markers.

The pediatric medical history usually documents frequent office visits for early feeding problems, middle ear

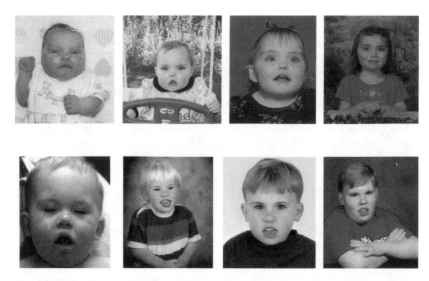

Figure 2 Characteristic facial features of Smith–Magenis syndrome in both males and females. Female shown (from top left to
top right) at birth; 8 months, 17 months, and 5 years of age, respectively. Male shown at ages 9 months, 5 years, 8 years, and 14 years
of age, respectively. Note the characteristic appearance to mouth
with open mouth posture, expressionless face, and tented upper
lip at younger ages. (*See color insert.*)

problems (chronic otitis media, conductive hearing loss),
upper respiratory illnesses, and/or sinusitis. Specific
questioning about the child's sleep patterns (daytime and
nighttime) should be pursued. Mothers often report a need
to awaken their infant for feeds, due to their child's generalized lethargy and complacency (54). Some mothers may even
express concern that something is different about their baby,
but are usually gratified to not have a cranky, upset, or crying
infant. Although the significant sleep disturbance is generally
not recognized by parents until 18 months of ages, recent actigraphy sleep data suggest the emergence of significant sleep
dysfunction from as early as 9 months of age (55). Despite
these early clinical signs, unfortunately a "wait-and-see"
approach is frequently taken unless cardiac and/or other
birth defects are identified. Failure to explore the early

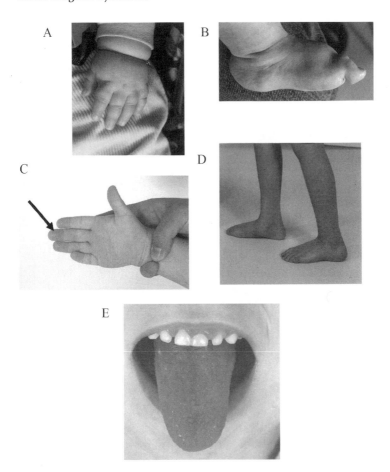

Figure 3 Clinical features of the extremities in Smith–Magenis syndrome. (A) Infant's left hand (note small, broad hands, dorsal edema/puffy appearance); (B) infant left foot (note dorsiflexed great toe, dorsal edema); (C) palmar appearance of child's hand demonstrating short 5th finger with clinodactyly and persistence of fetal pads on fingertips (arrow); (D) lower extremities from young child with SMS demonstrating characteristic thin lower legs with decreased muscle mass, pes planus, and prominent heels; and (E) exaggerated papillae of tongue. (*See color insert.*)

history may delay diagnostic pursuit to older ages, when the emerging sleep and behavioral disturbances are more readily apparent and subsequently prompt evaluation. However, the presence of early speech and motor delays, infantile hypotonia, and a quiet, placid demeanor in an infant with minimal vocalizations/babbling and/or diminished crying should strongly alert the clinician's suspicion for SMS.

III. CLINICAL DESCRIPTION

Smith–Magenis syndrome is associated with a distinct craniofacial appearance as well as other physical, developmental, and behavioral features. Some features may be subtle or nonspecific while others are more characteristic, especially at different developmental stages (Table 1). The core constellation of features that is present within the syndrome is discussed below.

A. Craniofacial Aspects

Craniofacial features in SMS are distinct across all ages (Fig. 2), but often subtle during infancy. The head is brachycephalic with a square-shaped face and prominent forehead. The eyes are close and deep set with upslanting palpebral fissures. Although the marked midface hypoplasia persists across all ages, it may not be fully appreciated in early infancy. In the infant/toddler stage, children with SMS have a smiling, almost angelic (cherubic) appearance, due to their rosy and pudgy cheeks, marked midface hypoplasia, and upslanting palpebral fissures. Their facial features have been described as reminiscent of the *Hummel* porcelain angel figurines. Eyebrows are usually heavy and dark with mild to complete synophrys that becomes more apparent with age. The nose is short (reduced nasal height) and broad with anteverted nares. The face may appear expressionless with an open mouth posture. The mouth is very distinct and characteristic of the syndrome, especially at younger ages. The upper lip is down-turned with a cupid's bow or "tented" appearance. Micrognathia changing to relative prognathism occurs with age. In a few instances, the micrognathia may lead to a clinical diagnosis of Pierre Robin sequence with/ without associated cleft palate (2,26). The facial appearance is most distinctive by mid-childhood (school age) and appears to coarsen with age (Fig. 2). The midface hypoplasia persists into adulthood, and the lower jaw grows, becomes more angulated and exhibits relative prognathia (56).

The skin and hair are generally fairer than other family members (Smith, personal observation). A range of ocular findings has been described, including iris anomalies (68%), microcornea (50%), strabismus (37%), myopia (42%), cataracts, and/or retinal detachment (6,9,25). The presence of heterochromatic irides (Wolfflin–Kruckmann spots) is reported which may be erroneously referred to as Brushfield spots as seen in DS. High myopia and retinal detachment appear to be age dependent. Other rare ocular anomalies reported in isolated cases include iris dysgenesis (25), congenital right Brown's syndrome (57), and visual loss caused by macular disciform scars (58).

B. Growth and Skeletal Aspects

Birth length, weight, and head circumference are usually within the normal range, though length tends to decelerate to less than the 5th percentile by 9–12 months of age. Short stature persists into adulthood with the majority in the low range of normal (5–10th percentile). Weight may decline in early infancy, but there is a tendency toward obesity with age. Even when failure to thrive is suspected, infants with SMS may appear healthy and robust. Body mass index (BMI) values have been reported in a group of 49 SMS children and found to be within the normal range in two-thirds of subjects (19). BMI values in females were not significantly different than normal, but males were slightly higher than expected (19).

Mild to moderate scoliosis occurs in approximately two-thirds of cases (>4 years of age), most commonly involving the midthoracic region (5). Vertebral anomalies are reported with low frequency (2,46). However, recent review of radiographs suggests at least a two-fold increase rate of spina bifida occulta in SMS (6/26; 23%) (Smith, personal observation) compared to the general population frequency (5–10%) (59).

A range of digital anomalies are seen in SMS that includes short broad hands (brachydactyly), cutaneous syndactyly of toes 2–3, clinodactyly, and/or polydacytly (3,8,40,60). Infants with SMS exhibit a characteristic appearance of the extremities (Fig. 3) with markedly small hands and feet that appear puffy due to dorsal edema and the redundant fat folds on the arms and legs, reminiscent of a "Michelin Man" appearance (2,47). The prominent fingertip fetal pads first reported by Kondo et al. (53) are also common. Metacarpophalangeal pattern profile analyses have confirmed brachydactyly (21,52,53). Though rare, short or bowed ulnae were reported in 12% of cases (5).

C. Otolaryngology, Speech/Language, and Hearing

Otolaryngologic abnormalities are a major feature of SMS, occurring in over 90% of cases (5,21,61). Chronic otitis media begin in early infancy and occur almost universally, often resulting in multiple PE tube placements. In a cross-sectional analysis of 48 individuals with SMS (age 5 months to 21 years), conductive hearing loss was common at all ages, but was most prevalent under age 5 (62). Over 95% of this group exhibited ear disease, tracheobronchial symptoms, and/or sinus infections. Middle ear dysfunction is a common cause of hearing loss in SMS. Over 64% of ears (right and left) show abnormal tympanograms (62) and associated conductive hearing loss. Only 26% of ears had normal tympanograms (62), while sensorineural deafness occured in 8–20% of cases (5,62), but may not occur until age 10 years (62).

Severe oral–sensori–motor dysfunction is characterized by decreased lingual movement and/or strength, lingual asymmetry, drooling, weak bilabial seal, palatal anomalies, and open mouth posture with anterior tongue carriage (61). Infants demonstrate significant difficulties related to poor suck reflex and persistent non-nutritive suckling pattern (61). Parents describe difficulties transitioning to solids and pureed and solid foods. Between 33% (5) and 84% (61) of persons with SMS are found to have laryngeal abnormalities including polyps, nodules, edema, plica ventricularis, and/or paralysis. Approximately two-thirds show signs of velopharyngeal insufficiency and a perceived nasal speech quality. Vocal impairments characterized by hoarse, wet, and harsh vocal qualities are evident in 84% (61). Exaggerated papillae of the tongue (Fig. 3) have been observed in about 50% of cases but without known clinical significance (61,63). Nevertheless, these findings highlight the relationship between dysfunctional ENT physiology and the impairments found in swallowing, speech/language development, and voice production (63).

Significant speech/language delays, with or without hearing loss, occur in over 90% of individuals with SMS. Early speech impairment with diminished vocalizations and babbling is a consistent feature in early childhood (61). Where tested, expressive language skills remain significantly more delayed than receptive and nonverbal communication skills in early childhood (5,64). In fact, most children with SMS do not show evidence of verbal language until about 4–5 years of age (Fig. 4) (61). Generally, vocal intensity is elevated, and has a rapid rate with moderate explosiveness (61,63). In contrast to extreme expressive speech/language delays in early childhood, older children and adults with SMS have sufficient speech to make themselves understood, although articulation problems usually persist.

Aggressive speech/language therapy consisting of a total communication program, including pictures and sign language, is integral to language development. The presence of some SIB, particularly head-banging, may be connected with delayed speech/language skills. Based upon personal observations, the onset of head-banging behaviors noted as early as age 18 months may relate to the child's generalized frustration and significant expressive language delays compared to receptive language function (13). The use of a total communication approach may positively impact early behavior by providing a

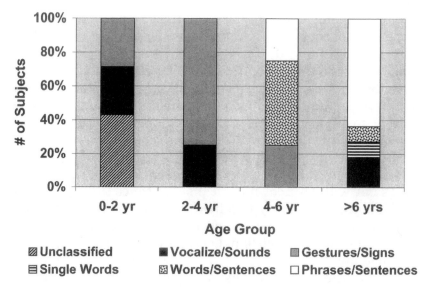

Figure 4 Primary communication modes by age. Comparison of the primary mode of communication used at the time of evaluation. Data shown are from 16 individuals with SMS undergoing comprehensive evaluation at the NIH (protocol 01-HG-0109). Note the use of gestures/signs less than 4 years of age, with decreased vocalizations in the first 2 years. (Solomon, personal communication). (Courtesy of Beth Solomon, M.S., SMS Research Team, Speech/Language Pathology, Clinical Center, Department of Rehabilitative Medicine, National Institutes of Health, HHS, Bethesda, MD.)

vehicle that helps to minimize frustration, thus diminishing early onset head-banging and other SIB (47).

D. Neurological Features

Persons with SMS exhibit features of both central and peripheral nervous system dysfunction (5,46). Structural anomalies of the CNS occur in about half of the cases studied to date, with ventriculomegaly being the most consistent finding (5,46). Using anatomical and functional brain imaging techniques, Boddeart et al. (65) found a high frequency of lenticulo-insular brain anomalies compared to normal age/sex matched controls among 5 males with SMS (<16 years of age).

There are only two known cases of SMS with published CNS neuropathological findings. The first (2) died 6 hr postoperatively of cardiogenic shock following repair of a ventricular septal defect. Notable CNS findings included microcephaly and foreshortened frontal lobes with depletion of neurons frontally and a small chorid plexus hemangioma in the lateral ventricle. The second case, a male born with cleft palate, died 2 days postoperatively following palatoplasty at 11 months of age (66). Clinically, he suffered respiratory arrest and hypotension, and died of apparent acute adrenal insufficiency that was confirmed at postmortem exam. On gross examination, the brain structures were normally formed (cerebrum, basal ganglia, midbrain, pons, and cerebellum) with widened gyri and narrowed sulci. Histological exam showed defined loss of the granular layer of cerebellum, but no evidence of dysplasia or lissencephaly.

The EEG abnormalities are reported in 20–50% of cases and occur independent of a history of clinical seizures (4,5,21,46). Based on recent reports, the frequency of EEG abnormalities is associated with deletion size, ranging from 49% in patients with the common deletion to 80% and 83% for patients with larger and smaller deletions, respectively (21). An isolated case of infantile spasms in a 9-month-old female is also reported (67). Recognition and treatment of seizures are important, since most individuals respond to traditional antiepileptic therapies that may also have a secondary effect on behavior and/or sleep (47). Clinical signs of peripheral neuropathy remain very common in SMS (5,46). Symptoms include mild to moderate infantile hypotonia (100%), hyporeflexia (84%), decreased sensitivity to pain, marked flat or highly arched feet (pes planus/cavus), and unusual broad-based flapping gait. Children with SMS often exhibit toe walking and distal muscle weakness in over 50% of cases. A previously undescribed peripheral neuropathy in the upper extremities was reported in 21% by Gropman et al. (64).

E. Endocrine/Biochemical Markers

Several biochemical and neuroendocrine abnormalties are found which may clinically assist in differential diagnosis. Low immunoglobulins (23%) and low thyroxine levels consistent with borderline hypothyroidism (29%) are reported (5). Low immunoglobuins, specifically IgA, are present in more than half of the cases (Smith, personal observation). Metabolic studies (amino acids, organic acids, and/or MPS screen) performed to date have been negative and/or nondiagnostic.

Haploinsufficiency for *SREBP1*, a gene located in the SMSCR involved in cholesterol homeostasis, may contribute to the increased frequency of hypercholesterolemia in SMS (19). An age and gender-controlled study of fasting lipid values in 49 children with SMS documented hypercholesterolemia in 57% (19). Only 16 (32%) were within normal limits. Hypercholesterolemia did not correlate significantly with BMI. Since the long-range implications of these findings are unknown, clinical management recommendations should be followed (68).

Remarkably, the circadian rhythm of melatonin is inverted in SMS (Fig. 5) (17,69–71). In contrast to the normal pattern in which melatonin is high at night and low during the day, a characteristic of all nocturnal and diurnal vertebrates and invertebrates, persons with SMS have high daytime and low nighttime melatonin levels. The mechanism(s) responsible for the inverse pattern is not understood but likely includes one of the 15–20 genes that reside in the critical region of the common deletion interval of chromosome 17. In contrast to the inverted pattern of melatonin, the circadian rhythms of cortisol and growth hormone appear not to be inverted, although their timing may be abnormal, and their levels somewhat diminished (70). Preliminary data also indicate that the body temperature in children with SMS is not inverted (Duncan and Smith, personal observation), consistent with the likelihood that the central circadian clock is not inverted. Rather, neural mechanisms that constitute output pathways of the clock, and which control melatonin production by the pineal gland, are suggested to be dysfunctional. The inverted melatonin rhythm may contribute to the disordered sleep pattern in SMS.

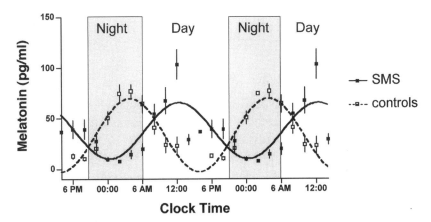

Figure 5 Circadian rhythm of melatonin in eight children with SMS (filled square with solid line) compared with 15 control children (open square with dotted line). Plasma melatonin levels were measured every 2 hr over a 24-hr period. Shown are the means ± SEM for the two groups. A sine wave was fit to the mean data of each group. The data are plotted twice to illustrate the circadian fluctuation of melatonin levels over the course of 2 days. Note that the peak melatonin occurs during the daytime in SMS and at night in the controls. The shaded dark rectangles correspond to the estimated hours of darkness, although this was not controlled in the study. (Modified from Ref. 71.)

F. Less Frequent Findings

Cardiovascular anomalies occur in ∼40% of cases, irrespective of deletion size (21). However, among the few reported cases with large deletions, all had cardiac anomalies (2,21). A variety of cardiac anomalies are seen, including valvular abnormalities and/or structural defects (2,5,72). An echocardiogram is recommended for all individuals with SMS (27).

The frequency of genitourinary anomalies in SMS is variable, with duplication of the collecting system the most common anomaly reported (5,21). Renal/GU anomalies were seen in 60% of those with a small deletion, in contrast to 15% of those with the common deletion (21). Infrequent genital anomalies are seen in both sexes, including cryptorchidism, shawl, or undeveloped scrotum in males and infantile cervix and/or hypoplastic uterus in females (2,3).

G. Life Expectancy Issues

Smith–Magenis syndrome does not appear to be associated with significant reduced lifespan or increased morbidity. The oldest known living case is now in her 80s (Case 8) (2). The only two reported cases of early demise included the original male (Case 1), reported by Smith et al. (1,2), who died at 6 months of postcardiogenic shock, and a second male who died unexpectedly from adrenal aplasia-hypoplasia after perioperative stress following palatoplasty at 11 months of age (66).

IV. NEUROBEHAVIORAL PHENOTYPE IN SMITH–MAGENIS SYNDROME

Delineating the neurobehavioral phenotype of rare syndromes that include MR demands a rigorous approach that builds on psychiatric nosology, psychometric methods, and detailed syndrome specific observations (73). Even with the same underlying molecular deletion, variability occurs in SMS (21). While behavioral aspects are prevalent in persons with MR, a striking neurobehavioral phenotype is recognized in SMS (Table 2) that includes significant and chronic sleep disturbance associated with an inverted melatonin pattern, stereotypies, hyperactivity, and aggression, and other maladaptive and SIB (5,7,10,11,14–17,71). Persons with SMS also exhibit major difficulties with eating and toileting. Understanding complex syndrome-specific features and their unique aspects is crucial to identifying the gene(s) that underlies the syndrome's pathogenetic etiology.

A. Sleep Disturbance in Smith–Magenis Syndrome

Sleep disturbance in SMS is a lifelong and severe problem that occurs in virtually all cases. Parent reports of their child's sleep behaviors consistently describe fragmented and shortened sleep cycles, frequent and prolonged nocturnal awakenings (particularly in the early morning hours), early morning awake times, and excessive daytime sleepiness and/or napping (4,5,14,17,54,70,71). These sleep behaviors were similar in three SMS cohorts living in the United States (14), France (71), and the United Kingdom (74,75). Due to nocturnal behaviors that often occur upon awakening, the sleep disorder also affects the parents and siblings who are often aroused at night by the child (14,74,76). The sleep disturbance is a significant contributing factor to the neurobehavioral phenotype (11,14,71). Although sleep disorders are commonly associated with neurological disorders in children (77), the inverted melatonin pattern is a unique feature of the sleep disorder in SMS. This pattern may, therefore, help distinguish the sleep disorder in SMS from that in other MR and neurologically related disorders.

Parent reports also suggest that increasing age is often accompanied by decreased total sleep time, earlier bedtimes, shorter nap lengths, and increased nap frequency (14). Nap lengths decline, and increase in frequency from 1.2 to 1.7 naps/day between ages 5–10 years. Sleep diaries also document a decline in total sleep with age and less total sleep in SMS compared to age group controls. As discussed next, objective measures of sleep, such as EEG or actigraphy, support and extend the age-related changes in sleep patterns.

1. Objective Measures of Sleep

The EEG sleep studies and wrist actigraphy studies provide more objective measures of sleep than parent reports. Clinical polysomnography can also be used to document primary sleep disorders such as sleep apnea and sleep stage-specific dysfunction within the clinical setting. Actigraphy is more tolerable and, therefore, can be used to estimate the dynamic relationship between behavior and sleep loss over a prolonged (weeks) duration at home. These EEG and actigraphy studies generally corroborate parental reports and show a significantly disrupted sleep pattern in SMS with frequent nocturnal

Table 2 35 High Frequency Behaviors and 12 Predictors

	SMS (%)	PWS (%)	Mixed MR (%)	Signif. ($p < 0.001$)	Predictor behavior
Attention-seeking	100	71	71	a	b
Disobedience at home	97	82	55	a	
Temper tantrums	94	91	43	a	
Hyperactivity	94	26	63	a	
Sleeps less than most children	94	16	6	a	b
Distractibility (cannot concentrate)	89	68	86	a	
Lability/sudden mood shifts	89	74	54	a	b
Speech problems	89	80	46	a	
Too dependent, "clingy"	89	48	43	a	
Destroys things	86	36	6	a	
Impulsivity	86	65	74		
Stubborn, sullen	86	89	52		
Argumentative	80	89	51	a	b
Bedwetting	80	30	0	a	
Easily jealous	74	54	37	a	
Whining	74	63	20	a	
Nail biting behaviors	72	60	17	a	b
Repetitive behavior	69	69	29		
Nervous, high strung	66	22	25		
Deliberately hurts self	63	14	3	a	
Obsessions	63	91	28	a	b
Physically attacks others	57	28	32		
Talks excessively	57	74	37		

Behavior				a	b
Daytime wetting	54	8	3	a	
Skin-picks	54	100	6	a	b
Overtired	51	91	20	a	
BM outside toilet (encopresis)	50	0	3	a	b
Teased a lot	44	60	22	a	
Overeating	40	80	14	a	b
Underactive, slow	34	94	23	a	b
Overweight	31	70	14	a	
Lying, cheating	31	65	34		
Sleeps more than most children	25 (day time)	83	6	a	b
Withdrawn	11	57	22	a	
Steals at home	11	50	6	a	b

[a]Behaviors with mean scores that differ significantly across groups per MANCOVA with Bonferroni correction. These can prove useful clinical markers in diagnostic assessment based on information regarding regulatory behaviors of sleep, affect, and activity level.

[b]Twelve predictors of group membership (100% accuracy).

Source: Unpublished table with data reported by Dykens and Smith (11). The data reflects a group of 35 children and adolescents with SMS and age/gender matched subjects with PWS and Mixed MR. Based on step-wise discriminant analysis of mean scores on CBCL (92). 35 behaviors occurred frequently, 12 behaviors emerged as predictors of group membership with 100% accuracy for SMS, PWS and/or Mixed MR.

arousals/awakenings and daytime sleepiness (4,5,17,55,71). Furthermore, REM-sleep abnormalities are present in over 60%, with the majority reported to have diminished REM sleep (5,17). Multiple sleep latency test (MSLT) findings indicate decreased sleep latency (<10 in) in 50% (13/26), indicative of a significant sleep debt in persons with SMS (17). Dinnertime "sleep attacks" (i.e., falling suddenly asleep during evening meal) are prevalent. The dinner sleep attacks may represent a phase advance of the central circadian clock or a dysfunction of the sleep homeostat. Early reports described difficulties in falling asleep at bedtime (5,14), but current studies fail to fully support this finding (55,71).

The lack of data about sleep patterns in infants with SMS is hindered by the failure to recognize SMS in infancy, and consequently, the paucity of infants for study. Parents frequently recall their infant as easy-going, happy, rarely fussy, generally good sleepers, compared to their siblings at the same age (47). In contrast to these parent reports, actigraphy-estimated sleep suggests that infants, 9–12 months old, sleep poorly (Fig. 6). Both total 24-hr and night sleep was less when compared with previously reported sleep amounts in healthy infants. A discrepancy may exist between the parent report of "good" sleep and the subjective report of "poor" sleep, which may attribute to diminished vocalization and crying (possibly due to the underlying oral–sensory–motor dysfunction), thus, the child does not signal to the parent that he/she is awake. Overall, from infancy to 8 years, actigraphy-estimated sleep suggests a progressive decline in sleep (55).

2. Relationship Between Sleep and Behavior

Sleep disturbance is the single greatest correlate of maladaptive behaviors in SMS (11). Individuals with SMS face an increased sleep debt due to disrupted sleep patterns and diminished total sleep. Frequent and prolonged nighttime arousals (>15 min) occur in 75% of cases. Insufficient night sleep translates into significant sleep debt during the day, a finding that is confirmed by MSLT studies (17,71) and actigraphy (55). Snoring and labored breathing at night were

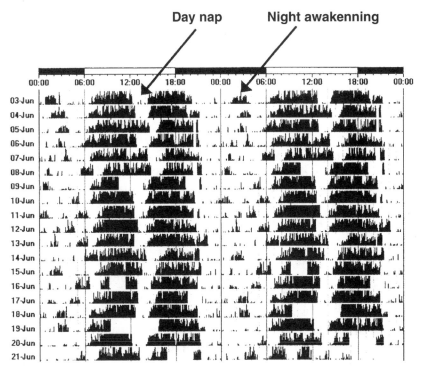

Figure 6 Activity-rest periods in a toddler with Smith–Magenis syndrome. Actigraphy, a noninvasive technique that measures rest and activity patterns, is used to estimate sleep behavior in Smith–Magenis syndrome in a young preschool age child with SMS. The actigraph illustrates elevated activity (dark vertical bars) and rest (white) for 19 consecutive days. The data are plotted both horizontally and vertically. The open and filled horizontal bar at the top corresponds to the estimated day (light) and night (dark) portions of the 24-hr cycle. Each horizontal line represents a 48-hr interval, with 2 consecutive days plotted on the same horizontal line. Successive days are also plotted vertically (beneath each other) for 19 consecutive days. Note nighttime awakenings and daytime naps (arrows), a feature common to SMS.

found to correlate with aggressive and acting out behaviors and attention problems (11). Awakening with bad dreams is often associated with acting out behavior, aggression, and anxiety/depression (11).

Daytime naps and sleepiness are a significant issue in SMS that affect learning and other aspects of social functioning. A significant inverse relationship is seen between daytime nap length and aggressive behavior and attention problems (11). This relationship may be due to the reduction in sleep debt that occurs as a result of prolonged napping. If correct, one might encourage naps—especially naps between late morning and noon—as a means for improving daytime behavior. In contrast, interrupting naps prematurely would serve to elevate sleep debt, aggressive behavior, and poor attention.

The hyperactivity and attention problems prevalent in SMS may be due to the child's struggle to stay awake in response to the combined effects of daytime melatonin (71) and the increased sleep debt. Melatonin has daytime soporific effects when given during the day to healthy volunteers (78). Not surprisingly, a relationship exists among elevated daytime melatonin levels, increased negative behaviors, and sleep attacks (71).

The connection between sleep regulation on the one hand, and behavioral and emotional problems on the other hand, has been described in children and adolescents (non-SMS) with diminished attention and impulse control (71,79). In a cross-sectional survey of 866 children scheduled at two general pediatric clinics, inattention and hyperactivity were associated with increased daytime sleepiness, snoring, and other symptoms of sleep disordered breathing (80). The relationship between disturbed sleep and ADHD symptoms raises questions for study in SMS. The ADHD features, specifically attention problems, impulsivity, and/or hyperactivity are reported in 50–100% of persons with SMS (11,74,81,82). Effective management and therapeutic strategies that improve nighttime sleep and reduce sleep debt may have a significant impact on the executive functioning, well-being, and quality of life for persons affected by this rare syndrome.

3. Management and Interventions Strategies

The therapeutic management of sleep disturbance in SMS is a challenge for both clinicians and parents. Fifty-nine percent of children take prescription or over-the-counter medications (e.g., melatonin) to facilitate sleep (14). Individual case reports suggest either improvement, no effect, or worsening of sleep disturbance after treatment with melatonin (83,84). There is not a controlled double-blind study to support the beneficial effects of these compounds on sleep in SMS, although two open label studies described below (85,86) offer some promising treatment possibilities.

Despite the sometimes-favorable anecdotal parental reports of beneficial effects, drug effects are highly variable. A major problem for assessing drug response in rare syndromes is the low number of patients available for designing a full clinical trial. However, there are several positive reports of melatonin treatment in several diagnostic groups, including neurological disabilities, mental retardation, DS, and other chromosome abnormalities (87–89). Two randomized double-blind studies (non-SMS) reported a significant decrease sleep latency with fast release (FR) capsules and sleep maintenance with controlled release capsules (79,89). However, children with SMS have little difficulty in falling asleep, the need for FR medication use in SMS is questionable.

Promising open label pilot studies suggest that a combined pharmacologic approach using beta blockers and melatonin may be effective in SMS. Specifically, parents report improvement in their children's daytime behavior and an increased ability to concentrate after daytime suppression of melatonin with beta 1-adrenergic antagonist, acebutolol (10 mg/kg at 8:00 am) combined with a nighttime dose of melatonin (controlled release dose of 6 mg at 8:00 pm) that elevates nighttime melatonin (85,86). Carefully controlled trials are needed to evaluate these findings.

4. Sleep and Home Environment Issues

For the primary caretaker, nighttime awakenings and early awakening are a challenging management issue. Frequent nighttime arousals/awakenings often lead to getting out of bed, wandering and related safety issues (14). Thus, shifting from a crib to a regular bed creates new possibilities for the restless child and dilemmas for the caretakers (14). Overall, in addition to medications, two general strategies are employed that attempt to "contain" and/or "entertain" the child who might awaken during the night. Most parents reported a general lack of effectiveness with medications. In U.K. studies, strategies that alter the sleep environment or modify behaviors showed greater efficacy for both child and adult groups with SMS (74,76). All parents who used cosleeping with their child found it effective (74). Eighty-one percent of caretakers reported reduced nighttime sleep problems of adult SMS sleep behaviors compared to childhood SMS sleep behaviors (74,76). Improvement of nighttime behavior appeared related to the ability of the person with SMS to entertain themselves during periods of nighttime wakefulness. Both caretakers, as well as and other family members, are at increased risk for sleep problems themselves, due to repeated nighttime awakenings by their child. Therefore, it is critical that the family with an SMS member be educated with regard to proper sleep hygiene to reduce the health risks of sleep loss while serving as caretaker.

B. Development and Cognitive Function

Developmental delay and variable levels of cognitive impairment are seen in all individuals with SMS. Some general observations can be made from studies that have systematically examined cognitive and adaptive function (5,90). Persons with SMS function below age level, with the majority functioning in the moderate to borderline/mild range of mental retardation. Published IQ scores (Table 3) range from 20 to 84, depending on the age group studied.

Dykens et al. (10) first reported on the strengths and weaknesses that characterize the cognitive and behavioral profile of SMS. Cognitive and behavioral strengths are found in long-term memory, attention to meaningful visual detail, reading/decoding (i.e., letter/word recognition), and alertness to the environment. Relative weaknesses are found in sequential processing, and auditory, visual, and motoric short-term auditory memory. More recently, a strikingly similar profile

Table 3 Developmental and Cognitive Function in Smith–Magenis Syndrome

Study	SMS subjects (gender)[a]	Mean age (range)	Mean IQ/DQ (range)	Instrument/scale
Greenberg et al. (5)	$N = 25$ (18F/9M) $N = 18$ $N = 18$	9.2 year (1–30 year)	Full scale 47.44 (SD 15.10) range 20–78 Verbal 55.83 (SD 11.45) range 30–73 Performance 55.17 (SD 13.43) range 30–88	BSID-II, MSCA, WISC-R, WAIS
Dykens et al. (10)	$N = 10$ (8F/2M)	27 year (14–51 yr)	44 (SD 6.41) range 35–44	
Madduri et al. (90)[a]	$N = 55$ (NG)	10 months to 31 year	44/55 (80%) range 40–70 (mild moderate) $1/55 < 30$ (profound)	BSID-II, MSCA, WISC-R, WAIS
Webber (74) Udwin et al. (75)	$N = 29$ (16F/13M)	9.7 year (6.3–16 year)	Full scale 48.5 ($N = 22$) range 42–60 (excludes $7 < 40$ basal floor) (range 41–50; $N = 15$) (range 51–60; $N = 7$) Verbal 53.9 ($N = 20$) range 48–62 (excludes $9 <$ test floor) Performance 52.6 ($N = 18$) range 47–64 (excludes $11 <$ test floor)	WISC-III ns v/p

(Continued)

Table 3 Developmental and Cognitive Function in Smith–Magenis Syndrome (*Continued*)

Study	SMS subjects (gender)[a]	Mean age (range)	Mean IQ/DQ (range)	Instrument/scale
Horn (76) Udwin et al. (75)	N = 21 (12F/9M)	26.8 year (16–51 year)	Full scale 56 (N=18) SD 6.65; range 46–68 (range <50; N=5) (range 50–69; N=14) Verbal 58 (N=18) SD 5.4; range 51–71 Performance 61 (N=18) SD 7.02; range 48–74	WAIS-R Ns verbal/perf
Martin et al. (82)	N = 19 (10F/9M)	5.7 year (2–12 year)	Full scale 62.5 +/− 14.4; range 29–84 Mild retardation N=6 Moderate retardation N=6 Borderline N=5 Low average N=1	BSID-II or SB-IV

[a]Madduri et al. (90) includes some of the same subjects reported by Greenberg et al. (5).
Abbreviations used: WISC-III, Wechsler intelligence scale for children-III; WAIS-R, Wechsler adult intelligence scale, revised-UK; BSID-II, Bayley scales of infant development; SB-IV, Stanford Binet intelligence scale-IV; MSCA, McCarthy scales of children's abilities; NG, not given; NA, not applicable.

of strengths (long-term memory, computer skills, and perceptual skills) and weaknesses (visuomotor coordination, sequencing, and response speed) was found in a large British/U.K. series of children and adults with SMS (16). Although reading was found to be a strength by Dykens et al. (10), this was not confirmed in the U.K. cohort (16).

Dual diagnosis is common in SMS. If a diagnosis of SMS has not been made prior to school age, then often the presence of stereotypies, maladaptive, and SIB usually leads to a functional diagnosis of pervasive developmental disorder, ADHD, obsessive–compulsive disorder, or autism. Furthermore, parental recognition of sudden mood shifts raise questions about bipolar spectrum or other neuropsychiatric diagnoses. The underlying genetic etiology for SMS and other neuropsychiatric illnesses remain to be clearly identified. It is possible that SMS and other neuropsychiatric syndromes may share a common gene(s). Interestingly, recent linkage data based on genome-wide scans of multigenerational ADHD families have identified several chromosome regions of interest, including a region overlapping the 17p11.2 SMSCR (91).

C. Maladaptive Behaviors

Maladaptive and SIB are generally not reported until after 1 year of age. Mild to moderate autistic-like behaviors are seen after 18 months of age, based on data derived from a group of toddlers with SMS (Wolters and Smith, personal observation). Head-banging is often first reported at 18–24 months of age (46,47) when emerging expressive language (babbling, single words) is expected, but remains delayed. Both sleep disturbance and undesired behaviors tend to escalate with pubertal onset. Unprovoked outbursts and/or aggression may become issues at home and through the school years into adulthood.

Despite clinical variability among individuals with SMS, certain behaviors appear to be prevalent and distinguish the SMS phenotype from other developmental disabilities. In 1998, Dykens and Smith (11) conducted the first age and gender matched comparative study examining maladaptive behaviors among 35 children and adolescents with SMS with a group of PWS and mixed MR subjects. Compared with both PWS (71%) and the mixed MR group (28%), the SMS group (89%) exhibited higher levels of clinically elevated externalizing maladaptive behaviors on the child behavior checklist (CBCL) (92). While 35 behaviors occurred more frequently across the three groups, 23 showed group differences (Table 2). Discriminant function analysis identified 12 behaviors (Table 2) that were able to predict group membership with 100% accuracy (11). Individuals with SMS have significantly more difficulties regulating basic bodily functions (especially sleeping), modulating activity (hyperactivity), and affect (emotional lability) as well as eating and toileting (enuresis and encopresis) compared to their counterparts. Within the SMS group alone, a variety of maladaptive behaviors have a high prevalence (Table 2). Thus, recognition of these syndrome-specific behaviors may be useful for the clinician when considering possible diagnosis.

Significant deficits in sensory processing appear to support Dykens and Smith's data (11) which indicates that differences in sensory input produce dysfunctional emotional and social responses. Evidence exists for vestibular dysfunction and proprioceptive difficulties (e.g., abnormal gait) and suspected problems of depth perception (e.g., difficulties climbing stairs). Overall, these observations suggest a major developmental defect impacting the sensory pathways.

1. Self-Injurious Behaviors

Self-injurious behaviors (SIB) are a major age-dependent issue in SMS (Table 4) (11,15). Behaviors seen in over half of cases include hand/wrist biting, head-banging, slapping/hitting oneself with the hand, and skin picking. Two behaviors that appear unique to SMS, onychotillomania (nail pulling) and polyembolokomania (object insertion into body orifices) also occur at older ages with increased frequency (15). A direct correlation has been found between frequency and severity of SIB with age and level of intellectual functioning. Nail pulling occurs at lower rates in children (~30%) compared to adults (86%) with SMS (11,15). Finucane et al.

Table 4   Self-Injurious Behaviors in Smith–Magenis Syndrome

	Dykens and Smith (11)	Finucane et al. (15)	
	$N=35$ Mean = 9 year (%)	$N=15$ Younger Mean = O6.46 year (%)	$N=14$ Older Mean = 25.01 year (%)
Self-injurious behavior	92	93	100
Bites self	77	87	
Hits/slaps self	71	40	86
Head-banging		47	64
Hits self against surface	40	NN	NN
Pulls hair or skin	31	NN	NN
Hits self with object	20	NN	NN
Skin picking/scratching	29	33	71
Nail pulling	29	27	86
Object insertion	25		
Ears	NN	20	43
Nose	NN	7	29
Rectum	NN	0	7
Vagina	NN	11	30

NN, not noted or differentiated.

(15) found a direct correlation between both the "repertoire" and number of SIB types and functional level.

Due to their relative insensitivity to pain, persons may cause self-injury due to persistent picking, biting, nail pulling, self hitting, and/or throwing themselves at objects (windows, walls, doors) during uncontrolled rages (11). Evidence of nail damage or scarring of skin due to persistent biting or picking is often visible on the extremities (hands/feet) or accessible body areas. Sometimes the self-inflicted injuries raise erroneously concern by social services for suspected child abuse (13). Self-extraction of teeth is also reported by parents. During sudden explosive outbursts, persons with SMS may thrust a fist/foot or throw their body against doors, walls, and/or through windows, risking potential personal injuries as well as structural damage to the home. Parents often use contrasting descriptors, i.e., "Jekyll and Hyde" or "Tasmanian Devil and Angel" to describe these sudden mood shifts and onset of rage behaviors that occur without warning or provocation.

2. Stereotypic Behaviors

All persons with SMS demonstrate one or more stereotypies, that include insertion of hands (69%) or objects (54%) into the mouth, teeth grinding (54%), self-hugging (46%), body rocking (43%), and spinning/twirling objects (40%) (11). For the practicing clinician, some stereotypic behaviors may serve to raise diagnostic suspicion of SMS. The spasmodic upper body squeeze, or "self-hug" originally described by Finucane et al. (7) is an upper body movement, accompanied by clasping of hands at the chest or chin level and squeezing, often with interlocked fingers. Among children with SMS, it is observed in almost 50% of cases (11). This movement appears to be involuntary with a tic-like quality and is usually exhibited when excited, happy, or pleased. A "face-hug," seen most frequently in children and adolescents, consists of the palms held tightly against the face (one parent refers to this as an angel-hug). Hugging others (people and pets), in addition to hugging themselves, with a perceptibly tight squeeze is sometimes observed. Being "hugged" to death (13) has unfortunately led to the demise of several family pets (gerbils, kitten), attesting to the under recognized physical strength often present in SMS. While the hugging behavior is socially acceptable at younger ages, at older ages it becomes less acceptable and may raise significant safety concerns. Since stranger anxiety or awareness does not appear to be well developed in persons with SMS, some will eagerly approach and hug strangers, often with force. Parents are encouraged to begin at a young age to modify this stereotypic behavior by promoting the use of an introductory handshake and/or standing an arm's length away.

Another stereotypy movement involving the face and hands, but associated with mild distress and/or anxiety, involves clasped hands held at the forehead while wiggling fingers, almost "shading" the eyes from view. This movement is reminiscent of dysfunctional social behavior of gaze aversion/avoidance commonly seen in fragile X syndrome (93). Additionally, page flipping behavior or "lick-and-flip" behavior is a stereotypic behavior that consists of flipping through pages or ruffling the page corners of a book or magazine in rapid succession (faster than speed reading) (10,11). Observed in 51% (11), such page flipping appears to have a calming effect. Some parents keep a magazine available for their child when behaviors escalate in public settings.

D. Adaptive Function in Smith–Magenis Syndrome

Adaptive function is significantly impaired in persons with SMS, regardless of IQ (16,21,82) and independent of gender. Communication and daily living skills pose a significant challenge for individuals with SMS. Independence in daily living skills, especially in those skills related to personal hygiene (bathing, brushing teeth), was significantly impaired. Research utilizing the Vineland Adaptive Behavior Scales found that scores were significantly below average on all domain subscales in a young group (<12 years) of SMS children: communication (mean 51.29), daily living skills (mean 44.33) and socialization (56.04) (82,90). Socialization skills appeared to be an area of relative strength and were more developed than daily living or communication skills. Socialization skills were significantly higher than IQ scores ($r = 0.63$; $p < 0.01$) (82) while the other domains (communication and daily living) were consistent with the cognitive level. There was a relative worsening of daily living activities compared with age-related peers (82). Thus, children with SMS require supervision and assistance in areas of personal hygiene, such as bathing, brushing teeth, and/or menstruation.

Consistent with the above observation in children, parental reports in the largest adult SMS study conducted to date (76) suggested that the need for supervision does not diminish in adulthood. Only 3 of 21 (14%) adults with SMS performed personal hygiene tasks independently. Nearly 25% required full supervision for bathing and brushing teeth

(76). The majority required a high degree of support and supervision. These adults with SMS had difficulties performing complex household tasks such as cooking a meal. Not surprisingly only a few have attained sufficient degree of personal autonomy to live independently (76). In contrast to these negative behaviors, there are many positive attributes and endearing qualities that merit recognition. Individuals with SMS exhibit loving and engaging personalities, have a well-developed sense of humor, and have excellent long-term memories, especially for faces, places, and events. Their affinity for computers and electronics, especially electronic games (e.g., Gameboy) can be used as positive motivators in the classroom and at home.

V. CONCLUSIONS

In 1982, the microdeletion, del (17)(p11.2p11.2), was first described in two infants born with multiple anomalies, and led to the description of a new syndrome recognized today as SMS. Scientific and technological advances in the field of human cytogenetics during the 1960–70s laid the foundation for this discovery. More recently, advances arising from Human Genome Project provided the necessary tools to narrow the SMS critical chromosome region to $\sim 1\,\text{Mb}$, with an estimated 20–30 genes. Individual case reports and larger clinical series published in the 1990s clarified the physical, developmental, and behavioral aspects of the complex phenotype. The inverted circadian rhythm of melatonin, unique to SMS, is a distinguishing aspect of the sleep disturbances in SMS. To the extent that the pattern might be normalized, inverted melatonin may be a target for therapeutic interventions to seek improvement in sleep quality.

The natural progression of the physical, developmental, and neurobehavioral features of SMS is poorly understood. To overcome this deficiency, a systematic longitudinal study of the developmental and neurobehavioral features of SMS was initiated at the NIH in 2001. This study plans to identify key areas to improve clinical management and treatment for both patient and families. For example, interventions are being identified to normalize the inverted circadian rhythm of melatonin, to improve nighttime sleep, reduce daytime drowsiness, and to improve daytime behaviors.

Numerous medications to control behaviors in SMS have been tried on an ad hoc basis by many parents with mixed results. Often adverse reactions have been reported (47). Two open label studies (85,86) that specifically target the melatonin abnormality have offered promising treatment possibilities. However, there are no controlled double-blind studies to support the beneficial effects of any medication(s) on sleep or behavior in SMS. The absence of controlled clinical trials makes predictions difficult and underscores the need for such research. Conventional anticonvulsant therapy has been effective in treating seizures; however, older stimulant drugs (e.g., Ritalin) are not particularly helpful in controlling behavior or increasing attention span. Newer medications (e.g., Strattera) have not been formally studied to deduce efficacy and are associated with a decline in sleep and escalation of aggression and outbursts.

Although there is not treatment with proven efficacy for managing the behavioral dysfunction in SMS, there are several promising developments that may in the future foster treatment possibilities. Controlled trials are needed to clearly document the efficacy of medication(s) used in therapeutic management of persons with SMS. Identification of the circadian dysfunction may lead to treatment(s) to improve sleep quality and secondarily the negative daytime behaviors and cognitive consequences.

At the frontier of basic research, transgenic technology is being used to develop SMS mouse models (94) based on the fact that genes deleted in the 1 Mb human SMSCR are syntenic to a region of murine chromosome 11. These heterozygous-deleted mice (Df(11)/+) exhibit craniofacial abnormalities, seizures, obesity, and behavioral features similarly seen in SMS (95,96). More specifically, homozygosity for *Myo15* (−/−) is associated with profound deafness and vestibular defects in mice (97), a phenotype that correlates with SMS. Circadian rhythm disruption in Del mutant mouse models

[*Df*(11)(17)] indicates that genes in this critical region likely contribute to the clinically observed sleep disruption in SMS (98). In contrast, several other gene(s) of interest in the SMS common deletion interval [*Pemt* (99), *Srebf1* (100), *Myo15* (97), *Top3a* (101), and *Fliih* (102), and *Csn3* (formerly *Cops3)* (96)] fail to demonstrate SMS phenotypic features in mice heterozygous $(+/-)$ for each of these genes. Such research efforts may someday lead to new treatment strategies as well as identification of specific genes that contribute to the SMS phenotype. However, advances in knowledge about SMS would not be possible without a dedicated cadre of researchers working in partnership with individuals with SMS and their families. The goal of researchers is to recognize the critical research questions as they seek to expand the SMS information base. Expanding the base of knowledge has major relevance not only for optimizing outcomes for the individuals affected by this rare syndrome, but also for expanding the scientific knowledge of biological processes that may also be present in other developmental disorders.

REFERENCES

1. Smith ACM, McGavran L, Waldstein G, Robinson J. Deletion of the 17 short arm in two patients with facial clefts. Am J Hum Genet 1982; 34:410A.

2. Smith ACM, McGavran L, Robinson J, et al. Interstitial deletion of (17)(p11.2p11.2) in nine patients. Am J Med Genet 1986; 24:393–414.

3. Stratton RF, Dobyns WB, Greenberg F, et al. Interstitial deletion of (17)(p11.2p11.2): report of six additional patients with a new chromosome deletion syndrome. Am J Med Genet 1986; 24:421–432.

4. Greenberg F, Guzzetta V, Montes de Oca-Luna R, et al. Molecular analysis of the Smith–Magenis syndrome: a possible contiguous gene syndrome associated with del(17)(p11.2). Am J Hum Genet 1991; 49:1207–1218.

5. Greenberg F, Lewis RA, Potocki L, et al. Multi-disciplinary clinical study of Smith–Magenis syndrome (deletion 17p11.2). Am J Med Genet 1996; 62:247–254.

6. Finucane BM, Jaeger ER, Kurtz MB, Weinstein M, Scott CI Jr. Eye abnormalities in the Smith–Magenis contiguous gene deletion syndrome. Am J Med Genet 1993; 45: 443–446.

7. Finucane BM, Konar D, Haas-Givler B, Kurtz MB, Scott C Jr. The spasmodic upper-body squeeze: a characteristic behavior in Smith–Magenis syndrome. Dev Med Child Neurol 1994; 36:78–83.

8. Chen KS, Potocki L, Lupski JR. The Smith–Magenis syndrome (del(17)(p11.2)): clinical review and molecular advances. Ment Retard Dev Disabil Res Rev 1996; 49:1207–1218.

9. Chen RM, Lupski JR, Greenberg F, Lewis RA. Ophthalmic manifestations of Smith–Magenis syndrome. Ophthalmol 1996; 103:1084–1091.

10. Dykens EM, Finucane BM, Gayley C. Brief report: cognitive and behavioral profiles in persons with Smith–Magenis syndrome. J Autism Dev Disord 1997; 27:203–211.

11. Dykens EM, Smith AC. Distinctiveness and correlates of maladaptive behaviour in children and adolescents with Smith–Magenis syndrome. J Intellect Disabil Res 1998; 42:481–489.

12. Allanson JE, Greenberg F, Smith AC. The face of Smith–Magenis syndrome: a subjective and objective study. J Med Genet 1999; 36:394–397.

13. Smith AC, Dykens E, Greenberg F. Behavioral phenotype of Smith–Magenis syndrome (del 17p11.2). Am J Med Genet 1998; 81:179–185.

14. Smith AC, Dykens E, Greenberg F. Sleep disturbance in Smith–Magenis syndrome (del 17p11.2). Am J Med Genet 1998; 81:186–191.

15. Finucane B, Dirrigl KH, Simon EW. Characterization of self-injurious behaviors in children and adults with Smith–Magenis syndrome. Am J Ment Retard 2001; 106:52–58.

16. Udwin O, Webber C, Horn I. Abilities and attainment in Smith–Magenis syndrome. Dev Med Child Neurol 2001; 43:823–828.

17. Potocki L, Glaze D, Tan DX, Park SS, Kashork CD, Shaffer LG, et al. Circadian rhythm abnormalities of melatonin in Smith–Magenis syndrome. J Med Genet 2000; 37: 428–433.

18. De Leersnyder H, De Blois MC, Claustrat B, et al. Inversion of the circadian rhythm of melatonin in the Smith–Magenis syndrome. J Pediatr 2001; 139:111–116.

19. Smith AC, Gropman AL, Bailey-Wilson JE, et al. Hypercholesterolemia in children with Smith–Magenis syndrome: del (17)(p11.2p11.2). Genet Med 2002; 4:118–125.

20. Vlangos CN, Yim DK, Elsea SH. Refinement of the Smith–Magenis syndrome critical region to approximately 950 kb and assessment of 17p11.2 deletions. Are all deletions created equally? Mol Genet Metab 2003; 79:134–141.

21. Potocki L, Shaw CJ, Stankiewicz P, Lupski JR. Variability in clinical phenotype despite common chromosomal deletion in Smith–Magenis syndrome [del(17)(p11.2p11.2)]. Genet Med 2003; 5:430–434.

22. Vlangos CN, Wilson M, Blancato J, Smith ACM, Elsea SH. Diagnostic FISH probes for del(17)(p11.2p11.2) associated with Smith–Magenis syndrome should contain the RAI1 gene. Am J Med Genet 2005; 132A(3):278–282.

23. Chen KS, Manian P, Koeuth T, et al. Homologous recombination of a flanking repeat gene cluster is a mechanism for a common contiguous gene deletion syndrome. Nat Genet 1997; 17:154–163.

24. Struthers JL, Carson N, McGill M, Khalifa MM. Molecular screening for Smith–Magenis syndrome among patients with mental retardation of unknown cause. J Med Genet 2002; 39:E59.

25. Barnicoat AJ, Moller HU, Palmer RW, Russell-Eggitt I, Winter RM. An unusual presentation of Smith–Magenis syndrome with iris dysgenesis. Clin Dysmorphol 1996; 5: 153–158.

26. Behjati F, Mullarkey M, Bergbaum A, Berry AC, Docherty Z. Chromosome deletion 17p11.2 (Smith–Magenis syndrome) in seven new patients, four of whom had been referred for fragile-X investigation. Clin Genet 1997; 5:171–174.

27. Smith ACM, Allanson J, Allen AJ, et al. Smith–Magenis syndrome. In: GeneReviews at GeneTests-GeneClinics: Medical Genetics Information Resource [database online]. Copyright. Seattle: University of Washington, 2001.

28. Slager RE, Newton TL, Vlangos CN, Finucane B, Elsea SH. Mutations in RAI1 associated with Smith–Magenis syndrome. Nat Genet 2003; 33:466–468.

29. Lucas RE, Vlangos CN, Das P, Patel PI, Elsea SH. Genomic organization of the approximately 1.5 Mb Smith–Magenis syndrome critical interval: transcription map, genomic contig, and candidate gene analysis. Eur J Hum Genet 2001; 9:892–902.

30. Elsea SH, Juyal RC, Jiralerspong S, et al. Haploinsufficiency of cytosolic serine hydroxymethyltransferase in the Smith–Magenis syndrome. Am J Hum Genet 1995; 57: 1342–1350.

31. Bi W, Yan J, Stankiewicz P, et al. Genes in a refined Smith–Magenis syndrome critical deletion interval on chromosome 17p11.2 and the syntenic region of the mouse. Genome Res 2002; 12:713–728.

32. Liburd N, Ghosh M, Riazuddin S, et al. Novel mutations of MYO15A associated with profound deafness in consanguineous families and moderately severe hearing loss in a patient with Smith–Magenis syndrome. Hum Genet 2001; 109:535–541.

33. Trask BJ, Mefford H, van den Engh G, et al. Quantification by flow cytometry of chromosome-17 deletions in Smith–Magenis syndrome patients. Hum Genet 1996; 98:710–718.

34. Shaw CJ, Bi W, Lupski JR. Genetic proof of unequal meiotic crossovers in reciprocal deletion and duplication of 17p11.2. Am J Hum Genet 2002; 71:1072–1081.

35. Lupski JR. Genomic disorders: structural features of the genome can lead to DNA rearrangements and human disease traits. Trend Genet 1998; 14:417–422.

36. Park SS, Stankiewicz P, Bi W, et al. Structure and evolution of the Smith–Magenis syndrome repeat gene clusters, SMS-REPs. Genome Res 2002; 12:729–738.

37. Potocki L, Chen KS, Park S, et al. Molecular mechanism for duplication 17p11.2—the homologous recombination reciprocal of the Smith–Magenis microdeletion. Nat Genet 2000; 24:84–87.

38. Howard-Peeples PH, Friedman JM, Harrod MJE, Brookshire GS, Lockwood JEA. A stable supernumerary chromosome derived from a deleted segment of 17p. Am J Hum Genet 1985; 37:A97.

39. Zori RT, Lupski JR, Heju Z, et al. Clinical, cytogenetic, and molecular evidence for an infant with Smith–Magenis syndrome born from a mother having a mosaic 17p11.2p12 deletion. Am J Med Genet 1993; 47:504–511.

40. Lockwood D, Hecht F, Dowman C, et al. Chromosome subband 17p11.2 deletion: a minute deletion syndrome. J Med Genet 1988; 25:732–737.

41. Hansen M, Kurinczuk JJ, Bower C, Webb S. The risk of major birth defects after intracytoplasmic sperm injection and in vitro fertilization. NEJM 2002; 346:725–730.

42. Williams CA, Dong HJ, Driscoll DJ. Angelman syndrome. GeneReviews at GeneTests-GeneClinics: Medical Genetics Information Resource [database online]. Copyright. Seattle: University of Washington, 2003.

43. Shuman C, Weksberg R. Beckwith–Wiedeman Syndrome. GeneReviews at GeneTests-GeneClinics: Medical Genetics Information Resource [database online]. Copyright. Seattle: University of Washington, 2003.

44. DeBaun MR, Niemitz EL, Feinberg AP. Association of in vitro fertilization with Beckwith–Wiedemann syndrome and epigenetic alterations of LIT1 and H19. Am J Hum Genet 2003; 72(1):156–160.

45. Maher ER, Brueton LA, Bowdin SC, et al. Beckwith–Wiedemann syndrome and assisted reproduction technology (ART). J Med Genet 2003; 40:62–64.

46. Gropman A, Smith ACM, Greenberg F. Neurologic aspects of the Smith–Magenis syndrome. Ann Neurol 1998; 44:561.

47. Smith ACM, Gropman A. Smith–Magenis syndrome. In: Allanson J, Cassidy S, eds. Clinical Management of Common Genetic Syndromes. New York: Wiley-Liss, 2001.

48. Thomson KA, Finucane BM, Bauer MS, Weinstein MB. Overlap of clinical features of Smith–Magenis syndrome in newborns and infants: implications for testing and diagnosis. Am J Hum Genet 1994; 55(3 suppl):529A.

49. Allanson JE, Ohara P, Farkas LG, Nair RC. Anthropometric craniofacial pattern profiles in Down syndrome. Am J Med Genet 1993; 47:748–752.

50. Sweeney E, Peart I, Tofeig M, Kerr B. Smith–Magenis syndrome and tetralogy of Fallot [letter]. J Med Genet 1999; 36:501–502.

51. Maddalena A, Richards CS, McGinniss MJ, et al. Technical standards and guidelines for fragile X: the first of a series of disease-specific supplements to the Standards and Guidelines for Clinical Genetics Laboratories of the American College of Medical Genetics. Genet Med 2001; 3:200–205.

52. Meinecke P. Confirmation of a particular but non-specific metacarpophalangeal pattern profile in patients with the Smith–Magenis syndrome due to interstitial deletion of 17p [letter; comment]. Am J Med Genet 1993; 45:441–442.

53. Kondo I, Matsuura S, Kuwajima K, et al. Diagnostic hand anomalies in Smith–Magenis syndrome: four new patients with del (17)(p11.2p11.2) [see comments]. Am J Med Genet 1991; 41:225–229.

54. Gropman A, Smith ACM, Allanson J, Greenberg F. Smith–Magenis Syndrome: aspects of the infant phenotype. Am J Hum Genet 1998; 63:A19.

55. Duncan WC, Gropman A, Morse R, Krasnewich D, Smith ACM. Good babies sleeping poorly: insufficient sleep in infants with Smith–Magenis syndrome. Am J Hum Genet 2003; 73(5 suppl):A896.

56. Hammond P, Hutton TJ, Allanson J, Smith ACM. The 3D face of Smith–Magenis syndrome (SMS): a study using dense surface models. Eur J Hum Genet 2003; 11:102.

57. Salati R, Marini G, Degiuli A, Dalpra L. Brown's syndrome associated with Smith–Magenis syndrome. Strabismus 1996; 4:139–143.

58. Babovic-Vuksanovic D, Jalal SM, Garrity JA, Robertson DM, Lindor NM. Visual impairment due to macular disciform scars in a 20-year-old man with Smith–Magenis syndrome: another opthalmologic complication. Am J Med Genet 1998; 80:373–376.

59. Spina Bifida Occulta and Open Spina Bifida—A Patient's Guide, 2004.

60. Yang SP, Bidichandani SI, Figuera LE, et al. Molecular analysis of deletion (17)(p11.2p11.2) in a family segregating a 17p paracentric inversion: implications for carriers of paracentric inversions. Am J Hum Genet 1997; 60(5):1184–1193.

61. Solomon B, McCullagh L, Krasnewich D, Smith ACM. Oral motor, speech and voice functions in Smith–Magenis syndrome children: a research update. Am J Hum Genet 2002; 71:271.

62. Brewer CC, Zalewski CK, Solomon B, McCullagh L, Smith ACM. Audiologic findings in patients with Smith–Magenis syndrome. Amer Speech Hearing Assoc 2003.

63. Sonies BC, Solomon B, Ondrey F, McCullagh L, Greenberg F, Smith ACM. Oral–motor and otolaryngologic findings in 14 patients with Smith–Magenis syndrome (del 17p11.2): results of an interdisciplinary study. Am J Hum Genet 1997; 61(4 suppl):A5.

64. Gropman A, Wolters P, Solomon B, Smith ACM. Neurodevelopmental assessment and functioning in five young children

with Smith–Magenis syndrome (SMS). Am J Hum Genet 1999; 65:A151.

65. Boddeart N, Zilbovicius M, Munnich A, Brunell F, De Leersnyder H. Anatomical and functional brain imaging evidence of lenticulo-insular anomalies in Smith–Magenis syndrome. Am J Hum Genet 2003; 73:A551.

66. Denny AD, Weik LD, Lubinsky MS, Wyatt DT. Lethal adrenal aplasia in an infant with Smith–Magenis syndrome, deletion 17p11.2. J Dysmorph Clin Genet 1992; 6(4): 175–179.

67. Roccella M, Parisi L. The Smith–Magenis syndrome: a new case with infant spasms. Minerva Pediatr 1999; 51:65–71.

68. AAP. Cholesterol in childhood. Policy Statement of the American Academy of Pediatrics, 1998.

69. Potocki L, Reiter RJ, Glaze D, Lupski JR. Twenty-four hour urinary excretion of 6-sulphatoxymelatonin in Smith–Magenis syndrome. American College of Medical Genetics 4th Annual Meeting, Fort Lauderdale, FL, 1997.

70. De Leersnyder H, Von Kleist-Retzow JC, Munnich A, Claustrat B, Lyonnet S, et al. Inversion of the circadian rhythm of melatonin in Smith–Magenis syndrome. Am J Hum Genet 1999; 65(suppl):A2.

71. De Leersnyder H, DeBois MC, Claustrat B, et al. Inversion of the circadian rhythm of melatonin in the Smith–Magenis syndrome. J Pediatr 2001; 139:111–116.

72. Thomas DG, Jacques SM, Flore LA, et al. Prenatal diagnosis of Smith–Magenis syndrome (del 17p11.2). Fetal Diagn Ther 2000; 15:335–337.

73. Dykens EM. Measuring behavioral phenotypes: provocations from the "new genetics". Am J Ment Retard 1995; 99:522–532.

74. Webber C. Cognitive and behavioural phenotype of children with Smith–Magenis syndrome. University of Leicester, 1999:139 (doctoral dissertation).

75. Udwin O. Williams and Smith–Magenis syndromes. In: Howlin P, Udwin O, eds. Outcomes in Neurodevelopmental and Genetic Disorders. Cambridge: Cambridge University Press, 2002.

76. Horn IA. The Cognitive and Behavioural Phenoytpe of Smith–Magenis Syndrome. London: University of London, 1999:113 (doctoral dissertation).

77. Kohrman MH, Carney PR. Sleep-related disorders in neurologic disease during childhood. Pediatr Neurol 2000; 23:107–113.

78. Dollins AB, Zhdanova IV, Wurtman RJ, Lynch HJ, Deng MH. Effect of inducing nocturnal serum melatonin concentrations in daytime on sleep, mood, body temperature, and performance. Proc Natl Acad Sci USA 1994; 91:1824–1828.

79. Dahl R. The regulation of sleep and arousal: development and psychopathology. Dev Psychopathol 1996; 8:3–27.

80. Chervin RD, Archbold KH, Dillon JE, et al. Inattention, hyperactivity, and symptoms of sleep-disordered breathing. Pediatrics 2002; 109:449–456.

81. de Rijk-van Andel JF, Catsman-Berrevoets CE, van Hemel JO, Hamers AJ. Clinical and chromosome studies of three patients with Smith–Magenis syndrome. Dev Med Child Neurol 1991; 33:343–347.

82. Martin S, Wolters P, Smith ACM. Adaptive and maladaptive behavior in children with Smith–Magenis syndrome. J Autism Develop Dis, 2005, In press.

83. Chou IC, Tsai FJ, Yu MT, Tsai CH. Smith–Magenis syndrome with bilateral vesicoureteral reflux: a case report. J Formos Med Assoc 2002; 101:726–728.

84. Hou JW. Smith–Magenis syndrome: report of one case. Acta Paediatr Taiwan 2003; 44:161–164.

85. De Leersnyder H, Bresson JL, de Blois MC, et al. Beta 1-adrenergic antagonists and melatonin reset the clock and restore sleep in a circadian disorder, Smith–Magenis syndrome. J Med Genet 2003; 40:74–78.

86. De Leersnyder H, deBlois MC, Bekemans M, et al. β1-adrenergic antogonists improve sleep and behavioral disturbances in a circadian disorder, Smith–Magenis syndrome. J Med Genet 2001; 38:586–590.

87. Jan JE, Hamilton D, Seward N, Fast DK, Freeman RD, Laudon M. Clinical trials of controlled-release melatonin in children with sleep–wake cycle disorders. J Pineal Res 2000; 29:34–39.

88. Jan JE, O'Donnell ME. Use of melatonin in the treatment of paediatric sleep disorders. J Pineal Res 1996; 21:193–199.

89. Dodge NN, Wilson GA. Melatonin for treatment of sleep disorders in children with developmental disabilities. J Child Neurol 2001; 16:581–584.

90. Madduri NS, Turcich M, Lupski JR, Potocki L. Low adaptive behavior and cognitive functioning in patients with Smith–Magenis syndrome [del(17)(p11.2p11.2)]. Am J Hum Genet 2002; 71:A109.

91. Arcos-Burgos M, Castellanos X, Pineda D, et al. Attention-deficit/hyperactivity disorder in a population isolate: linkage to loci at 4q13.2, 5q33.3, 11q22, and 17p11. Am J Hum Genet 2004;75(6):998–1014.

92. Achenbach TM. Manual for the Child Behavior Checklist/4–18 and 1991 Profile. Burlington: University of Vermont, Department of Psychiatry, 1991.

93. Levitas A. Neuropsychiatric aspects of fragile syndrome X. Semin Clin Neuropsychiatry 1996; 1:154–167.

94. Walz K, Caratini-Rivera S, Bi W, et al. Modeling del(17)(p11.2p11.2) and dup(17)(p11.2p11.2) contiguous gene syndromes by chromosome engineering in mice: phenotypic consequences of gene dosage imbalance. Mol Cell Biol 2003; 23:3646–3655.

95. Fonseca P, Walz K, Lupski JR. Identifying dosage-sensitive genes in the Smith–Magenis syndrome region. Am J Hum Genet 2003; 73(suppl):A2350.

96. Yan J, Walz K, Nakamura H, et al. COP9 signalosome subunit 3 is essential for maintenance of cell proliferation

in the mouse embryonic epiblast. Mol Cell Biol 2003; 23:6798–6808.

97. Probst FJ, Fridell RA, Raphael Y, et al. Correction of deafness in shaker-2 mice by an uncoventional myosin in a BAC transgene [see comments]. Science 1998; 280: 1444–1447.

98. Walz K, Spencer C, Kaaisk K, Lee CC, Lupski JR, Paylor R. Behavioral characterization of mouse models for Smith–Magenis syndrome and dup(17)(p11.2p11.2). Hum Mol Genet 2004; 13(4):367–378.

99. Walkey CJ, Donohue LR, Bronson R, Agellon LB, Vance DE. Disruption of the murine gene encoding phosphatidylethanolamine *N*-methyltransferase. Proc Natl Acad Sci USA 1997; 94:12880–12885.

100. Shimano H, Shimomura I, Hammer RE, Herz J, Goldstein JL, Horton JD. Elevated levels of SREBP-2 and cholesterol synthesis in livers of mice homozygous for a targeted disruption of the SREBP-1 gene. J Clin Invest 1997; 100:2115–2124.

101. Li W, Wang JC. Mammalian DNA topoisomerase IIIalpha is essential in early embryogenesis. Proc Natl Acad Sci USA 1998; 95:1010–1013.

102. Campbell HD, Fountain S, McLennan IS, et al. Fliih, a gelsolin-related cytoskeletal regulator essential for early mammalian embryonic development. Mol Cell Biol 2002; 22: 3518–3526.

103. Colley AF, Leversha MA, Voullaire LE, Rogers JG. Five cases demonstrating the distinctive behavioural features of chromosome deletion 17(p11.2 p11.2) (Smith–Magenis syndrome). J Paediatr Child Health 1990; 26:17–21.

104. Al-Qudah AA, El-Khateeb MS, Abu-Hamour W, Bulos NK. Smith–Magenis syndrome: report of two cases and review of the literature. Annu Saudi Med 1994; 14:417–419.

105. Juyal RC, Finucane B, Shaffer LG, et al. Apparent mosaicism for del(17)(p11.2) ruled out by fluorescence in situ hybridization in a Smith–Magenis syndrome patient. Am J Med Genet 1995; 59:406–407.

106. Fischer H, Oswald HP, Duba HC, et al. Constitutional interstitial deletion of 17(p11.2)(Smith–Magenis syndrome): a
clinically recognizable microdeletion syndrome. Report of
two cases and review of the literature. Klin Padiatr 1993;
205:162–166.

107. Salati R, Marini G, Degiuli A, Dalpra L. Brown's syndrome
associated with Smith–Magenis syndrome. Strabismus
1996; 4:139–143.

14

Rett Syndrome

THIERRY BIENVENU
Institut Cochin, INSERM, Paris, France

I. HISTORY

In 1966, Andreas Rett, an Austrian pediatrician in Vienna, first described a peculiar disorder in girls characterized by global deceleration of psychomotor development and subsequent loss of acquired cognitive and motor skills, occurring after 6–18 months of apparently normal development (1). However, the condition was not brought to the attention of the English-speaking world (clinicians and researchers worldwide) until 1983, when Hagberg and his colleagues described 35 patients, all girls from three different countries (France, Portugal, and Sweden), with a uniform and striking, progressive encephalopathy. After development up to the age of 6–18 months, developmental stagnation occurs, followed by rapid deterioration of higher brain functions. Within the

477

following 1.5 years, this deterioration progresses to severe dementia with loss of speech, autistic features (poor eye contact, lack of sustained interest, speech disturbances, and repetitive truncal rocking), loss of purposeful use of the hands (repetitive, purposeless, usually midline, and stereotypic hand movements) (Fig. 1), jerky truncal ataxia, postnatal microcephaly, and also irregular breathing while awake, with hyperventilation. Thereafter, there is a period of apparent stability lasting for decades. However, profound mental retardation persists, with marked motor dysfunction and jerky truncal

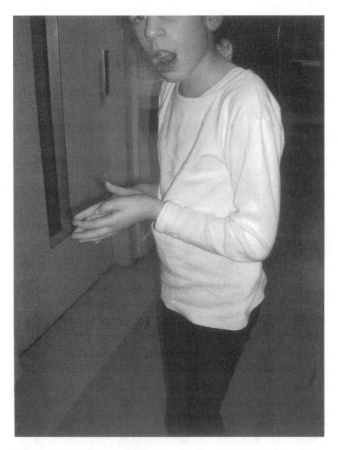

Figure 1   Clinical picture of a Rett patient showing typical positions of the hands. (Kindly provided by Dr. Nadia Bahi.) (*See color insert.*)

ataxia. Additional neurologic abnormalities intervene insidiously, mainly spastic paraparesis, vasomotor disturbances of the lower limbs, and epilepsy. Scoliosis is also very common, and the feet may be trophic and cyanotic. Emotional contact tends to improve with age (2).

In 1984, a panel of international experts developed diagnostic criteria for Rett syndrome (RS) (MIM no. 312750). These diagnostic criteria were restricted to include only typical patients (3) (Table 1). In 1986, Hagberg and Witt-Engerström

Table 1 Diagnostic Criteria for Rett Syndrome

Necessary criteria (diagnosis tentative until 2–5 years of age)
  Apparently normal pre- and perinatal history
  Psychomotor development largely normal through the first 6 months of
    life or may be delayed from birth
  Normal head circumference at birth
  Postnatal deceleration of head growth in the majority
  Loss of achieved purposeful hand skill between ages 6 and 30 months
  Stereotypic hand movements such as hand wringing/squeezing,
    clapping/tapping, mouthing, and "washing"/rubbing automatisms
  Emerging social withdrawal, communication dysfunction, loss of learned
    words, and cognitive impairment
  Impaired (dyspraxic) or failing locomotion
Supportive criteria
  Awake disturbances of breathing (hyperventilation, breath-holding,
    forced expulsion of air or saliva, and air swallowing)
  Bruxism
  Impaired sleep pattern from early infancy
  Abnormal muscle tone successively associated with muscle wasting and
    dystonia
  Peripheral vasomotor disturbances
  Scoliosis, kyphosis progressing through childhood
  Growth retardation
  Hypotrophic small and cold feet; small and thin hands
Exclusion criteria
  Organomegaly or other signs of storage disease
  Retinopathy, optic atrophy, or cataract
  Evidence of perinatal or postnatal brain damage
  Existence of identifiable metabolic or other progressive neurological
    disorder
  Acquired neurological disorders resulting from severe infections or head
    trauma

Source: Ref. 108.

suggested a staging system for describing the impairment profile with increasing age. This system, which is characterized by four clinical stages [I, early destructive deceleration stage at 6–18 months; II, rapid destructive stage at 1–4 years; III, pseudo-stationary stage in preschool years (age 4–7 years) with persistent mental retardation; and IV, late motor deterioration stage from the teen years], was adopted by the international RS diagnostic criteria work group in 1988 (Table 2) (4–6).

However, during the 1980s, increasing experiences indicated that a number of clinical variants do exist and that the RS concept represents a broader and larger group than previously imagined. The first atypical RS to be added was the "forme frustre" (FF) defined with an inclusion age of greater than 13 years (usually with less severe regression, milder mental retardation, and no seizures) and presented at the International Rett Conference in Baltimore in November 1985. At the same conference, a variety of other atypical RS case reports were discussed. Over the years, an array of more atypical RS presentations has been established [including "formes frustres," early seizure onset type, late childhood regression, preserved speech variant (PSV), and congenital variant]. Among the variants, PSV is probably the most common. Atypical RS constitutes a wide range of different phenotypes, some quite difficult to recognize and diagnose (7). In 1994, Hagberg and Skjeldal suggested a model for the clinical delineation of atypical RS cases. It was postulated that these atypical RS girls should have, at age of 10 or more years, mental retardation of unexplained origin and at least three of six primary criteria such as loss of acquired fine finger skills in early childhood, stereotypes such as wringing of hands, and deceleration of head growth. In addition, these girls were expected to have at least five out of 11 supportive manifestations appearing through childhood with advancing age, like breathing irregularities, grinding of teeth, and intensive eye communication (Table 3). Reviewing a Swedish series of 170 affected females, aged 2–52 years, Hagberg (8) showed that the well-recognized classic phenotype was found in 75% of cases and that atypical variant forms were still a minority, but constituted an expanding cohort.

Table 2 Rett Syndrome: Clinical Characteristics and Differential Diagnosis by Stage

Stages defined by Hagberg and Witt-Engerström	Clinical characteristics	Differential diagnosis
Early onset deceleration stage Onset: 6–18 months Duration: months	Developmental stagnation Deceleration of head/brain growth Disinterest in play activity Hypotonia	Benign congenital hypotonia Prader–Willi syndrome Cerebral palsy
Rapid destructive stage Onset: 1–3 years Duration: weeks to months	Rapid developmental regression Irritability Loss of hand use Hand stereotypies Autistic manifestations Loss of expressive language Insomnia Self-abusive behavior	Autism Psychosis Hearing or visual disturbance Encephalitis Infantile spasms Tuberous sclerosis Ornithine transcarbamylase deficiency Phenylketonuria Infantile neuronal ceroidlipofuscinosis
Pseudostationary stage Onset: 2–10 years Duration: months to years	Severe mental retardation Apparent dementia Amelioration of autistic features Seizures Typical hand stereotypies Prominent ataxia and apraxia Spasticity Hyperventilation Apnea during wakefulness	Spastic ataxia cerebral palsy Spinocerebellar degeneration Leukodystrophies Neuroaxonal dystrophy Lennox–Gastaut syndrome Angelman syndrome

(Continued)

Table 2 Rett Syndrome: Clinical Characteristics and Differential Diagnosis by Stage (*Continued*)

Stages defined by Hagberg and Witt-Engerström	Clinical characteristics	Differential diagnosis
Late motor deterioration stage Onset: > 10 years Duration: years	Weight loss with excellent appetite Early scoliosis Bruxism Combined upper and lower motor neuron signs Progressive scoliosis, muscle wasting, and rigidity Decreasing mobility, wheel-chair bound Growth retardation Improved eye contact Staring, unfathomable gaze Virtual absence of expressive and receptive language Trophic disturbance of feet Reduced seizure frequency	Unknown degenerative disorder

Source: Ref. 109.

Table 3 Diagnostic Criteria for Variant Phenotypes

Inclusion criteria: meet at least three of the six following primary criteria and at least five of the following 11 RS supportive manifestations

Primary criteria

A1	Absence or reduction of hand skills
A2	Reduction or loss of babble speech
A3	Monotonous pattern to hand stereotypies
A4	Reduction or loss of communication skills from first years of life
A5	Deceleration of head growth
A6	RS disease profile: a regression period followed by a recovery of interaction contrasting with slow neuromotor regression

Supportive criteria

B1	Breathing irregularities (hyperventilation and/or breath-holding)
B2	Bloating/marked air swallowing
B3	Characteristic RS teeth grinding
B4	Gait dyspraxia
B5	Neurogenic scoliosis or high kyphosis (amulant girls)
B6	Development of lower limb neurologic abnormalities
B7	Small blue/cold impaired feet, autonomic/trophic dysfunction
B8	Characteristic RS electroencephalographic development
B9	Unprompted sudden langhing/screaming spells
B10	Impaired/delayed nociception
B11	Intensive eye communication—"eye pointing"

Exclusion criteria

	According to the Diagnostic Criteria Work Group (See Table 1)

Source: Ref. 108.

In 1998, Leonard and Bower retrospectively studied the neonatal characteristics and early development of Australian girls with RS and showed that their mean birth weight and head circumference are slightly below the average for normal control infants of the same gestational age. They suggested that using normal development in the first 6 months and normal neonatal head circumference as diagnostic criteria may cause missed or delayed diagnoses (Table 4) (9). In common with this study that examined early (preregressive) development in detail, Charman and colleagues suggested that

Table 4 Parental Description of Abnormal
Behaviors and Development in First 6 months of
Life in Girls with Rett Syndrome

Description of behavior	%
Placid	15.7
Floppy	8.7
Feeding problems/poor weight	8.7
Developmental problems	6.3
Colic/constipation	5.5
Problems with eye contact/focusing	4.7
Night screaming	3.9
Seizures/shakiness	3.9

Source: Ref. 9.

normal development prior to the onset of regression appeared
to be the exception and not the norm in RS. Only 30% of cases
were considered to have no clear signs of abnormality prere-
gression, and sometimes there was insufficient information
to definitely record an abnormality suspected to have been
present (10). Close attention in the recording of early developmental history may lead to the identification of early warning
signs (low tone and delay in motor milestones) that, once
accompanied by a period of regression, will indicate a possible
case of RS, requiring genetic investigation. In fact, in the fall
of 1999, using the positional candidate cloning strategy, Amir
et al. (11) identified mutations in the methyl-CpG-binding
protein 2 (*MECP2*) gene in several girls with RS (5/21 sporadic cases and 1/8 familial cases), a first major step in the
understanding of this enigmatic disorder.

II. CLINICAL FEATURES AND DIAGNOSTIC
CRITERIA

Diagnostic criteria have been separated into three categories:
necessary criteria, supportive criteria, and exclusion criteria
(Table 1). In general, cases were categorized as classical if
all eight necessary criteria were met. Although most RS
patients will meet many, if not all, of the supportive criteria,

diagnosis is possible in the absence of all of the supportive criteria, especially in young patients. The presence of one or more of the exclusion criteria excludes the diagnosis of RS, regardless of whether all of the necessary criteria have been met in an individual patient. The clinical characteristics and differential diagnosis of RS vary according to the stage of the disease (Table 2).

Although these are not considered necessary criteria for diagnosis, most patients have seizures, abnormal electroencephalograms (EEGs), and respiratory dysfunction. Complex partial, atypical absence, generalized tonic–clonic, atonic, and/or myoclonic seizures occur in up to 80% of patients (6). After the age of 2 years, the EEG is typically abnormal, usually with a slow, poorly organized waking background. Glaze et al. (12) correlated the EEG with clinical staging. In stage II, the EEG frequently shows slowing of background rhythms, rare focal spike or sharp wave discharges while awake, and progressive loss of sleep characteristics like spindles and vertex transients. In stage III, further slowing is noted with appearance of delta waves, and generalized spike–wave patterns may first be seen during sleep. In stage IV, the EEG may improve to some extent, with fewer epileptiform discharges and frequent fronto-central theta activity. Central spikes tend to decrease after the age of 10 years. The frequency of epileptiform findings ranged from 60% of patients in stage IV to 97% in patients in clinical stage III (13,14). Osteopenia is also a common feature, despite apparently normal homeostasis of calcium, phosphate, and the endocrine systems that regulate bone density. In addition, about half of the girls with RS have prolonged QTc intervals, possibly related to the eventual sudden death seen in certain children with RS.

The diagnostic criteria of atypical RS were defined by Hagberg and Skjeldal in 1994 (see Table 3) (7). Although the diagnostic criteria are clearly defined, nevertheless diagnosis remains difficult. A first differential diagnosis can be infantile autism, which also shows significant deterioration in the second year. Autistic children may have mild ataxia, but less than RS girls aged 1 year or older. Another condition

difficult to distinguish from RS is Angelman (or happy puppet) syndrome. These retarded children may also develop seizures. However, in this syndrome, both sexes are involved
equally and they have a fairly characteristic phenotype and
a different underlying genetic defect. A child neurologist
may wish to look further to exclude congenital metabolic
defects and possible brain injury from anoxia, ischemia, or
trauma. Neuroimaging may also be required, including
magnetic resonance imaging (MRI), with volumetric studies,
single photon emission computed tomography (SPECT), cerebral proton magnetic resonance spectroscopy, and positron
emission tomography (PET). In RS, volumetric MRI studies
have shown an overall decrease in brain volume, affecting
gray matter more than white matter (15,16).

III. NEUROPATHOLOGY

Neuropathological studies have shown no consistent site of
gross neuronal degeneration and no evidence of abnormal
neuronal migration. However, slowing of head growth usually
becomes definite from the age of about 3 months. Jellinger
et al. (17) found that in nine RS girls aged 3–17 years, brain
weight was decreased to 66–88% of expected values for the
age. In accumulated autopsy studies of over 50 cases, the Rett
brain consistently weighed less than controls when matched
for both age and height. The weight of the average classic
Rett brain at autopsy is 950 g, which is the brain weight for
a normal 1-year-old child (18). It should be noted though that
in the formes frustres of RS, in which there is preservation
of speech and hand use, the head circumference (and presumably, the brain weight) is within the low normal range (19). In
RS, the brain weight does not continue to decrease with age
(16). This stable brain size and the absence of markers for
degenerative disorders support the idea that the decreased
brain size in RS is the result of arrested brain development.

Subramaniam et al. (16) compared volumetric MRI brain
analysis of 20 RS girls with those of age matched normal girls.
They observed a global reduction in gray and white matter

volumes that is predominantly present within the prefrontal, posterior frontal, and anterior temporal regions. They also observed a preferential reduction in the volume of the caudate nucleus. The midbrain, which had previously been reported to be reduced in area showed no reduction when volume was determined. There was no age-related change in the overall size of the cerebellum or the cerebrum that differed from that of controls.

It is clear that there are regional differences in the state of maturation or malformation in the RS brain. The volumes of frontal and temporal lobes and of the caudate nucleus are smaller than the rest of the cerebrum and cerebellum. The poor development of the pyramidal neurons in cortical layers III and V suggests that a delay in maturation coincides with the second stage of cortical development proposed by Poliakov (20). In this time period, from birth to 2 years of age, there is a reorganization of the thalamic input into layers III and V of the cortex, a growth of dendrites and a maturation of inter-neurons. Thus, it seems that the pathogenic process is not one of simple developmental arrest. It involves a selective change in specific brain regions during a critical period of brain development. This produces a brain deprived of its capacity to regulate independent speech and hand use.

Neuropathologists have further attempted to understand why the brain is small. There is no apparent alteration in the myelin, no consistent evidence of cell loss or atrophy, no ventriculomegaly, and no obvious malformations. Bauman et al. (21) observed a global decrease in the size of individual neurons in RS, associated with increased packing density (neurons per 0.1 mm^3 area) in the two areas which were examined, the hippocampus and entorhinal cortex. Dendritic trees were found to be significantly diminished in the following areas of RS brains: the basal branches of pyramidal neurons in layers III and V of the prefrontal and motor cortex and the apical branches of pyramidal neurons of layer V and the basilar branches of layer IV neurons of the subicular cortex (subiculum) (22). The dendrites of hippocampal and occipital regions were found not to be significantly reduced. The reduction in dendritic arborization may account for some of the decrease in brain size. In general, the decrease in brain size was most marked in the frontal lobe, the caudate, and the midbrain. Kitt and Wilcox (23) further reported preliminary results showing abnormalities in the substantia nigra, including decreased numbers of neurons, ubiquitin-stained neuronal inclusion bodies, decreased immunostaining for transmitter markers, and histochemical evidence for cell death. The decreased dendritic branching in RS suggests that the synaptic input is reduced. This has been confirmed in the frontal cortex. In fact, in 1997, Belichenko et al. (24), using special techniques and confocal laser scanning microscopy in the affected focal areas, showed greatly thinned dendrites with reduced spines in RS girls and concluded that RS might best be explained by postnatal deficiency of synaptogenic development. A decrease in the numbers of synapses is also suggested by the decrease in synaptophysin staining observed by Belichenko and Dahlstrom in the speech areas (25).

Many studies have reported an altered expression of specific proteins in certain cerebral neurons. Parvalbumin immunoreactivity in the speech areas is reduced suggesting a reduction of gamma amino-butyric acid (GABA) ergic interneurons (25). Cyclo-oxygenase and microtubule-associated protein 2 (MAP2), an important cytoskeletal component of neuronal dendrites, were altered in the motor and frontal cortex and MAP2 was absent in the subplate neurons, particularly in the prefrontal cortex (26). However, these abnormalities could still indicate maldevelopment. In addition, some RS neurons have been shown to have an altered expression of neurotransmitters. Many studies have been performed, but the results are often inconsistent, because the performance of neurotransmitter assays seems problematic. Moreover, there are important normal age-related changes in the neurotransmitters and their receptors, and these are difficult to define in RS girls of various stages and ages. A review by Wenk et al. (26) summarizes some of the alterations that have been observed in different brain regions using various techniques. The only consistent changes observed were a reduction in the cholinergic system. Since Wenk's review, Blue et al. (27,28) reported an alteration in amino acid receptors in the frontal cortex of nine RS patients. The youngest girls (aged from 4 to 15 years) exhibited a slightly higher density of N-methyl-D-aspartate (NMDA), α-amino-3-hydroxy-4-isoxazole propionic acid (AMPA), GABA, and metabotropic type glutamate receptors and a decreased density was observed in the older RS patients (aged from 15 to 39 years). Yamashita et al. (29) found benzodiazepine receptor binding to be decreased in the fronto-temporal cortex in three adult RS patients, suggesting a decrease in GABA receptors in RS. Moreover, substance P, an 11-amino acid neuropeptide that has been shown to stimulate neurite extension in cultured neuroblastoma cells, is significantly decreased in the CSF (30–32). This decrease of the substance P level reflects the autonomic dysfunction, including constipation, small and cold feet, progressive limb muscle weakness, and muscle atrophy in RS (30). Many studies also reported a decrease of substance P immunoreactivity in RS brain tissues (33,34), especially in the dorsal horns, the intermediolateral column of the spinal cord, the spinal trigeminal tract, the solitary tract and nucleus, the parvocellular and pontine reticular nuclei, and in the locus coerelus (33). Sleep abnormalities, frequently observed in RS patients, could be influenced by the decreased level of substance P in the reticular formation and locus coerelus. Deguchi et al. (33) suggested that the sleep abnormalities were not a primary defect of substance P in RS, but may be secondary to an abnormality in the serotonin system that is co-localized with substance P at some sites.

IV. POPULATION GENETICS

Rett syndrome was initially thought to be a rare disorder. However, in independent studies from Sweden (3,35) and Scotland (18,19), investigators estimated the prevalence of RS to be about 1/10,000 girls, about twice the sex-specific prevalence of phenylketonuria in these countries. Moreover, among girls aged 0–18 years in North Dakota, Burd et al. (36) found the frequency of RS to be 1 in 19,786. Miyamoto et al. (37) quoted data suggesting that RS has a frequency of 1 in 20,000 girls in metropolitan Tokyo (38). Thus, RS represents one of the more frequent causes of severe mental retardation in girls.

V. INHERITANCE AND IDENTIFICATION OF THE GENE

The earliest hypothesis on the inheritance of RS was founded on the seemingly exclusive appearance of the disorder in females. Most of the cases of RS are isolated, apart from some cases of affected identical twins (39). It was thus believed to be an X-linked dominant disorder in which every case represented a new mutation, with male lethality. The identification of males who harbored an extra X chromosome (47, XXY) and bore features identical to those of RS in girls was also compatible with X-linked inheritance (40). Moreover, occasionally a brother of a RS girl was born with a severe encephalopathy which proved to be fatal (41,42). However, there was no such gross deficiency of males among the siblings of RS girls as might be expected. In the course of a systematic high-resolution chromosome analysis on patients with RS, Zoghbi et al. (43) and Journel et al. (44) found two distinct translocations t(X;22) (p11.22;p11) and t(X;3) (p22.1;q13.31). The reason for the discrepancy between the two breakpoint localizations in these cases was not clear. Subsequently, linkage studies were used in rare familial cases. In 1992, Ellison et al. (45) performed genotypic analysis using 63 DNA markers from the X chromosome in two families with maternally related, affected half-sisters. They excluded the region from Xp21.2 to Xq21–q23. Curtis et al. (46) did linkage studies in four families, each with two individuals affected by RS. They excluded much of the short arm of the X chromosome. In a family with recurrence of RS in a maternal aunt and niece, Schanen et al. (47), using combined exclusion mapping data, excluded the region between DXS1053 in Xp22.2 and DXS1222 in Xq22.3. Xiang et al.(48) presented haplotype analysis of nine families with at least two closely related females affected by classic RS. They concluded that the RS locus is likely to lie within Xq28, close to marker DXS15. At the same time, Webb et al. (49) presented a study of six

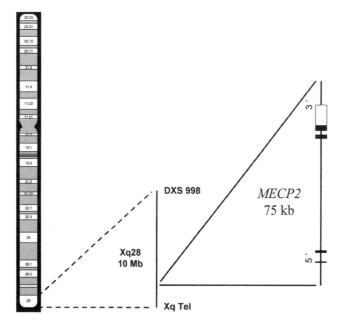

Figure 2 Localization of the *MECP2* gene in the long arm of the X chromosome.

families with more than one female affected with RS. They showed weak linkage to loci in Xq28, with a maximum lod score of 1.935 at theta = 0.0 at DXYS154. Sirianni et al. (50), using a family with three female sibs affected with RS, confirmed X-linked dominant inheritance of RS and the localization to Xq28. These studies suggested a critical region at Xq28, the telomeric part of the long arm of the X chromosome (Fig. 2). After systematic exclusion of several candidate genes within Xq27.3–Xqter, in 1999, Amir et al. (11) found several mutations in the X-linked *MECP2* gene encoding the methyl-CpG-binding protein 2 (MeCP2) [MIM 300005] in a proportion of RS patients.

VI. MeCP2 PROTEIN

Methyl-CpG-binding protein 2 is an abundant chromosome-binding protein that selectively binds 5-methylcytosine

residues in symmetrically positioned CpG dinucleotides in
mammalian genomes (51). It is thought to function as a transcriptional repressor in methylated regions of DNA via two
distinct domains, a methyl-CpG-binding domain (MBD) and
a transcriptional repression domain (TRD) (52,53). The
MBD consists of an 85-amino acid (aa) stretch (aa 78–162)
at the N-terminal end of the protein, which is both necessary
and sufficient to bind DNA in the presence or absence of
assembled chromatin. The TRD was delineated by Nan and
colleagues in 1997, who mapped the domain to amino acids
207–310 by replacing the MBD with the GAL4DNA-binding
domain fused to various *MECP2* deletion constructs and
assayed for repression of a reporter gene containing the
GAL4-binding element. In addition to the MBD and the
TRD, there are two other domain motifs in MeCP2 associated
with specific functions (53). First, lying within the TRD is a
nuclear localization signal (NLS) (aa 255–271) (Fig. 3), which
is sufficient for transportation of the protein into the nucleus
(54). Second, the last 63 aa of MeCP2 have been shown to
facilitate binding of the protein to both naked and nucleosomal DNA (55). Many proteins have been shown to contain
MBDs, but so far, MeCP2 is unique in its ability to bind to
a single symmetrical pair of methyl-CpG dinucleotides both
in naked DNA and within chromatin (51,53). The TRD of
MeCP2 represses transcription through its interaction with
the Sin3A complex containing histone deacetylases 1 and 2
(HDAC1 and HDAC2), which remodel the chromatin structure
such that it becomes refractory to transcription (56) (Fig. 4).
Methyl-CpG-binding protein 2 also interacts with two other
corepressors, the proto-oncoprotein of the Sloan–Kettering
virus named after the Sloan–Kettering Institute (c-Ski) and
the nuclear receptor corepressor (N-CoR) (57). c-Ski and N-
CoR are components of histone deacetylase complexes that
can, but do not always, function together (58). However, the
inhibition of histone deacetylase activity using drugs such as
Trichostatin A only partially relieves MeCP2-mediated transcriptional repression. This partial relief indicates that
additional mechanisms of repression by MeCP2 likely exist
aside from the recruitment of histone deacetylase. Beside

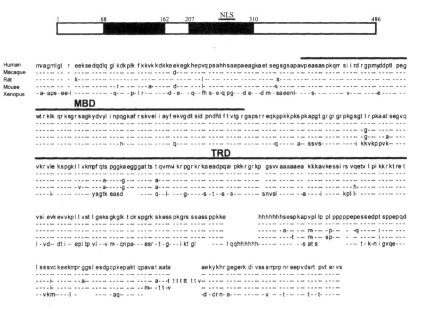

Figure 3 Sequence alignment of MeCP2 from human, macaque, rat, mouse, and *Xenopus*. Identities are indicated with a dash, gaps with a blank; different aa are shown. Methyl-CpG-binding protein 2 with its two functional domains MBD and TRD are indicated. The NLS is marked.

histone deacetylation, histone methylation is emerging as another key post-translational modification of histones and represents an important epigenetic mechanism for the organization of chromatin structure and the regulation of gene expression. In particular, methylation at lysine 9 of histone H3 is associated with gene silencing and several enzymes that catalyze the addition of methyl groups to lysine 9 have been identified (59). Recently, it has been shown that MeCP2 is associated with histone methylation in vitro as well as in vivo. The MeCP2-associated methylation activity is found to be specific for lysine 9 of histone H3. Methyl-CpG-binding protein 2 facilitates H3 K9 methylation of the *H19* gene, a bona fide MeCP2-regulated gene. All the data indicate that MeCP2 acts as a mechanistic bridge between DNA methylation and histone methylation and shows the repressive

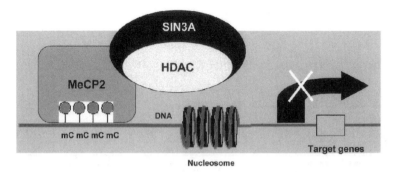

Figure 4 Normal function of MeCP2. Methyl-CpG-binding protein 2 binds methylated cytosine residues (mC) in CpG islands and recruits Sin3A and histone deacetylases HDACs. Deacetylation of the histone tails compacts the chromatin and silences transcription. (*See color insert.*)

function of these two distinct methylation events (60). Moreover, MeCP2 has been demonstrated to inhibit the assembly of the basal transcriptional machinery onto methylated promoters in the absence of chromatin assembly and to associate with TFIIB and E2F (61,62). It is clear that the role of MeCP2 in the nucleus is complex and it is likely to mediate transcriptional silencing through several overlapping mechanisms.

By immunohistochemistry, it has been shown that MeCP2 expression is high in brain, lung, and spleen, moderate in kidney and heart, and low in liver, stomach, and small intestine. In the brain, MeCP2 expression was not detected in glial cells and was abundant in mature neurons. Methyl-CpG-binding protein 2 was found in nuclear compartments but also in at least a subset of neurons in postsynaptic compartments (63). These data suggest that the delayed onset and other characteristics of RS may be partially explained by the preferential function of MeCP2 in mature rather than in immature neurons (64). It is possible that MeCP2 primarily represses genes that are important during neuronal development but that are detrimental for mature neurons. For example, developing neurons progress through a sequence of stages characterized by the expression of specific neurotransmitters and neuropeptides. The complement of signaling molecules expressed by the mature neuron may be entirely different from that during the embryonic stages. It could therefore be the case that MeCP2 represses genes coding for certain transmitters or peptides that are expressed only early in neuronal development.

Methyl-CpG-binding protein 2 has been implicated in the regulation of imprinted genes. For example, MeCP2 binds selectively to the parental allele of the differentially methylated domain of the *H19* gene (65) and to the maternal (methylated) allele of the imprinted *U2af1-rs* gene (65,66). It is interesting that several imprinted genes have been implicated in neurological functions such as *Ube3A* and *Peg1* (67,68). Moreover, in an effort to identify the MeCP2-target genomic regions, Kubota and colleagues performed immunofluorescence analysis with an anti-MeCP2 antibody on metaphase chromosomes of normal lymphoblasts and showed that MeCP2 staining was dispersed throughout the chromosome arms (Kubota et al., personal communication). This staining pattern was similar to that seen in rats, but was different from that in mice, where staining was predominantly localized to the heterochromatin regions. Thus, the authors performed a chromatin immunoprecipitation assay with the same anti-MeCP2 antibody using normal lymphoblasts. Sequence analysis of cloned MeCP2-binding genomic DNA fragments showed that 53 of the 93 fragments (57%) fulfilled the criteria of CpG island (over 50% G + C content and high CpG frequency). Of these, only two fragments were identified in a BLAST search (12q13 and 14q32) of which one was matched with a CpG island of a known gene. These results suggest that the MeCP2-target genomic regions should be identified in the near future.

VII. MUTATIONS OF *MECP2* IN RETT SYNDROME

The *MECP2* gene spans 76 kb in Xq28 and lies between the interleukin-1 receptor-associated kinase 1 (IRAK1) and red opsin loci, a region of conserved synteny with mouse ChrXC. The *MECP2* gene is composed of four exons that are transcribed from telomere to centromere, with the 1461-nucleotide coding sequence in exons 2–4 (exon 2 from bp 1 to 26, exon 3 bp 27 to 377, and exon 4 bp 378 to 1461). The 3′-untranslated region (3′-UTR) in exon 4 is unusually long (8.5 kb) and well conserved between human and mouse, although its functional significance has not been clearly elucidated. This gene is generally considered as a housekeeping gene because it has a CpG island associated with the 5′ end and is ubiquitously expressed. There are several potential Sp1-binding sites in the CpG island and indirect evidence that Sp1 at least partially regulates its expression. The gene is subject to X inactivation in mouse and human cells (69).

In mammals, MeCP2 protein is widely expressed in embryonic and adult tissues, although at low levels early in development. There are three transcripts detected in most tissues in humans which vary in length (1.8, 7.5, and 10 kb) and result from different polyadenylation signals present in the 3′-UTR. In most human and rodent tissues, short (1.8 kb) and long (10 kb) transcripts are equally present, but in adult brain and spinal cord the long transcript is predominantly expressed (70).

Since the discovery of the gene, numerous studies have found a variety of mutations in the coding region of *MECP2* in patients with RS, identifying mutations for as many as 55–90% of patients (for example, 55% in China and 87% in Denmark) (61–63,71,72). The remaining 10–45% of cases may have mutations in other regions of this gene, such as in regulatory elements and in noncoding regions, but this remains to be determined. Moreover, the PCR-based genomic screening strategy currently used in clinical laboratories would not be expected to detect large deletions or intragenic inversions. It is highly probable that large deletions could account for some cases in which no mutation has been identified.

An alternative hypothesis to explain the absence of *MECP2* mutation in a number of RS patients, that takes into account the exclusive involvement of females, could be the involvement of a putative second X-linked gene. This hypothesis is reinforced by the absence of identified mutations in some RS families. Moreover, the absence of sister–brother pairs would implicate a second X-linked gene if indeed there exists a second locus. Translocations also support this hypothesis. It is also likely that the inclusion criteria of patients in the study play an important role in determining the detection rate.

To date, more than 190 different mutations in the *MECP2* gene have been reported for RS all over the world (see *MECP2* variation database at http://mecp2.chw.edu.au) (73). A large proportion of mutations (67%) involve C → T transitions at CpG mutation hot spots and were found in unrelated patients, reflecting the hypermutability of these sites. A third of these mutations lead to single amino acid substitutions. These missense mutants cluster essentially in the methyl-binding domain (MBD). Truncating mutations make up about two-thirds. They are either nonsense mutations or insertions/deletions that lead to frameshifts and premature stop codons. Several small deletions, ranging between 10 and 26 bp and localized in the region between 1150 and 1200 of the coding sequence of the cDNA have been identified in numerous studies (Fig. 5). These deletions are probably the result of recombination between the four CCACC direct repeat sequences present in this C-rich region. Most of these deletions are distal to the MBD. One hypothesis holds that the truncated protein still binds methylated DNA but cannot interact with the corepressor Sin3A, though it is still possible that mutations in the C-terminus of the protein disable DNA binding. This would prevent proper assembly of the silencing complex. Another hypothesis is that deletions within the C-terminus of MeCP2 significantly decrease protein stability (74).

According to the mutation frequencies, four groups of mutations (A–D) can be distinguished as follows. Group A (most common mutations) includes 7 mutations with relative frequencies >5% (R106W, T158M, R168X, R255X, R270X, R294X, and R306C). Group B comprises 3 mutations whose respective frequencies range from 5% to 2% (R133C, P152R, and 806delG). Together, these 10 mutations account for 65% of 191 RS mutation alleles in France (75). The third group, Group C, comprises 9 mutations which were identified thus

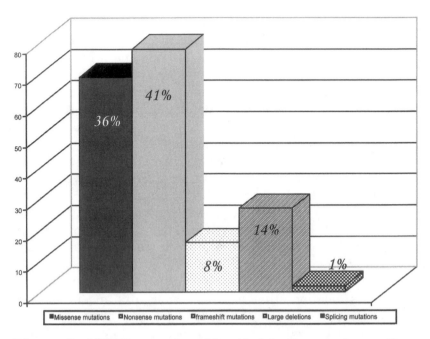

Figure 5 *MECP2* mutations identified in Rett syndrome. Data obtained from 191 mutations identified in 301 Rett patients.

far only twice (R106Q, D156E, P302R, X487C, 608insA, 1194insT, 1156del41, 1164del43, and 378-2T → G). Finally, 50 mutations were identified only once. Analysis of the data in comparison to the area of residence of the different families revealed no significant regional differences in the relative frequencies of the most common RS mutations (75).

The most common mutation found in RS is R168X, followed by two other nonsense mutations, R255X and R270X. Laccone et al. (76) found in the German population that the most frequent mutation is R294X. In the Danish population, the most common mutation is the R255X (72). The most frequent mutation in an American cohort is the missense mutation T158M (77). The great majority of the mutations are located in exon 4 (third coding exon). Few mutations (5%) are located in exon 3 (second coding exon) and rarely have mutations been identified in exon 2 (first coding exon).

Two MBD mutations observed in RS (R106W and R133C) are both located in the β-sheets comprising the wedge-shaped domain and have a greatly reduced affinity for methylated DNA in unassembled chromatin (78). Other missense mutations within the MBD (R111G, Y123A, I125A, and F155S) also significantly reduce the affinity of MeCP2 for methylated DNA (74,78). Consistent with these observations, MeCP2 containing the R106W or F155S mutation, when transfected into cells, is impaired in its ability to localize to heterochromatic domains and to repress transcription of a reporter (79). However, another common MBD mutation T158M, which replaces the threonine residue in the loop structure outside of the DNA-binding domain by a methionine, shows only a small reduction in binding affinity to methylated DNA and intermediary binding to native heterochromatin. The missense mutation in the TRD (R306C) does not reduce repressive activity of MeCP2 in a transfection assay, although it may have stronger effects in vivo (74).

VIII. PRENATAL DIAGNOSIS

Following requests from several families in which a *MECP2* mutation was identified in an index case, some laboratories have performed prenatal tests for *MECP2* mutations. The de novo status of the *MECP2* mutation was confirmed by DNA analysis of the mother in each family. In fact, in most cases, no mutations or other abnormalities were detected in the parents. Prenatal diagnosis and direct sequencing performed on amniotic fluid and cultured amniocytes was negative for the mutation in all cases. In view of these results as well as the very rare familial and germline mosaicism cases, it has been suggested that prenatal diagnosis should not be encouraged in any family with a sporadic case of RS syndrome. However, if the mutation is inherited from a healthy mother, the family should be informed about the high risk of occurrence in further generations and appropriate genetic counseling should be provided to the family. In fact, when a normal mother was found to carry a potentially

disease-causing mutation but escapes clinical symptoms
because of nonrandom skewing of X inactivation, the carrier
has a 50% risk of transmitting the mutant allele.

IX. CORRELATION BETWEEN PHENOTYPE
AND GENOTYPE

Two different genetic factors are likely to influence the phenotype in RS: X inactivation and the type and location of the
mutations. There is no clear correlation between the type
and position of the mutations and the phenotypic features of
classic and variant RS patients. However, X-chromosome
inactivation (XCI) appears to be a major determinant of
phenotypic severity. In three cases of familial RS, skewed X
inactivation was found on maternal investigation. The
mothers were either clinically normal or exhibited only minor
neurological symptoms (80,81). However, XCI (when studied
on peripheral lymphocytes) did not give the full explanation
for the clinical differences between patients with identical
mutations. For example, three patients with similar deletions
were phenotypically quite different: one patient with "forme
frustre" had random XCI as had the two other patients with
the classical form (72).
        The spectrum of clinical phenotypes caused by *MECP2*
mutations is wide, including milder preserved speech variants and the severe congenital Rett variant. Studies have
shown that atypical and classical RS syndrome can be caused
by the same *MECP2* mutations, indicating a variable phenotype. It remains, however, difficult to classify the severity of
individual features in a disorder that evolves over time.
        Conflicting results have been found as to whether the
type of mutation influences the phenotype. Amir and Zoghbi
(82) found no correlation between their composite clinical
severity score and the type of mutation. The same result
was found by Nielsen et al. (72), Auranen et al. (83), and
Huppke et al. (84). However, Cheadle et al. (85), in their study
of 44 patients, found that girls with truncating mutations present with higher severity scores. Zappella et al. (86) and

De Bona et al. (87) reported mutations in both classic and pre-served speech (PSV) variant RS. Approximately 55% (10/18) had an *MECP2* mutation (72). All mutations found in PSV were either missense or late-truncating mutations. In parti-cular, they did not find the four early-truncating hot spot mutations: R168X, R255X, R270X, and R294X. These results suggested that early-truncating mutations lead to a poor prognosis, while late-truncating or missense mutations lead either to classic RS or PSV. Moreover, Huppke et al. (88) found that mutations that lead to a complete or partial truncation of the region that codes for the NLS lead to a more severe phenotype than other mutations in the TRD and truncating mutations located downstream of the NLS (88).

The relationship between type of *MECP2* mutation, X-inactivation status, and clinical phenotype of RS is complex and likely involves other environmental and polygenic modi-fiers (89). Further research focuses on the pathogenic conse-quences of these mutations along the hypothesis of loss of transcriptional repression of a small number of genes that are essential for neuronal function in the maturing brain (90).

In future, papers relating phenotypes to genotypes involving mutations in *MECP2* should provide a minimum data set reporting the range of disturbances frequently encoun-tered in RS. A simple scoring system has been suggested which facilitate comparison among the various clinical profiles (91).

X. *MECP2* MUTATIONS IN MALE PATIENTS

Male patients with RS are extremely rare suggesting that RS causing mutations in the *MECP2* gene might be lethal in hemizygous males. However, in 1998, two studies described three males born into RS families with encephalopathies with neonatal onset. Two of the males had congenital hypotonia, respiratory distress requiring mechanical ventilation, sei-zures, and severe intestinal dysfunction (42,50). All died in infancy. Moreover, it has previously been demonstrated that an excess of paternally derived mutations might account for the nearly exclusive occurrence of RS in females (92,93).

Clayton-Smith et al. (94) described the first male with somatic mosaicism for a *MECP2* mutation leading to a progressive but nonfatal neurodevelopmental disorder. The patient was born at term with height and weight parameters within the normal range. He was a placid baby who never crawled, but walked at 15 months and learned to say some single words in the second year of life. At age 3 years, he began to have generalized seizures, and magnetic resonance imaging revealed atrophy of the brainstem and of the frontal and temporal lobes. At 6 years, he had a thoracic scoliosis and poor-limb musculature and he walked with an ataxic gait. He had abnormal muscle tone with rigidity of the limbs and truncal hypotonia. His feet were small, blue, and puffy. His hand use was very limited, but there were no obvious hand-wringing movements. Recently, a second case of somatic mosaicism was also described (95).

Affected males can be divided into two groups according to the type of their mutation (Table 5). The first group carries mutations in the *MECP2* gene either already described in RS females or mutations of unquestionable pathological value (frameshift mutations or nonsense mutations) (Fig. 6). These patients are characterized by early onset of the disease and a severe encephalopathy (81). However, recently a de novo mutation (P225L) was identified in a 21-year-old male with severe mental retardation, spastic tetraplegia, dystonia, apraxia, and neurogenic scoliosis (96). An additional subgroup are males with a (47,XXY) Klinefelter karyotype who present with the typical RS symptoms (34,97). The second group includes patients carrying mutations inherited from their mother, which have never been found in Rett females (98–100). These patients feature mental retardation of different degrees and possibly additional symptoms. For example, the A140V mutation has been identified in sporadic and familial cases of mental retardation (98,100). More recently, the same mutation was found in all affected individuals with PPM-X syndrome, an X-linked syndrome of psychosis, pyramidal signs, and macro-orchidism (101). Another example is the Q406X mutation which eliminates the last 80 aa of the protein. This mutation was found in two males with delayed development, macrocephaly, seizures, ataxia, and absence of

Table 5 Male *MECP2* Mutations and Predicted Effect on MeCP2: A: Mutations Already Described in RS Females or Mutations of Unquestionable Pathological Value; B: Mutations Never Found in RS Females but Described in Males with MR or Other Clinical Phenotypes

Mutation	Type	Comments	Domain	Family	Male phenotype
A					
166del2	Truncating	mosaic	Before MBD	–	RS-like
241del2	Truncating	mosaic	MBD	–	RS-like
R133H	Missense	mosaic	MBD	–	RS-like
Y141X	Truncating	47,XXY; de novo	MBD	–	RS-like
T158M	Missense		MBD	+	Severe, neonatal, early death
T158M	Missense	47,XXY/46,XY	MBD	–	RS-like
T158M	Missense	47,XXY	MBD	–	RS-like
488del2	Truncating		After MBD	+	Congenital encephalopathy
754insC	Truncating		TRD	+	Congenital encephalopathy
806del1	Truncating		TRD	+	Severe, neonatal, early death
R270X	Truncating	mosaic	TRD	–	RS-like
R270X	Truncating	47,XXY/46,XY	TRD	–	RS-like
816dep7	Truncating		TRD	–	RS-like
1154del32	Truncating	46,XY,inv(X) (q27;q28)	After TRD	+	Severe, neonatal, early death

(Continued)

Table 5 Male *MECP2* Mutations and Predicted Effect on MeCP2: A: Mutations Already Described in RS Females or Mutations of Unquestionable Pathological Value; B: Mutations Never Found in RS Females but Described in Males with MR or Other Clinical Phenotypes (*Continued*)

Mutation	Type	Comments	Domain	Family	Male phenotype
B					
E137G	Missense	MBD		+	Non specific MR
A140V	Missense	MBD		+	Non specific MR; PPM-S
R167W	Missense		After MBD	+	Mild non specific MR
A181V	Missense		After MBD	–	Autism
P225L	Missense	de novo	TRD	–	Severe MR, neurologic features
P376S	Missense		After TRD	+	Autism
P402L	Missense		After TRD	+	Autism
Q406X	Truncating		After TRD	+	Severe MR, progressive spasticity
G428S	Missense		After TRD	+	Non progressive encephalopathy
R453Q	Missense		After TRD	?	Non specific MR
1161del240	Truncating		After TRD	+	Mild MR
1415–1416del	Truncating	de novo	After TRD	?	Moderate MR

Source: From Refs. 34, 80,81,94–98,100,102,103,110–113.

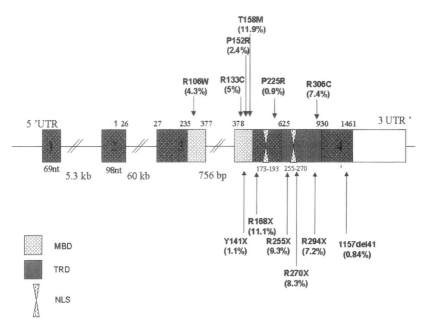

Figure 6 The genomic organization of the *MECP2* gene. It is comprised of four exons (1–4), and nucleotide positions relative to the ATG codon are indicated. The 5'-UTR is short (167 nucleotides), and contained exon 1 (69 nucleotides) and part of exon 2 (98 nucleotides). Position of the common mutations and their relative frequencies are indicated above (missense) and below (nonsense and frameshift). (See *MECP2* variation database at http://mecp2.chw.edu.au.)

language (102). Females with this same mutation were, even with balanced XCI patterns, unaffected.

At present, based on the analysis of the *MECP2* gene in sporadic mental retardation, it has been suggested that the frequency of *MECP2* in the fragile-X negative mentally retarded males is 0.2–0.4% (103).

XI. RETT SYNDROME ANIMAL MODELS

In 2001, two independent groups Guy et al. (104) and Chen et al. (105) reported studies in mice in which the X-linked *MECP2* gene has been deleted using the Cre–Lox system

(104,105). The mice display a neurologic phenotype similar to human RS, and therefore are useful models for studying this disease. To obtain MeCP2-null animals, both groups generated mice in which *MECP2* was flanked by loxP sites, and crossed these mice with deleted animals that ubiquitously express the Cre enzyme. The Cre–Lox approach allowed them to make null mice as well as spatially and temporally specific mutants, and thus circumvent the problem of potential embryonic lethality in males. Surprisingly, the null mice, both male hemizygotes and female homozygotes are viable and are phenotypically normal at birth. However, between 3 and 8 weeks after birth, these null mice develop uncoordinated motor behavior, reduced activity, breathing irregularities, and usually die within 10 weeks. Heterozygous females also develop ataxia and respiratory abnormalities, closely paralleling the condition of human; however, the onset of symptoms was found to be delayed until 4 months of age or later.

Jaenisch and colleagues reported that MeCP2-null mice have smaller brains, and that neurons in the hippocampus, cerebellum, and cortex have smaller somas, smaller nuclei and are more densely packed. Other abnormalities seen included undescended testes in MeCP2-null males and changes in body weight (105).

To accomplish CNS-specific *MECP2* deletions, mice carrying the loxed *MECP2* allele were crossed with mice carrying Cre driven by the nestin promoter. Because nestin is expressed in neural precursor cells, *MECP2* is deleted in the nervous system in the offspring of these mice. Both groups show that when *MECP2* is deleted in this way, the mice exhibit a phenotype similar to that of a global *MECP2* deletion. This result indicates that the behavioral and neuropathological disorders in these mice result from a lack of MeCP2 protein in the nervous system and not in other tissues, suggesting that neurons have a special requirement for MeCP2. To determine whether MeCP2 is specifically required in postmitotic neurons, Jaenisch and colleagues used mice in which Cre was driven by the Cam kinase promoter to delete *MECP2* specifically from postmitotic neurons (105).

They observed that these mice develop the same behavioral phenotype and neuropathology as mice with a global *MECP2* deletion, indicating that postmitotic neurons have an ongoing requirement for MeCP2. Mutations in *MECP2* thus are likely to lead to uncontrolled target gene expression in neurons while perhaps expression in other tissues remains repressed. An alternative hypothesis is that neurons are less tolerant of background transcriptional noise than other cell types.

Comparison of global gene expression in wild-type and *MECP2* mutant mice by microarray analyses revealed no dramatic changes in transcription even in mice displaying overt disease symptoms, although statistical power analyses of the data indicated that even a small number of relatively subtle changes in transcription would have been detected if present (106).

More recently, mice with a truncating mutation similar to those found in RS patients have been created (107). These mice appeared normal and exhibited normal function for about 6 weeks, but then developed a progressive neurological disease that includes many features of RS such as tremors, motor impairments, hypoactivity, increased anxiety-related behavior, seizures, kyphosis, and stereotypic forelimb motions. The authors showed that although the truncated MeCP2 protein in these mice localizes normally to heterochromatic domains in vivo, histone H3 is hyperacetylated, providing evidence that the chromatin architecture is abnormal and that gene expression may be misregulated in this model of RS.

XII. CONCLUSIONS

Rett syndrome, the most common cause of profound cognitive impairment in females, is a developmental neurologic disorder characterized by postnatal deceleration of head growth, autistic behavior, stereotypic hand movements, and frequently seizures. The disorder is associated in the majority of cases with mutations of the coding region of the gene encoding methyl-CpG-binding protein 2. More recently, other neurologic syndromes different from RS have also been reported to be associated with *MECP2* mutations. Methyl-CpG-binding protein 2, a protein originally thought of as a global transcriptional repressor, is actually specialized for a function in neurons of the CNS. It is remarkable that mouse models have reproduced virtually every aspect of RS, including the highly specialized hand-wringing behaviors, suggesting that the pathways leading from dysfunctional MeCP2 to each of these features are conserved between humans and mice. Gene expression analyses in these mouse models may help elucidate the neuronal-specific functions of MeCP2 that are misregulated in RS.

ACKNOWLEDGMENTS

The author thanks Assistance Publique–Hôpitaux de Paris (AP–HP), Institut National de la Santé et de la Recherche Médicale (INSERM), and the Association Française du syndrome de Rett (ASFR). The author is grateful to F. Francis, H. Van Hesch, and N. Bahi for their helpful comments.

REFERENCES

1. Rett A. On a unusual brain atrophy syndrome in hyperammonemia in childhood. Wien Med Wochenschr 1966; 116:723–726.

2. Hagberg B, Aicardi J, Dias K, Ramos O. A progressive syndrome of autism, dementia, ataxia, and loss of purposeful hand use in girls: Rett's syndrome: report of 35 cases. Ann Neurol 1983; 14:471–479.

3. Hagberg B. Rett's syndrome: prevalence and impact on progressive severe mental retardation in girls. Acta Paediatr Scand 1985; 74:405–408.

4. Hagberg B, Witt-Engerström I. Rett syndrome: a suggested staging system for describing impairment profile with increasing age towards adolescence. Am J Med Genet Suppl 1986; 1:47–59.

5. The Proceedings of the 5th International Conference on the Rett Syndrome, Vienna, Nov 4–7, 1988. Dedicated to Professor Andreas Rett. Brain Dev 1990; 12:1–183.

6. The Rett Syndrome Diagnostic Criteria Work Group. Diagnostic criteria for Rett syndrome. Ann Neurol 1988; 23:425–428.

7. Hagberg BA, Skjeldal OH. Rett variants: a suggested model for inclusion criteria. Pediatr Neurol 1994; 11:5–11.

8. Hagberg B. Clinical delineation of Rett syndrome variants. Neuropediatrics 1995; 26:62.

9. Leonard H, Bower C. Is the girl with Rett syndrome normal at birth? Dev Med Child Neurol 1998; 40:115–121

10. Charman T, Cass H, Owen L, Wigram T, Slonims V, Weeks L, Wisbeach A, Reilly S. Regression in individuals with Rett syndrome. Brain Dev 2002; 24:281–283.

11. Amir RE, Van den Veyver IB, Wan M, Tran CQ, Francke U, Zoghbi HY. Rett syndrome is caused by mutations in X-linked *MECP2*, encoding methyl-CpG-binding protein 2. Nat Genet 1999; 23:185–188.

12. Glaze DG, Frost JD Jr, Zoghbi HY, Percy AK. Rett's syndrome. Correlation of electroencephalographic characteristics with clinical staging. Arch Neurol 1987; 44:1053–1056.

13. Glaze DG, Schultz RJ, Frost JD. Rett syndrome: characterization of seizures versus non-seizures. Electroencephalogr Clin Neurophysiol 1998; 106:79–83.

14. Niedermeyer E, Rett A, Renner H, Murphy M, Naidu S. Rett syndrome and the electroencephalogram. Am J Med Genet Suppl 1986; 1:195–199.

15. Reiss AL, Faruque F, Naidu S, Abrams M, Beaty T, Bryan RN, Moser H. Neuroanatomy of Rett syndrome: a volumetric imaging study. Ann Neurol 1993; 34:227–234.

16. Subramaniam B, Naidu S, Reiss AL. Neuroanatomy in Rett syndrome: cerebral cortex and posterior fossa. Neurology 1997; 48:399–407.

17. Jellinger K, Armstrong D, Zoghbi HY, Percy AK. Neuropathology of Rett syndrome. Acta Neuropathol (Berl) 1988; 76:142–158.

18. Kerr AM, Stephenson JB. Rett's syndrome in the west of Scotland. Br Med J (Clin Res Ed) 1985; 291:579–582.

19. Kerr AM, Stephenson JB. A study of the natural history of Rett syndrome in 23 girls. Am J Med Genet Suppl 1986; 1: 77–83.

20. Poliakov GI. Development and complication of the cortical part of the coupling mechanism in the evolution of vertebrates. J Hirnforsch 1964; 7:253–273.

21. Bauman ML, Kemper TL, Arin DM. Microscopic observations of the brain in Rett syndrome. Neuropediatrics 1995; 26: 105–108.

22. Armstrong DD. The neuropathology of Rett syndrome—overview 1994. Neuropediatrics 1995; 26:100–104.

23. Kitt CA, Wilcox BJ. Preliminary evidence for neurodegenerative changes in the substantia nigra of Rett syndrome. Neuropediatrics 1995; 26:114–118.

24. Belichenko PV, Hagberg B, Dahlstrom A. Morphological study of neocortical areas in Rett syndrome. Acta Neuropathol (Berl) 1997; 93:50–61.

25. Belichenko PV, Dahlstrom A. Studies on the 3-dimensional architecture of dendritic spines and varicosities in human cortex by confocal laser scanning microscopy and Lucifer yellow microinjections. J Neurosci Methods 1995; 57: 55–61.

26. Wenk GL. Rett syndrome: neurobiological changes underlying specific symptoms. Prog Neurobiol 1997; 51:383–391.

27. Blue ME, Naidu S, Johnston MV. Altered development of glutamate and GABA receptors in the basal ganglia of girls with Rett syndrome. Exp Neurol 1999; 156:345–352.

28. Blue ME, Naidu S, Johnston MV. Development of amino acid receptors in frontal cortex from girls with Rett syndrome. Ann Neurol 1999; 45:541–545.

29. Yamashita Y, Matsuishi T, Ishibashi M, Kimura A, Onishi Y, Yonekura Y, Kato H. Decrease in benzodiazepine receptor binding in the brains of adult patients with Rett syndrome. J Neurol Sci 1998; 154:146–150.

30. Matsuishi T, Nagamitsu S, Yamashita Y, Murakami Y, Kimura A, Sakai T, Shoji H, Kato H, Percy AK. Decreased cerebrospinal fluid levels of substance P in patients with Rett syndrome. Ann Neurol 1997; 42:978–981.

31. Satoi M, Matsuishi T, Yamada S, Yamashita Y, Ohtaki E, Mori K, Riikonen R, Kato H, Percy AK. Decreased cerebrospinal fluid levels of beta-phenylethylamine in patients with Rett syndrome. Ann Neurol 2000; 47:801–803.

32. Lappalainen R, Lindholm D, Riikonen R. Low levels of nerve growth factor in cerebrospinal fluid of children with Rett syndrome. J Child Neurol 1996; 11:296–300.

33. Deguchi K, Antalffy BA, Twohill LJ, Chakraborty S, Glaze DG, Armstrong DD. Substance P immunoreactivity in Rett syndrome. Pediatr Neurol 2000; 22:259–266.

34. Armstrong DD. Rett syndrome neuropathology review 2000. Brain Dev 2001; 23:S72–S76.

35. Witt-Engerström I, Gillberg C. Rett syndrome in Sweden. J Autism Dev Disord 1987; 17:149–150.

36. Burd L, Vesley B, Martsolf JT, Kerbeshian J. Prevalence study of Rett syndrome in North Dakota children. Am J Med Genet 1991; 38:565–568.

37. Suzuki H, Hirayama Y, Arima M. Prevalence of Rett syndrome in Tokyo. No To Hattatsu 1989; 21:430–433.

38. Miyamoto A, Yamamoto M, Takahashi S, Oki J. Classical Rett syndrome in sisters: variability of clinical expression. Brain Dev 1997; 19:492–494.

39. Tariverdian G. Follow-up of monozygotic twins concordant for the Rett syndrome. Brain Dev 1990; 12:125–127.

40. Vorsanova SG, Demidova IA, Ulas V, Soloviev IV, Kazantzeva LZ, Yurov Yu B. Cytogenetic and molecular-cytogenetic investigation of Rett syndrome: analysis of 31 cases. Neuroreport 1996; 8:187–189.

41. Schanen C, Francke U. A severely affected male born into a Rett syndrome kindred supports X-linked inheritance and allows extension of the exclusion map. Am J Hum Genet 1998; 63:267–269.

42. Schanen NC, Kurczynski TW, Brunelle D, Woodcock MM, Dure LSt, Percy AK. Neonatal encephalopathy in two boys in families with recurrent Rett syndrome. J Child Neurol 1998; 13:229–231.

43. Zoghbi HY, Ledbetter DH, Schultz R, Percy AK, Glaze DG. A de novo X;3 translocation in Rett syndrome. Am J Med Genet 1990; 35:148–151.

44. Journel H, Melki J, Turleau C, Munnich A, de Grouchy J. Rett phenotype with X/autosome translocation: possible mapping to the short arm of chromosome X. Am J Med Genet 1990; 35:142–147.

45. Ellison KA, Fill CP, Terwilliger J, DeGennaro LJ, Martin-Gallardo A, Anvret M, Percy AK, Ott J, Zoghbi H. Examination of X chromosome markers in Rett syndrome: exclusion mapping with a novel variation on multilocus linkage analysis. Am J Hum Genet 1992; 50:278–287.

46. Curtis AR, Headland S, Lindsay S, Thomas NS, Boye E, Kamakari S, Roustan P, Anvret M, Wahlstrom J, McCarthy G, et al. X chromosome linkage studies in familial Rett syndrome. Hum Genet 1993; 90:551–555.

47. Schanen NC, Dahle EJ, Capozzoli F, Holm VA, Zoghbi HY, Francke U. A new Rett syndrome family consistent with X-linked inheritance expands the X chromosome exclusion map. Am J Hum Genet 1997; 61:634–641.

48. Xiang F, Zhang Z, Clarke A, Joseluiz P, Sakkubai N, Sarojini B, Delozier-Blanchet CD, Hansmann I, Edstrom L, Anvret M. Chromosome mapping of Rett syndrome: a likely candidate region on the telomere of Xq. J Med Genet 1998; 35:297–300.

49. Webb T, Clarke A, Hanefeld F, Pereira JL, Rosenbloom L, Woods CG. Linkage analysis in Rett syndrome families suggests that there may be a critical region at Xq28. J Med Genet 1998; 35:997–1003.

50. Sirianni N, Naidu S, Pereira J, Pillotto RF, Hoffman EP. Rett syndrome: confirmation of X-linked dominant inheritance, and localization of the gene to Xq28. Am J Hum Genet 1998; 63:1552–1558.

51. Lewis JD, Meehan RR, Henzel WJ, Maurer-Fogy I, Jeppesen P, Klein F, Bird A. Purification, sequence, and cellular localization of a novel chromosomal protein that binds to methylated DNA. Cell 1992; 69:905–914.

52. Nan X, Meehan RR, Bird A. Dissection of the methyl-CpG binding domain from the chromosomal protein MeCP2. Nucleic Acids Res 1993; 21:4886–4892.

53. Nan X, Campoy FJ, Bird A. MeCP2 is a transcriptional repressor with abundant binding sites in genomic chromatin. Cell 1997; 88:471–481.

54. Nan X, Tate P, Li E, Bird A. DNA methylation specifies chromosomal localization of MeCP2. Mol Cell Biol 1996; 16:414–421.

55. Chandler SP, Guschin D, Landsberger N, Wolffe AP. The methyl-CpG binding transcriptional repressor MeCP2 stably associates with nucleosomal DNA. Biochemistry 1999; 38: 7008–7018.

56. Jones PL, Veenstra GJ, Wade PA, Vermaak D, Kass SU, Landsberger N, Strouboulis J, Wolffe AP. Methylated DNA and MeCP2 recruit histone deacetylase to repress transcription. Nat Genet 1998; 19:187–191.

57. Kokura K, Kaul SC, Wadhwa R, Nomura T, Khan MM, Shinagawa T, Yasukawa T, Colmenares C, Ishii S. The Ski protein family is required for MeCP2-mediated transcriptional repression. J Biol Chem 2001; 276:34115–34121.

58. Nomura T, Khan MM, Kaul SC, Dong HD, Wadhwa R, Colmenares C, Kohno I, Ishii S. Ski is a component of the histone deacetylase complex required for transcriptional repression by Mad and thyroid hormone receptor. Genes Dev 1999; 13:412–423.

59. Kouzarides T. Histone methylation in transcriptional control. Curr Opin Genet Dev 2002; 12:198–209.

60. Fuks F, Hurd PJ, Wolf D, Nan X, Bird AP, Kouzarides T. The methyl-CpG-binding protein MeCP2 links DNA methylation to histone methylation. J Biol Chem 2003; 278:4035–4040.

61. Kaludov NK, Wolffe AP. MeCP2 driven transcriptional repression in vitro: selectivity for methylated DNA, action

at a distance and contacts with the basal transcription machinery. Nucleic Acids Res 2000; 28:1921–1928.

62. Di Fiore B, Palena A, Felsani A, Palitti F, Caruso M, Lavia P. Cytosine methylation transforms an E2F site in the retinoblastoma gene promoter into a binding site for the general repressor methylcytosine-binding protein 2 (MeCP2). Nucleic Acids Res 1999; 27:2852–2859.

63. Aber KM, Nori P, MacDonald SM, Bibat G, Jarrar MH, Kaufmann WE. Methyl-CpG-binding protein 2 is localized in the postsynaptic compartment: an immunochemical study of subcellular fractions. Neuroscience 2003; 116:77–80.

64. Shahbazian MD, Antalffy B, Armstrong DL, Zoghbi HY. Insight into Rett syndrome: MeCP2 levels display tissue- and cell-specific differences and correlate with neuronal maturation. Hum Mol Genet 2002; 11:115–124.

65. Drewell RA, Goddard CJ, Thomas JO, Surani MA. Methylation-dependent silencing at the *H19* imprinting control region by MeCP2. Nucleic Acids Res 2002; 30:1139–1144.

66. Gregory RI, Randall TE, Johnson CA, Khosla S, Hatada I, O'Neill LP, Turner BM, Feil R. DNA methylation is linked to deacetylation of histone H3, but not H4, on the imprinted genes *Snrpn* and *U2af1-rs1*. Mol Cell Biol 2001; 21:5426–5436.

67. Matsuura T, Sutcliffe JS, Fang P, Galjaard RJ, Jiang YH, Benton CS, Rommens JM, Beaudet AL. De novo truncating mutations in E6-AP ubiquitin-protein ligase gene (UBE3A) in Angelman syndrome. Nat Genet 1997; 15:74–77.

68. Lefebvre L, Viville S, Barton SC, Ishino F, Keverne EB, Surani MA. Abnormal maternal behaviour and growth retardation associated with loss of the imprinted gene *Mest*. Nat Genet 1998; 20:163–169.

69. Dragich J, Houwink-Manville I, Schanen C. Rett syndrome: a surprising result of mutation in *MECP2*. Hum Mol Genet 2000; 9:2365–2375.

70. Coy JF, Sedlacek Z, Bachner D, Delius H, Poustka A. A complex pattern of evolutionary conservation and alternative polyadenylation within the long 3″-untranslated region of the methyl-CpG-binding protein 2 gene (*MECP2*) suggests a

regulatory role in gene expression. Hum Mol Genet 1999; 8:1253–1262.

71. Pan H, Wang YP, Bao XH, Meng HD, Zhang Y, Wu XR, Shen Y. *MECP2* gene mutation analysis in Chinese patients with Rett syndrome. Eur J Hum Genet 2002; 10:484–486.

72. Nielsen JB, Henriksen KF, Hansen C, Silahtaroglu A, Schwartz M, Tommerup N. *MECP2* mutations in Danish patients with Rett syndrome: high frequency of mutations but no consistent correlations with clinical severity or with the X chromosome inactivation pattern. Eur J Hum Genet 2001; 9:178–184.

73. Christodoulou J, Grimm A, Maher T, Bennetts B. RettBASE: The IRSA *MECP2* variation database—a new mutation database in evolution. Hum Mutat 2003; 21:466–472.

74. Yusufzai TM, Wolffe AP. Functional consequences of Rett syndrome mutations on human MeCP2. Nucleic Acids Res 2000; 28:4172–4179.

75. Bienvenu T, Villard L, De Roux N, Bourdon V, Fontes M, Beldjord C, Tardieu M, Jonveaux P, Chelly J. Spectrum of *MECP2* mutations in Rett syndrome. Genet Test 2002; 6:1–6.

76. Laccone F, Huppke P, Hanefeld F, Meins M. Mutation spectrum in patients with Rett syndrome in the German population: evidence of hot spot regions. Hum Mutat 2001; 17: 183–190.

77. Buyse IM, Roa BB. Denaturing high-performance liquid chromatography and sequence analyses for *MECP2* mutations in Rett syndrome. Methods Mol Biol 2003; 217:119–130.

78. Ballestar E, Yusufzai TM, Wolffe AP. Effects of Rett syndrome mutations of the methyl-CpG binding domain of the transcriptional repressor MeCP2 on selectivity for association with methylated DNA. Biochemistry 2000; 39:7100–7106.

79. Kudo S, Nomura Y, Segawa M, Fujita N, Nakao M, Dragich J, Schanen C, Tamura M. Functional analyses of MeCP2 mutations associated with Rett syndrome using transient expression systems. Brain Dev 2001; 23:S165–S173.

80. Wan M, Lee SS, Zhang X, Houwink-Manville I, Song HR, Amir RE, Budden S, Naidu S, Pereira JL, Lo IF, Zoghbi HY,

516 Bienvenu

Schanen NC, Francke U. Rett syndrome and beyond: recurrent spontaneous and familial MECP2 mutations at CpG hotspots. Am J Hum Genet 1999; 65:1520–1529.

81. Villard L, Kpebe A, Cardoso C, Chelly PJ, Tardieu PM, Fontes M. Two affected boys in a Rett syndrome family: clinical and molecular findings. Neurology 2000; 55:1188–1193.

82. Amir RE, Zoghbi HY. Rett syndrome: methyl-CpG-binding protein 2 mutations and phenotype–genotype correlations. Am J Med Genet 2000; 97:147–152.

83. Auranen M, Vanhala R, Vosman M, Levander M, Varilo T, Hietala M, Riikonen R, Peltonen L, Jarvela I. MECP2 gene analysis in classical Rett syndrome and in patients with Rett-like features. Neurology 2001; 56:611–617.

84. Huppke P, Laccone F, Kramer N, Engel W, Hanefeld F. Rett syndrome: analysis of MECP2 and clinical characterization of 31 patients. Hum Mol Genet 2000; 9:1369–1375.

85. Cheadle JP, Gill H, Fleming N, Maynard J, Kerr A, Leonard H, Krawczak M, Cooper DN, Lynch S, Thomas N, Hughes H, Hulten M, Ravine D, Sampson JR, Clarke A. Long-read sequence analysis of the MECP2 gene in Rett syndrome patients: correlation of disease severity with mutation type and location. Hum Mol Genet 2000; 9:1119–1129.

86. Zappella M, Meloni I, Longo I, Hayek G, Renieri A. Preserved speech variants of the Rett syndrome: molecular and clinical analysis. Am J Med Genet 2001; 104:14–22.

87. De Bona C, Zappella M, Hayek G, Meloni I, Vitelli F, Bruttini M, Cusano R, Loffredo P, Longo I, Renieri A. Preserved speech variant is allelic of classic Rett syndrome. Eur J Hum Genet 2000; 8:325–330.

88. Huppke P, Held M, Hanefeld F, Engel W, Laccone F. Influence of mutation type and location on phenotype in 123 patients with Rett syndrome. Neuropediatrics 2002; 33:63–68.

89. Hoffbuhr KC, Moses LM, Jerdonek MA, Naidu S, Hoffman EP. Associations between MeCP2 mutations, X-chromosome inactivation, and phenotype. Ment Retard Dev Disabil Res Rev 2002; 8:99–105.

90. Van den Veyver IB, Zoghbi HY. Genetic basis of Rett syndrome. Ment Retard Dev Disabil Res Rev 2002; 8:82–86.

91. Kerr AM, Nomura Y, Armstrong D, Anvret M, Belichenko PV, Budden S, Cass H, Christodoulou J, Clarke A, Ellaway C, d'Esposito M, Francke U, Hulten M, Julu P, Leonard H, Naidu S, Schanen C, Webb T, Engerstrom IW, Yamashita Y, Segawa M. Guidelines for reporting clinical features in cases with *MECP2* mutations. Brain Dev 2001; 23:208–211.

92. Trappe R, Laccone F, Cobilanschi J, Meins M, Huppke P, Hanefeld F, Engel W. *MECP2* mutations in sporadic cases of Rett syndrome are almost exclusively of paternal origin. Am J Hum Genet 2001; 68:1093–1101.

93. Girard M, Couvert P, Carrie A, Tardieu M, Chelly J, Beldjord C, Bienvenu T. Parental origin of de novo *MECP2* mutations in Rett syndrome. Eur J Hum Genet 2001; 9:231–236.

94. Clayton-Smith J, Watson P, Ramsden S, Black GC. Somatic mutation in *MECP2* as a non-fatal neurodevelopmental disorder in males. Lancet 2000; 356:830–832.

95. Topcu M, Akyerli C, Sayi A, Toruner GA, Kocoglu SR, Cimbis M, Ozcelik T. Somatic mosaicism for a *MECP2* mutation associated with classic Rett syndrome in a boy. Eur J Hum Genet 2002; 10:77–81.

96. Moog U, Smeets EE, van Roozendaal KE, Schoenmakers S, Herbergs J, Schoonbrood-Lenssen AM, Schrander-Stumpel CT. Neurodevelopmental disorders in males related to the gene causing Rett syndrome in females (*MECP2*). Eur J Paediatr Neurol 2003; 7:5–12.

97. Leonard H, Silberstein J, Falk R, Houwink-Manville I, Ellaway C, Raffaele LS, Engerstrom IW, Schanen C. Occurrence of Rett syndrome in boys. J Child Neurol 2001; 16:333–338.

98. Couvert P, Bienvenu T, Aquaviva C, Poirier K, Moraine C, Gendrot C, Verloes A, Andres C, Le Fevre AC, Souville I, Steffann J, des Portes V, Ropers HH, Yntema HG, Fryns JP, Briault S, Chelly J, Cherif B. *MECP2* is highly mutated in X-linked mental retardation. Hum Mol Genet 2001; 10: 941–946.

99.   Dotti MT, Orrico A, De Stefano N, Battisti C, Sicurelli F, Severi S, Lam CW, Galli L, Sorrentino V, Federico A. A Rett syndrome *MECP2* mutation that causes mental retardation in men. Neurology 2002; 58:226–230.

100. Orrico A, Lam C, Galli L, Dotti MT, Hayek G, Tong SF, Poon PM, Zappella M, Federico A, Sorrentino V. *MECP2* mutation in male patients with non-specific X-linked mental retardation. FEBS Lett 2000; 481:285–288.

101. Klauck SM, Lindsay S, Beyer KS, Splitt M, Burn J, Poustka A. A mutation hot spot for nonspecific X-linked mental retardation in the *MECP2* gene causes the PPM-X syndrome. Am J Hum Genet 2002; 70:1034–1037.

102. Meloni I, Bruttini M, Longo I, Mari F, Rizzolio F, D'Adamo P, Denvriendt K, Fryns JP, Toniolo D, Renieri A. A mutation in the Rett syndrome gene, *MECP2*, causes X-linked mental retardation and progressive spasticity in males. Am J Hum Genet 2000; 67:982–985.

103. Yntema HG, Kleefstra T, Oudakker AR, Romein T, de Vries BB, Nillesen W, Sistermans EA, Brunner HG, Hamel BC, van Bokhoven H. Low frequency of *MECP2* mutations in mentally retarded males. Eur J Hum Genet 2002; 10:487–490.

104. Guy J, Hendrich B, Holmes M, Martin JE, Bird A. A mouse Mecp2-null mutation causes neurological symptoms that mimic Rett syndrome. Nat Genet 2001; 27:322–326.

105. Chen RZ, Akbarian S, Tudor M, Jaenisch R. Deficiency of methyl-CpG binding protein-2 in CNS neurons results in a Rett-like phenotype in mice. Nat Genet 2001; 27:327–331.

106. Tudor M, Akbarian S, Chen RZ, Jaenisch R. Transcriptional profiling of a mouse model for Rett syndrome reveals subtle transcriptional changes in the brain. Proc Natl Acad Sci USA 2002; 99:15536–15541.

107. Shahbazian M, Young J, Yuva-Paylor L, Spencer C, Antalffy B, Noebels J, Armstrong D, Paylor R, Zoghbi H. Mice with truncated MeCP2 recapitulate many Rett syndrome features and display hyperacetylation of histone H3. Neuron 2002; 35: 243–254.

108. Hagberg B, Hanefeld F, Percy A, Skjeldal O. An update on clinically applicable diagnostic criteria in Rett syndrome. Comments to Rett Syndrome Clinical Criteria Consensus Panel Satellite to European Paediatric Neurology Society Meeting, Baden Baden, Germany, Sep 11, 2001. Eur J Paediatr Neurol 2002; 6:293–297.

109. Hagberg B, Witt-Engerström I. Rett syndrome: epidemiology and nosology—progress in knowledge 1986—a conference communication. Brain Dev 1987; 9:451–457.

110. Hoffbuhr K, Devaney JM, LaFleur B, Sirianni N, Scacheri C, Giron J, Schuette J, Innis J, Marino M, Philippart M, Narayanan V, Umansky R, Kronn D, Hoffman EP, Naidu S. MeCP2 mutations in children with and without the phenotype of Rett syndrome. Neurology 2001; 56:1486–1495.

111. Schwartzman JS, Bernardino A, Nishimura A, Gomes RR, Zatz M. Rett syndrome in a boy with a 47,XXY karyotype confirmed by a rare mutation in the *MECP2* gene. Neuropediatrics 2001; 32:162–164.

112. Imessaoudene B, Bonnefont JP, Royer G, Cormier-Daire V, Lyonnet S, Lyon G, Munnich A, Amiel J. *MECP2* mutation in non-fatal, non-progressive encephalopathy in a male. J Med Genet 2001; 38:171–174.

113. Yntema HG, Oudakker AR, Kleefstra T, Hamel BC, van Bokhoven H, Chelly J, Kalscheuer VM, Fryns JP, Raynaud M, Moizard MP, Moraine C. In-frame deletion in *MECP2* causes mild nonspecific mental retardation. Am J Med Genet 2002; 107: 81–83.

15

Microdeletion Syndromes

GOPALRAO V. N. VELAGALETI

Division of Genetics, Departments
of Pediatrics and Pathology, University
of Texas Medical Branch,
Galveston, Texas, U.S.A.

NANCY J. CARPENTER

Center for Genetic Testing,
Saint Francis Health Sysem, Tulsa,
Oklahoma, U.S.A.

I. INTRODUCTION

Chromosome rearrangements that result in interstitial or terminal deletions or unbalanced translocations lead to disturbances in gene dosage. The rearrangements may be relatively large, one to several million bases in length, and involve a large number of genes. Disorders in which loss of multiple genes at closely linked loci result in diverse phenotypic effects are known as microdeletion or contiguous gene syndromes.

The nine well-known clinical entities associated with developmental disabilities and physical anomalies reviewed in this chapter can be classified as microdeletion syndromes.

521

For some, such as Alagille syndrome and Rubinstein–Taybi syndrome (RTS), the loss of one gene may be the major factor in producing the disorder, but other genes deleted from the critical region may also play a role in some features of the phenotype. In others, such as cri du chat and Wolf–Hirschhorn syndromes, the abnormal phenotypes observed are considered to be due to the combined loss of many genes from a given region of the genome.

Studies of the natural history and the cognitive and behavioral aspects of some of these disorders have been published, but more studies are warranted, particularly of adolescent and adult patients. Recently, the application of new molecular technologies, such as fluorescence in situ hybridization (FISH), microsatellite analysis by PCR, and automated DNA sequencing, has resulted in the development of specific diagnostic assays. In addition, these techniques have made possible studies of the molecular extent of the deletions and genotype–phenotype correlations leading to more accurate prognostic information for families and physicians. Current molecular research is focusing on the identification of genes in the deleted regions and their function in determining the phenotype. Eventually, understanding mechanisms leading to chromosome rearrangements and the function of genes within critical regions of the genome may lead to new therapies.

II. ALAGILLE SYNDROME

Alagille syndrome (AGS) (OMIM #118450) (http://www.ncbi. nlm.nih.gov/omim/) was first described in 1969 (1) and to date more than 300 cases have been reported. Alagille syndrome (syndromic bile duct paucity or arteriohepatic dysplasia) is a clinically distinct syndrome with variable clinical expression. The prevalence is reported to be 1 in 100,000 live births (2). However, this might be an underestimate because it is based only on the number of children with hepatic manifestations.

A. Clinical Presentation

The clinical diagnosis of AGS is based on the criteria established by Alagille et al. (1,3). These criteria are: (i) the histologic finding of paucity of the interlobular bile ducts on liver biopsy, and (ii) at least three of these five major clinical features: chronic cholestasis, cardiac disease, skeletal abnormalities, ocular abnormalities, and characteristic facial features (Fig. 1). The clinical features associated with the syndrome can be classified into five major groups.

1. Hepatic Manifestations

Most symptomatic patients present in infancy with manifestations of hepatic disease ranging from mild cholestasis, jaundice, and pruritus to progressive liver failure and ultimately failure to thrive. Jaundice can present as conjugated hyperbilirubinemia in the neonatal period. Cholestasis manifests as pruritus, elevated serum bile acid concentrations, xanthomas, and growth failure. Progression to cirrhosis and liver failure occurs in the majority of patients, and ~15% of the patients require transplantation. Growth failure has been reported in 50–90% of patients (1–4).

2. Cardiac Manifestations

Approximately 90% of patients with AGS have congenital heart defects. Abnormalities of pulmonary valve or artery or its branches are most commonly involved, with peripheral pulmonary stenosis being the most common feature. Tetralogy of Fallot, seen in about 7–16% of the patients, is the most common complex malformation. Other cardiac defects include ventricular septal defects, atrial septal defects, aortic stenosis, and coarctation of the aorta. Most cardiac malformations are hemodynamically insignificant, but the severity of the malformation is directly proportional to the mortality (1–5).

3. Ophthalmologic Manifestations

Defects of the anterior chamber, such as posterior embryotoxon, Axenfeld anomaly, and Rieger anomaly, are the most common eye abnormalities (6). One of the important diagnostic features is the posterior embryotoxon (a prominent, centrally positioned Schwalbe ring). This feature is present in

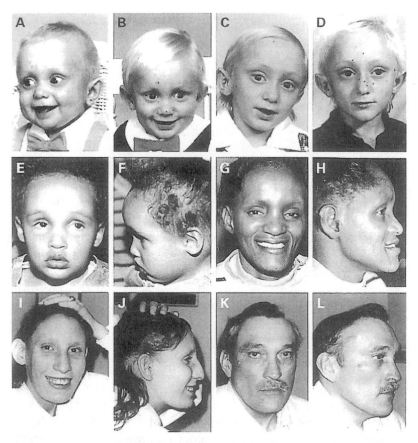

Figure 1   Characteristic facial features of AGS. Figures (A)–(D) show the same patient at 1, 2, 4, and 6 years, respectively. Note evolution of features with loss of baby fat, as well as excoriations secondary to severe pruritus as a result of cholestasis. Figures (E)–(H) show full face and profile views of an affected mother and daughter, whereas figures (I)–(L) depict a father and daughter with AGS. (Reprinted from Krantz et al. J Med Genet 1997; 34:152–157.)

89% of patients with AGS and can be seen on slit-lamp examination. In some children with AGS, ocular ultrasonographic examination showed optic disk drusen and this may aid in clinical diagnosis (7). Most patients have good visual prognosis, although mild decreases in acuity have been reported.

4. Skeletal Manifestations

Butterfly vertebrae resulting from clefting abnormalities of the vertebral body are characteristic for AGS. The frequency of such vertebral anomalies ranges from 22% to 87% (8). Other skeletal anomalies include narrowing of interpeduncular spaces in the lumbar spine, pointed anterior process of C1, spina bifida occulta, fusion of adjacent vertebrae, hemivertebrae, and bony connections between ribs and short fingers (9).

5. Facial Features

The characteristic facial features are prominent forehead, deep-set eyes with moderate hypertelorism, pointed chin, and saddle or straight nose with a bulbous tip. The combination of these features gives the face a triangular appearance (1,2).

Another major feature is pancreatic insufficiency (4) and recently, digital crease abnormalities have been reported (10). With more than 35% of patients displaying supernumerary flexion creases, this finding might aid in the diagnosis. Less commonly seen features of AGS include functional and structural renal abnormalities (23–74%), neurovascular accidents, significant mental retardation (10%), delayed puberty, high-pitched voice, and hearing loss (3,4).

B. Clinical Management

About 15–20% of patients with AGS die due to abnormalities of liver and/or heart. Congenital heart disease is the single greatest cause of neonatal mortality, whereas liver failure accounts for later morbidity and mortality. The overall outcome and prognosis are highly variable and are directly correlated with the severity of heart and liver anomalies (2,3). One of the most important clinical management issues is nutrition. All patients with AGS should be advised to consume a high-energy diet with an adequate protein intake to prevent malnutrition and growth failure. Fat intake needs to be monitored, as its tolerance varies with severity of cholestasis (11). To avoid deficiencies, every effort should be made to ensure that patients ingest at least 5% of their total energy intake in the form of essential fatty acids.

Malnutrition, growth failure, disfiguring xanthomatosis, and progressive portal fibrosis and cirrhosis are commonly seen in AGS patients with severe and prolonged cholestasis beyond 1 year of age. Liver transplantation must be considered for such patients.

C. Chromosomal and Molecular Basis

On the basis of several published reports showing cytogenetically visible deletions (Fig. 2) or translocations involving the short arm of chromosome 20, AGS was mapped to 20p12 (12). A cell surface protein that functions as a key signaling molecule called Jagged 1 (*JAG1*) was identified by two groups to be physically located within this region, commonly deleted on chromosome 20p. Mutations in *JAG1* were found in AGS patients in multiple families and thus confirming that *JAG1* is the AGS disease gene (13,14).

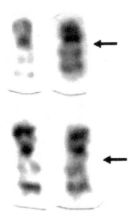

Figure 2 Partial karyotypes showing chromosome 20 deletion seen in AGS in a patient (top panel) and his mother (bottom panel). Arrow shows the deleted chromosome. (Courtesy of Dr. Nancy Spinner, Children's Hospital, Philadelphia, PA.)

JAG1 is a cell surface protein and functions as a ligand for the Notch transmembrane receptor, a key-signaling molecule found on the surface of a variety of cells. *JAG1* and Notch, both play a significant role in the highly conserved Notch signaling pathway. This pathway functions in many cell types during development and regulates the cell fate decisions. In a large series of AGS patients, *JAG1* mutations were found in about 70% (15). Of these, frameshift and nonsense mutations leading to protein truncation accounted for 49% of the patients, splicing and missense mutations accounting for 9% each, deletion of the entire *JAG1* gene accounting for 4%, while 31% of the patients had no detectable mutation. Two possible mechanisms, haploinsufficiency of *JAG1* and a dominant negative effect due to the mutations in *JAG 1*, are proposed as the cause of AGS. No phenotypic differences based on the type or location of the mutation have been seen.

D. Genetic Testing

The best method for diagnosis of AGS is the clinical examination and histological confirmation of a paucity of interlobular bile ducts (11). Chromosome analysis and/or FISH may detect 7% of the AGS patients by showing a visible deletion on chromosome 20p (Fig. 2). Direct mutation analysis of *JAG1* will detect more than 70% of patients. In a recent study of 300 patients with AGS, the spectrum of mutations in AGS patients was broad with the majority (72%) being frame shift mutations and a few (3–7%) with complete gene deletions (15). The majority of the mutations are de novo in origin. The mutations appear to cluster at the 5' end of the gene that is highly conserved, and the spectrum of mutations identified is consistent with haploinsufficiency for *JAG1* being the mechanism for AGS (15). Approximately 30% of the AGS patients tested showed no identifiable mutations in the *JAG1* gene. Thus, other genes or loci might be involved in the pathogenesis of AGS. There is at least one case of prenatal diagnosis of AGS in a fetus with severe pulmonary stenosis and progressively severe intrauterine growth retardation, whose mother was also affected (16).

E. Genetic Counseling

Since the first description of AGS, its familial nature has been well recognized. On the basis of the published reports, it is clear that AGS follows an autosomal dominant inheritance pattern with reduced penetrance and variable expressivity (17). In theory, the risk for recurrence is 50%, but one must take into account the reduced penetrance and variable expressivity. It should also be stressed that phenotypically normal individuals may carry the mutant gene and can transmit it to their offspring.

F. Resources

Information can be obtained online through computer searches of key words or syndrome names. Parent or family support groups are also available for most syndromes or disorders. The following is a list of organizations or support groups where pertinent information about this syndrome can be found:

Alagille Syndrome Alliance.
American Liver Foundation: www.liverfoundation.org.

III. CRI DU CHAT SYNDROME

The name of the syndrome, cri du chat (OMIM #123450), is derived from the first description in 1963 by Lejeune et al. (18) of patients with a characteristic cry resembling the mewing of a cat. The incidence of the syndrome is estimated to be 1 in 50,000 with slightly fewer males than females (19,20).

A. Clinical Presentation

Infants with this condition have low birth weight and often fail to thrive due to sucking problems and gastroesophageal reflux. The distinctive cry is high pitched and thought to be due to a small, hypoplastic larynx. There is microcephaly and a round face with hypertelorism, epicanthal folds, and a

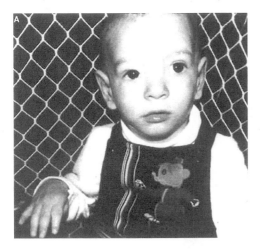

Figure 3 A young child with cri du chat syndrome. Note the round face, hypertelorism, broad nasal bridge, and down-slanting palpebral fissures. (From Ref. 21.)

broad nasal bridge (Fig. 3). Often the philtrum is short and the eyes have down-slanting palpebral fissures. The ears are low set and there may be preauricular skin tags. Hypotonia and strabismus are common. Various types of heart disease including atrial septal defects, ventricular septal defects, tetralogy of Fallot, and persistent ductus Botalli are found in approximately one-third of the patients (19,20).

With increasing age, the phenotype changes and becomes less distinctive (21). The cry disappears during the first two years. The face lengthens and the eyes may become deep set. The hypertelorism and epicanthal folds disappear and the palpebral fissures are normally placed (Fig. 4). In adult patients, the mouth is large with a high-arched palate and there is severe dental malocclusion and decay. They may have a wide-based or ataxic-like gait. Sometimes hypertonia replaces the hypotonia seen in childhood. Premature graying of the hair and scoliosis are commonly seen in adults. A CT scan of the brain in one adult with this syndrome showed dilatation of the lateral ventricles and widened basal cisternae (21). Additional studies of malformations of the

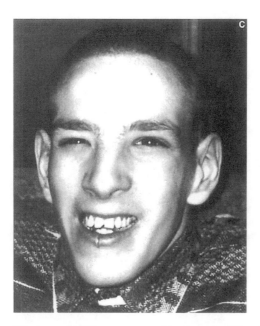

Figure 4 The same patient as in Fig. 3 at 16 years of age. Note the changes in the facial features with the long face and wide mouth and the absence of hypertelorism and a broad nasal bridge. (From Ref. 21.)

cranial base in patients with this syndrome suggested the presence of a developmental field between the brainstem and the laryngeal region (22).

Early development is significantly delayed with head control being achieved at about 1 year, sitting at 2 years, and walking at 4 years. Poor growth persists throughout childhood due to feeding difficulties and constitutional factors. This results in a slender shape particularly in males and in short stature with microcephaly in adulthood. Growth charts specific for this syndrome have been compiled to assist in monitoring growth in affected individuals and for evaluating the impact of treatment (23).

About 10% of the patients die during the first year of life due to respiratory problems or heart defects (19). Many patients live well into adulthood, although the mortality curve probably increases after the age of 35.

Early descriptions indicated that patients with cri du chat syndrome had profound mental retardation, very limited communicative abilities, and slow psychomotor development. However, a study by Wilkins et al. (20) showed a broader array of abilities in 80 home-reared children with cri du chat syndrome. In a more recent study of cognitive functioning and language skills, Cornish et al. (24) found that, while cognitive abilities as measured on the WISC-III consistently showed low performance, patients had better receptive than expressive skills. Many were able to communicate their needs using nonverbal methods or formal signs. In terms of motor skills, most children (> 90%) had unimpaired gross hand movements such as waving, whereas fewer children (65%) were competent in fine motor skills such as holding a pencil (25). Behavioral characteristics included hypersensitivity to sensory stimuli, repetitive movements, clumsiness, and self-injurious behavior. A low incidence of hyperactivity was reported by Cornish and Pigram (25), whereas Wilkins et al. (26) found hyperactivity to be a major problem in their patients.

B. Clinical Management

Recommendations for clinical management of patients with cri du chat syndrome have been published (27). Growth parameters should be closely monitored. Some children may require gastrostomy because of feeding difficulties and poor nutrition. Echocardiograms are warranted to detect congenital heart defects. Most defects can be repaired, but these children may have problems with anesthesia due to their hypoplastic larynx and respiratory abnormalities. Patients with this condition are also prone to recurrent upper respiratory infections and otitis media that require treatment. Early assessment of developmental delays should include evaluation of cognitive abilities, gross and fine motor skills, and speech and language. Developmental disabilities should be addressed through early intervention programs. Psychological evaluation and early treatment of behavior problems including sleep disorders and hyperactivity are recommended. Because of the limited communicative abilities of children with cri du chat syndrome, it has been suggested that interventions emphasizing nonverbal commands may help reduce behavior problems.

C. Chromosomal and Molecular Basis

Cri du chat syndrome is caused by a deletion of the short arm of chromosome 5 (del 5p). The majority of cases are due to terminal deletions or interstitial deletions, but unbalanced translocations with partial loss (monosomy) of 5p and partial gain (trisomy) of another chromosome may also occur. The deletions are usually de novo, although a few familial cases have been described. Unbalanced translocations result from segregation of a balanced translocation in one of the parents and passed to the child. Mosaicism for the deletion has been reported in several affected patients and in one unaffected parent (28).

Breakpoints occur throughout the short arm of chromosome 5, and therefore the deletions vary in size and location from patient to patient. Studies using FISH and polymorphic DNA markers have been helpful in determining the size of the deletion and the parent of origin of the deleted chromosome for investigation of genotype–phenotype correlations (29–31). Several studies have showed that in 80–90% of the cases, the paternal chromosome was deleted (32).

Deletion of the 5p15.2 region is necessary for the cri du chat phenotype (the Cdc critical region) except for the cat-cry which is located in the proximal part of the 5p15.3 band (30). Church et al. (33) also proposed a region for speech delay to be in the distal part of 5p15.3 and distinct regions for childhood and adult facial features to be located in 5p15.2. Deletions of other regions of 5p result in mild to severe MR but are not associated with the typical cri du chat phenotype. Three members of one family with a deletion of part of 5p14 were reported to have a normal phenotype, whereas deletion of this region was also reported in a normal father and his son with microcephaly and developmental delay (34,35). In addition, a study by Marinescu et al. (36) showed that there was no correlation between the size of the deletion and the level of developmental delay.

A few genes of interest have been localized to chromosome 5p. Two genes that have been mapped to the cri du chat region and could possibly play a role in cognition are the semaphorin F gene that has a role in neuronal migration during development and the δ-catenin gene (*CTNND2*) that codes a neuronal-specific protein involved in cell motility (37,38). The telomerase reverse transcriptase (*hTERT*) gene that is located at 5p15.33 was also shown to be insufficient for maintaining telomere length in cri du chat patients and may contribute to the phenotype (39).

D. Genetic Testing

Although cri du chat syndrome may be suspected from clinical features, conventional chromosome analysis is used for diagnosis in the majority of patients. Some patients have very small deletions or translocations that are recognized by FISH analysis, and a few patients have been identified by use of a subtelomeric FISH probe. Subtelomeric FISH probes are useful in determining whether a deletion is interstitial or terminal. It is important to test the parents of an affected child to determine if the deletion is caused by an inherited deletion or translocation. Prenatal diagnosis by conventional cytogenetic analysis and FISH analysis is available for familial cases.

E. Genetic Counseling

In the case of de novo deletions, the recurrence risk is negligible (<0.5%). However, if the parent is a carrier of a deletion, the risk may be as high as 50%. If the parent is a carrier of a balanced translocation, the risk is about 10–15% (40). Individuals with cri du chat syndrome are fertile and have produced affected offspring (41). It is important to note that not all patients with deletions of 5p have typical cri du chat syndrome and that the phenotype may vary greatly depending on the region of the chromosome deleted. Clinical evaluation combined with molecular analysis may someday provide a more individualized prognosis for patients. However, studies with polymorphic DNA markers are available for research purposes only.

F. Resources

Information can be obtained through computer searches of key words or syndrome names. Parent or family support groups are also available for most syndromes or disorders. The following is a list of organizations or support groups where pertinent information about this syndrome can be found:

5p- Society: A national support group for families with members with cri du chat syndrome. The group sponsors an annual national conference (www.fivepminus.org).

IV. DELETION 1p36 SYNDROME

Deletion chromosome 1p36 syndrome is a newly recognized syndrome characterized by specific craniofacial features, growth retardation and microcephaly, and severe mental retardation (42–44). This disorder is one of the most common deletion syndromes with an estimated prevalence of 1 in 5000 (45).

A. Clinical Presentation

The craniofacial features include a large anterior fontanel, midface hypoplasia, flat nasal bridge, small nose, deep-set eyes, pointed chin, and low-set or asymmetric ears (Fig. 5). Other features are cleft lip and/or palate, clinodactyly, visual impairment, sensorineural hearing loss, hypotonia, seizures, and precocious puberty. Structural heart defects, most commonly patent ductus arteriosus, and infantile cardiomyopathy have been reported. Some patients have hypothyroidism. The majority of patients have significant growth retardation, and microcephaly occurs in about 60% (44). However, a few individuals developed obesity in childhood after having poor weight gain in infancy.

Development is invariably delayed, and the vast majority of patients have severe mental retardation. Speech is also severely affected. However, three patients with the smallest deletions have complex speech abilities and mild mental retardation. Formal studies of cognitive abilities in older children

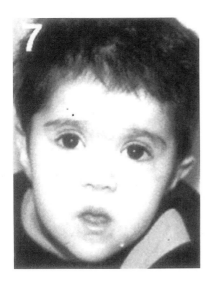

Figure 5 A young child with the facial features of the deletion 1p36 syndrome including large anterior fontanelle, flat nasal bridge, and pointed chin. (From Ref. 42.)

and adults have not been performed. Behavior abnormalities include temper tantrums, throwing objects, and self-injurious and autistic behaviors (43).

There is reported mortality in infancy; three of 39 patients reviewed by Slavotinek et al. (43) died between 2 days and 2 months of age. However, most patients live into adulthood with the oldest patient reported at 47 years of age (43).

B. Clinical Management

On the basis of clinical findings, Heilstedt et al. (44) suggested selected evaluations for patients diagnosed with a deletion of chromosome 1p36. Audiometric evaluation that includes testing at high frequencies should be done. Hearing impairment is very common (82%), and many patients have sensorineural hearing loss at high frequencies that would be missed with more basic testing procedures. Echocardiograms, ophthalmologic evaluations, and thyroid function tests are warranted because of structural heart defects (43%), visual problems (83%), and hypothyroidism (20%) (44). The palate should be evaluated, because 17% of patients have palatal abnormalities that affect feeding, as well as speech development. Patients should also be monitored for seizure activity, as 48% may have seizures.

C. Chromosome and Molecular Basis

The p36 band at the terminus of chromosome 1 is G-negative and lightly stained, therefore difficult to visualize. The first cases reported had visible abnormalities due to unbalanced translocations. Patients have been identified through high-resolution chromosome analysis (42). However, the introduction of FISH analysis has improved the detection of this deletion. Fluorescence in situ hybridization probes specifically for 1p36 have been used to confirm the diagnosis in patients suspected of having the deletion because of their craniofacial features (46). Other patients have been identified by screening patients with mental retardation for subtelomeric deletions using FISH or molecular marker analysis (47,48).

In a recent study of 61 patients, the disorder was caused by de novo terminal deletions in 72%, interstitial deletions in 7%, and de novo and familial unbalanced rearrangements in 17% (44). The deletion sizes were determined by analysis using microsatellite markers and FISH (44,49). The deletions vary in size from 1.5 to >10.5 Mb, and breakpoints occur throughout the 1p36 band rather than occurring at a single site. About 60% of the de novo terminal deletions are on the maternal chromosome (44). In general, the more severely affected individuals have larger deletions. Critical regions for certain clinical findings such as clefting, hypothyroidism, cardiomyopathy, hearing loss, large fontanel, and hypotonia have been proposed (44).

More than 90 genes are thought to be located in the 1p36 band including several putative tumor suppressor genes. The *SKI* proto-oncogene is deleted in individuals with this syndrome and may contribute to the phenotype, particularly facial clefting (50).

D. Genetic Testing

The deletion of 1p36 is difficult to detect and requires high-resolution chromosome analysis at the 650–850 band level. For individuals suspected of having this deletion, FISH analysis with probes in the subtelomeric region of 1p should be performed. However, approximately 7–10% of the cases have interstitial deletions that would be interpreted as normal if only subtelomeric FISH analysis was done. In about 5% of cases, the loss of 1p36 has been found to be due to segregation of a balanced translocation in a parent (44). Because an unbalanced translocation may also be difficult to detect, chromosome and FISH analysis should be performed on all parents of 1p36 deletion patients.

E. Genetic Counseling

In the case of de novo deletions, the recurrence risk is negligible (<0.5%). However, if the parent is a carrier of a balanced translocation, the risk is about 10–15% (40). It is not known if individuals with the deletion 1p36 syndrome are fertile, as no offspring of affected individuals have been reported to date.

F. Resources

No syndrome-specific resources are available for the deletion 1p36 syndrome. However, there are general resources for chromosome abnormalities. Information about the disorder can be obtained by searching databases online through your computer service network and from the following sources:

Unique: The largest source of information, mutual support, and self-help to families with children with any rare chromosome disorder.

Contact a Family (CaF): Based in London, CaF has information on over 1000 rare syndromes and can put families in touch with each other.

Family Village: A global community of disability-related resources.

Chromosome deletion outreach: An international support group for families with chromosome abnormalities in U.S.A.

Med Help International: An organization helping patients find the highest quality medical information.

V. JACOBSEN SYNDROME

Jacobsen syndrome (OMIM #147791), also referred to as deletion 11q syndrome, was first described in 1973 (51), and to date more than 75 cases have been reported (52). Jacobsen syndrome is a rare, yet clinically recognizable entity with a broad spectrum of phenotypic variability. The prevalence is estimated to be < 1 in 100,000 live births (53). The proportion of males to females is 1–2. In order to explain the preponderance of female patients with Jacobsen syndrome, it has been proposed that the expression of 11q terminal deletion is some how determined by the sex chromosome complement, which contributes to a differential survival depending on the sex of the patient (54).

A. Clinical Presentation

Jacobsen syndrome is characterized by intrauterine growth retardation, failure to thrive, and severe to moderate mental retardation. Hypotonia, which is seen in the neonatal period, leads to spasticity later on. The most consistent phenotypic features are trigonocephaly, microcephaly, and facial dysmorphism, including telecanthus, down-slanting palpebral fissures, epicanthal folds, ocular hypertelorism, ptosis, strabismus, depressed nasal bridge, large carp-shaped mouth, micrognathia, and ear abnormalities (Fig. 6). More than half of the patients present with cardiac abnormalities such as a single ventricle or hypoplasia of the left ventricle with or without stenosis or atresia of the aortic and mitral valve. Joint contractures appear to be common and about half of the patients also have genital abnormalities such as hypospadias and/or cryptorchidism.

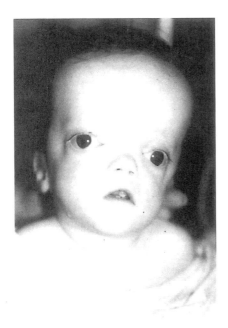

Figure 6 A 11-month-old girl with Jacobsen syndrome. Note the characteristic features of ocular hypertelorism, telecanthus, downward slanting palpebral fissure, colobomas, and short nose. (From Ref. 52.)

Patients with distal 11q deletions have been reported with an unusual thrombocytopenia with platelet inclusion bodies, dysmegakaryopoiesis, mild congenital anomalies, and mental retardation termed "Paris–Trousseau syndrome" (55). Upon electron microscopic examination, the platelet inclusion bodies were found to be giant α granules. Recent reports suggest that Paris–Trousseau syndrome is a variant of the Jacobsen syndrome, and the thrombocytopenia observed in all cases of chromosome 11q23.3 deletion is due to dysmegakaryopoieses (56).

There are several reports of occasional abnormalities including macrocephaly, hydrocephalus, holoprosencephaly, ocular coloboma, abnormality of supratentorial white matter on CT scan, short neck, digital anomalies, pyloric stenosis, inguinal hernias, renal malformations such as hydronephrosis, cystic kidneys, horse shoe-shaped kidneys, duplication of kidneys, and hypoplasia of labia and clitoris. Other abnormalities reported are supernumerary nipples, absent ribs, and clubfeet.

B. Clinical Management

About one-fourth of the patients die within the first days of life due to cardiac and respiratory failure. The oldest surviving subject is 25 years old (57). The rare individuals that do not have major cardiac and respiratory anomalies may have normal life spans. Almost all patients with Jacobsen syndrome have mental retardation ranging from moderate to severe.

C. Chromosomal and Molecular Basis

Jacobsen syndrome is caused by a deletion on the long arm of chromosome 11 extending from q23 to the terminus. More than 85% of the deletions are terminal in nature, whereas the remainder are interstitial deletions. The majority of the deletions are de novo in origin, with a few cases resulting from familial balanced translocations and ring chromosomes (52). Fryns et al. (58) suggested that the deletion of sub-band 11q24.1 is crucial for the full expression of the phenotype. Unlike some of the other microdeletion syndromes, no parent-of-origin effect has been shown for the deleted chromosome 11 in Jacobsen syndrome. Interestingly, deletion break points that are proximal seem to have a bias towards the maternally derived chromosome 11, whereas those that are distal are often paternally derived (53). However, there appears to be no clinical significance as yet associated with this bias. Recent studies have shown that the break points in Jacobsen syndrome patients cluster within CCG-trinucleotide repeats, thus indicating a common mechanism for the chromosome breakage in this region of chromosome 11, leading to Jacobsen syndrome (59).

No genes directly responsible for the Jacobsen phenotype have yet been identified or cloned, but several genes localized to the distal 11q23 to qter region are postulated to play a role. The genes *ETS1* and *NFRKB* encode proteins that interact with several genes in hematopoietic cells and thus might play a role in thrombocytopenia seen in several Jacobsen syndrome patients. Similarly, the *FLI1* gene, localized distal to *ETS1*, is expressed in hematopoietic cells. The *THY1* gene, localized to distal 11q23.3, encodes a T-cell surface glycoprotein that is shown to stimulate neuronal growth and development (53). The recently cloned *BARX2* homeobox protein gene, localized to 11q25 region, has been suggested as a candidate, as its murine homolog, *barx2*, has been reported to be expressed in neural and craniofacial development (60,61).

D. Genetic Testing

Genetic testing for Jacobsen syndrome is carried out by conventional chromosome analysis. The deletion causing this syndrome, even when it is interstitial, is very large and thus can be detected with routine chromosome analysis (Fig. 7). There are no reports of patients with Jacobsen syndrome phenotype without a visible chromosome deletion. However, FISH studies with locus-specific DNA probes might help detect submicroscopic deletions (Fig. 8). As yet, no DNA probes are available from commercial sources to be used in the cytogenetic laboratories.

Prenatal diagnosis of Jacobsen syndrome is possible. Wax et al. (62) demonstrated that some of the hallmarks of Jacobsen syndrome, such as trigonocephaly, hydronephrosis, dysmorphic features such as hypertelorism, micrognathia, and prominent anteverted nares, and unusually short femurs were apparent on ultrasound examination at 29 weeks gestation in a fetus with 11q monosomy.

E. Genetic Counseling

Because the majority of the deletions are de novo in origin, the risk for recurrence is often negligible ($<0.5\%$). In those cases where the deletion is the result of a balanced translocation found in the parents, the recurrence risk is the same as

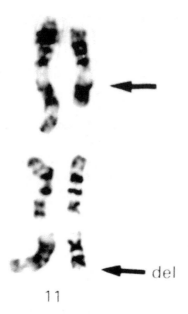

11

Figure 7 Partial karyotypes showing chromosome 11 deletion seen in Jacobsen syndrome. Arrows show the deleted chromosome. (From Ref. 52.)

for other translocation carriers (about 10–15%) (40). There is no documentation of fertility in affected persons.

F. Resources

Information can be obtained through computer searches of key words or syndrome names. Parent or family support groups are also available for most syndromes or disorders. The following is a list of organizations or support groups where pertinent information about this syndrome can be found:

> Jacobsen syndrome (www.11q.net).
> **The European Chromosome 11q Network:** Support for families of children with any chromosome 11q-related disorder.
> **11q Canada:** Database of Canadian families who have children with 11q deletion.

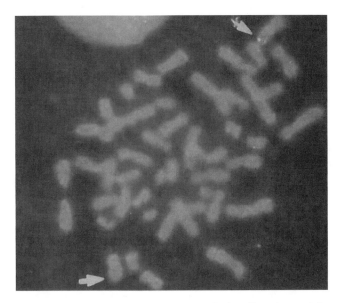

Figure 8 Fluorescence in situ hybridization with a locus-specific probe showing a submicroscopic deletion in a patient with Jacobsen syndrome. The shorter deleted chromosome is marked by an arrow (bottom) and the normal chromosome by an arrowhead (top). (From Ref. 52.) (*See color insert.*)

VI. LANGER–GIEDION SYNDROME

Langer–Giedion syndrome (LGS) (OMIM #150230) is also known as trichorhinophalangeal syndrome, type 2. In 1974, Hall et al. (63) outlined the diagnostic criteria, and Langer et al. (64) more fully delineated the phenotype in a review of 36 cases in 1984.

A. Clinical Presentation

Minimal diagnostic criteria for LGS include a typical facial appearance and two specific skeletal abnormalities—cone-shaped epiphyses and multiple cartilaginous exostoses. The typical craniofacial features include sparse scalp hair, bushy eyebrows, bulbous nose, long philtrum, long upper lip with thin upper vermillion border, and prominent ears (Fig. 9).

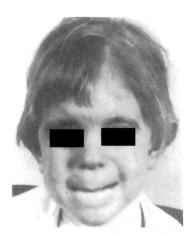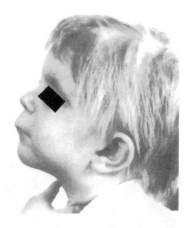

Figure 9 A 3-½-year-old child with Langer–Giedion syndrome. The child has sparse hair, a bulbous nose, and long upper lip. (From Ref. 64.)

Malocclusion and dental abnormalities are common. There is marked laxity of the skin in infancy and early childhood, which diminishes with age. Cone-shaped epiphyses, particularly in the hands, are noted in radiographs in early childhood (Fig. 10). Multiple cartilaginous exostoses (bony growths from the surfaces of various bones) first develop between 1 and 5 years of age. They can occur on the ribs, flat bones, tubular bones, and the vertebrae. Other frequent abnormalities include hyperextensible joints, winged scapulae, pes planus and/or other foot deformities, scoliosis, narrow posterior ribs, and abnormal or brittle nails. Heart defects and bilateral tibial hemimelia have been reported in a few patients (65). Birth weights and lengths are in the range of 15–20% of normal, and the head circumference at birth is also normal (64). Feeding difficulties occur in infancy. Slow postnatal growth results in short stature in all patients, and microcephaly is seen in 85% of the patients (64).

In terms of cognitive development, about 75% are intellectually impaired (64). The levels of mental retardation range from mild to severe or profound. Conductive and neurosensory hearing loss have also been reported. At least half of the patients have severe speech delay (64). Patients may have

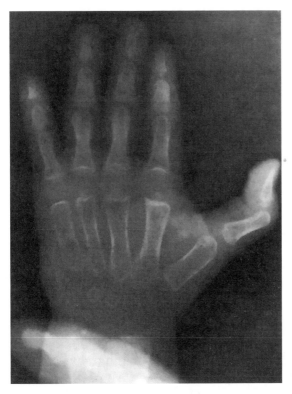

Figure 10 Radiograph of the hand of the patient in Fig. 9. Note the cone-shaped epiphyses in the middle phalanges 2–5 and the proximal phalanx of the thumb. (From Ref. 64.)

significant psychological problems due to their unusual facial appearance and short stature. Manipulative, disruptive, and oppositional behaviors have been reported in some patients (64).

Langer–Giedion syndrome can be distinguished from two other disorders with similar features. Trichorhinophalangeal syndrome, type 1 (TRPS1) is associated with similar facial features and cone-shaped epiphyses but with no cartilaginous exostoses. These patients are usually not mentally retarded. On the other hand, patients with the hereditary multiple exostoses (HME) syndrome have exostoses but not the other features seen in TRPS1 and LGS.

B. Clinical Management

Early assessment of speech and appropriate treatment of speech and language delays should be performed. Hearing evaluations and early intervention in individuals with hearing loss are also necessary. Growth parameters should be monitored. Plastic surgery may be considered for the facial abnormalities such as the nasal deformity, prominent ears, and fatty infiltration of the upper lip. Dislocation or subluxation of the hips may be managed by nonsurgical or surgical treatment. Surgical removal of the exostoses may be necessary if they are deforming, impinge on nerves or blood vessels, or interfere with joint function. Early assessment of developmental delays and intellectual impairment and early intervention are appropriate to achieve an optimal cognitive outcome. Psychological evaluation and treatment may be necessary for some patients who experience difficulties due to abnormal facial appearance, learning disabilities, and short stature.

C. Chromosomal and Molecular Basis

Most subjects with LGS are sporadic, although a few familial cases showing an autosomal dominant pattern of inheritance have been reported (66,67). Langer–Giedion syndrome is associated with deletions of the long arm of chromosome 8 which are usually visible by conventional cytogenetic analysis. Early reports of patients included those with terminal and interstitial deletions involving the 8q22–q24 region (68). In 1984, Buhler and Malik (69) reported the shortest region of overlap of the deletions as part of band q24.1. This finding was subsequently confirmed by reports of other patients with small interstitial deletions (70,71). Deletion maps were subsequently constructed for the 8q23–q24 region using polymorphic DNA markers (72,73). A study by Ludecke et al. (74) of chromosome abnormalities in TRPS1 patients using YAC cloning, Southern blotting, PCR analysis, and FISH analysis demonstrated that the *TRPS1* gene was located about 1000 kb from a gene for HME. Because patients with LGS have deletions encompassing both genes, LGS is a true contiguous gene syndrome and is not due to the pleiotropic effects of a single gene. Subsequently, the genes *EXT1* and *TRPS1* were cloned (75,76), and mutations in these genes were reported in patients with HME and TRPS1 (77).

D. Genetic Testing

Fluorescence in situ hybridization analysis using two probes for the *TRPS1* and *EXT1* genes is available for detection of the deletion in patients suspected of having LGS.

E. Genetic Counseling

Most subjects with LGS are due to de novo deletions. Because the parents are not affected, the risk of recurrence is low (<0.1%). However, in familial cases, the risk to inherit the deletion and to be affected is 50%.

F. Resources

Information can be obtained online through computer searches of key words or syndrome names. Parent or family support groups are also available for most syndromes or disorders. The following is a list of organizations or support groups where pertinent information about this syndrome can be found:

Langer–Giedion Syndrome, University of Houston: Information and resources for clinicians and families (http://wimp. nsm.uh.edu/LGS.html).

Langer–Giedion Syndrome Association: A family support group (http://lgsa.net).

VII. MILLER–DIEKER SYNDROME

Miller–Dieker syndrome (MDS) (OMIM #247200), originally thought to be an autosomal recessive condition, was first described by Miller (78) and later by Dieker et al. (79). The name "Miller–Dieker" syndrome was coined by Jones et al. (80) to distinguish this syndrome from other related brain malformation syndromes. The prevalence of MDS is estimated to be 1 in 50,000, whereas the incidence of lissencephaly, one of the major characteristics of MDS, is estimated to be 1 in 13,000 to 1 in 20,000 (81).

A. Clinical Presentation

Miller–Dieker syndrome is characterized by type I lissence-phaly (agyria with thick cortex and normal cerebellum), characteristic facial anomalies (Fig. 11), severe developmental delay, and seizures (82). In patients with MDS, the most characteristic finding on computerized tomography is complete failure of opercularization of the frontal and temporal lobes leading to bitemporal hollowing (83). The brain malformation results from arrest of neuronal migration at about 10–14 weeks of embryonic development. Some of the brain malformations include absent or hypoplastic corpus callosum (74% of the patients), large cavum septi pellucidi (77%), small midline calcifications in the region of the third ventricle (45%), whereas the brain stem and cerebellum appear grossly normal. Infants with MDS are present with hypotonia, opisthotonos, spasticity, and failure to thrive. The facial anomalies include a high, prominent, and wrinkled forehead, bitemporal hollowing, short and pointed nose with anteverted nares, long upper lip with thin upper vermilion border, and micrognathia. In some cases, congenital heart disease, clino-dactyly, camptodactyly, cryptorchidism, and sacral dimple may be present. Some of the occasional abnormalities also include intrauterine growth retardation, decreased fetal activity, omphalocele, pelvic kidneys, cystic dysplasia of kidney, and lipomen-ingocele with tethered cord, sacral tail, cleft palate, and cataracts (84).

B. Clinical Management

The prognosis for patients with MDS is generally poor. All patients with this syndrome are severely retarded and have no speech. Affected patients may walk by 3–5 years of age, but spastic diplegia with spastic gait is evident. Death usually occurs before 2 years of age and often within the first 3 months. Infants may require gastrostomy because of poor

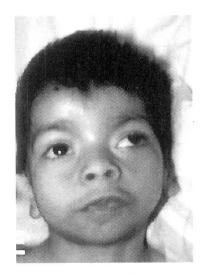

Figure 11 Characteristic features of MDS. Notice the small jaw, microcephaly, tall square forehead, vertical forehead furrow, flattened midface, short upturned nose, frontal bossing, low-set posteriorly rotated ears, and diffuse agyria. (From Ref. 87.)

feeding and poor nutrition. Antiepileptic treatment often is not effective for seizure control.

C. Chromosomal and Molecular Basis

Miller–Dieker syndrome is a contiguous gene disorder caused by haploinsufficiency of genes having a major role in the development of brain and face. In 1983, the first case of chromosome 17 deletion [del(17)(p13)] was reported in a patient with MDS (83). Subsequently, several reports narrowed the chromosomal region responsible for MDS to 17p13.3 (81,85). Recent studies with different DNA probes showed that at least 90% of patients with MDS and 38% of patients with isolated lissencephaly (ILS) have a microdeletion of a 350 kb region of chromosome 17p13.3, and a gene, termed *LIS1* (lissencephaly 1), was mapped to this critical region (81,82,86). Lissencephaly is a heterogeneous disorder that can result from nongenetic causes such as intrauterine infection with cytomegalovirus or rubella and poor perfusion, as well as from genetic causes such as chromosome abnormalities. Lissencephaly type I, characterized by agyria with thick cortex and normal cerebellum, is the hallmark of two distinct genetic conditions, namely, MDS and ILS. Unlike its appearance in MDS, lissencephaly in a related condition, ILS, appears with no other dysmorphic features. Apparent nonoverlapping deletions of *LIS1* in both MDS and ILS patients suggested that *LIS1* is responsible for both these disorders (86). However, deletions in MDS patients always extended more distally than those in the deleted ILS patients, thus suggesting that additional genes telomeric to *LIS1* are involved in MDS. Recent studies concluded that MDS is truly a contiguous gene deletion syndrome caused by haploinsufficiency of at least eight critical genes, *PRP8, RILP, SREC, PITPNα, SKIP, MYO1C, 14-3-3ε,* and *LIS1,* that contribute to the facial and brain phenotype (87).

D. Genetic Testing

About 90% of patients with MDS have either a visible deletion or a submicroscopic deletion of 17p13.3. This can be demonstrated by high-resolution chromosome analysis in about 50% of the patients, by DNA polymorphisms in 70%, or by FISH in 90% (Fig. 12). In the remaining 10% of the patients, no deletion has been detected with the current methods (88,89).

Prenatal diagnosis of MDS is possible using all the methods mentioned earlier. However, some of the fetal ultrasound findings such as mild ventriculomegaly, polyhydramnios, intrauterine growth retardation, and cardiac abnormalities are nonspecific, and routine chromosome analysis might not detect the smaller deletions of chromosome 17p13.3. Some reports suggest that whenever kidney anomalies, dilated occipital horns, and polyhydramnios are observed during prenatal ultrasound, a possible diagnosis of MDS should be considered and prenatal chromosome studies should include FISH analysis (90).

E. Genetic Counseling

The majority of cases with MDS have de novo deletions with a low risk of recurrence (< 0.5%). However, there have been a

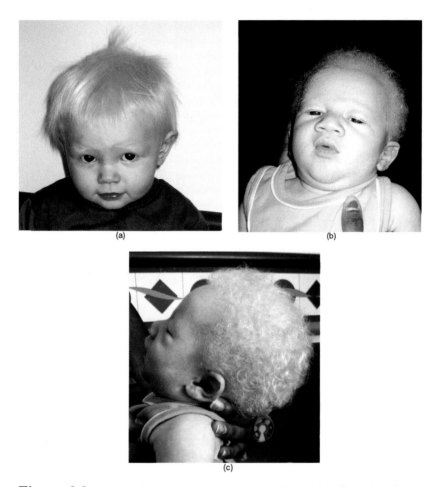

Figure 2.8 Two infants, ages 9 and 2 months, each affected with an autosomal recessive form of oculocutaneous albinism and from different ethnic backgrounds.

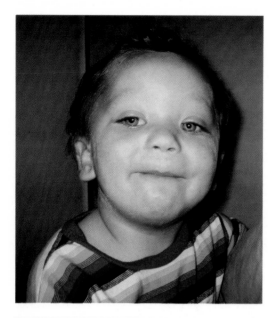

Figure 2.15 Two-year-old white male with developmental and speech delay due to fragile X syndrome. Note pale blue eyes, flattened nasal bridge, and prominent appearing ears.

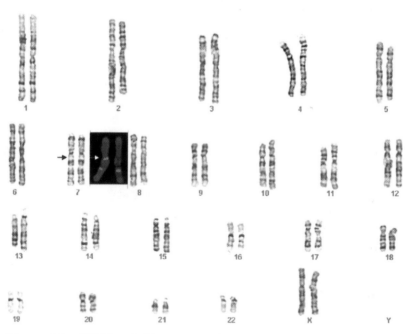

Figure 3.3 GTG-banded karyotype of a cell from a female with Williams syndrome (WS). An interstitial deletion of one chromosome 7q11.23 is evident by FISH (colored inset) where the WS critical region DNA probe (red color, white arrow) is absent. The chromosome 7s appear normal by GTG banding. Chromosome 7q11.23 is indicated by arrows.

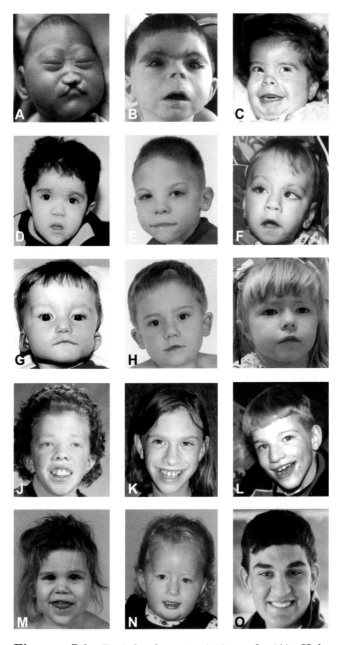

Figure 5.1 Facial characteristics of: (A) Holoprosencephaly.
(B) Cornelia de Lange syndrome. (C) Miller–Dieker syndrome.
(D) Chromosome 1p36 deletion syndrome. (E) Smith–Lemli–Opitz
syndrome. (F) Kabuki syndrome. (G) CHARGE association. (H)
Smith–Magenis syndrome. (I) Chromosome 22q11 deletion syndrome.
(J) Noonan syndrome. (K) Williams–Beuren syndrome. (L) Angelman
syndrome. (M) Beckwith–Wiedemann syndrome. (N) Prader–Willi
syndrome. (O) Fragile X syndrome. (See p. 137 for full legend.)

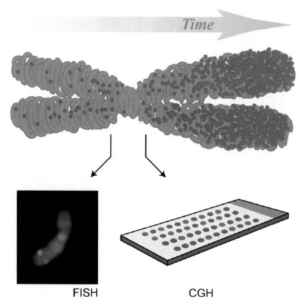

Figure 5.2 Bacterial artificial chromosomes (BACs) mapped to a human chromosome. (See p. 141 for full legend.)

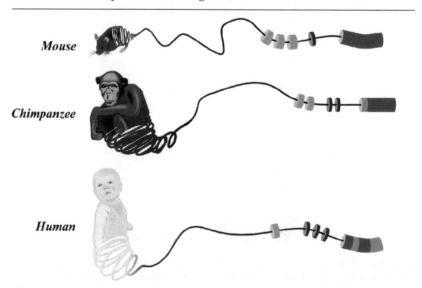

Figure 5.3 Comparative genomics. Comparison of mouse and chimpanzee genomes with human genome identified a similar number of genes. However, large variations are created by duplicated genes and/or chromosomal segments. Differences are also seen in the way genes are processed. These variations lead to new insight into human gene function and dysfunction. (See p. 144 for full legend.)

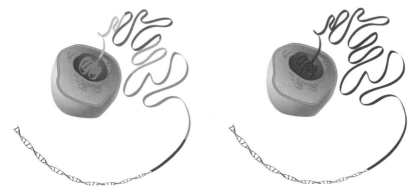

Figure 5.4 Haplotype blocks across the genome. Variation across the genome has been conserved through evolution in large, shared lengths of DNA referred to as "haplotype blocks." The discovery that sequence variation occurs in large units, rather than randomly across the genome, allows large-scale association studies to screen for fewer variations by identifying the shared haplotype blocks. Complex diseases such as developmental disabilities may be studied by tracking these blocks with specific phenotypes.

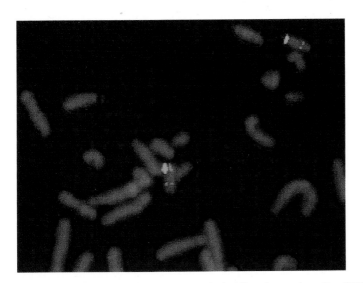

Figure 9.3 Fluorescence in situ hybridization using the SNRPN probe (red color) from the proximal 15q11–q13 region, a centromeric probe (green color) from chromosome 15, and a distal control probe (red color) from the distal end of the long arm of chromosome 15. The lack of the red SNRPN signal close to the centromere on the deleted chromosome 15 (shown at the top) is demonstrated from a PWS subject with the 15q11–q13 deletion.

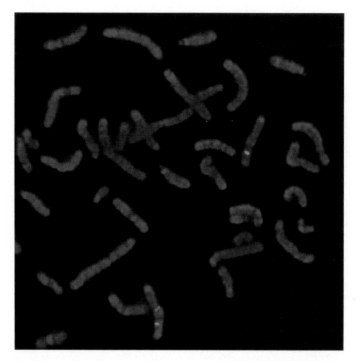

Figure 11.3 Fluorescence in situ hybridization (FISH) using the elastin probe (red color) from the 7q11.23 chromosome band and a control probe from 7q31 (green color) showing the absence of the elastin signal in the deleted chromosome 7 (at upper right) from an individual with Williams–Beuren syndrome.

Figure 13.1 *(Facing page)* Smith–Magenis syndrome critical chromosome region. Refinement of the SMS critical chromosome interval, transcription map, and unusual 17p deletions. The SMS deletions important to the refinement of the SMS critical interval are indicated by the open/closed bars. Deleted DNA is represented by the open portion of the bars, while the closed portion represents nondeleted DNA. The common SMS deletion is labeled and represented by the largest openbar (bottom) includes the locations of the three SMS-REPs in relation to genomic markers mapped to this region of 17p. The SMS critical deletion region is represented by the pink bar. The current SMS transcription map (modified from Ref. 29 using the GenomeBrowser at UCSC and Unigene at NCBI information) is shown; genes, ESTs, and markers mapping to the critical interval are represented by pink circles. The *RAI1* gene is indicated by a blue circle. The green bars above the transcription map represent the currently available FISH probes from Vysis and Cytocell, the blue bar represents the PAC RP1-253P07 used in our FISH experiments, and the previously available FISH probes from Oncor are indicated by yellow bars. This figure is not to scale. (Courtesy of Sarah Elsea, Ph.D., Virginia Commonwealth University, Richmond, Virginia.)

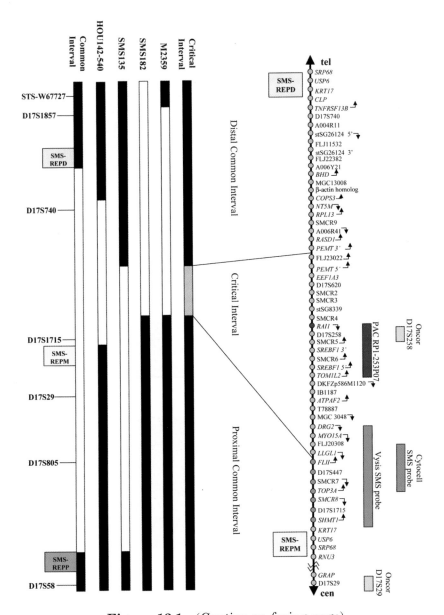

Figure 13.1 *(Caption on facing page)*

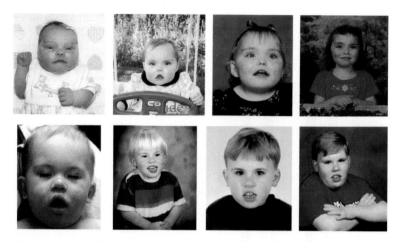

Figure 13.2 Characteristic facial features of Smith–Magenis syndrome in both males and females. Female (top row): birth, 8 months, 17 months, and 5 years; male: 9 months, 5 years, 8 years, and 14 years, respectively. (See p. 436 for full legend.)

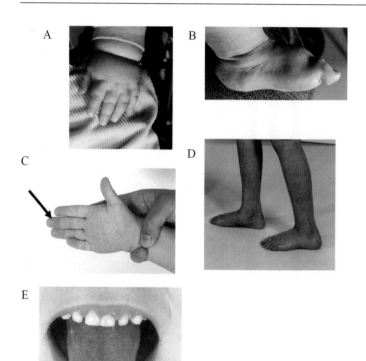

Figure 13.3 Clinical features of the extremities and tongue in Smith–Magenis syndrome. (See p. 437 for full legend.)

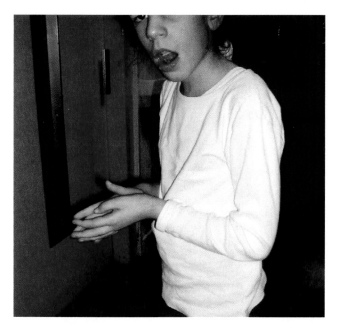

Figure 14.1 Clinical picture of a Rett patient showing typical positions of the hands. (Kindly provided by Dr. Nadia Bahi.)

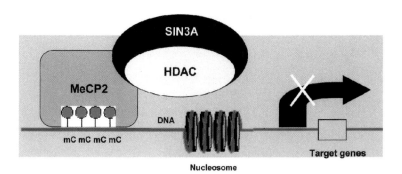

Figure 14.4 Normal function of MeCP2. Methyl-CpG-binding protein 2 binds methylated cytosine residues (mC) in CpG islands and recruits Sin3A and histone deacetylases HDACs. Deacetylation of the histone tails compacts the chromatin and silences transcription.

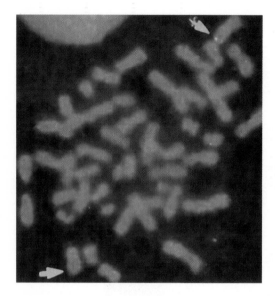

Figure 15.8 Fluorescence in situ hybridization with a locus-specific probe showing a submicroscopic deletion in a patient with Jacobsen syndrome. The shorter deleted chromosome is marked by an arrow (bottom) and the normal chromosome by an arrowhead (top). (See p. 543 for full legend.)

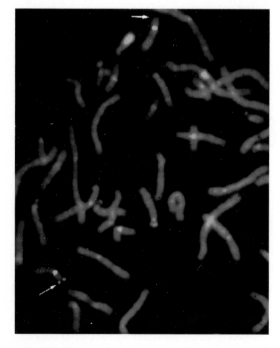

Figure 15.12 Fluorescence in situ hybridization with locus-specific probes showing a submicroscopic deletion (chromosome at top designated by arrow) in a patient with MDS. The locus-specific probe is labeled with spectrum orange; the control probe in spectrum green. The control probe facilitates identification of the deleted chromosome (notice only the bluish-green signal present on the deleted chromosome) (Courtesy of Dr. William Dobyns.)

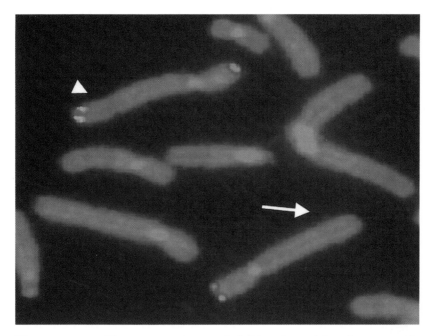

Figure 15.15 Fluorescence in situ hybridization with a locus-specific probe for the NSD1 gene showing a submicroscopic deletion in a patient with Sotos syndrome. Deleted chromosome is marked by an arrow; normal chromosome by an arrowhead.

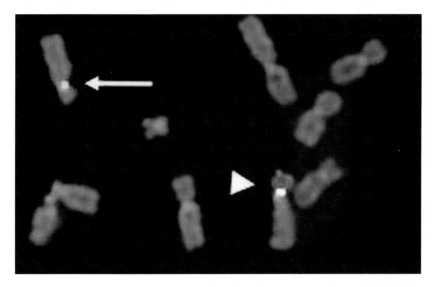

Figure 15.18 Fluorescence in situ hybridization with a locus-specific probe showing deletion in a patient with Wolf–Hirschhorn syndrome. Deleted chromosome is marked by an arrow; normal chromosome by an arrowhead. The locus-specific probe is labeled with spectrum orange; control probe in spectrum green. The control probe facilitates identification of the deleted chromosome (notice only the green signal present on the deleted chromosome).

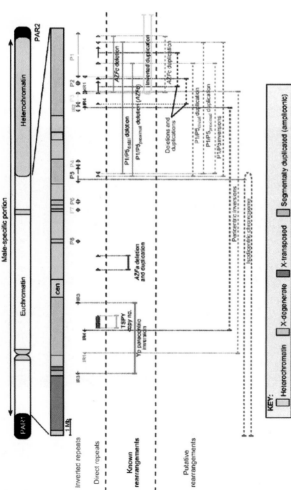

Figure 16.1   Sequence organization of the human Y chromosome. The mosaic of three main classes is shown together with the principal inverted and direct repeats on the MSY. Eight palindromes (P1–P8) and four dispersed inverted repeats (IR1–IR4) are labeled. Beneath these are the known rearrangements, and a representative subset of putative rearrangements that are associated with these repeats.

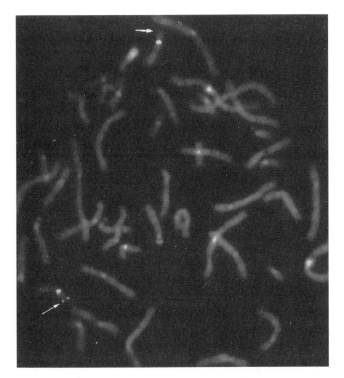

Figure 12 Fluorescence in situ hybridization with locus-specific probes showing a submicroscopic deletion (chromosome at top designated by arrow) in a patient with MDS. The locus-specific probe is labeled with spectrum orange, and the control probe is labeled in spectrum green. The control probe facilitates identification of the deleted chromosome (notice only the bluish-green signal present on the deleted chromosome). (Courtesy of Dr. William Dobyns, University of Chicago, Illinois.) (*See color insert.*)

few reports of familial cases due to parental balanced translocations (91) and inversions (92) leading to an unbalanced chromosome rearrangement in the child, which results in higher recurrence risk. Therefore, it is essential to perform chromosome and FISH analysis for the affected individuals and their family members to characterize the abnormality, so that accurate risk assessment can be made. Carriers of balanced translocations with breakpoints in 17p13 ascertained because of a relative with MDS should be counseled

for a high recurrence risk of offspring with abnormal phenotypes. According to the estimates, the recurrence risk is
~26% of all recognized pregnancies and 33% in pregnancies
that remain viable into or after the second trimester (93).

F. Resources

Information can be obtained through computer searches of key
words or syndrome names. Parent or family support groups
are also available for most syndromes or disorders. The following is a list of organizations or support groups where pertinent
information about this syndrome can be found:

> Lissencephaly Network, Inc. (http://www.lissencephaly.
> org).
> Lissencephaly Network.
> Lissencephaly Launch Pad
> (hompage.ntlworld.com/foliot/liss).
> Lissencephaly Contact Group, UK
> (http://www.lissencephaly.org.uk/).

VIII. RUBINSTEIN–TAYBI SYNDROME

In 1963, Rubinstein and Taybi (94) first described a syndrome
with congenital malformations, distinctive facial features,
and mental retardation. The prevalence of RTS (OMIM #
180849) is estimated to be 1 in 125,000 (94).

A. Clinical Presentation

Patients with RTS are usually recognized in infancy or early
childhood because of their facial appearance and broad
thumbs and great toes (Fig. 13). The distal phalanges of the
fingers also may be broadened. The craniofacial features
include microcephaly, large or late closing anterior fontanel,
down-slanting palpebral fissures, beaked nose, columella
extending below the nares, high-arched palate, and small
mouth (95–97). Eye abnormalities include refractive errors,
strabismus, ptosis, cataracts, colobomas, obstruction of the
nasolacrimal duct, and corneal abnormalities (97,98). An
easily collapsible larynx may lead to sleep apnea and

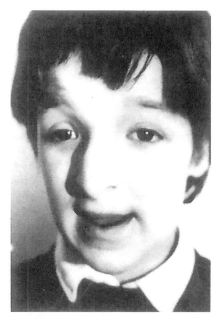

Figure 13 A 11-½-year-old boy with facial features of RTS such as prominent beaked nose. (From Ref. 96.)

problems with anesthesia (99). Renal abnormalities are common and males usually have undescended testes. About one-third of the patients have congenital heart defects (100). Orthopedic problems include dislocated patellas, scoliosis, and lax joints (101). Dental abnormalities include malocclusion and talon cusps on the permanent upper incisors. There seems to be an increased risk of neoplasia, as there are a number of reports of tumors in RTS patients, including leukemia, meningioma, and rhabdomyosarcoma (95,102).

Prenatal growth is usually normal, whereas postnatal growth retardation begins within the first 6 months of life. Parameters for height, weight, and head circumference fall below the fifth percentile during infancy. Patients often become obese in childhood or in adolescence. As adults, the patients have short stature. Growth curves specific for RTS patients have been published to assist in monitoring the growth (103). Puberty and sexual development are normal.

Patients with RTS are mentally retarded, but IQ scores have been reported to vary from 25 to 80. The performance IQ is generally higher than the verbal IQ (97). Attention deficit, impulsivity, moodiness, sensitivity to noise, and autism are frequently observed in RTS patients (97,104,105).

B. Clinical Management

Recommendations for clinical management of individuals with RTS have been published (106). The evaluation of infants with RTS includes examinations for congenital malformations, such as echocardiogram, ophthalmologic and audiologic exams, and renal ultrasound. There should be monitoring of growth, orthopedic assessment of significantly angulated thumbs, and examination of the joints and spine. Assessment for gastroesophageal reflux and aggressive management of constipation are recommended. Developmental evaluations should include assessment of cognitive abilities, speech and language, and gross and fine motor skills. Developmental disabilities should be addressed through early intervention programs and special education. Behavior assessment is recommended and behavior management programs and medication are used when warranted.

C. Chromosomal and Molecular Basis

Reports of several patients with RTS and chromosome translocations or inversions lead to the recognition of a consistent breakpoint on chromosome 16 (16p13.3) (107,108). In 1993, Breuning et al. (109) reported the finding of submicroscopic deletions in 16p13.3 in six of 24 patients with RTS using FISH analysis. Subsequently, the gene encoding the CREB-binding protein (CBP) located at 16p13.3 was cloned and mutations in this gene were reported to cause RTS (110). The CBP is found virtually in all tissues and has histone acetyltransferase activity that is necessary for gene transcription (111,112). Mutations in CBP may lead to cancer, because the gene plays a role in tumor suppression.

Regarding genotype–phenotype correlations, no phenotypic differences have been observed between individuals with deletions, protein truncating mutations, or missense mutations (112,113). However, Bartsch et al. (114) suggested that patients with deletions have a more severe phenotype and Hennekam et al. (115) found that microcephaly, partial duplication of the hallux, and angulation of the first rays of the hands and feet were increased in patients with deletions.

D. Genetic Testing

The diagnosis of RTS is generally made from a clinical evaluation, but the finding of a defect in the CBP gene by genetic testing can confirm the diagnosis. Fluorescence in situ hybridization analysis is available for detection of microdeletions of the CBP gene that occur in about 10% of the patients with RTS (114). The RT1 probe, which covers the 3' end of the gene, has been commonly used for these studies, but Petrij et al. (112) and Blough et al. (113) have emphasized the need to use all five FISH probes that are available in order to detect all possible microdeletions. Direct DNA analysis using northern blotting, Southern blotting, and sequencing is available on a research basis and may detect CBP mutations in another 35% of patients (114–116).

E. Genetic Counseling

Rubinstein–Taybi syndrome usually occurs sporadically but in familial cases is inherited as an autosomal dominant disorder. Most parents are not affected and do not need to be tested. Affected individuals are assumed to have new mutations and therefore, the risk of recurrence is low (0.5%). Although there is the possibility of germline mosaicism, no instances have been reported. Prenatal diagnosis by FISH analysis or direct DNA testing is possible for families in which a deletion or CBP mutation is identified in a previous child.

F. Resources

Information can be obtained online through computer searches of key words or syndrome names. Parent of family support groups are also available for most syndromes or disorders. The following is a list of organizations or support groups where pertinent information about this syndrome can be found:

> Rubinstein–Taybi Syndrome: A web site for families who have members diagnosed with RTS (www.Rubinstein–Taybi.org).
> Rubinstein–Taybi Parent Group.
> Rubinstein–Taybi Syndrome Support Group—England.
> RTS Canada.

IX. SOTOS SYNDROME

First described in 1964, Sotos syndrome (OMIM #117550) is a relatively common condition with more than 300 cases reported (117,118). The prevalence is not known, but it is estimated to be between 1 in 10,000 and 1 in 50,000 (119).

A. Clinical Presentation

Sotos syndrome (cerebral gigantism) is a pleiotropic syndrome of multiple congenital anomalies, developmental delay, and overgrowth. The syndrome is characterized by macrocephaly, dolichocephaly (prominent forehead), conductive hearing loss, variable mental deficiency, hypotonia, hyper-reflexia, prenatal onset of excessive size, large hands and feet, advanced bone age, down-slanting palpebral fissures, nystagmus, strabismus, high hairline, prominent jaw, high and narrow palate, and psychomotor delay (Fig. 14). Other abnormalities include congenital heart defects such as atrial and ventricular septal defects and patent ductus arteriosus, skeletal malformations including joint laxity, genu valgus, pes planus, disharmonic maturation of phalanges and carpal bones, thin, brittle fingernails, and sparse hair in frontoparietal area (117–122).

Several types of neoplasms in patients with Sotos syndrome prompted the theory that patients with Sotos syndrome have a slightly increased risk for malignancy (123). Gorlin et al. (124) estimated a risk of 3.9% of benign or malignant tumors in Sotos syndrome.

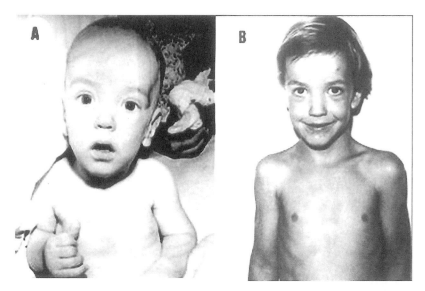

Figure 14 Characteristic facial features of Sotos syndrome. Figures (A) and (B) show the same patient at 6 months and 4.6 years of age, respectively. Note the prominent forehead, telecanthus, epicanthic folds, flat nasal bridge, down-slanting palpebral fissures, and pointed chin. (From Melo DG et al. Arq Neuropsiquiatr 2002; 60:234–238, with permission from Arquivos de Neuro-Psiquiatria.)

Sotos patients and their sibs are known to have increased risk for spontaneous abortions and/or stillbirths. Other authors have reported "subfertility" and delayed menarche/ oligomenorrhea (118). Although infants with Sotos syndrome may have feeding difficulties in the early neonatal period, they later develop voracious appetites, but without any evidence of diencephalic disturbance, resulting in overweight (118). Sotos patients are also known to exhibit behavioral disturbances including ritualistic behavior and little awareness of danger (125,126).

B. Clinical Management

Individuals with Sotos syndrome appear to have normal life span and are fertile (121). The two most important features in Sotos patients for clinical management are excessive height and increased risk for tumor development. The height is not considered as a handicap for males, but girls diagnosed with Sotos syndrome might benefit from treatment with high doses of estrogen or octreotide to curtail the linear growth (119). Early assessment of developmental delays should include evaluation of cognitive abilities, gross and fine motor skills, and speech and language. Developmental disabilities should be addressed through early intervention programs. Physical therapy may improve balance, gait, and posture, and psychological counseling may help in coping with social and behavioral problems during adolescence. To improve speech development, augmentative communication is recommended in addition to speech therapy (127).

C. Chromosomal and Molecular Basis

For a long time, the etiology of Sotos syndrome was not known. Several patients with chromosome abnormalities involving chromosomes 2, 3, 6, and 12 have been reported, although the majority of the patients showed normal karyotypes. Recent studies have shown that haploinsufficiency for *NSD1* (nuclear receptor binding Su-var, enhancer of zeste, and trithorax domain protein 1) gene, cloned from the 5q35 breakpoint in a patient with a chromosomal translocation (128) is one of the genes responsible for Sotos syndrome. *NSD1* consists of 23 exons and encodes at least six functional domains that are thought to be related to chromatin regulation in addition to 10 putative nuclear localization signals. *NSD1* is expressed in several tissues including fetal and adult brain, kidney, skeletal muscle, spleen, and thymus. Analysis of the *NSD1* gene in sporadic cases of Sotos syndrome showed that the majority of the patients had submicroscopic deletions (Fig. 15), while a small number of patients showed frame shift and nonsense mutations (128). As a common ~2.2 Mb deletion accounts for the majority of the *NSD1* deletions in Sotos syndrome patients, it is hypothesized that unequal crossing over or intrachromosomal recombination between low copy repeats is responsible for the deletions (129).

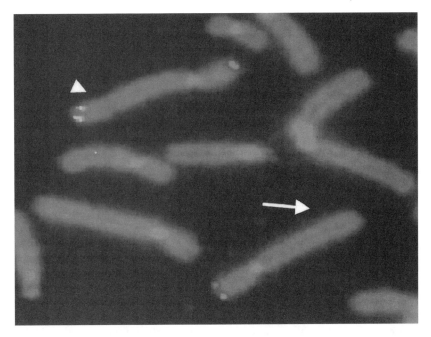

Figure 15 Fluorescence in situ hybridization with a locus-specific probe for the NSD1 gene showing a submicroscopic deletion in a patient with Sotos syndrome. The deleted chromosome is marked by an arrow and the normal chromosome by an arrowhead. (From Ref. 128.) (*See color insert.*)

Comparative analysis of clinical features between patients with intragenic mutations and submicroscopic deletions suggested that certain clinical features are more or less associated with the type of abnormality. For example, features like overgrowth, advanced maturation, performance disturbance, slowing of growth, and amelioration of mental development in later stages are ascribed to *NSD1* haploinsufficiency due to submicroscopic deletions (129). Development of large ventricles, brain atrophy, neonatal asphyxia, and hypoglycemia may also be due to deletions. Features like agenesis or hypoplasia of the corpus callosum, cardiovascular and urinary anomalies, neonatal jaundice, and recurrent convulsions are thought to be due to some other genes and are not related to *NSD1* haploinsufficiency, because patients with *NSD1* mutations do not manifest these features. In addition, the body size tends to be smaller and mental development tends to be more retarded in patients with deletions than those with point mutations.

D. Genetic Testing

Because *NSD1* haploinsufficiency has been identified as one of the major factors contributing to the Sotos syndrome, it is possible to screen the affected individuals for mutations and/or submicroscopic deletions of the *NSD1* gene. Fluorescence *in situ* hybridization analysis to detect deletions is clinically available (Fig. 15), and DNA mutation analysis is available on a research basis. Because some of the features are thought to be due to other genes within the deleted region, Sotos syndrome may be a contiguous gene deletion syndrome. The deleted region is known to contain 21 genes in addition to *NSD1* and is yet to be characterized.

There is at least one report of prenatal diagnosis of Sotos syndrome (130). The authors reported that fetuses at risk for Sotos syndrome might present with abnormal sonographic findings of the brain and skull in association with overgrowth, unilateral hydronephrosis, and polyhydramnios in the third trimester.

E. Genetic Counseling

Although the majority of subjects with Sotos syndrome are sporadic in nature, familial cases have been reported. In familial cases, the most likely mode of inheritance is autosomal dominant with variable expressivity. Reports of children affected with Sotos syndrome with normal parents suggest the possibility of reduced penetrance (131). Theoretically, the risk for recurrence is 50%, but one must take into account reduced penetrance and variable expressivity. Therefore, carriers of *NSD1* mutations could be phenotypically normal.

F. Resources

Information can be obtained online through computer searches of key words or syndrome names. Parent or family support groups are also available for most syndromes or disorders. The following is a list of organizations or support groups where pertinent information about this syndrome can be found:

> Sotos Syndrome Support Association (www.well.com/user/sssa).
> Child Growth Foundation.
> Sotos Association—L'Eveil.
> Eltern-Initiative Sotos-Syndrom (EISS), Germany (www.sotossyndrom.de/).

X. WOLF–HIRSCHHORN SYNDROME

Wolf–Hirschhorn syndrome (WHS) (OMIM #194190), also referred to as deletion 4p syndrome, was first described in 1965 (132,133). Wolf–Hirschhorn syndrome is a well-known congenital malformation syndrome with a distinct clinical phenotype. The prevalence is estimated to be about 1 per 50,000 births, with a female predilection of 2:1 (134).

A. Clinical Presentation

"Greek warrior helmet appearance" of the nose is the most striking feature in patients with Wolf–Hirschhorn syndrome (132–135). This feature is easily recognizable in childhood but is much less evident at puberty (136). Other clinical features present in almost all WHS patients include microcephaly, high forehead, prominent glabella, hypertelorism, epicanthal folds, high-arched eyebrows, short philtrum, distinct mouth, and micrognathia (135–138). The distinctive appearance of the mouth is similar to that seen after repair of cleft lip. The facial features of WHS (Fig. 16) are currently proposed as the minimum criteria for its clinical diagnosis (137). About 60% of the WHS patients show some degree of craniofacial asymmetry. Ear anomalies, such as poorly differentiated, posteriorly angulated, or low-set, or lobeless pinnae, or extremely underdeveloped or absent cartilage of the outer ear or pits and tags, are seen in ~80% of the patients. Cleft lip and palate appear in

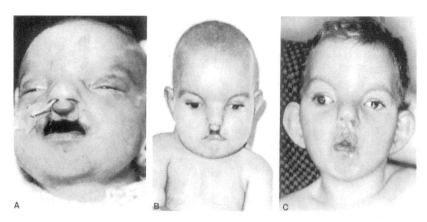

Figure 16 Characteristic facial features of individuals with Wolf–Hirschhorn syndrome. A–C, a 2-week-old, 11-month-old, and 33-month-old child, respectively. (Reprinted from Jones KL, ed. *Smith's Recognizable Patterns of Human Malformation.* 5th ed. 1997:39, with permission from Elsevier.)

slightly more than one-third of the patients; about 40% have eye/optic nerve defects such as coloboma. About 50% show bilateral ptosis of the eyelid and, occasionally, eyelid hypoplasia requiring skin graft. Facial angiomas are recognized in about 50% of the patients. Midline scalp defects seem to be an occasional finding in WHS with the frequency varying from 0% to 50% (135).

All patients with WHS show marked growth deficiency of prenatal onset and continue to have short stature and slow weight gain (137–139). Infants with WHS may have a higher risk for failure to thrive and respiratory distress due to gastroesophageal reflux (135).

Skeletal anomalies are common in WHS occurring in 60–70% (135). The most common anomalies are craniostenosis with brachycephalic skull, underdevelopment of ossification centers in the cervical spine, anomalies of the sternal ossification, split hand, clinodactyly, finger-like appearance of the thumb, and thin fingers with bilateral over-riding of the second finger onto the third. Absence of the ossification nucleus for the ulnar styloid apophysis, proximal radioulnar synostosis, severely delayed bone age, club feet, malformed toes, scoliosis and kyphosis, hip dislocation, and lack of pubic bone ossification is also observed. In about 50% of the WHS patients, dental anomalies such as agenesis of lower lateral incisors or upper canines, peg-shaped teeth, delayed teeth eruption with persistence of deciduous teeth, and taurodontism are observed (135). Sacral dimple and other skin anomalies, such as cutis marmorate, dry skin, and hemangiomas of the forehead, are also common in WHS patients. Congenital heart defects are seen in about 30–50% (135). The most common heart defect is atrial septal defect, followed by pulmonary stenosis, ventricular septal defect, patent ductus arteriosus, and aortic insufficiency. Tetralogy of Fallot is also reported. Genitourinary abnormalities are present in about 25% of the patients with WHS (135). Renal abnormalities mostly include renal agenesis, cystic dysplasia and/or hypoplasia, and oligomeganephroma (135). Abnormalities of the genitalia include hypospadias and cryptorchidism in about 50% of the males and absent uterus and streak gonads in females. Sensorineural hearing loss has been reported in a few children.

Generalized hypotonia is present in all children with WHS (137). Unilateral clonic or tonic seizures with or without secondary generalization or generalized tonic–clonic seizures are common in 50–100% of children with WHS (137). Mental retardation with minimal communication skills is a universal feature in patients with WHS (135,137). There have been reports that children with WHS and deletion of 4p are predisposed to develop malignant conditions, especially myelodysplastic syndrome (140).

B. Clinical Management

Wolf–Hirschhorn syndrome is reported to have a high mortality rate with one-third of the patients dying during infancy. Children with large 4p deletions were more likely to die than those with smaller deletions, and it has been shown that there is a statistically significant relationship between the deletion size and the overall risk of death in de novo deletion cases

(141). However, there are other reports suggesting that the
life span of individuals with WHS is similar to that of the
general population (135).

Seizures and feeding difficulties are the two most severe
complications encountered in the management of children
with WHS. Gastrostomy, occasionally associated with gastroesophageal fundoplication, was suggested to be the best way
to deal with feeding difficulties (135). Children who underwent
this procedure were reported to have satisfactory weight gain,
became more responsive to stimuli, and showed improvement
in motor abilities. Seizures, though difficult to control, are
reported to eventually disappear with age, provided they are
treated with appropriate antiepileptic drugs (135,139).
Administration of valproic acid soon after the first seizure
is indicated, as 95% of WHS children suffer from multiple
seizures, most often triggered by fever accompanying frequent
infections, and almost 60% later show atypical absences.
Congenital heart defects are usually not complex in WHS
and can be repaired. In order to check for hearing impairment,
it is recommended that WHS children be studied with brainstem auditory-evoked responses, otoacoustic emissions, or
both, as early diagnosis is vital for appropriate interventions.
Though not common, children with WHS must be tested
for renal function to rule out kidney disease. It is also
recommended that WHS children should receive appropriate
psychometric, speech, and motor evaluations, and these
children should be enrolled in personalized rehabilitation
programs that cover motor aspects, cognition, communication,
and social skills. Such an effective intervention should
lead to a slow but constant improvement in psychomotor
development.

C. Chromosomal and Molecular Basis

Wolf–Hirschhorn syndrome is caused by a deletion of the short
arm of chromosome 4 extending from 4p16 to the terminus.
About 75% of the deletions are uncomplicated and de novo,
about 12% are due to unusual chromosomal rearrangements
such as ring chromosomes or mosaicism for the deletion, and

the remaining 13% result from segregation of balanced translocations in the parents (134). According to one report, there are at least 20 cases of WHS that are inherited (135). Among the de novo deletions, there appears to be a preponderance of paternal deletions (142,143). Because the majority of the unbalanced translocations are maternal in origin (144) and the de novo cases are paternal in origin, it was suggested that imprinting might play a role in the phenotypic expression of WHS (143).

Recent studies have shown that even in those WHS patients with apparently normal chromosomes, a microdeletion involving the chromosome 4p16.3 region can be demonstrated by molecular techniques including FISH (144). The WHS critical region has been narrowed to a region of 165 kb in 4p16.3 by overlapping deletion analysis (145). Two candidate genes named *WHSC1* (Wolf–Hirschhorn syndrome candidate 1) (146) and *WHSC2* (Wolf–Hirschhorn syndrome candidate 2) (147) were identified within this region, though no mutations have been identified in either of the genes as yet. A third gene in the region, *LETM1* (leucine zipper/EF-hand-containing transmembrane), was considered as an excellent candidate gene for WHS, in particular for seizures (148). However, recent evidence suggests that some of the patients with distinctive WHS phenotype have deletions that are outside the proposed WHS critical region (149) and may be a new critical region for WHS termed *WHSCR-2*, which lies within a 300–600 kb interval in 4p16.3. There is no consensus on whether the size of the deletion is correlated with the severity of the phenotype (150).

D. Genetic Testing

Genetic testing for WHS can be carried out by conventional chromosome analysis. In most patients, the deletion is large and thus can be detected on routine chromosome analysis (Fig. 17). Fluorescence in situ hybridization is extremely useful in identifying WHS patients with submicroscopic deletions (Fig. 18). Chromosome analysis is recommended for the parents of children with a deletion to detect the presence of

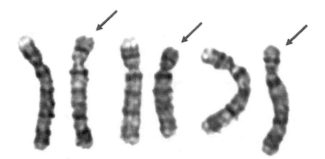

Figure 17 Partial karyotypes showing chromosome 4 deletion seen in Wolf–Hirschhorn syndrome. Arrow shows the deleted chromosome.

balanced translocations or other cryptic rearrangements. Fluorescence in situ hybridization studies are also very useful in families or parents with more than one affected child with WHS.

There have been several reports of prenatal diagnosis of WHS (151). Several features such as intrauterine growth retardation, Greek helmet facies, cleft lip/palate, diaphragmatic hernia, heart defect, and hypospadias can be diagnosed with fetal ultrasonography and should prompt karyotyping.

E.   Genetic Counseling

As the majority of deletions are de novo in origin, the risk for recurrence is often negligible (<0.5%). In cases where the deletion is the result of translocation in a parent, the recurrence is about 10–15% (40). It is not known whether WHS is associated with infertility, as there are no reports of affected person reproducing it.

F.   Resources

Information can be obtained online through computer searches of key words or syndrome names. Parent or family support groups are also available for most syndromes or disorders. The following is a list of organizations or support

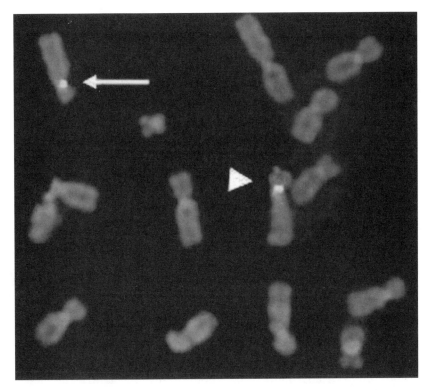

Figure 18 Fluorescence in situ hybridization with locus-specific probe showing deletion in a patient with Wolf–Hirschhorn syndrome. The deleted chromosome is marked by an arrow and the normal chromosome by an arrowhead. The locus-specific probe is labeled with spectrum orange, and the control probe is labeled in spectrum green. The control probe facilitates identification of the deleted chromosome (notice only the green signal present on the deleted chromosome). (*See color insert.*)

groups where pertinent information about this syndrome can be found:

> 4p-Support Group (Wolf–Hirschhorn Syndrome)
> (www.4p-supportgroup.org).
> Wolf–Hirschhorn Syndrome Support Group.
> Wolf–Hirschhorn Syndrome Support Group
> (www.netdoctor.co.uk).

REFERENCES

1. Alagille D, Habib EC, Thomassin N. L'atresie des voies biliaires intrahepatiques avec voies bilaires extrahepatiques permeables chez l'enfant. A Propos de 25 Observations. Paris: Editions Mëdicales Flammarion, 1969:301–318.

2. Krantz ID, Piccoli DA, Spinner NB. Clinical and molecular genetics of Alagille syndrome. Curr Opin Pediatr 1999; 11: 558–564.

3. Alagille D, Estrada A, Hadchouel M, Gautier M, Odievre M, Dommergues JP. Syndromic paucity of interlobular bile ducts. J Pediatr 1987; 110:195–200.

4. Emerick KM, Rand EB, Goldmuntz E, Krantz ID, Spinner NB, Piccoli DA. Features of Alagille syndrome in 92 patients: frequency and relation to prognosis. Hepatology 1999; 29: 822–829.

5. Silberbach M, Lashley D, Reller MD, Kinn WF, Terry A, Sunderland CO. Arteriohepatic dysplasia and cardiovascular malformations. Am Heart J 1994; 127:695–699.

6. Puklin JE, Riely CA, Simon RM, Cotlier E. Anterior segment and retinal pigmentary abnormalities in arteriohepatic dysplasia. Ophthalmology 1981; 88:337–347.

7. Nischal KK, Hingorani M, Bentley CR, Vivian AJ, Bird AC, Baker AJ, Mowat AP, Mieli-Vergani G, Aclimandos WA. Ocular ultrasound in Alagille syndrome. Ophthalmology 1997; 104:79–85.

8. Deprettere A, Portman B, Mowat A. Syndromic paucity of the intrahepatic bile ducts: diagnostic difficulty; severe morbidity throughout early childhood. J Pediatr Gastroenterol Nutr 1987; 6:865–871.

9. Rosenfield NS, Kelley MJ, Jensen PS, Cotlier E, Rosenfield AT, Riley CA. Arteriohepatic dysplasia: radiologic features of a new syndrome. Am J Radiol 1980; 135:1217–1223.

10. Kamath BM, Loomes KM, Oakey RJ, Krantz ID. Supernumerary digital flexion creases: an additional clinical manifestation of Alagille syndrome. Am J Med Genet 2002; 112: 171–175.

11. Alagille D. Alagille syndrome today. Clin Invest Med 1996; 19:325–330.

12. Krantz ID, Rand EB, Genin A, Hunt P, Jones M, Louis AA, Graham JM, Bhatt S, Piccoli DA, Spinner NB. Deletions of 20p12 in Alagille syndrome: frequency and molecular characterization. Am J Med Genet 1997; 70:80–86.

13. Li L, Krantz ID, Den Y, Genin A, Banta AB, Collins CC, Qi M, Trask BJ, Kuo WL, Cochran J, Costa T, Pierpont ME, Rand EB, Piccoli DA, Hood L, Spinner NB. Alagille syndrome is caused by mutations in human Jagged 1, which encodes a ligand for Notch 1. Nat Genet 1997; 16:243–251.

14. Oda T, Elkahloun AG, Pike BL, Okajima K, Krantz ID, Genin A, Piccoli DA, Meltzer PS, Spinner NB, Collins FS, Chandrasekharappa SC. Mutations in the human Jagged 1 gene are responsible for Alagille syndrome. Nat Genet 1997; 16: 235–242.

15. Spinner NB, Colliton RP, Crosnier C, Krantz ID, Hadchouel M, Meunier-Rotival M. *Jagged 1* mutations in Alagille syndrome. Hum Mutat 2001; 17:18–33.

16. Albayram F, Stone K, Nagey D, Schwarz KB, Blakemore K. Alagille syndrome: prenatal diagnosis and pregnancy outcome. Fetal Diagn Ther 2001; 17:182–184.

17. Spinner NB, Rand EB, Fortina P, Genin A, Taub R, Semeraro A, Piccoli DA. Cytologically balanced t(2;20) in a two-generation family with Alagille syndrome: cytogenetic and molecular studies. Am J Hum Genet 1994; 55:238–243.

18. Lejeune J, Lafourcade J, Berger R, Vialatte J, Boeswillwald M, Seringe P, Turpin R. Trois cas de deletion partielle du bras court d'un chromosome 5. C R Acad Sci (D) 1963; 257: 3098–3102.

19. Niebuhr E. The cri du chat syndrome: epidemiology, cytogenetics, and clinical features. Hum Genet 1978; 44:227–275.

20. Wilkins LE, Brown JA, Nance WE, Wolf B. Clinical heterogeneity in 80 home-reared children with cri du chat syndrome. J Pediatr 1983; 102:528–533.

21. Van Buggenhout GJCM, Pijkels E, Holvoet M, Schaap C, Hamel BCJ, Fryns JP. Cri du chat syndrome: changing phenotype in older patients. Am J Med Genet 2000; 90:203–215.

22. Kjaer I, Niebuhr E. Studies of the cranial base in 23 patients with cri-du-chat syndrome suggest a cranial developmental field involved in the condition. Am J Med Genet 1999; 82:6–14.

23. Marinescu RC, Mainardi PC, Collins MR, Coucourde G, Pastore G, Eaton-Evans J, Overhauser J. Growth charts for cri-du-chat syndrome. Am J Med Genet 2000; 91:153–162.

24. Cornish KM, Bramble D, Munir F, Pigram J. Cognitive functioning in children with typical cri du chat (5p-) syndrome. Devel Med Child Neurol 1999; 41:263–266.

25. Cornish KM, Pigram J. Developmental and behavioral characteristics of cri du chat syndrome. Arch Dis Child 1996; 75:448–450.

26. Wilkins LE, Brown JA, Wolf B. Psychomotor development in 65 home-reared children with cri du chat syndrome. J Pediatr 1980; 97:401–405.

27. Cornish KM, Bramble D. Cri du chat syndrome: genotype–phenotype correlations and recommendations for clinical management. Dev Med Child Neurol 2002; 44:494–497.

28. Perfumo C, Cerruti Mainardi P, Cali A, Coucourde G, Zara F, Cavani S, Overhauser J, Dagna Bricarelli F, Pierluigi M. The first three mosaic cri di chat syndrome patients with two rearranged cell lines. J Med Genet 2000; 37:967–972.

29. Marinescu RC, Johnson EI, Grady D, Chen X-N, Overhauser J. FISH analysis of terminal deletions in patients diagnosed with cri-du-chat syndrome. Clin Genet 1999; 56:282–288.

30. Overhauser J, Huang X, Gersh M, Wilson W, McMahon J, Bengtsson U, Rojas K, Meyer M, Wasmuth JJ. Molecular and phenotypic mapping of the short arm of chromosome 5: sublocalization of the critical region for the cri-du-chat syndrome. Hum Mol Genet 1994; 3:247–252.

31. Gersh M, Goodart SA, Pasztor LM, Harris DJ, Weiss L, Overhauser J. Evidence for a distinct region causing a cat-like cry in patients with 5p deletions. Am J Hum Genet 1995; 56: 1404–1410.

32. Mainardi PC, Perfumo C, Cali A, Coucourde G, Pastore G, Cavani S, Zara F, Overhauser J, Pierluigi M, Dagna Bricarelli F. Clinical and molecular characterization of 80 patients with 5p deletion: genotype–phenotype correlation. J Med Genet 2001; 38:151–158.

33. Church DM, Bengtsson U, Nielsen KV, Wasmuth JJ, Niebuhr E. Molecular definition of deletions of different segments of distal 5p that result in distinct phenotypic features. Am J Hum Genet 1995; 56:1162–1172.

34. Overhauser J, Golbus MS, Schonberg SA, Wasmuth JJ. Molecular analysis of an unbalanced deletion of the short arm of chromosome 5 that produces no phenotype. Am J Hum Genet 1986; 39:1–10.

35. Johnson EI, Marinescu RC, Punnett H, Tenenholz B, Overhauser J. 5p14 deletion associated with microcephaly and seizures. J Med Genet 2000; 37:125–127.

36. Marinescu RC, Johnson EI, Dykens EM, Hodapp RM, Overhauser J. No relationship between the size of the deletion and the level of developmental delay in cri-du-chat syndrome. Am J Med Genet 1999; 86:66–70.

37. Simmons AD, Pueschel AW, McPherson JD, Overhauser J, Lovett M. Molecular cloning and mapping of human semaphorin F from the cri-du-chat candidate interval. Biochem Biophys Res Commun 1998; 242:685–691.

38. Medina M, Marinescu RC, Overhauser J, Kosik SK. Hemizygosity of δ-catenin (CTNND2) is associated with severe mental retardation in cri-du-chat syndrome. Genomics 2000; 63:157–164.

39. Zhang A, Zheng C, Hou M, Lindvall C, Li K-J, Erlandsson F, Bjorkholm M, Gruber A, Blennow E, Xu D. Deletion of the telomerase reverse transcriptase gene and haploinsufficiency of telomere maintenance in cri cu chat syndrome. Am J Hum Genet 2003; 72:940–948.

40. Simpson JL, Globus MS. Genetics in Obstetrics and Gynecology. 2d ed. Philadelphia: WB Sanders, 1992:26.

41. Martinez JE, Tuck-Miller CM, Superneau D, Wertelecki W. Fertility and the cri du chat syndrome. Clin Genet 1993; 43: 212–214.

42. Shapira SK, McCaskill C, Northrup H, Spikes AS, Elder FFB, Sutton VR, Korenberg JR, Greenberg F, Shaffer LG. Chromosome 1p36 deletions: the clinical phenotype and molecular characterization of a common newly delineated syndrome. Am J Hum Genet 1997; 61:642–650.

43. Slavotinek A, Shaffer LG, Shapira SK. Monosomy 1p36. J Med Genet 1999; 36:657–663.

44. Heilstedt HA, Ballif BC, Howard LA, Lewis RA, Stal S, Kashork CD, Bacino CA, Shapira SK, Shaffer LG. Physical map of 1p36, placement of breakpoints in monosomy 1p36, and clinical characterization of the syndrome. Am J Hum Genet 2003; 72:1200–1212.

45. Shaffer LG, Lupski JR. Molecular mechanisms for constitutional chromosomal rearrangements in humans. Ann Rev Genet 2000; 34:297–329.

46. Zenker M, Rittinger O, Grosse K-P, Speicher MR, Kraus J, Rauch A, Trautmann U. Monosomy 1p36—a recently delineated, clinically recognizable syndrome. Clin Dysmorph 2002; 11:43–48.

47. Giraudeau F, Aubert D, Young I, Horsley S, Knight S, Kearney L, Vergnaud G, Flint J. Molecular-cytogenetic detection of a deletion of 1p36.3. J Med Genet 1997; 34:314–317.

48. Riegel M, Castellan C, Balmer D, Brecevic L, Schinzel A. Terminal deletion, del(1) (p36.3), detected through screening for terminal deletions in patients with unclassified malformation syndromes. Am J Med Genet 1999; 82:249–253.

49. Wu Y-Q, Heilstedt HA, Bedell JA, May KM, Starkey DE, McPherson JD, Shapira SK, Shaffer LG. Molecular refinement of the 1p36 deletion syndrome reveals size diversity and a preponderance of maternally derived deletions. Hum Mol Genet 1999; 8:313–321.

50. Colmenares C, Heilstedt HA, Shaffer LG, Schwartz S, Berk M, Murray JC, Stavnezer E. Loss of the SKI proto-oncogene in individuals affected with 1p36 deletion syndrome is predicted

by strain-dependent defects in Ski$^{-/-}$ mice. Nat Genet 2002; 30:106–109.

51. Jacobsen P, Hauge M, Henningen K. An (11;22) translocation in four generations with chromosome 11 abnormalities in the offspring. Hum Hered 1973; 23:368–385.

52. Pivnick EK, Velagaleti GVN, Wilroy RS, Smith ME, Rose SR, Tipton RE, Tharapel AT. Jacobsen syndrome: report of a patient with severe eye anomalies, growth hormone deficiency, and hypothyroidism associated with deletion 11(q23q25) and review of 52 cases. J Med Genet 1996; 33:772–778.

53. Michaelis RC, Velagaleti GVN, Jones C, Pivnick EK, Phelan MC, Boyd E, Tarleton J, Wilroy RS, Tunnacliffe A, Tharapel AT. Most Jacobsen syndrome deletion breakpoints occur distal to FRA11B. Am J Med Genet 1998; 76:222–228.

54. Frank J, Riccardi VM. The 11q-syndrome. Hum Genet 1977; 35:241–246.

55. Favier R, Douay L, Esteva B, Partnoi MF, Gaulard P, Lecompte T, Perot C, Adam M, Lecrubier C, Van den Akker J, Lasfurgues G, Najean Y, Breton-Gorius J. A Novel genetic thrombocytopenia (Paris–Trousseau) associated with platelet inclusions, dysmegakaryopoiesis and chromosome deletion at 11q23. C R Acad Sci Paris 1993; 316:698–701.

56. Krishnamurti L, Neglia JP, Nagarajan R, Berry SA, Lohr J, Hirsch B, White JG. Paris–Trousseau syndrome platelets in a child with Jacobsen's syndrome. Am J Hematol 2001; 66:295–299.

57. Schinzel A. Catalogue of unbalanced chromosome aberrations in man. 2nd ed. New York: Walter de Gruyter, 2001:496.

58. Fryns JP, Kleczkowska A, Buttiens M. Distal 11q monosomy. The typical 11q monosomy syndrome is due to deletion of subband 11q24.1. Clin Genet 1986; 30:255–260.

59. Jones C, Mullenbach R, Grossfeld P, Auer R, Favier R, Chien K, James M, Tunnacliffe A, Cotter F. Co-localization of CCG repeats and chromosome deletion breakpoints in Jacobsen syndrome: evidence for a common mechanism of chromosome breakage. Hum Mol Genet 2000; 9:1201–1208.

60. Krasner A, Wallace L, Thiagalingam A, Jones C, Lengauer C, Minahan L, Ma Y, Kalikin L, Feinberg AP, Jabs EW, Tunnacliffe A, Baylin SB, Ball DW, Nelin BD. Cloning and chromosomal localization of the human BARX2 homeobox protein gene. Gene 2000; 250:171–180.

61. Jones FS, Kioussi C, Copertino DW, Kallunki P, Holst BD, Edelman GM. Barx2, a new homeobox gene of the Bar class, is expressed in neural and craniofacial structures during development. Proc Natl Acad Sci USA 1997; 94:2632–2637.

62. Wax JR, Smith JF, Floyd RC, Eggleston MK. Prenatal ultrasonographic findings associated with Jacobsen syndrome. J Ultrasound Med 1995; 14:256–258.

63. Hall BD, Langer LO, Giedion A, Smith DW, Cohen MM, Beals RK, Brandner M. Langer–Giedion syndrome. Birth Defects Orig Art Ser 1974; 12:147–164.

64. Langer LO, Krassikoff N, Laxova R, Scheer-Williams M, Lutter LD, Gorlin RJ, Jennings CG, Day DW. The tricho-rhino-phalangeal syndrome with exostoses (or Langer–Giedion syndrome): four additional patients without mental retardation and review of the literature. Am J Med Genet 1984; 19:81–112.

65. Stevens CA, Moore CA. Tibial hemimelia in Langer–Giedion syndrome—possible gene location for tibial hemimelia at 8q. Am J Med Genet 1999; 85:409–412.

66. Murachi S, Nogami H, Oki T, Ogino T. Familial tricho-rhino-phalangeal syndrome type II. Clin Genet 1981; 19:149–155.

67. Brenholz P, Swayne L, Twersky S, Arbeitel B, Singer N. Dominant inheritance of the Langer–Giedion syndrome. Am J Hum Genet 1989; 45:A41.

68. Buhler EM, Buhler UK, Stalder GR, Jani L, Jurik LP. Chromosome deletion and multiple cartilaginous exostoses. Eur J Pediatr 1980; 133:163–166.

69. Buhler EM, Malik NJ. The tricho-rhino-phalangeal syndrome(s): chromosome 8 long arm deletion: is there a shorted region of overlap between reported cases? TRPI and

TRPII syndromes: are they separate entities? Am J Med Genet 1984; 19:113–119.

70. Bowen P, Biederman B, Hoo JJ. The critical segment for the Langer–Giedion syndrome:8q24.11q24.12. Ann Genet 1985; 28:224–227.

71. Okuno T, Inoue A, Asakura T, Nakao S. Langer–Giedion syndrome with del 8(q24.13–q24.22). Clin Genet 1987; 32: 40–45.

72. Ludecke HJ, Johnson C, Wagner MJ, Wells DE, Turleau C, Tommerup N, Latos-Bielenska A, Sandig K-R, Meinecke P, Zabel B, Horsthemke B. Molecular definition of the shortest region of deletion overlap in the Langer–Giedion syndrome. Am J Hum Genet 1991; 49:1197–1206.

73. Parrish JE, Wagner MJ, Hecht JT, Scott CI, Wells DE. Molecular analysis of overlapping chromosomal deletions in patients with Langer–Giedion syndrome. Genomics 1991; 11:54–61.

74. Ludecke HJ, Wagner MJ, Nardmann J, LaPillo B, Parrish PJ, Willems JE, Haan EA, Frydman M, Hamers GJH, Wells DE, Horsthemke B. Molecular dissection of a contiguous gene syndrome: localization of the genes involved in the Langer–Giedion syndrome. Hum Mol Genet 1995; 4:31–36.

75. Ahn J, Ludecke HJ, Lindow S, Horton WA, Lee B, Wagner MJ, Horsthemke B, Wells DE. Cloning of the putative tumour suppressor gene for hereditary multiple exostoses (EXT1). Nat Genet 1995; 11:137–143.

76. Momeni P, Glickner G, Schmidt O, von Holtum D, Albrecht B, Gillessen-Kaesbach G, Hennekam R, Meinecke P, Zabel B, Riosenthal A, Horsthemke B, Ludecke HJ. Mutations in a new gene, encoding a zinc-finger protein, cause tricho-rhino-phalangeal syndrome type I. Nat Genet 2000; 24:71–64.

77. Hilton MJ, Sawyer JM, Gutierrez L, Hogart A, Kung TC, Wells DE. Analysis of novel and recurrent mutations responsible for the tricho-rhino-phalangeal syndromes. J Hum Genet 2002; 47:103–106.

78. Miller JQ. Lissencephaly in 2 siblings. Neurology 1963; 13: 841–850.

79. Dieker H, Edwards RH, ZuRhein G, Chou SM, Hartman HA, Opitz JM. The lissencephaly syndrome. In: Bergsma D, ed. The Clinical Delineation of Birth Defects: Malformation Syndromes. New York: National Foundation—March of Dimes (pub) II, 1969:53–64.

80. Jones KL, Gilbert EF, Kaveggia EG, Opitz JM. The Miller–Dieker syndrome. Pediatrics 1980; 66:277–281.

81. Dobyns WB, Reiner O, Carrozzo R, Ledbetter DH. Lissencephaly—a human brain malformation associated with deletion of the LIS1 gene located at chromosome 17p13. J Am Med Assoc 1993; 270:2838–2842.

82. Dobyns WB, Curry CJR, Hoyme HE, Turlington L, Ledbetter DH. Clinical and molecular diagnosis of Miller–Dieker syndrome. Am J Hum Genet 1991; 48:584–594.

83. Dobyns WB, Stratton RF, Parke JT, Greenberg F, Nussbaum RL, Ledbetter DH. Miller–Dieker syndrome: lissencephaly and monosomy 17p. J Pediatr 1983; 102:552–558.

84. Dobyns WB, Stratton RF, Greenberg F. Syndromes with lissencephaly I: Miller–Dieker and Norman–Robert syndromes and isolated lissencephaly. Am J Med Genet 1984; 18: 509–526.

85. Stratton RF, Dobyns WB, Airhart SD, Ledbetter DH. New chromosomal syndrome: Miller–Dieker syndrome and monosomy 17p13. Hum Genet 1984; 67:193–200.

86. Reiner O, Carrozo R, Shen Y, Wehnert M, Faustinella F, Dobyns WB, Caskey CT, Ledbetter DH. Isolation of a Miller–Dieker lissencephaly gene containing G protein beta-subunit-like repeats. Nature 1993; 364:717–721.

87. Cardoso C, Leventer RJ, Ward HL, Toyo-oka K, Chung J, Gross A, Martin CL, Allanson J, Pilz DT, Olney AH, Mutchinick OM, Hirotsune S, Wynshaw-Boris A, Dobyns WB, Ledbetter DH. Refinement of a 400-kb critical region allows genotypic differentiation between isolated lissence-phaly, Miller–Dieker syndrome, and other phenotypes secondary to deletion of 17p13.3. Am J Hum Genet 2003; 72: 918–930.

88. Ledbetter SA, Kuwano A, Dobyns WB, Ledbetter DH. Microdeletions of chromosome 17p13 as a cause of isolated lissencephaly. Am J Hum Genet 1992; 50:182–189.

89. Kuwano A, Ledbetter SA, Dobyns WB, Emanuel BS, Ledbetter DH. Detection of deletions and cryptic translocations in Miller–Dieker syndrome by in situ hybridization. Am J Hum Genet 1991; 49:707–714.

90. Van Zelderen-Bhola SL, Breslau-Siderius EJ, Beverstock GC, Stolte-Dijkstra I, de Vries LS, Stoutenbeek PH, de Pater JM. Prenatal and postnatal investigation of a case with Miller–Dieker syndrome due to a family cryptic translocation t(17;20) (p13.3;q13.3) detected by fluorescence in situ hybridization. Prenat Diagn 1997; 17:173–179.

91. Alvarado M, Bass HN, Caldwell S, Jamehdor M, Miller AA, Jacobs PA. Miller–Dieker syndrome: detection of a cryptic chromosome translocation using in situ hybridization in a family with multiple affected offspring. Am J Dis Child 1993; 147:1291–1294.

92. Yokoyama Y, Narahara K, Teraoka M, Koyama K, Seino Y, Yagi S, Konishi T, Miyawaki T. Cryptic pericentric inversion of chromosome 17 detected by fluorescence in situ hybridization study in familial Miller–Dieker syndrome. Am J Med Genet 1997; 71:236–237.

93. Pollin TI, Dobyns WB, Crowe CA, Ledbetter DH, Bailey-Wilson JE, Smith ACM. Risk of abnormal pregnancy outcome in carriers of balanced reciprocal translocation involving the Miller–Dieker syndrome (MDS) critical region in chromosome 17p13.3. Am J Med Genet 1999; 85:269–375.

94. Rubinstein JH, Taybi H. Broad thumbs and toes and facial abnormalities. Am J Dis Child 1963; 105:588–608.

95. Hennekam RC, Van Den Boogaard MJ, Sibbles BJ, van Spijker HG. Rubinstein–Taybi syndrome in The Netherlands. Am J Med Genet Suppl 1990; 6:17–29.

96. Rubinstein JH. Broad thumb-hallux (Rubinstein–Taybi) syndrome 1957–1988. Am J Med Genet Suppl 1990; 6:3–16.

97. Stevens CA, Carey JC, Blackburn BL. Rubinstein–Taybi syndrome: a natural history study. Am J Med Genet Suppl 1990; 6:30–37.

98. van Genderen MM, Kinds GF, Riemslag FC, Hennekam RC. Ocular features in Rubinstein–Taybi syndrome: investigation of 24 patients and review of the literature. Br J Ophthalmol 2000; 84:1177–1184.

99. Zucconi M, Ferini-Strambi L, Erminio C, Pestalozza G, Smirne S. Obstructive sleep apnea in the Rubinstein–Taybi syndrome. Respiration 1993; 60:127–132.

100. Stevens CA, Bhakta MG. Cardiac abnormalities in the Rubinstein–Taybi syndrome. Am J Med Genet 1995; 59: 246–348.

101. Moran R, Calthorpe D, McGoldrick F, Fogarty E, Dowling F. Congenital dissociation of the patella in Rubinstein–Taybi syndrome. Ir Med J 1993; 86:34–35.

102. Miller RW, Rubinstein JH. Tumors in Rubinstein–Taybi syndrome. Am J Med Genet 1995; 56:112–115.

103. Stevens CA, Hennekam RC, Blackburn BL. Growth in the Rubinstein–Taybi syndrome. Am J Med Genet Suppl 1990; 6:51–55.

104. Hennekam RC, Baselier AC, Beyaert E, Bos A, Blok JB, Jansma HB, Thorbecke-Nilsen H Veerman VV. Psychological and speech studies in Rubinstein–Taybi syndrome. Am J Ment Retard 1992; 96:645–660.

105. Stevens CA, Schmitt C, Speraw S. Behavior in Rubinstein–Taybi syndrome. Proc Gr Genet Ctr 1999; 18:144–145.

106. Wiley S, Swayne S, Rubinstein JH, Lanphear NE, Stevens CA. Rubinstein–Taybi syndrome medical guidelines. Am J Med Genet 2003; 119A:101–110.

107. Imaizumi K, Kuroki Y. Rubinstein–Taybi syndrome with de novo reciprocal translocation t(2;16) (p13.3;p13.3). Am J Med Genet 1991; 38:636–639.

108. Tommerup N, van der Hagen CB, Heiberg A. Tentative assignment of a locus for Rubinstein–Taybi syndrome to

16p13.3 by a de novo reciprocal translocation, t(7;16) (q34;p13.3). Am J Med Genet 1992; 44:237–241.

109. Breuning MH, Dauwerse HG, Fugazza G, Saris JJ, Spruit L, Wijnen H, Tommerup N, van der Hagen CB, Imaizumi K, Kuroki Y, van den Boogaard M-J, de Pater JM, Mariman ECM, Hamel BCJ, Himmelbauer H, Frischauf A-M, Stalling RL, Beverstock G, van Ommen G-J, Hennekam RCM. Rubinstein–Taybi syndrome caused by submicroscopic deletions within 16p13.3. Am J Hum Genet 1993; 52:249–254.

110. Petrij F, Giles RH, Dauwerse HG, Saris JJ, Hennekam RC, Masuno J, Tommerup N, van Ommen G-J, Goodman RH, Peters DJM, Breuning MH. Rubinstein–Taybi syndrome caused by mutations in the transcriptional co-activator CBP. Nature 1995; 376:248–351.

111. Murata T, Kurokawa R, Krones A, Tatsumi K, Ishii M, Taki T, Masuno M, Ohashi H, Yanagisawa M, Rosenfeld MG, Glass CK, Hayashi Y. Defect of histone acetyltransferase activity of the nuclear transcriptional coactivator CBP in Rubinstein–Taybi syndrome. Hum Mol Genet 2001; 10:1071–1076.

112. Petrij F, Dauwerse HG, Blough RI, Giles RH, van der Smagt JJ, Wallerstein R, Maaswinkel-Mooy PD, van Karnebeek CD, van Ommen G-J, van Haeringen A, Rubinstein JH, Saal HM, Hennekam RCM, Peters DJM, Breuning MH. Diagnostic analysis of the Rubinstein–Taybi syndrome: five cosmids should be used for microdeletion detection and low number of protein truncating mutations. J Med Genet 2000; 37: 168–176.

113. Blough RI, Petrij F, Dauwerse JG, Milatovich-Cherry A, Weiss L, Saal HM, Rubinstein JH. Variation in microdeletions of the cyclic AMP-responsive element-binding protein gene at chromosome band 16p13.3 in Rubinstein–Taybi syndrome. Am J Med Genet 2000; 90:29–34.

114. Bartsch O, Wagner A, Hinkel GK, Krebs P, Stumm M, Schmalenberger B, Bohm S, Balci S, Majewski F. FISH studies in 45 patients with Rubinstein–Taybi syndrome: deletions associated with polysplenia, hypoplastic left heart and death in infancy. Eur J Hum Genet 1999; 7:748–756.

115. Hennekam RC, Tilanus M, Hamel BCJ, Voshart-van Heeren H, Mariman ECM, van Beersum SEC, van den Boogard M-JH, Breuning MH. Deletion at chromosome 16p13.3 as a cause of Rubinstein–Taybi syndrome: clinical aspects. Am J Hum Genet 1993; 52:255–262.

116. Coupry I, Roudaut C, Stef M, Delrue M-A, Marche M, Burgelin I, Taine L, Cruaud C, Lacombe D, Arveiler B. Molecular analysis of the CBP gene in 60 patients with Rubinstein–Taybi syndrome. J Med Genet 2002; 39:415–421.

117. Sotos JF, Dodge PR, Muirhead D, Crawford JD, Talbot NB. Cerebral gigantism in childhood. N Engl J Med 1964; 271: 109–116.

118. Opitz JM, Weaver DW, Reynolds JF Jr. The syndromes of Sotos and Weaver: reports and review. Am J Med Genet 1998; 79:294–304.

119. Sotos JF. Overgrowth. Clin Pediatr 1997; 36:89–103.

120. Allanson JE, Cole TRP. Sotos syndrome: evolution of facial phenotype subjective and objective assessment. Am J Med Genet 1996; 65:13–20.

121. Cole TRP, Hughes HE. Sotos syndrome: a study of the diagnostic criteria and natural history. Am J Med Genet 1994; 31:20–32.

122. Noreau DR, Al-Ata J, Jutras L, Teebi AS. Congenital heart defects in Sotos syndrome. Am J Med Genet 1998; 79:327–328.

123. Yule SM. Cancer in Sotos syndrome. Arch Dis Child 1999; 80:193–194.

124. Gorlin RJ, Cohen MM, Levin LS. Overgrowth syndromes and postnatal onset obesity syndromes. In: Syndromes of the Head and Neck. New York: Oxford University Press, 1990:323–352.

125. Finegan JK, Cole TRP, Kingwell E, Smith ML, Smith M, Sitarenios G. Language and behavior in children with Sotos syndrome. J Am Acad Child Adolesc Psychiatry 1994; 33: 107–115.

126. Rutter SC, Cole TRP. Psychological characteristics of Sotos syndrome. Dev Med Child Neurol 1991; 33:898–902.

127. Battaglia A, Ferrari AR. Cognitive and psychological profiles in dysmorphic syndromes. Pediatric Med Chir 1993; 15:23–25.

128. Kurotaki N, Imaizumi K, Harada N, Masuno M, Kondoh T, Jagai T, Ohashi H, Naritomi K, Tsukahara M, Makita Y, Sugimoto T, Sonoda T, Hasegawa T, Chinen Y, Tomita HS, Kinoshita A, Mizuguchi T, Yoshiura K, Ohta T, Kishino T, Fukushima Y, Niikawa N, Matsumoto N. Haploinsufficiency of NSD1 causes Sotos syndrome. Nat Genet 2002; 30:365–366.

129. Nagai T, Matsumoto N, Kurotaki N, Harada N, Niikawa N, Ogata T, Imaizumi K, Kurosawa K, Kondoh T, Ohashi H, Tsukahara M, Makita Y, Sugimoto T, Sonoda T, Yokoyama T, Uetake K, Sakazume S, Fukushima Y, Naritomi K. Sotos syndrome and haploinsufficiency of NSD1: clinical features of intragenic mutations and submicroscopic deletions. J Med Genet 2003; 40:285–289.

130. Chen C-P, Lin S-P, Chang T-Y, Chiu N-C, Shih S-L, Lin C-J, Wang W, Hsu H-C. Perinatal imaging finding of inherited Sotos syndrome. Prenat Diagn 2002; 22:887–892.

131. Boman H, Nilsson D. Sotos syndrome in two brothers. Clin Genet 1980; 18:421–427.

132. Wolf U, Reinwein H, Porsch R, Schrotter R, Baitsch H. Defizienz an den kurzen armen eines chromosomes nr. 4. Humangenetik 1965; 1:397–413.

133. Hirschhorn K, Cooper HL, Firschein IL. Deletion of the short arms of chromosome 4–5 in a child with defects of midline fusion. Humangenetik 1965; 1:479–482.

134. Laurie IW, Lazjuk CL, Ussova YL, Pressman EB, Gurevich DB. The Wolf–Hirschhorn syndrome. I. Genetics. Clin Genet 1980; 17:375–384.

135. Battaglia A, Carey JC, Wright TJ. Wolf–Hirschhorn (4p–) syndrome. Adv Pediatr 2001; 48:75–113.

136. Battaglia A, Carey JC, Viskochil DH. Wolf–Hirschhorn syndrome (WHS): a history in pictures. Clin Dysmorpol 2000; 9:25–30.

137. Battaglia A, Carey JC, Cederholm P, Viskochil DH, Brothman AR, Galasso C. Natural history of Wolf–Hirschhorn syndrome: experience with 15 cases. Pediatrics 1999; 103:830–836.

138. Estabrooks LL, Breg WR, Hayden DH, Ledbetter MR, Myers RM, Wyandt HE, Yang-Feng TL, Hirschhorn K. Summary of the 1993 ASHG ancillary meeting "Recent research on chromosome 4p syndromes and genes". Am J Med Genet 1995; 55:453–458.

139. Battaglia A, Carey JC. Health supervision and anticipatory guidance of individuals with Wolf–Hirschhorn syndrome. Am J Med Genet (Semin Med Genet) 1999; 89:111–115.

140. Sharathkumar A, Kirby M, Freedman M, Abdelhaleem M, Chitayat D, Teshima IE, Dror Y. Malignant hematological disorders in children with Wolf–Hirschhorn syndrome. Am J Med Genet 2003; 119A:194–199.

141. Shannon NL, Maltby EL, Rigby AS, Quarrell OWJ. An epidemiological study of Wolf–Hirschhorn syndrome: life expectancy and cause of mortality. J Med Genet 2001; 38:674–679.

142. Tupler R, Bortotto L, Buhler E, Alkan M, Malik NJ, Bosch-Al Jadooa N, Memo L, Maraschio P. Paternal origin of de novo deleted chromosome 4 in Wolf–Hirschhorn syndrome. J Med Genet 1992; 29:53–55.

143. Dallapiccola B, Mandich P, Bellone E, Selicorni A, Mokin V, Ajmar F, Novelli G. Parental origin of chromosome 4p deletion in Wolf–Hirschhorn syndrome. Am J Med Genet 1993; 47:921–924.

144. Zollino M, Stefano CD, Zampino G, Mastroiacovo P, Wright TJ, Sorge G, Selicorni A, Tenconi R, Zappala A, Battaglia A, Rocco MD, Palka G, Pallotta R, Altherr MR, Neri G. Genotype–phenotype correlations and clinical diagnostic criteria in Wolf–Hirschhorn syndrome. Am J Med Genet 2000; 94:254–261.

145. Wright TJ, Ricke DO, Denison K, Abmayr S, Cotter PD, Hirschhorn K, Keinanen M, McDonald-McGinn D, Somer M, Spinner N, Yang-Feng T, Zackai E, Altherr MR. A transcript map of the newly defined 165 kb Wolf–Hirschhorn syndrome critical region. Hum Mol Genet 1997; 6:317–324.

146. Stec I, Wright TJ, van Ommen G-JB, de Boer PAJ, van Haeringen A, Moorman FM, Altherr MR, den Dunnen JT. WHSC1, a 90 kb SET domain-containing gene, expressed in early development and homologous to a *Drosophila* dysmor-

phy gene maps in the Wolf–Hirschhorn syndrome critical region and is fused to IgH in t(4;14) multiple myeloma. Hum Mol Genet 1998; 7:1071–1082.

147. Wright TJ, Costa JL, Naranjo C, Francis-West P, Altherr MR. Comparative analysis of a novel gene from the Wolf–Hirschhorn/Pitt–Rogers–Danks syndrome critical region. Genomics 1999; 59:203–212.

148. Endele S, Fuhry M, Pak SJ, Zabel BU, Winterpacht A. *LETM1* a novel gene encoding a putative EF-hand Ca^{2+}-banding protein, flanks the Wolf–Hirschhorn syndrome (WHS) critical region is deleted in most WHS patients. Genomics 1999; 60:218–225.

149. Zollino M, Lecce R, Fischetto R, Murdolo M, Faravelli F, Selicorni A, Butte C, Memo L, Capovilla G, Neri G. Mapping the Wolf–Hirschhorn syndrome phenotype outside the currently accepted WHS critical region and defining a new critical region WHSCR-2. Am J Hum Genet 2003; 72:590–597.

150. Estabrooks LL, Rao KW, Driscoll DA, Candrall BF, Dean JCS, Ikonen E, Korf B, Aylsworth S. Preliminary phenotypic map of chromosome 4p16 based on 4p deletions. Am J Med Genet 1995; 57:581–586.

151. Tapper JK, Zhang S, Harirah HM, Panova NI, Merryman LS, Hawkins JC, Lockhart LH, Gei AB, Velagaleti GVN. Prenatal diagnosis of a fetus with unbalanced translocation (4;13) (p16;q32) with overlapping features of Patau and Wolf–Hirschhorn syndromes. Fetal Diagn Ther 2002; 17:347–351.

16

Sex Chromosome Anomalies

JOHN L. HAMERTON

Departments of Biochemistry and
Medical Genetics; Pediatrics and Child
Health, University of Manitoba,
Winnipeg, Manitoba, Canada

JANE A. EVANS

Departments of Biochemistry and
Medical Genetics; Pediatrics and
Child Health; and Community Health
Sciences, University of Manitoba,
Winnipeg, Manitoba, Canada

I. INTRODUCTION

Anomalies of the X and Y chromosomes form a significant part of the total load of chromosome mutations carried by the human species (1–3). Fortunately, most sex chromosome aberrations (SCA) lead to fewer developmental disabilities than autosomal aneuploidy. Follow up of children identified with SCA in several consecutive newborn studies worldwide has revealed that, when identified as newborn infants and followed through to late adolescence, most children are not dysmorphic nor do they suffer from major developmental disabilities (4,5).

585

The discovery by Barr and Bertram (6) of sex chromatin—otherwise known as the Barr body and now known to represent the condensed inactive X chromosome in somatic cell nuclei—led to renewed interest in a number of syndromes that had been described earlier including Klinefelter syndrome (7) and Turner syndrome (8). Sex chromatin studies showed that a proportion of males with clinical features of Klinefelter syndrome were chromatin positive and thus were initially thought to be sex-reversed females; while a high proportion of females with the clinical features of Turner syndrome were shown to be chromatin negative. Later, following the development of modern cytogenetic techniques, it was shown that a patient with Klinefelter syndrome had a 47,XXY chromosome complement (9,10) while four patients with Turner syndrome were 45,X (11,12).

Sex chromosome aneuploidy has been shown to be relatively common. Males may have XXY or XYY karyotypes. Females may have trisomy X (47,XXX) or monosomy X (45,X). Individuals with four and five sex chromosomes have also been described, as well as individuals with sex chromosome mosaicism (e.g., 45,X/46,XX; 46,XY/47,XXY) or structural rearrangements of the X and Y chromosomes. Such abnormalities may result in infertility or hypogonadism, and perhaps lower intelligence, but usually cause little morbidity or mortality. The one exception is the 45,X karyotype that results in a 99% fetal loss during gestation (3).

Painter (13) was the first to report that the sex chromosome constitution of humans involved heteromorphic X and Y chromosomes. After 1956, when the human chromosome number was confirmed as 46 rather than the 48 that had previously been reported, studies of subjects with SCA demonstrated that the Y chromosome was essential for determination of the male sex. Normally, in the presence of the Y chromosome, the fetal primordial gonad differentiates into a testis, leading to a developmental cascade that results in a male phenotype. In the absence of the Y, the gonad develops into an ovary, and the phenotype is female. The Y chromosome is one of the smallest human chromosomes. A complete physical map and sequence of the Y is now available (14,15).

Sequencing data have revealed that the male specific region (MSY, formerly named NRY or nonrecombining region) of the Y is a mosaic of heterochromatic sequences, and three classes of euchromatic sequences, X-transposed, X-degenerate, and segmented and duplicated (referred to as "ampliconic") (Fig. 1). The X-transposed sequences exhibit 99% identity to the X chromosome, the X-degenerate are remnants of ancient autosomes from which the modern X and Y evolved, while the segmented and duplicated region includes about 30% of the MSY euchromatin where sequence pairs show greater than 99.9% identity. Skaletsky and colleaques postulate that this structure is maintained by frequent gene conversion (nonreciprocal transfer) between the arms of eight massive palindromes at least six of which contain testis genes

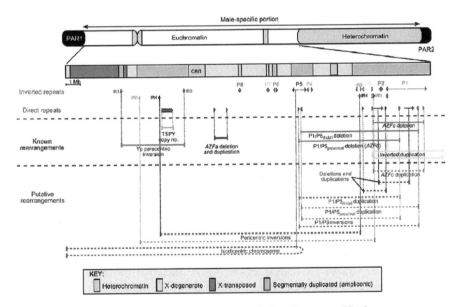

Figure 1 Sequence organization of the human Y chromosome. The mosaic of three main classes is shown together with the principal inverted and direct repeats on the MSY. Eight palindromes (P1–P8) and four dispersed inverted repeats (IR1–IR4) are labeled. Beneath these are the known rearrangements, and a representative subset of putative rearrangements that are associated with these repeats. (From Ref. 16.) (*See color insert.*)

(15). They suggest that this protects against the degeneration that is the inevitable consequence of haploidy (16). Sequencing of the MSY region identified 156 transcription units 78 of which are MSY genes that seem to encode proteins. Of these, 60 are members of nine MSY specific gene families with >98% nucleotide identity among family members in both introns and exons. The remaining 18 protein-coding units are present in one copy each. Thus, the MSY seems to encode at least 27 distinct proteins or protein families (15). The major testis-determining gene, *SRY*, is present in single copy and is mapped to the most distal region of the short arm adjacent to the boundary of the PAR1 or major pseudoautosomal region on the short arm. This gene has been cloned (17) and has been shown to be essential for initiating testicular development. The Y chromosome also carries a series of genes affecting male fertility. Deletions, duplications, and inversions (Fig. 1) of these genes result in failure of sperm development (Sec. VI). The high degree of rearrangement detected may be a direct consequence of gene conversion resulting from crossover within the arms of the palindromes leading to inversion, dele-tion, and duplication (18).

The X chromosome is a much larger chromosome carry-ing approximately 1100 genes. Both the X and Y have small pseudoautosomal pairing regions (PAR1 and PAR2), which allow pairing of the X and Y during male meiosis and the occasional exchange of the sex determining region (SRY) from the Y to the X chromosome resulting in rare XX males (see below). The phenotypic effect of X chromosome aneuploidy is modified by the phenomenon of X inactivation (19–21), a process of random inactivation of all X chromosomes but one, so that genes carried on the X chromosomes are usually expressed as single copies, ensuring similar gene dosage in males and females. Genes on the X chromosome (XIST) mediate this process (OMIM 314670).

The terms used to describe abnormalities in chromosome number have been clearly defined elsewhere (22). Most SCA arise as a result of errors in the distribution of the chromosomes at meiosis I (MI) or meiosis II (MII) or at a postzygotic mitotic division (PZM). Such a process is termed nondisjunction, which may simply be defined as the failure of two chromosomes or sister chromatids to pass to opposite poles of the cell at cell division, resulting in daughter cells with abnormal chromosome numbers. Early in the study of SCA, attempts were made to determine where such errors occurred, initially using an X-linked blood group (Xga) and other X-linked conditions such as red-green color blindness. The application of molecular biology to cytogenetic studies has resulted in the determination not only of the erroneous cell division, but also potential factors that may be involved in nondisjunction. For example, mosaicism of the sex chromosomes is relatively frequent and must result from postzygotic errors. Bean et al. (23), based on studies of the mouse WtY chromosome, have suggested that the earliest postzygotic cell divisions in mammals are highly nondisjunction prone and that the malsegregation is both chromosome specific as well as dependent on the genetic background. The authors suggest the early cleavage divisions in both mice and humans may be nondisjunction prone thus providing a possible explanation for the frequency of mosaics among sex chromosome anomalies as well as an explanation for the high level of mosaicism in preimplantation embryos derived from in vitro fertilization (24,25).

In this chapter, we will review the clinical features, mode of origin, epidemiology, and impact on fertility of the major forms of SCA caused by nondisjunctional events. We will also outline the effects of certain structural aberrations of the sex chromosomes. We will not, however, deal with X-autosome translocations.

II. SEX CHROMOSOME ABNORMALITIES IN THE FEMALE

A. Turner Syndrome

The eponym Turner syndrome (TS) was coined to describe a new syndrome of sexual infantilism, webbing of the neck, short stature, and cubitus valgus (wide carrying angle at the elbows) first described by Turner in 1938 (8). The syndrome is highly variable and includes many clinical features besides those originally described by Turner. To add to the confusion, the term Turner syndrome is frequently used when patients do not have these classical features. Polani (26) and Robinson and De la Chapelle (27) have attempted to clarify the nomenclature suggesting that the term ovarian dysgenesis or gonadal dysgenesis is more appropriate when the classical stigmata of TS are absent. In the majority of cases, the underlying cause is a chromosome abnormality—usually 45,X—but many types of mosaicism as well as structural anomalies of the X chromosome have been reported. Gonadal or ovarian dysgenesis may occur in individuals with normal 46,XX or 46,XY karyotypes. These cases are caused by single gene mutations or small structural deletions of the Y chromosome (Sec. V).

1. Prevalence

The 45,X karyotype is found in approximately 1 in 10,000 newborn infants (1,3). This is in direct contrast to other sex chromosome abnormalities such as 47,XXX, 47,XXY, and 47,XYY all of which occur at frequencies of about 1 in 1000 live births (1,3). The situation is quite different when fetal loss is considered, as 45,X is the most frequent karyotype seen in chromosomally abnormal abortuses. Hamerton (3) estimated that about 99.8% of 45,X fetuses were lost during gestation. Evans et al. (28) reviewed the frequency of sex chromosome abnormalities among unselected amniocenteses and found an incidence of SCA of 1 in 235, of which 18% were 45,X in nonmosaic or mosaic form. Among amniocenteses carried out because of low maternal serum alpha-fetoprotein, the frequency of sex chromosome abnormalities was 1 in 290 with 58% being either 45,X or mosaics with a 45,X cell line.

2. Clinical Features

The clinical features of patients with the complete Turner phenotype are summarized in Table 1. This diagnosis is often made at birth due to low birth weight, webbing of the neck, pitting edema of the hands and feet, a shield-shaped chest

Table 1 Clinical Abnormalities Associated with a 45,X Karyotype[a]

Skeletal
  Short stature frequently < 5 feet (150 cm)
  Cubitus valgus (abnormal carrying angle of the elbow (54%)[b]
  Short metacarpals or metatarsals, usually IV (48%)
  Deformities of the median tibial condyle
  Osteoporosis
Craniofacial
  Epicanthic folds (25%)
  High-arched palate (36%)
  Abnormal teeth
  Visual abnormalities, usually strabismus (22%)
  Auditory defects, usually due to inner ear defects
  Abnormal facies—large mouth, squashed flat nose[b]
Neck
  Pterygium colli (webbing of the neck)(46%)[b]
  Short broad neck with low hairline (74%)[b]
Chest
  Shield chest with wide spaced nipples (53%)
Cardiovascular
  Congenital heart defects often coarctation of the aorta or
    ventricular septal defect (10–16%)[b]
Renal
  Horseshoe kidney
  Duplicated or otherwise anomalous ureters
  Unilateral renal aplasia or hypoplasia
Gastrointestinal
  Telangiectases
Skin and lymphatic system
  Pigmented naevi (63%)
  Pitting lymphoedema of hands and feet (38%)[b]
Nails
  Hypoplastic or malformed (66%)
Reproductive system and genitalia
  Primary amenorrhoea
  Streak gonads, composed of ovarian stroma, but lacking
    follicles after birth
  Slight breast development
  Scant to absent pubic hair
  Infantile external genitalia

[a]The abnormalities listed here represent the extremes of the phenotype. Many patients with Turner syndrome lack many of the somatic features of the syndrome.
[b]Characteristic features of the phenotype in the newborn.
Source: Adapted and modified from Refs. 27,62.

and cubitus valgus (Fig. 2). Congenital heart disease, either coarctation of the aorta or ventricular septal defect, and renal anomalies such as horseshoe kidney are also common (29). Such infants are, however, manifesting the most severe form of the syndrome seen in live births. Other patients may not be diagnosed until later because of short stature and failure to enter puberty (Fig. 3). The ovaries of 45,X females contain

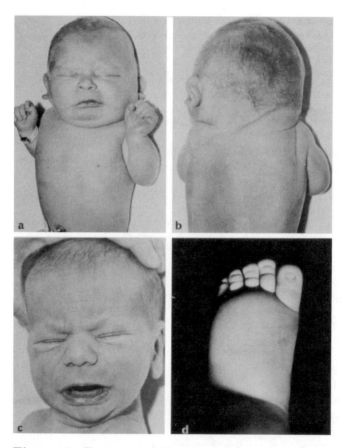

Figure 2 Features of Turner syndrome in the newborn. Note abnormal facies, consisting of large mouth and squashed flat nose, short broad neck with loose skin folds, low hair line, and edema of the feet. (From Ref. 38.)

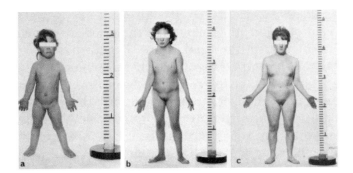

Figure 3 Clinical features of patients with various degrees of Turner syndrome (a) Turner syndrome, 45,X age 4 years, note gross webbing of the neck, abnormal facies, and short stature. (b) Turner syndrome 45,X age 14 years, note webbing of the neck, short stature, cubitus valgus, and absence of secondary sexual characteristics. (c) Turner syndrome 45,X age 22 years, note short stature and absence of somatic malformations. (From Ref. 38.)

primordial follicles during prenatal life and at birth, but these follicles degenerate during childhood to be replaced by thin yellowish white streaks that contain ovarian-like stroma and hilar cells of indeterminate origin. Thus, most of these individuals do not experience natural menarche and are infertile. A minority (5–10%) have relatively regular menses until an early menopause. A few women have gone on to bear children. Such events are exceptional, but the number of reported cases now exceeds 20. Children born to these women have been chromosomally and clinically normal (27). Estrogen production is usually very low and gonadotropin excretion is high indicating primary ovarian failure. Secondary sexual characteristics usually remain infantile, but, as with other features, there is wide variation in the spontaneous occurrence of pubic hair and the development of external genitalia and breasts (Fig. 3). Cyclic estrogen therapy can result in the development of relatively normal secondary sexual characteristics and menstruation indicating that the organs in question are normal in their response to hormone therapy (27).

Dean (30) summarized the growth patterns of girls with Turner syndrome as (i) a normal growth rate from 0 to 3 years, (ii) a progressive decline in growth from age 3 to 14 years and (iii) a prolonged adolescent growth period. The most important variable affecting final adult height has been shown to be the mid-parental height (31). It was hypothesized that low-level estrogen therapy might increase growth hormone (GH) secretion and secondarily increase the growth rate. Ross et al. (32) found that 100 ng/kg estrogen daily in young children with Turner syndrome resulted in a significant increase in short-term growth rate, but this waned with time (32). Several randomized clinical trials are currently in progress examining the effect of GH alone or in combination with estrogen. Preliminary results of two of these trials have been published. An early trial by Rosenfeld et al. (33,34) indicated that both oxandrolone and hGH separately and combined can significantly stimulate short-term skeletal growth and potentially increase final adult height. A more recent trial (35) concluded that early treatment with GH results in a modest increase in final height gain, and that younger and shorter girls gain the greatest height advantage from GH. Low-dose estrogen supplementation before planned induction of puberty was not beneficial. Ranke et al. (36) examined the final adult height of 346 near adult patients who had been treated with GH in the late 1980s. The conclusions were that GH doses used at this time were too low, that height gain and final height are determined by age and height at start of GH treatment, and that little gain in height is achieved after spontaneous or induced puberty. The results of a recent randomized trial from the Netherlands (37) involving 68 patients with Turner syndrome randomized into four groups, confirmed the findings that GH treatment in sufficient dose (6–8 iu/m^2 day) and begun early during development (6.6 years) results in normal final heights reached by the age of 15.8 years with a bone age of 15.5 years. Estrogen treatment begun at 12 years stabilized height velocity and did not have a negative effect on final height. In conclusion, it seems that there is now ample evidence that GH treatment begun at an early age and at adequate dose should significantly improve final height in patients with Turner syndrome.

3. Intelligence and Personality

Turner syndrome patients usually have normal intelligence (27,38,39). Verbal abilities are generally normal; however, 45,X patients as a group have specific intellectual deficits when compared with 46,XX females matched for age, height, IQ, and socioeconomic status. Romans et al. (40) found that they performed significantly less well on measures of spatial/ perceptual skills, visual motor integration, affect recognition, visual memory, attentional abilities, and executive function. Decreased performance in some of these areas persists through late adolescence and early adulthood while improvement occurs in others. Some of these girls experience difficulties in social development and social functioning (41). McCauley et al. (42) found that girls with TS were characterized by immature social relationships, poor school performance, and lower self-esteem in adolescence.

4. Origin

Using molecular techniques to determine the origin of the X chromosome, researchers have found that 74–80% of individuals with monosomy X carry a maternal X and 20–26% a paternal X, with no differences noted between live births and spontaneous abortions (43–45). Studies of the relationship between parental age and X chromosome origin have shown a reduction in maternal age for cases involving a maternal error, i.e., carrying a paternal X. Among spontaneous abortions, there was some indication of an increase in paternal age when the abortus was carrying a maternal X chromosome, thus implicating paternal nondisjunction. These differences did not exist among liveborns (43).

5. Pathogenesis

Since X inactivation ensures that females normally have only one functioning X chromosome from an early stage in embryonic development, why do females with a single X display specific physical and intellectual differences? The answer

surely rests with the fact that the pseudo-autosomal regions
(PAR1 and PAR2) of the X chromosome escape inactivation
and that genes located there are required in double dosage
for normal development. Two aspects of the phenotype—short
stature and the TS associated neurocognitive phenotype—
have been associated with PAR1. Ellison et al. (46) and Rao
et al. (47) reported the isolation of a gene from PAR1 that they
called pseudoautosomal homeobox-containing osteogenic gene
(*PHOG*) alternatively *SHOX* (short stature homeobox). They
suggested that this gene may be associated with the short
stature in TS. The gene product is a transcription factor,
the expression of which is restricted to osteogenic cells, trabe-
cular bone cells, and bone marrow stromal fibroblasts. Several
mutations of *SHOX* have been shown to be associated with
short stature (OMIM 312865). Ross et al. (48) used Xp deletions to identify a critical ~10 Mb region of DNA associated
with the specific TS associated neurocognitive phenotype.
The mapping and sequencing of the Y chromosome (14,15)
have revealed several genes expressed ubiquitously or in
tissues other than the testis, many of which have X-linked
homologues, which may be required in double dose for normal
development. Haplo-insufficiency of one or more of these
genes may lead to specific features of Turner syndrome (15)
and the identity of these genes will now, no doubt, be pursued.
Clearly, for normal development, either an X and a Y chromosome need to be present, or both X chromosomes need to be
active prior to X inactivation. Inactivation occurs early in
embryogenesis, roughly coinciding with the differentiation
of pluripotent cells to restricted lineages (49) and is initiated
at a region initially called XIC for X-inactivation center (50)
(for review see Ref. 51). Brown et al. (52) localized the XIST
(X inactivation-specific transcript) gene, expressed specifically from the inactive and not the active X chromosome,
to the XIC region between Xq13 and Xq21.1. The XIST gene
has now been isolated and sequenced (53). Cytogenetic
analyses have shown that the region Xq11.2-q21 is retained
in structurally abnormal X chromosomes, supporting the
observation that most structurally abnormal X chromosomes
are preferentially inactivated. Structurally abnormal X

chromosomes lacking an inactivation center could not be inactivated. Thus, nonpseudoautosomal genes on the X could potentially be expressed in more than one copy, a presumably nonviable state. The exception to this rule would appear to be females with tiny ring X chromosomes that are unable to inactivate; they have severe mental retardation and multiple congenital malformations.

6. Karyotypes

The most frequent karyotype in Turner syndrome is 45,X, which accounts for most spontaneous abortions and 40–60% of live births. However, a wide range of mosaic karyotypes are also observed, including those where the second X chromosome is structurally altered to form an isochromosome, a ring or a deletion of the long or short arm. The second most common karyotype is 46,X,i(Xq) denoting an isochromosome for the long arm. These patients have a phenotype similar to the 45,X cases. Deletions of the short arm of the X chromosome, 46,X,del(Xp), are commoner than deletions of the long arm, 46,X,del(Xq). Banding studies have shown that deletions can vary in length and position and may be both terminal and interstitial. The phenotype is variable, but includes many of the features of Turner syndrome, including streak ovaries, short stature, and primary amenorrhoea. Patients with del(Xp) tend to be taller than 45,X patients and the proportion who menstruate and may be fertile is also increased. A greater proportion of patients with del(Xq) also have menses and are possibly fertile (27). Invariably, with the exception of the small rings referred to earlier, the abnormal X chromosome is inactivated.

Observations on both ring chromosomes and deletions suggest a preferential involvement of the paternal X in structural abnormalities of the X chromosome potentially due to the absence of pairing along the XY bivalent during paternal MI. This would result in susceptibility to both structural and nondisjunctional errors during male gametogenesis. These results, together with data from previous studies, suggest that the majority of TS karyotypes are caused by paternal meiotic errors that generate abnormal sex chromosomes and that most 45,X cell lines result from mitotic loss of these abnormal sex chromosomes (45,54,55).

Patients with an isochromosome for the long arm of the X chromosome [i(Xq)] show a relatively similar distribution of male and female meiotic errors (45,56). Neither maternally or paternally derived isochromosomes are associated with an increase in parental age and at least 90% of i(Xq) contain proximal Xp sequences suggesting that centromere misdivision is not a frequent mechanism for i(Xq) formation (57). The majority of isochromosomes originate from a single X chromosome with breakpoints on the short arm ranging from the centromeric alpha-satellite to distal UBE1, a distance spanning 12 Mb. As many isochromosomes are dicentric, the most reasonable explanation is that they arise by breakage and reunion of sister-chromatids over a wide region of proximal DNA (56–60).

One group of patients requires special mention: the 45,X/46,XY mosaics who have a birth prevalence of about 1 in 25,000 (61). Their phenotype ranges from normal males, through males with cryptorchidism or penile hypospadias, and individuals with ambiguous genitalia, to females indistinguishable from Turner syndrome patients with 45,X (62). Internally, the gonads may vary from normal testes to a streak on one side and contralateral dysgenetic testis on the other to bilateral streak gonads. Gonadoblastomas or dysgerminomas occur in about 15–20% of 45,X/46,XY individuals (62). 45,X/46,XY has also been detected among true hermaphrodites. It is clear, however, from prenatally diagnosed cases that most individuals with 45,X/46,XY mosaicism are normal males. Chang et al. (63) reviewed 92 such cases. Seventy-six of these had physical examinations following delivery or termination; 75 (99%) were male and one female; four had significant genital anomalies, three males with hypospadias, and the one female, who had clitoromegaly. Three out of 11 cases, all with normal male external genitalia, had abnormal gonadal histology. These authors concluded that 95% of 45X/46,XY fetuses will have normal male external genitalia, but that a significant number will have abnormal gonadal histology. Sher et al. (64) studied two subjects with 45,X/ 46,X,r(Y); both had short stature, and subnormal linear growth rates; both had normal male external genitalia. Molecular studies showed two copies of the PAR1 gene, MIC2; SRY and other Yp genes were also present. However, significant portions of the long arm were missing suggesting breaks in Yq distal to region 5B and PAR1, and consequent rearrangement.

7. Ring X Chromosomes

The phenotype of patients with a ring X chromosome may be either severe or mild, depending on whether or not the ring contains the XIST locus and can be inactivated. Most patients with TS who have a structurally abnormal X have a mild phenotype similar to that of 45,X subjects. Patients with ring X, however, often have a more severe phenotype including mental retardation and other congenital abnormalities, which can often be ascribed to lack of inactivation of the abnormal X chromosome. Wolff et al. (65) reported absence of the X-inactivation center in patients with small marker X chromosomes and postulated that the abnormal phenotype was due to failure of dosage compensation for genes in the pericentromeric region of the X chromosome. Migeon (66) found that some rings lacked the XIST locus while others had sequences homologous to XIST probes. In the latter group, XIST was either not expressed or only minimally expressed perhaps due to a mutation. These researchers further showed that three X-linked loci, AR, TIMP, and PHK1, were expressed in rings from two patients, indicating activity of these genes. They suggested that the severe phenotype associated with these tiny rings is due to functional disomy resulting from lack of dosage compensation of genes present within the ring. Turner et al. (67) studied females with 45,X/46,X,r(X) and found 15% to have an XIST negative ring. However, only one had a severe phenotype; the rest had phenotypes consistent with TS presumably due to the mosaic nature of the karyotype. Migeon et al. (68) examined the transcriptional activity of ring X chromosomes lacking XIST expression (XISTe-) in three females. In two cases, XIST was absent from the ring chromosome; in one case, it was present but not expressed. They looked at five loci, three on the short arm and two on the long arm that were normally silent in inactivated X chromosomes and demonstrated their expression in the small ring X chromosomes. In a further study, Migeon (69) reported a patient with severe mental retardation and multiple congenital abnormalities with 45,X/46,X,del(X) (q21.3-qter)/46,X,r(X). All of the X chromosomes originated from the same maternal X, and all were shown to be transcriptionally active. None expressed XIST, although the locus and region (XIC) were present on both normal and deleted X chromosomes. Yorifuji et al. (70) analysed parental origin and inactivation status in six TS patients with mar(X) or r(X) in one cell line. Two of these patients were mentally retarded. All of the mar(X) and r(X) retained the X centromere and the XIST locus. Both patients with MR were shown to have uniparental X disomy (both X chromosomes originating from a single parent). These authors suggest that uniparental X disomy may not be uncommon in TS patients with unexplained MR.

B. 47,XXX

1. Prevalence

Jacobs et al.(71,72) were the first to report patients with trisomy for the X chromosome (47,XXX). Such females have two sex chromatin bodies in their somatic cells and invariably all of the X chromosomes in excess of one are inactivated. There is no clear-cut phenotype and no major congenital malformations. There are, however, a number of reports of renal anomalies in association with the 47,XXX karyotype (73,74). Hoang et al. (75) reported a 22-week stillborn fetus with multiple lower mesodermal defects including imperforate anus, a multicystic dysplastic horseshoe kidney, single umbilical artery, dysplastic ovaries, and uterine hypoplasia. Chromosome studies of consecutive newborn infants indicates that about 1:1000 newborn females have a 47,XXX chromosome complement (1,3).

2. Clinical Features

Follow up of 47,XXX girls detected in newborn surveys into early adolescence or young adulthood demonstrated the absence of a specific clinical phenotype (76). Of these girls, 80% were 15 years or older. Most reported good health, although about 25% had episodes of recurrent nonorganic abdominal pain as teenagers. 47,XXX girls are tall adolescents and adults with final heights generally at or above the 90th centile (171 cm). Subjects are generally underweight for height and cluster near the 60–70th centiles (59–62 kg), resulting in a tall thin appearance. Head circumference is generally reduced to the 25–35th centiles (53–54 cm), a trend that had been noted since birth. Motor milestones were delayed and the poor coordination and awkwardness seen in childhood persisted. Few 47,XXX girls participated in sports in school or in athletic activities as young adults. Menarche was established in all subjects between the ages of $11\frac{1}{2}$ and $13\frac{1}{2}$ years and they had regular periods. Nine out of 37 (24%) had become pregnant. Chromosome analysis of seven of the resulting fetuses showed all with normal chromosomes.

Most women with 47,XXX karyotypes are fertile, and many have had children. When the karyotypes of the offspring have been studied, the majority have normal 46,XY or XX karyotypes (27,38). However, there are several reports of premature ovarian failure (POF) and recurrent spontaneous abortion (RSA) in women with 47,XXX or mosaic karyotypes (77–80). Castillo et al. (81) showed that 15% of patients referred for POF (menopause prior to the age of 40 years) were mosaics with a normal cell line and an additional aneuploid line (45,X, 47,XXX, 48,XXXX) two subjects were 47,XXX and in one, there was a reciprocal translocation. Wu et al. (78) reviewed couples with a history of RSA and women with POF; X chromosome mosaicism was found in 3% of women in the group with RSA, and 8% with POF. Five women had a karyotype of 45,X/46,XX/47,XXX, four were 45,X/46,XX, and two were 46,XX/47,XXX. These last two women both had POF and RSA. Whether or not there is an increased frequency of such events in these women will have to await further long-term follow up of the consecutive series of subjects identified as newborns. However, evidence of POF among 47,XXX mosaics appears firm and should be stressed in counseling sessions (78). Several authors have suggested that this increase in POF may be due to an increased rate of germ cell attrition in women with sex chromosome anomalies (81,82). A recent study of couples who were candidates for intra-cytoplasmic sperm injection (ICSI) (83) demonstrated female as well as male constitutional chromosome abnormalities. Out of 1012 females studied, 42 out of 49 (5%) with a constitutional chromosome abnormality were mosaics for the sex chromosomes. As would be expected the majority had a 45,X cell line; however, three were 46,XX/47,XXX and one was 46,XX/48,XXXX.

3. Intelligence and Personality

Full scale IQ scores in these females tends to be around 85–90 with a range from 50 to 115. Scores are generally lower than those of sibs. Verbal language problems usually persist into adult years and a paucity of expressive language is common. Learning difficulties are frequent, with 59% of one sample (76) placed in special education classes in high school. Several girls dropped out of high school and only 8% attended college. Of the girls not in school or college, most were either unemployed or in jobs requiring unskilled labor.

Behavior among this sample was variable. Twenty-five (68%) reported no behavioral problems while the others were described as being mildly depressed, having conflict disorders or being under-socialized. Concerns for interpersonal relationships were noted and the girls appeared more vulnerable to a stressful home life than their peers or sibs. Independence from their families was achieved later than their sibs. One girl had married, many reported boyfriends, and most seemed to be adapting to their somewhat lower IQ without major problems.

A further follow up of 11 47,XXX girls as young adults (mean age 23.8 years) showed persistence of behavioral problems in some, a higher level of psychosocial stressors as compared to sibs, an increased number of psychiatric diagnoses, a lower mean full scale IQ (81 vs. 103), and a less positive relationship with their extended family. There were no significant differences between cases and sibs with respect to sexual experiences, marriage, number of pregnancies, number of living children, and incestuous experiences (84). These researchers, however, noted some trends (early consensual intercourse, <13 years, teenage pregnancies) that suggested greater sexual promiscuity in the 47,XXX group. In addition, the 47,XXX group, while showing no differences in the number of pregnancies (1.18 vs. 1.33), appeared to suffer greater reproductive casualties. Two of the 47,XXX women had been married twice in contrast to none in the sibling group (84).

The frequency of current psychiatric disorders was much higher in the 47,XXX group than among sibs (11 vs. 2) both during adolescence and in early adulthood. There was no clear trend as to a particular disorder, although affective and substance abuse disorders were predominant (84).

In summary, longitudinal follow up of women with 47,XXX during adolescence and young adulthood showed them to be less well adapted with more stressful lives; more work, leisure, and relationship problems; a lower mean full scale IQ, and more evidence of psychopathology when contrasted with a comparison group composed of female siblings. However, while many case reports have emphasized severe psychopathology and antisocial behavior in individuals with a 47,XXX karyotype, longitudinal studies such as those of Harmon et al. (84) and Evans et al. (5) suggest that extreme outcomes are rare and that variability of the behavioral phenotype is much greater than would have been expected from clinical case reports. A study by Rovet et al. (85) on an similar longitudinal sample identified through screening of a cohort of newborns, found that adaptation of 47,XXX women was better than that described by Harmon et al. (84). It should be noted, however, that the subjects in the former study were from families with a higher socioeconomic status and had higher IQ scores. The small sample size of the longitudinal studies is of concern, and it is unlikely that further such studies will be carried out in the future.

The results of these studies on 47,XXX females identified at birth in consecutive newborn studies seem to confirm the observations made on sex chromatin and chromosome studies of special populations (see Ref. 38 for review) of an increased frequency of these women in mental hospitals and in institutions for the mentally retarded. Changes in social policy regarding the care of mentally handicapped individuals over the past several decades suggests that many of these women, who would previously have been incarcerated in institutions or hospitals, will now be cared for in the community and be able to lead relatively normal lives.

4. Origin

Most 47,XXX females (65%) result from nondisjunction at maternal MI with fewer (18–26%) occurring at maternal MII or involving maternal X chromosome errors postzygotically (16%); only 4–10% are paternally derived (43,86,87). Maternal age is increased in maternal MI events, but not in paternal, MII or PZM events. Abnormalities in the number of recombination events and distribution are implicated in the etiology of 47,XXX cases (86,87).

III. SEX CHROMOSOME ABNORMALITIES IN THE MALE

A. Klinefelter Syndrome

Klinefelter et al. (7) described a syndrome in nine male patients who had gynecomastia (breast enlargement), hypogonadism with hyalinized seminiferous tubules and absent spermatogenesis, but with intact Leydig cells. There was increased secretion of urinary gonadotrophins to levels found in castrated males, but no increase in estrogen production. This syndrome is now well established in clinical practice and is one of the most frequent causes of male infertility. The phenotype is variable with the most outstanding feature being the presence of small testes with hyalinized tubules that fail to enlarge at puberty (88).

Numerous studies in the late 1950s and early 1960s demonstrated that the frequency of a chromatin positive finding among male newborns was approximately 1 in 500 (38). Similar studies in mentally subnormal and mental hospital populations showed the frequency ranged from about 1 in 80 to 1 in 170 men studied. It was originally suggested that these chromatin positive males were sex-reversed females with a 46,XX chromosome complement. The observation that chromatin positive males with small testes had a 47,XXY chromosome complement (9,10) demonstrated clearly that these were true males with an aneuploid sex chromosome complement and not sex-reversed females.

1. Prevalence

More reliable data based on karyotyping of 56,952 unselected newborn infants in six studies worldwide indicate that approximately 1 in 1000 newborn males have a 47,XXY sex chromosome complement (1,3). Since most of these studies confined their analysis to two cells (2), some instances of mosaicism will have been missed. A recent analysis of data in the Danish Cytogenetic Central Registry for the period 1970–2000 showed that the frequency of 47,XXY in prenatally karyotyped male fetuses was 1 in 470 (89). Postnatally, only 1 in 2500 had a 47,XXY karyotype (89). Fewer than 10% of cases anticipated by the newborn frequency data were diagnosed before puberty, indicating a significant under diagnosis of Klinefelter syndrome. This is not surprising given that the major features of the syndrome only become apparent at puberty.

2. Clinical and Behavioral Phenotype

The original clinical description by Klinefelter et al. (7) is now known to be the most extreme phenotype that results from a 47,XXY karyotype (Fig. 4). Follow up of 105 boys with a 47,XXY karyotype, identified in six newborn studies worldwide, provides the best series of unselected patients (76). The boys and young men, who ranged in age from 10 to 24

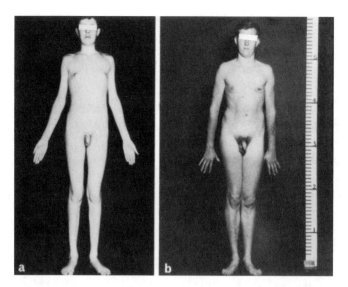

Figure 4   Two patients with Klinefelter syndrome, 47,XXY. (a) Age 15 years: Note absence of pubic hair, eunuchoid proportions and slight breast development, otherwise normal external genitalia. (b) Age 21 years: Feminine distribution of pubic hair, mastectomy scar under left nipple, and slight gynecomastia on right. (From Ref. 38.)

years, tended to be taller than sib controls with mean heights at the 75th centile. Individual heights ranged from the 25th to the 99th centile. Weight and head circumference were closer to the 50th centile. These individuals tended to be awkward and have mild neuromotor deficits. Most of these boys entered puberty normally; however, there was a tendency for testosterone levels to drop off in late adolescence and early adulthood. In all cases, the testes were small, but penis size was within normal limits. At the time of the study, no evidence of fertility had been reported in any of these subjects. Eleven were reported to have gynecomastia. An accurate assessment of the frequency of this feature will become available as the remainder pass through adolescence and into adulthood.

47,XXY boys generally have lower IQs than controls with average full scale IQs falling between 85 and 90. A wide range of IQs has been noted extending from well below to well above average. Verbal IQ is often lower than performance IQ. Lower IQs tend to be associated with learning problems, and are consistent across all studies. 47,XXY boys have tended to require special help at school, especially in reading and spelling. Not all learning problems were severe, and at the time of the follow up (1991), 10 (~10%) of the young men were in college or planning to attend college. These XXY males were described as shy, immature, restrained, and reserved, and the formation of peer relationships had been problematic. In early adulthood, none were yet married although several reported having girl friends. Most did not have any significant psychiatric disturbance, although difficulties with psychosocial adjustment appeared to be increased.

Further follow up of 19 boys from the Edinburgh series by Ratcliffe (90) found an increased growth spurt between 5 and 8 years owing to greater leg growth, and 75% had some degree of central obesity. A minority had a small penis at birth. Testes were initially normal in size and consistency, but failed to grow normally. At the onset of puberty at 11.9 years, testes enlarged to only around 5 mL in volume except for two boys where there was enlargement to 12 mL. By the end of puberty, the penis was of normal size in 77% of boys and pubic hair had progressed to Tanner stage 6 (91). Adolescent gynecomastia was observed in 56%, but was usually transient lasting 1–3 years; as expected, it was also frequent in controls (36%). Testosterone levels were normal during childhood and started to rise at puberty; however, by age 16, they were significantly lower than controls. Gonadotrophins became elevated 6 months after the onset of puberty. Delayed speech development was more common than in controls with 42% requiring speech therapy. The mean WISC verbal scores of 94 (range 65–129) and performance scores of 98 (range 75–128) were significantly lower than controls. Reading difficulties were experienced by 77%, requiring remedial help. Mathematical ability was also poorer, as was short and long-term memory. The two boys with the highest IQ scores had obtained university degrees. This potential for high performance bears out Becker's observations from a clinic-based population of Klinefelter syndrome males that included physicians, engineers, ministers, and accountants (92).

Kamischke et al. (93) evaluated 309 patients suspected of having Klinefelter syndrome: 28% were 47,XXY and 72% had a normal male chromosome complement. Higher proportions of patients with 47,XXY had lower educational backgrounds, were taller, and had smaller testis volume, higher levels of FSH and LH, a less androgenic phenotype and secondary hair distribution than patients with 46,XY. No differences were found in testosterone, estradiol, sex hormone binding globulin (SHBG), prostate specific antigen (PSA) levels, or prostate volume between the two groups. In the group with XXY, 93% were azoospermic compared to 54% of those with 46,XY.

In summary, the original description of the Klinefelter phenotype fits only a relatively small proportion of those with a 47,XXY karyotype. The majority of patients will, however, have low testicular volume with specific histology, azoospermia, and elevated gonadotrophins. A proportion will have gynecomastia. Individuals with Klinefelter syndrome may have learning difficulties, require special help in school and have a slightly lower IQ than their peers. However, most will lead normal adult lives, marry and have children through donor insemination. Boys with a supportive and understanding family background are likely to do better than those living in a less structured environment. With the advent of assisted reproductive technologies such as ICSI, patients who produce a few sperm may be able to father children. Patients suspected on clinical grounds to have Klinefelter syndrome, but who prove to be 46,XY, require further evaluation of their male infertility. In appropriate cases, this could include additional cytogenetic studies to rule out mosaicism or Y-chromosome microdeletions.

3. Origin

Jacobs et al. (94) studied nondisjunction in males with 47,XXY karyotypes. Fifty-three percent were attributable to paternal MI errors, 34% to maternal MI errors, and 9% to maternal MII errors. Three percent were due to PZM events. In the majority of maternal errors, there was clear evidence of recombination involving the nondisjoined chromosomes, suggesting that failure to recombine is not a major factor in nondisjunction of the X chromosomes in female meiosis. Maternal age was significantly increased among the maternally derived XXY cases, associated primarily with those with MI errors. Paternal age was not increased in paternally derived cases. Thomas et al. (95) investigated the nondisjunctional event in paternally derived 47,XXY males using polymorphisms within PAR1. Among informative results, 16% showed single crossovers, 2% had a double crossover, and 83% had no evidence of a crossover. Thus, most XXY males of paternal origin result from a meiosis in which the X and Y chromosomes fail to recombine. There was no association with recombination frequencies in the smaller PAR2 region, or with the presence of microdeletions within PAR1.

4. Treatment of Patients with Klinefelter
   Syndrome

There are three potential areas of treatment that may be important in enabling men with 47,XXY to lead normal lives. These are (i) treatment of endocrine problems starting before and continuing through puberty, (ii) treatment of behavioral problems and learning difficulties during adolescence, and (iii) treatment of infertility. Winter (96) suggested that, from the beginning of adolescence around 12 years, all 47,XXY males should receive supplementary androgen therapy, in increasing dosage sufficient to maintain age-appropriate serum concentrations of testosterone, estradiol, FSH, and LH. Benefits should include prevention of pathological gynecomastia and eunuchoid body habitus, together with more subtle effects on osteoporosis, autoimmune disease, self-esteem, energy, interpersonal relationships, and libido. Winter (96) cautioned that this recommendation should be balanced against the difficulty of evaluating the degree of benefit that may be achieved given the variable expression and persistence of adolescent gynecomastia, and the strong placebo effect of any form of therapy on the psychosexual parameters. Manning and Hoyme (97) consider treatment options to include testosterone replacement for the correction of androgen deficiency and the tailoring of school curricula to address specific learning problems. They point out that, while most boys with Klinefelter syndrome do not differ much from their peers, several features of the syndrome should be carefully monitored. Visootsak et al. (98) in a review aimed at the primary care giver, point out that the primary care physician has an important role in the care of patients with Klinefelter syndrome and their families by providing anticipatory guidance on issues relating to endocrinology, behavior, development, and preventative medical care, and can serve as a valuable source of support for the family of a boy with Klinefelter syndrome.

Behavioral problems and learning difficulties often, but not always, accompanied by a lower IQ need to be recognized and treated by appropriate remedial action and assistance in school. Appropriate referrals to psychological or psychiatric services should be provided where necessary. However, as shown by Bojesen et al. (89) and Abramsky and Chapple (99) many patients with Klinefelter syndrome are not diagnosed until well after puberty when the main features of the syndrome become apparent. Such patients are likely to be diagnosed due to psychosocial or behavioral problems or because of infertility. Failure to achieve early diagnosis in a significant number of patients makes the initiation of treatment at the most appropriate time difficult.

Klinefelter syndrome is one of the commoner causes of male infertility, occurring in about 8% of patients (96). Males with 47,XXY are invariably infertile, either as the result of azoospermia or oligospermia. In some cases, small numbers of sperm are produced, but only rarely has there been indisputable evidence of paternity (27) without the aid of assisted reproductive techniques. The advent of ICSI has allowed a few patients with Klinefelter syndrome to father biological children (100–108). Most of the children conceived after assisted fertilization have normal chromosomes; however,

Ron-El et al. (101) reported a 47,XXY fetus following ICSI using spermatozoa from a 47,XXY nonmosaic patient. Kitamura et al. (108) reported two fetal losses following ICSI in addition to one healthy infant with normal chromosomes. Several authors have assessed the level of sex chromosome aneuploidy in sperm nuclei using FISH. Foresta et al. (109) showed an abnormal distribution of sperm chromosome complements in an XXY male with an increase in 24,XY disomic sperm and a reduction in 23,Y sperm. Rives et al. (103) showed that the frequency of XX and YY disomic, XY hyperhaploid and diploid spermatozoa was significantly increased in the 47,XXY male compared to both infertile and fertile 46,XY males. There was also an increase in chromosome 12 disomy. Hennebicq et al. (110) observed a similar increase in XX and YY sperm in a 47,XXY male, but also showed an increase in sperm with 21 disomy, suggesting a possibly higher risk for Down syndrome following ICSI using sperm from this individual. It is clear from these studies that the use of ICSI to alleviate the infertility problems of males with Klinefelter syndrome may carry other genetic risks to the fetus. Such procedures should be accompanied by appropriate genetic counseling and monitoring of subsequent pregnancies or the use of preimplantation genetic diagnosis so that only blastocysts with normal chromosomes are implanted.

Yamamoto et al. (111) used the sensitive quantitative telomerase assay (SQTA) to assess sperm production in nonmosaic 47,XXY males and demonstrated that men with higher levels of protein had a greater chance of producing testicular spermatozoa than those with lower protein levels. Mroz et al. (112) examined the expression of X-linked genes in the germ cells from male XXY mice and showed expression of both parental alleles in germ cell enriched cell populations. They concluded that correct X chromosome dosage is essential for normal fertility of male mammals and demonstrated abnormalities in germ cell development in an XXY testis within several days of X reactivation. Germ cells that survived in the postnatal XXY testis were exclusively XY and resulted from secondary nondisjunctional events giving rise to clones of XY cells.

B. 47,XYY Males

Interest in 47,XYY was initially stimulated by reports of an increased frequency of XYY males in institutions for the criminally insane (113,114). These observations led to significant controversy and discussion as to whether the Y chromosome conferred susceptibility to criminal behaviour (115–118). It is now clear that this is not so. In fact, the XYY state results in little phenotypic change and most such males lead normal lives.

1. Prevalence and Phenotype

Newborn chromosome studies revealed that about 1 in 1000 males carry an extra Y chromosome (1,3). Follow up of 39 boys and young men between the ages of 10 and 22 years (76) revealed a normal phenotype, with the majority being tall and thin with heights over the 75th centile. Head circumferences were closer to the 50th centile. A tendency to awkwardness and minor motor deficits was noted. Puberty was slightly later than controls (+6 months). Pubertal development was normal and one young man had fathered a child with normal chromosomes. Full scale IQ was within normal limits between 80 and 140, but was slightly lower than in sibs and controls. Speech delay was common and learning difficulties were present in about half of the boys. Distractibility, hyperactivity, and temper tantrums have been present in some cases during childhood. In adolescence, 47,XYY boys frequently have low frustration tolerance, but as they get older they learn to control anger. Evidence from this relatively small unselected sample suggests that the phenotype is variable and is readily influenced by the kind of environment and the support systems to which these individuals are exposed.

Several studies have examined the existence of a relationship between the 47,XYY karyotype and a tendency to criminal behavior. Witkin et al. (118,119) examined a large cross-section of the Danish male population born in Copenhagen. They identified 31,436 males born in 1944–1947, of whom 28,884 (92%) were still alive at the commencement of the study. Studying the surviving men with a height

≥184 cm, they detected 12 with 47,XYY (1 in 345) and 16 with 47,XXY (1 in 256). Danish laws allowed examination of criminal records, army selection test results (BPP) undergone by all Danish males by the age of 26, an educational index, and a seven point parental socioeconomic index (SES). A significantly higher proportion ($p < 0.01$) of both the XYY (42%) and XXY (19%) men had criminal records, mainly for minor property related offenses unrelated to aggression, compared to 9% of XY controls. XYY and XXY males showed lower scores on the BPP and educational index than did controls. No difference was observed in the parental SES between the groups. Both XYY and XXY males were taller than the controls ($p < 0.001$), but there was no evidence that this increase in height was related to the increase in criminality. As both XYY and XXY males showed lower BBP and educational index scores, it seems plausible that lower intellectual abilities may be related to the increase in what might be termed petty criminality. Additional studies on this same population (120) showed that the XYY males had higher levels of LH, FSH, and testosterone than controls, while XXY males had higher LH and FSH, but lower levels of testosterone. No differences were found in testicular volume and in numbers of children between XYY males and controls, while, as expected, XXY males had smaller testes and fewer children. Fryns et al. (121) reviewed 75 patients with an extra Y chromosome diagnosed among 98,725 male and female patients referred for chromosome studies largely because of mental retardation or multiple congenital anomalies. Fifty of these had an XYY karyotype, a similar frequency to the newborn studies. The main indication for karyotyping in this group was the presence of mental retardation or problems of psychosocial integration and psychiatric problems. Hunter (122) found 12 males with XYY karyotypes in 1811 male patients (1 in 151) in hospitals for the mentally handicapped. The main psychiatric findings were diminished intelligence, delay in development of secondary sexual characteristics, and poor emotional control leading to inadequate social adaptive patterns.

In conclusion, it seems that 47,XYY males generally show lower mean intelligence scores and poorer social adaptation, although IQ scores overlap the normal range. There is some evidence of speech delay and learning difficulties. While distractibility, hyperactivity, and temper tantrums may occur in childhood and XYY adolescents frequently have low frustration tolerance, there seems to be little evidence of aggressive tendencies as reported in the original studies. Criminal tendencies, when present, are of a relatively minor nature involving acts against property rather than persons and are most likely related to the overall lower intelligence and social functioning.

2. Origin

Nondisjunction that results in 47,XYY males can occur at only two times during development: paternal meiosis II (pat MII) or as a PZM (123). In theory, there are three types of disjunctional error: (i) nondisjunction at pat MII following a normal MI with recombination between the X and Y (MII-C), (ii) nondisjunction at pat MII after a failure of chiasma formation at MI (MII-NC), or (iii) postzygotic mitotic nondisjunction (PZM). By analyzing DNA polymorphisms at the distal tip of PAR1, Robinson and Jacobs (123) showed that in 84% of XYY males, nondisjunction occurred at MII-C, while three were either MII-NC or PZM. For an additional nine cases where no parental DNA was available, at least four were due to MII-C events. Thus, most 47,XYY males result from nondisjunction of the two Y chromatids at MII, following normal PAR1 recombination of the X and Y chromosomes during MI.

IV. X AND Y CHROMOSOME POLYSOMY
IN MALES AND FEMALES

Examples of patients with sex chromosome tetrasomy and pentasomy (48,XXXX, 49,XXXXX, 48,XXYY, 48,XXXY, 49,XXXXY, 49,XXXYY, 48,XYYY, 49,XYYYY) are rare and have been reviewed recently by Linden et al. (124) (Fig. 5). In general, patients with multiple sex chromosome anomalies are more severely affected than trisomic individuals. The fact

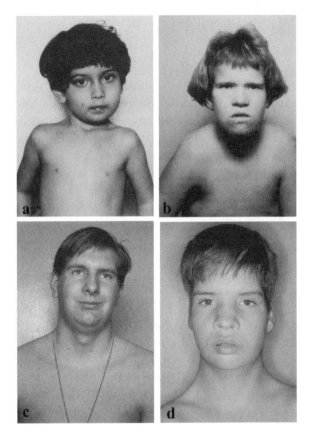

Figure 5 Patients with X chromosome polysomy (a) 48,XXXX; (b) 49,XXXXX; (c) 48,XXXY; (d) 49,XXXXY. (From Ref. 124.)

that all of these patients survived gestation and that sex chromosome polysomies are not found in any significant numbers among spontaneous abortions indicates a lower level of genetic imbalance than that found in autosomal trisomies, the majority of which are eliminated during gestation. Presumably, this is due to inactivation of all the X chromosomes in excess of one. All of these patients have been ascertained as clinical referrals due to their disabilities. This results in a potential for ascertainment bias towards more severely affected patients. These are rare conditions occurring in fewer than 1 in 10,000 births and, in some cases, perhaps as low as 1 in 100,000 births.

A. Tetrasomy X

Carr (125) described the first two cases of 48,XXXX (Fig. 5a). Approximately 40 cases were described up to 1995 (124). As with 47,XXX, there is no consistent clinical or behavioral phenotype in these cases. Patients had a mean height of 169 cm; facial dysmorphism was usually minor with reports of epicanthic folds, hypertelorism, and nystagmus. Genitalia were usually normal, but development of secondary sexual characteristics was incomplete in some cases. About one-half of the adult women reported normal menarche and menopause, while the other one-half had menstrual dysfunction. Three women have reproduced, two with healthy children, one with a child with trisomy 21.

Mental retardation was frequent with a mean IQ of 60 (range 30–75). Speech and language defects were common with articulation defects and delays in both expressive and receptive language. There was no consistent behavioral phenotype, but about one-half, the women were reported to have had periods of unstable behavior, described as angry, disruptive, and inappropriate (124).

B. Pentasomy X

Patients with five X chromosomes (49,XXXXX) are less common than those with four and are more severely affected (see Fig. 5b). The first such patient was reported in 1963 (126) and up to 1995 about 25 additional patients had been described, none older than 16 years of age (124). All patients were mentally retarded, had short stature, coarse facial features and skeletal and limb anomalies. Intrauterine and postnatal growth retardation were common. Craniofacial anomalies included microcephaly, hypertelorism, epicanthic folds, upslanting palpebral fissures, a depressed and/or broad nasal bridge and a short broad neck. Congenital heart defects, usually patent ductus arteriosus or ventricular septal defect, were common. Skeletal defects included bilateral clinodactyly of the hands and feet, radio-ulnar synostosis, generalized joint laxity with multiple dislocations, and talipes equinovarus. Several girls have been noted to have a small uterus.

All of these girls were mentally retarded with an average IQ of 50 (range 20–75). Speech was delayed and communication difficult. No distinctive behavioral profile has emerged. Most were said to be shy and cooperative.

C. Klinefelter Variants

The 48,XXYY karyotype is the most common variant of Klinefelter syndrome (124). It was first reported by Muldahl and Ockey (127), and Court Brown et al. (128) and subsequently several 48,XXYY males were found in institutions for the criminally insane (113,114,129,130). Approximately 120 cases worldwide had been reported up to 1995, with about one-third being ascertained during institutional surveys. The incidence is estimated to be about 1 in 50,000 male births (131). 48,XXYY males are usually tall with an adult height >171 cm and a eunuchoid habitus with long thin legs. Hypergonadotrophic hypogonadism is similar to XXY men. Serum FSH and LH levels are increased, and testosterone levels decreased. Small testes and sparse body hair are common. About one-half have a micropenis. Testicular histology is similar to Klinefelter syndrome (124).

Mild mental retardation is a common finding, with IQs ranging from 60 to 80. However, about 10% have IQs above 80 and values ranging up to 110 have been reported. Speech delay is often noted with receptive skills better than expressive skills. Behavior is often shy and reserved, but reports of impulsive and aggressive tendencies are more typical. However, it should be noted that many of the karyotypes were performed because of behavioral problems, leading to a potential ascertainment bias (124). It is generally assumed, however, that psychosocial development and behavior are more disturbed than in 47,XXY males.

Five cases of 49,XXXYY have been reported (124), one of which was diagnosed prenatally and terminated (132). Three adult males were all moderate to severely mentally retarded.

Physical features include normal to tall stature, facial dysmorphism, gynecomastia, and hypogonadism. Behavior was described as generally passive with occasional outbursts and aggression. A fifth case was diagnosed at 12 months because of hypotonia and developmental delay. His height was at the 75th centile, weight at the 50th centile and head circumference at the 98th centile. Dysmorphic features included a prominent forehead, broad nasal bridge, epicanthic folds, posteriorly rotated ears, and micrognathia. Magnetic resonance imaging indicated ventricular enlargement and deficient white matter in the frontal lobes. There were some skeletal abnormalities and genitalia were small. Behavioral concerns included some repetitive autistic-like behaviors, low frustration tolerance, and resultant temper tantrums (124).

48,XXXY males (Fig. 5c) were first reported in 1959 by Barr et al. (133) and, until 1995, about 50 cases had been described (124). Most were ascertained in the 1960s and 1970s through studies of patients in hospitals for the mentally retarded or mentally ill, and thus there may be significant bias in ascertainment. Few cases have been reported in recent years. Patients are considered to be a variant of Klinefelter syndrome with generally more pronounced features. Stature is normal to tall; hypertelorism and epicanthic folds are common. Skeletal anomalies include clinodactyly, abnormalities of the elbows, and radio-ulnar synostosis. Subjects are infertile with hypogonadotrophic hypogonadism and testicular histology similar to 47,XXY. About a quarter of the patients have a micropenis. Patients are usually mildly to moderately retarded with IQs in the 20–76 range, most in the 40–60 range (124). Behavior is often immature for chronological age, but consistent with the level of intelligence. Patients are described as passive, placid, pleasant, and cooperative. Aggressive behaviour is rarely observed (124).

After the first case was reported in 1960 (134), about 100 other 49,XXXXY males (Fig. 5d) had been reported by 1995 (124). The phenotype is more severe than other Klinefelter variants with coarse facies, skeletal anomalies, cardiac anomalies, hypogonadism, and small genitalia (124). Severe mental retardation is also characteristic of 49,XXXXY males with a mean IQ estimated to be 35 (135). Generally, there is severe retardation of language development characterized by poor speech fluency. Nonverbal skills are greater than verbal.

Behavior of these males is described as shy to friendly. However, periods of irritability are not uncommon and episodic temper tantrums may occur. They may have a low frustration tolerance. Some of these men have been able to function in semisupervised settings, but most were ascertained through institutional surveys.

D. Males with Three or Four Y Chromosomes

Polysomy Y conditions are rare. In total, 12 cases have been reported in the literature; eight 48,XYYY, three 49,XYYYY, and one 49,XXYYY (124). The first case of 48,XYYY reported was a five-year-old boy, ascertained because of psychomotor retardation (136). As with 47,XYY, there is no consistent phenotype. Most of the adults are tall, and have minor malformations such as transverse palmar creases, clinodactyly, and abnormal teeth. Genitalia are normal, but five out of the six adults had hypogonadism with azoospermia. Development was delayed, especially with respect to motor and speech development. IQs were in the low normal range with a range of 60–86. Behavior has been characterized by impulsivity and low frustration tolerance, with occasional aggressive outbursts and poor emotional stability (124).

The three 49,XYYYY boys were ascertained at birth because of the presence of dysmorphic features, including facial anomalies, skeletal anomalies, mental retardation, motor retardation with hypotonia, and speech delay. Similar behavioral characteristics to 48,XYYY have been recorded. Three additional cases have been reported since 1995 (137–139). Recently, DesGroseilliers et al. (139) reported a two-year-old boy with a mosaic karyotype 45,X/47,X,idic(Y)(q12),idic(Y)(q12), the predominant cell line having two isodicentric Y chromosomes. This boy was referred because of global psychomotor delay. He had an atrioseptal defect, brachycephaly, epicanthic folds, bilateral radio-ulnar synostosis, clinodactyly, and premature closure of the anterior fontanelle. The breakpoints were at Yq12 at probe DYZ1, Yp telomeres were shown to be present, but not Yq telomeres, suggesting a U type exchange. One similar case has been reported (137). The single 49,XXYYY boy reported had facial dysmorphism and mental retardation (140). Most recently, a case of 49,XYYYY was diagnosed prenatally and terminated at 24 weeks gestation. Postmortem examination showed a male fetus measuring 34 cm in length with no major abnormalities. The gonads were described as normal male. Brain weight was 115 gm with a hypoplastic corpus callosum and small cerebellum containing a large cyst blocking the aqueduct of Sylvius. The ventricular system was symmetrically enlarged (141).

E. Origin

Hassold et al. (142) used DNA markers to determine the origin of the extra X chromosomes in eight individuals with four or five sex chromosomes. With one exception, each parent contributed a single sex chromosome, either X or Y, while the other parent contributed three or four sex chromosomes, suggesting that many of these cases may be due to successive nondisjunctional events in one parent. The single exception was a case of uniparental maternal tetrasomy in a 48,XXXX individual in which all the X chromosomes were derived from the mother; no paternal sex chromosome was detected.

V. SEX CHROMOSOMES AND SEX DETERMINATION

The initial observation that individuals with a 45,X chromosome constitution were females (11) and that subjects carrying a Y chromosome, no matter how many X chromosomes were present, were males (10), clearly implicated genes carried by the Y chromosome in the process of sex determination in humans. Similar findings in the mouse and other mammalian species indicated that mammals, unlike *Drosophila*, had an XX/XY sex determining mechanism.

A. 46,XX Males and 46,XY Females

Originally described by De la Chapelle et al. (143), sex-reversed 46,XX males are important variants of Klinefelter syndrome, but, along with 46,XY females with gonadal dysgenesis, have been valuable in the molecular dissection of the genetic pathways that normally lead the bipotential embryonic gonad to develop into either a testis or an ovary (OMIM 480000) (144–146).

De la Chapelle (27) suggested that 1 in 25,000 newborn males has a 46,XX karyotype and that, in series of patients with Klinefelter syndrome, the incidence is 1 in 25. The clinical phenotype is similar to that of Klinefelter syndrome, except that XX males are shorter than XXY males and perhaps less prone to mental impairment (Fig. 6). Otherwise, the features are similar, with normal external genitalia and small testes with the same histological changes. Secondary sexual characteristics, hormonal status, and rates of gynecomastia and sterility are similar to 47,XXY subjects. Some 46,XX individuals are true hermaphrodites with both infertile testes and ovaries or ovotestis. In some males, there may be some ambiguity in the external genitalia.

Females with pure gonadal dysgenesis can have either XY or XX sex chromosomes. They have dysgenesis of the gonads, sexual infantilism, normal to tall stature, and lack the other stigmata of Turner syndrome. A study of 299 patients evaluated for primary amenorrhoea (62) identified 125 patients with gonadal dysgenesis (42%). Most of this group were 45,X or 45,X mosaics, but 29% of were XX and 9% were XY. Thus, over one-third of patients with primary ovarian hypergonadotrophic hypogonadism had gonadal dysgenesis with 46,XX or 46,XY karyotypes.

Ferguson-Smith (147) was the first to suggest a reciprocal X–Y chromosome interchange as the mode of origin of these 46,XX males. De la Chapelle et al. (148) reported a Finnish pedigree with three affected males. These men and their mother were found to express the H-Y antigen, which, at that time, was postulated to be the testis-determining gene. Their father expressed an excess of H-Y, suggesting that the H-Y

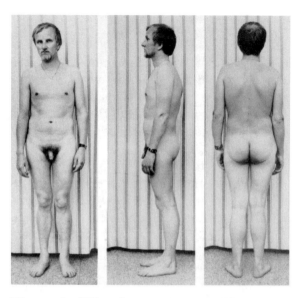

Figure 6 XX male, age 29 years. Note normal appearance, small testes, ascertainment infertility. (From Ref. 27.)

structural loci constituted a family of testis-determining genes, and that either dominant or recessive modes of XX sex reversal can be produced by Y-autosome or Y–X translocations (OMIM 278850). In 1986, Andersson et al. (149) demonstrated transfer of Y-specific DNA sequences to Xpter in three XX males. By studying XX males with a translocation of Yp material to Xp and XY females with a deletion of Yp, Simpson et al. (150) were able to separate the loci for H-Y, now known to map near the centromere or proximal Yq, from the testis-determining factor mapping distally to Yp. Molecular examination of sex-reversed subjects in the early 1990s led to the identification of the sex-determining region (SRY) in a 35 kb region of Y-specific DNA adjacent to the PAR1 boundary (17,151) (Fig. 1). It is now clear that a majority of human 46,XX males have a trans-location of Y sequences, including SRY, that are located close to the boundary of PAR1, to the tip of the X chromosome (146, 152,153). However, 10–20% of 46,XX males lack any evidence of Y sequences in their genomes so that some other cause for their sex reversal must be sought (154–157). Cotinot et al. (153) and Vilain (158) identify no fewer than 10 loci, all transcription factors, growth factors, or signaling molecules, on eight different chromosomes that are directly responsible for the decision to form either a testis or ovary, four of which—SRY, SOX9, DMRT1, and FGF9—are considered crucial for testis formation and seminiferous cord organization. Even less is known about the origin of 46,XY females (Fig. 7). Cotinot et al. (153) estimates that about 15% of 46,XY females carry mutations in SRY or more rarely in SOX9, SF1, DMRT1, or DAX1 (158).

SRY is a transcription factor whose function is to initiate testicular differentiation in mammalian embryogenesis. The protein contains a high mobility group box (HMG), a DNA binding motif conserved among a broad class of nuclear proteins. Almost all of the published mutations associated with sex reversal in 46,XY females are located in the HMG box and affect the structure of the DNA binding domain (146). Other loci involved in XY sex reversal include SOX9 at 17q24, a transcription factor whose duplication leads to XX sex reversal, while mutations lead to XY gonadal dysgenesis and campomelic dysplasia. Mutations in SF1 at 9q33 result in adrenal insufficiency and XY gonadal dysgenesis. Mutations in DMRT1 at 9p24 result in XY gonadal dysgenesis. Mutations at the DAX1 locus, an antitestis gene at Xp21.3, result in congenital adrenal hypoplasia, while duplications of a 160 kb region result in XY gonadal dysgenesis (158). Clearly, extensive genetic heterogeneity exists in both XX and XY sex reversal. The process of sex determination is clearly highly complex and only partially understood (153,158–160).

VI. Y CHROMOSOME ABNORMALITIES AND FERTILITY

Sex chromosome aneuploidy, with the exception of 47,XXX and 47,XYY, generally leads to impaired fertility. Clearly, either two X chromosomes or one X and one Y are required for normal sexual development. Having a single X chromosome leads to significant lethality during gestation and those

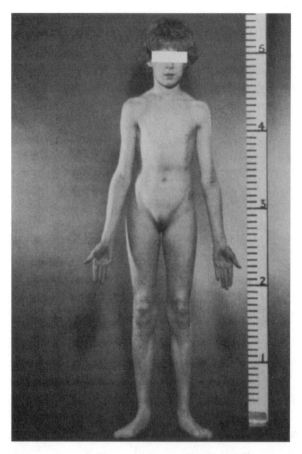

Figure 7 Patient with 46,XY gonadal dysgenesis: Age 17 years, normal stature, absence of secondary sexual characteristics. (From Ref. 38.)

fetuses that do survive to term are generally infertile as adults. The Y chromosome is not required for survival, but is essential for the normal development of the testis, including the formation of seminiferous tubules, the migration of the germ cells into the tubules, and their maturation to form spermatozoa. Initially, it was thought that the Y chromosome was only required to ensure that the bipotential gonad developed into a testis. In 1976, however, Tiepolo and Zuffardi (161) reported that the Y chromosome was also involved in the control of spermatogenesis. They observed deletions including Yq12–Yq11 in six sterile males. Two of the fathers had normal Y chromosomes suggesting a de novo event and a causal relationship. These authors postulated that a genetic factor located at Yq11 was important in male germ cell development. This gene or gene cluster was named the "azoospermia factor" (AZF). Molecular mapping of the Y chromosome in infertile men has revealed three nonoverlapping deletions, termed *AZFa* in Yq11.21, *AZFb* in Yq11.22, and *AZFc* in Yq11.23 in the euchromatic portion of the long arm (162–164). Several candidate genes for the AZF phenotype have now been identified in these regions (165).

Foresta et al. (165) reported that of 4868 infertile men studied between 1991 and 2000, 1 in 12 carried a Y chromosome microdeletion, compared to only 1 in 221 of 2663 fertile males. Among the studies cited, the prevalence varied from 1% to 35% reflecting different patient selection criteria. The highest frequencies of deletions were found in idiopathic oligospermia ($< 5 \times 10^6$ per mL) (14%), idiopathic azoospermia (18%), idiopathic severe hypospermatogenesis (24.7%), and idiopathic Sertoli cell only syndrome (35%). Thus, careful selection of patients to include only idiopathic cases will increase the likelihood of finding Yq deletions. No correlation was observed between the location of the deletion (*AZFa,b,c,*) and the clinical phenotype. The variability of the phenotype may be explained by the size of the deletions, the deletion of specific genes or gene clusters affecting different testicular or spermatogenic functions, the role of homologous genes located elsewhere in the genome, and the genetic background. The recent discovery of eight massive palindromic sequences in the MSY which are recombinogenic and appear to be maintained by frequent gene conversion—"the nonreciprocal transfer of information between one DNA duplex to another" (166)—has already allowed investigators to identify four distinct classes of recurrent MSY deletions, identify the absent genes as a result of these deletions, typically members of testis-specific gene families, and demonstrate that most such deletions are due to homologous recombination between near-identical segments of DNA (15,167–171). Evidently, microde-

letions and other rearrangements of Yq (Fig. 1) are relatively
frequent and play a significant role in male infertility.
Furthermore, these deletions have little effect on general
health, and would normally behave as classical genetic lethal
dominant mutations arising de novo in each generation, only
rarely being transmitted to male offspring.

The advent of assisted reproduction techniques means
that many couples, who would otherwise be infertile, are
now able to have children (165,172–174). Infertility is a major
health problem affecting 10–15% of couples attempting to conceive. About one-half of these situations result from a problem
in the male partner (175). The advent of ICSI and testicular
sperm extraction (TESA) allows transmission of these Y
microdeletions to males in the next generation, potentially
causing an increase in their frequency and a concomitant rise
in infertility in future generations. It is becoming increasingly
accepted that candidates for these assisted reproductive techniques should be screened for these deletions. When deletions
are found, families should be counseled that any male
offspring will be carrying the same deletion and therefore
likely to be infertile. This whole area raises a number of
ethical issues that will be discussed below.

VII. SEX CHROMOSOME ANOMALIES AND NEOPLASIA

With a few key exceptions, malignancy rates are not
increased in patients with SCA. One of these exceptions is
the risk for breast cancer among patients with 47,XXY.
Hulthorn et al. (176) showed a prevalence rate of 7.5% of
Klinefelter syndrome among males with breast cancer in
western Sweden and estimated the relative risk of XXY males
to be 49 times that of XY males and 0.3 times that of females.
This is a much higher figure than that reported in other
studies, which suggested an increased risk of about three to
four percent (177–179), i.e., a relative risk of about 20 times
that of XY males and about one-fifth of that of women (177).
Price et al. (180) reviewed the causes of death among 466

chromatin positive males who had been studied prospectively over 25 years. Among other causes of mortality was a small but nonsignificant increase in the numbers of deaths from breast cancer. Deaths from cardiovascular and respiratory diseases were also greatly increased ($p < 0.01$–0.0001); this was particularly evident in 47,XXY males first ascertained in psychiatric hospitals.

46,XY females with gonadal dysgenesis also have a significantly increased risk of developing tumors in the streak gonads, particularly gonadoblastomas, dysgerminomas, and juvenile granulosa cell tumors. Hamerton (38) reviewed the clinical findings in 20 patients with 46,XY gonadal dysgenesis and reported eight to have some form of gonadal malignancy, most frequently a gonadoblastoma. More recently, Radakovic (181) performed bilateral gonadectomies on 20 patients with 46,XY gonadal dysgenesis, and found 11 with gonadoblastomas or other streak gonad tumors. Based on the high frequency of gonadoblastomas in 46,XY females, the presence of a gonadoblastoma susceptibility gene (GBY) on the Y chromosome has been postulated (182,183). Molecular analysis of the Y chromosome in patients with XY gonadal dysgenesis and gonadal tumors found various deletions, missense mutations, or nucleotide substitutions in SRY in four of six patients (184,185). However, as deletions or mutations of SRY are known to be one of the etiological factors in XY gonadal dysgenesis, it is probable that the association between SRY and a high frequency of gonadoblastoma and other germ cell tumors is indirect. A more promising candidate for GBY may lie in a 4 Mb region in the proximal part of Yq that Salo et al. (186) identified as a region of overlap in two patients with gonadoblastoma who were carrying small marker chromosomes. While the precise molecular basis for their increased risk of gonadal tumors remains unknown, patients with XY gonadal dysgenesis obviously require detailed counseling and should be offered preventative gonadectomy.

Association of the 47,XYY state with various forms of leukemia have been reported in the literature (187–192), although there is little evidence that these are more than chance associations.

VIII. GENETIC COUNSELING AND SEX CHROMOSOME ANOMALIES

Sex chromosome anomalies are perhaps the most common form of chromosome anomaly detected in clinical practice. They are likely to be diagnosed at several stages in life for different reasons: before birth as the result of prenatal diagnosis; at birth as a result of clinical findings; during childhood due to abnormal growth, learning difficulties, or behavioral problems; in adolescence due to failure to enter puberty; or as adults due to infertility, behavioural problems, or psychiatric disturbance. Counseling and support needs to be directed to the parents when SCA is detected prior to birth or during childhood, and to the patient and family in adolescence and adult life. When an SCA is detected by prenatal testing, parents need to be given full, accurate, and detailed information about the prognosis, based on the most reliable data available, to enable them to reach the most appropriate decision for their family. Linden et al. (193) provide detailed guidelines that include the provision of accurate information and recognition of the variability and imprecise prognosis for SCA. Counseling strategies include contact with other families whose child has the same condition, viewing of photographs of SCA children, and the utilization of support groups when this seems appropriate. Issues of disclosure of the karyotype to others need to be addressed. Follow up should stress familial understanding and acceptance of the condition, provision of support, and opportunities for anticipatory guidance (98).

Experience with the counseling of parents following the detection of a SCA by prenatal diagnosis is now fairly extensive and it is clear that, while most prenatal testing is carried out for other reasons, the possibility that an SCA might be detected should be discussed during the pretest session. It has also been shown that the counseling provided following the diagnosis of an SCA can have a great influence on the decision to terminate or not. Sagi et al. (194) reported a termination rate of 80% of SCA pregnancies in Israel. The major reasons for termination were fear of a nonspecific abnormality in the child and concerns about abnormal sexual development in the child. In fact, 56% of the women interviewed felt that the counseling they received was directive towards termination. Christian et al. (195) found a significant correlation between the decision to continue the pregnancy and the type of SCA detected. The finding of fetal abnormalities on ultrasound significantly increased the likelihood of a decision to terminate. They also observed a statistically significant temporal trend with a higher rate of pregnancies being continued in the more recent years (40% in 1995–1998 vs. 0% in 1976–1979). Meschede et al. (196) found that after comprehensive genetic counseling, only 7 of 55 (13%) women carrying a fetus with an SCA elected for termination. Hall et al. (197) found differences between the counseling provided by geneticists and that provided by obstetricians following prenatal diagnosis of Klinefelter syndrome in five European countries. They found that geneticists were more likely to provide positive information than obstetricians, and that the perception of quality of life greatly influenced the decision to terminate. They concluded that the information provided to parents by counselors reflected personal, cultural, and professional differences between health professionals, rather than the provision of unbiased information based on the best data available. The DADA (Decision making After Diagnosis of a fetal Abnormality) group recently reported similar findings (198). This group examined the outcome of pregnancies following the diagnosis of Klinefelter syndrome prenatally and observed that the only predictor for the continuation of the pregnancy was the specialty of the health care professional providing postdiagnosis counseling: the affected pregnancy was more likely to continue when postdiagnosis counseling involved only a genetics specialist (relative risk 2.42, CI 1.14–5.92) (198). Counseling and support of patients with SCA later in life should reflect problems associated with the condition and should provide support and appropriate medical management, referral to appropriate agencies, specific help with learning difficulties, and psychiatric and psychological support, when this is required. Where possible and when the diagnosis is made early enough, hormonal regimens should be commenced at appropriate times to alleviate growth problems in Turner syndrome and other endocrine problems in Klinefelter syndrome. It is clear that people with SCA who grow and develop in the most supportive environments do better than their peers who have less support. As Linden et al. (193) conclude "utilization of counseling strategies unique to these conditions can provide parents with the necessary information to make informed decisions about the pregnancies and to assist families dealing with a child with SCA."

Genetic counseling of candidates for ICSI or TESA requires special attention. Patients with Klinefelter syndrome or XYY chromosomes should be informed that they may be at greater risk of sperm carrying abnormal chromosome complements, and that follow up should include prenatal diagnosis or, where available, preimplantation diagnosis. Patients with idiopathic oligospermia, azoospermia, or hypospermatogenesis should be screened for cryptic Y-chromosome deletions. If one is detected, they should be counseled that male fetuses resulting from these assisted reproductive technologies will be carrying the same Y chromosome and may therefore be infertile. The issue of fetal sex selection, perhaps by preimplantation diagnosis, needs to be carefully discussed.

IX. CONCLUSIONS

Sex chromosome anomalies are common at birth and frequently diagnosed during prenatal diagnosis. As careful clinical and epidemiological investigations have shown, with the exception of Turner syndrome and some rare X and Y polysomies, SCA rarely lead to major congenital malformations or developmental disabilities due largely to the fact that the additional X chromosomes are usually inactivated and the Y chromosome is not required for survival, but only to ensure male development and fertility. In those instances where the abnormal X is not inactivated, the degree of physical and mental impairment is increased. We have also learned that normal sexual development of both the male and the female requires the presence of two X chromosomes or an X and a Y chromosome early in embryogenesis to ensure normal fetal development. Molecular approaches have led to the identification of genes affecting stature and neurocognitive development on the X chromosome, genes controlling testicular development on the Y chromosome, the identification of two pseudoautosomal regions on the tips of both the X and the Y chromosomes and the demonstration of recombination between these regions, as well as informing us of the nondisjunctional events that usually lead to these anomalies. Most recently, the Y chromosome has been sequenced and a unique recombinogenic structure identified. This will may lead to identification of genes involved in the TS phenotype and has already led to the identification of the probable mechanisms involved in Y chromosome rearrangements leading to male infertility.

Research has taken our understanding of the nature and impact of SCA a long way from the days when patients with SCA were committed to institutions or considered criminally insane to the realization that the majority of these individuals can and do lead productive and healthy lives. Appropriate medical management, behavioral modification, and remedial education strategies have seen amelioration of many of the physical and mental problems of those who do come to medical attention. Counseling of families with SCA remains a complex issue, especially when such cases are ascertained by prenatal diagnosis. Thus, it is crucial that SCA patients or their families, as appropriate, receive accurate and unbiased information. It is just as vital that the health professionals who are responsible for their care are also well educated about these not infrequent conditions.

REFERENCES

1. Hook EB, Hamerton JL. The frequency of chromosome abnormalities detected in consecutive newborn studies. Differences between studies: results by sex and by severity of phenotypic involvement. In: Hook E, Porter IH, eds. Population Cytogenetics. New York: Academic Press, 1977:63–79.

2. Jacobs PA. The incidence and etiology of sex chromosome abnormalities in man. In: Robinson A, Lubs HA, Bergsma D, eds. Sex Chromosome Aneuploidy: Prospective Studies on Children. New York: Alan R Liss, 1979:3–14.

3. Hamerton JL. Population cytogenetics: a perspective. In: Adinolfi M, Benson P, Ganelli F, Sewer M, eds. Pediatric Research: A Genetic Approach. London: William Heinemann Medical Books Ltd, 1982:99–121.

4. Ratcliffe A, Paul N, eds. Prospective Studies on Children with Sex Chromosome Aneuploidy. In: Bergsma D, ed. Birth Defects, Original Art Series. Vol 22. New York: Academic Press, 1986.

5. Evans JA, de von Flindt R, Greenberg CR, Hamerton JL. Physical and psychological findings in adolescents with sex chromosome abnormalities ascertained in the Winnipeg cytogenetic study of newborns (1970–1973). In: Evans JA, Hamerton JL, Robinson A, eds. Children and Young Adults with Sex Chromosome Aneuploidy. New York: Wiley-Liss, 1991:189–200.

6. Barr ML, Bertram EG. Morphological distinction between neurons of the male and female, and the behaviour of the nucleolar satellite during accelerated nucleoprotein synthesis. Nature 1949; 163:676–677.

7. Klinefelter HF, Reifenstein EC, Albright F. A syndrome characterised by gynecomastia, aspermatogenesis without a-leydigism and increased excretion of follicle stimulating hormone. J Clin Endocr 1942; 2:615–627.

8. Turner HH. A syndrome of infantilism, congenital webbed neck, and cubitus valgus. Endocrinology 1938; 23:566–574.

9. Ford CE, Jones KW, Miller OJ, Mittwoch U, Penrose LS, Roberson JR. Chromosomes in a patient showing both mongolism and the Klinefelter syndrome. Lancet 1959; I:709–710.

10. Jacobs P, Strong JA. A case of human intersexuality having a possible XXY sex determining mechanism. Nature 1959; 183:303.

11. Ford CE, Polani PE, De Almeida JC, Briggs JH. A sex chromosome anomaly in a case of gonadal dysgenesis (Turner's Syndrome). Lancet 1959; I:709–710.

12. Fraccaro M, Kaijser J, Lindsten J. Sex chromosome complement in continuously cultured cells of two individuals with gonadal dysgenesis. Ann Hum Genet 1960; 24:45–61.

13. Painter TS. Studies in mammalian spermatogenesis: the spermatogenesis of man. J Exp Zool 1923; 37:291–335.

14. Tilford CA, Kuroda-Kawaguchi T, Skaletsky H, Rozen S, Brown LG, Rosenberg M. A physical map of the human Y chromosome. Nature 2001; 409:943–945.

15. Skaletsky H, Kuroda-Kawaguchi T, Minx PJ, Cordum HS, Hillier L, Brown LG. The male-specific region of the human Y chromosome is a mosaic of discrete sequence classes. Nature 2003; 423:825–837.

16. Hurles ME, Jobling MA. A singular chromosome. Nat Genet 2003; 34:246–247.

17. Sinclair AH, Berta P, Palmer MS, Hawkins JR, Griffiths BL, Smith MJ. A gene from the human sex-determining region encodes a protein with homology to a conserved DNA-binding motif. Nature 1990; 346:240–244.

18. Stankiewicz P, Lupski JR. Genome architecture, rearrangements and genomic disorders. Trends Genet 2002; 18: 74–82.

19. Lyon MF. Gene action in the X-chromosome of the mouse. Nature 1961; 190:372–373.

20. Lyon MF. X-chromosome inactivation: pinpointing the centre. Nature 1996; 379:116–117.

21. Lyon MF. X-chromosome inactivation: a repeat hypothesis. Cytogenet Cell Genet 1998; 80:133–137.

22. Hamerton JL. Human Cytogenetics–General Cytogenetics Vol.1.. New York: Academic Press, 1971.

23. Bean CJ, Hunt PA, Millie EA, Hassold TJ. Analysis of a malsegregating mouse Y chromosome: evidence that the earliest cleavage divisions of the mammalian embryo are non-disjunction-prone. Hum Mol Genet 2001; 10:963–972.

24. Delhanty JD, Harper JC, Ao A, Handyside AH, Winston RM. Multicolour FISH detects frequent chromosomal mosaicism

and chaotic division in normal preimplantation embryos from fertile patients. Hum Genet 1997; 99:755–760.

25. Munne S, Weier HU, Grifo J, Cohen J. Chromosome mosaicism in human embryos. Biol Reprod 1994; 51:373–379.

26. Polani PE. Sex chromosome anomalies in Man. In: Hamerton JL, ed. Chromosomes in Medicine. London: Heinemann Medical Books, 1962:72–130.

27. Robinson A, de la Chapelle A. Sex chromosome abnormalities. In: Emery A, Rimoin DL, eds. Principles and Practice of Medical Genetics. Edinburgh: Churchill Livingstone, 1997: 973–997.

28. Evans JA, MacDonald K, Hamerton JL. Sex chromosome anomalies: prenatal diagnosis and the need for continued prospective studies. In: Evans JA, Hamerton JL, Robinson A, eds. Children and Young Adults with Sex Chromosome Aneuploidy. New York: Wiley-Liss, 1991:273–281.

29. Cunniff C. Turner syndrome. Adolesc Med 2002; 13:359–366.

30. Dean HJ. Growth hormone therapy in girls with Turner syndrome. In: Evans JA, Hamerton JL, Robinson A, eds. Children and Young Adults with Sex Chromosome Aneuploidy. New York: Wiley-Liss, 1991:229–234.

31. Brook CGD, Murser G, Zachman M, Prader A. Growth in children with 45,XO Turner's syndrome. Arch Dis Child 1974; 49:789–794.

32. Ross JL, Long LM, Loriaux DL, Cutler GB. Growth hormone secretory dynamics in Turner syndrome. J Pediatr 1985; 106:202–206.

33. Rosenfeld RG, Hintz RL, Johanson AJ, Brasel JA, Burstein S, Chernausek SD. Methionyl human growth hormone and oxandrolone in Turner syndrome: preliminary results of a prospective randomized trial. J Pediatr 1986; 109:936–943.

34. Rosenfeld RG, Hintz RL, Johanson AJ, Sherman B, Brasel JA, Burstein S. Three-year results of a randomized prospective trial of methionyl human growth hormone and oxandrolone in Turner syndrome. J Pediatr 1988; 113:393–400.

35. Johnston DI, Betts P, Dunger D, Barnes N, Swift PG, Buckler JM. A multicentre trial of recombinant growth hormone and low dose oestrogen in Turner syndrome: near final height analysis. Arch Dis Child 2001; 84:76–81.

36. Ranke MB, Partsch CJ, Lindberg A, Dorr HG, Bettendorf M, Hauffa BP. Adult height after GH therapy in 188 Ullrich–Turner syndrome patients: results of the German IGLU follow-up study 2001. Eur J Endocrinol 2002; 147:625–633.

37. van Pareren YK, de Muinck Keizer-Schrama SM, Stijnen T, Sas TC, Jansen M, Otten BJ. Final height in girls with Turner syndrome after long-term growth hormone treatment in three dosages and low dose estrogens. J Clin Endocrinol Metab 2003; 88:1119–1125.

38. Hamerton JL. Human Cytogenetics–Clinical Cytogenetics Vol.2. New York: Academic Press, 1971.

39. Van Dyke DL, Wiktor A, Palmer CG, Miller DA, Witt M, Babu VR. Ullrich–Turner syndrome with a small ring X chromosome and presence of mental retardation. Am J Med Genet 1992; 43:996–1005.

40. Romans SM, Stefanatos G, Roeltgen DP, Kushner H, Ross JL. Transition to young adulthood in Ullrich–Turner syndrome: neurodevelopmental changes. Am J Med Genet 1998; 79: 140–147.

41. McCauley E, Kay T, Ito J, Treder R. The Turner syndrome: cognitive deficits, affective discrimination, and behavior problems. Child Dev 1987; 58:464–473.

42. McCauley E, Ross JL, Kushner H, Cutler G Jr. Self-esteem and behavior in girls with Turner syndrome. J Dev Behav Pediatr 1995; 16:82–88.

43. Hassold TJ, Arnovitz K, Jacobs P, May K, Robinson D. The parental origin of the missing or additional chromosome in 45,X and 47,XXX females. In: Evans JA, Hamerton JL, Robinson A, eds. Children and Young Adults with Sex Chromosome Aneuploidy. New York: Wiley-Liss, 1991:297–304.

44. Mathur A, Stekol L, Schatz D, MacLaren NK, Scott ML, Lippe B. The parental origin of the single X chromosome in

Turner syndrome: lack of correlation with parental age or clinical phenotype. Am J Hum Genet 1991; 48:682–686.

45. Jacobs P, Dalton P, James R, Mosse K, Power M, Robinson D. Turner syndrome: a cytogenetic and molecular study. Ann Hum Genet 1997; 61:471–483.

46. Ellison JW, Wardak Z, Young MF, Gehron RP, Laig-Webster M, Chiong W. PHOG, a candidate gene for involvement in the short stature of Turner syndrome. Hum Mol Genet 1997; 6: 1341–1347.

47. Rao E, Weiss B, Fukami M, Rump A, Niesler B, Mertz A. Pseudoautosomal deletions encompassing a novel homeobox gene cause growth failure in idiopathic short stature and Turner syndrome. Nat Genet 1997; 16:54–63.

48. Ross JL, Roeltgen D, Kushner H, Wei F, Zinn AR. The Turner syndrome-associated neurocognitive phenotype maps to distal Xp. Am J Hum Genet 2000; 67:672–681.

49. Monk M, Harper MI. Sequential X chromosome inactivation coupled with cellular differentiation in early mouse embryos. Nature 1979; 281:311–313.

50. Brown CJ, Willard HF. Localization of the X-inactivation centre (XIC) to Xq13. Cytogenet Cell Genet 1989; 51:971.

51. Plath K, Mlynarczyj-Evans S, Nusinow DA, Panning B. Xist RNA and the mechanism of X chromosome inactivation. Annu Rev Genet 2002; 36:233–278.

52. Brown CJ, Lafreniere RG, Powers VE, Sebastio G, Ballabio A, Pettigrew AL. Localization of the X inactivation centre on the human X chromosome in Xq13. Nature 1991; 349: 82–84.

53. Brown CJ, Hendrich BD, Rupert JL, Lafreniere RG, Xing Y, Lawrence J. The human XIST gene: analysis of a 17 kb inactive X-specific RNA that contains conserved repeats and is highly localized within the nucleus. Cell 1992; 71:527–542.

54. Monroy N, Lopez M, Cervantes A, Garcia-Cruz D, Zafra G, Canun S. Microsatellite analysis in Turner syndrome: parental origin of X chromosomes and possible mechanism of formation of abnormal chromosomes. Am J Med Genet 2002; 107:181–189.

55. Uematsu A, Yorifuji T, Muroi J, Kawai M, Mamada M, Kaji M. Parental origin of normal X chromosomes in Turner syndrome patients with various karyotypes: implications for the mechanism leading to generation of a 45, X karyotype. Am J Med Genet 2002; 111:134–139.

56. James RS, Dalton P, Gustashaw K, Wolff DJ, Willard HF, Mitchell C. Molecular characterization of isochromosomes of Xq. Ann Hum Genet 1997; 61:485–490.

57. Wolff DJ, Miller AP, Van Dyke DL, Schwartz S, Willard HF. Molecular definition of breakpoints associated with human Xq isochromosomes: implications for mechanisms of formation. Am J Hum Genet 1996; 58:154–160.

58. Callen DF, Mulley JC, Baker EG, Sutherland GR. Determining the origin of human X isochromosomes by the use of DNA sequence polymorphisms and detection of an apparent i(Xq) with Xp sequences. Hum Genet 1987; 77:236–240.

59. Harbison M, Hassold T, Kobryn C, Jacobs PA. Molecular studies of the parental origin and nature of human X isochromosomes. Cytogenet Cell Genet 1988; 47:217–222.

60. Lorda-Sanchez I, Binkert F, Maechler M, Schinzel AA. A molecular study of X isochromosomes: parental origin, centromeric structure, and mechanisms of formation. Am J Hum Genet 1991; 49:1034–1040.

61. Hamerton JL, Canning N, Ray M, Smith S. A cytogenetic survey of 14,069 newborn infants. I. Incidence of chromosome abnormalities. Clin Genet 1975; 8:223–243.

62. Simpson JL. Disorders of Sexual Differentiation. New York: Academic Press, 1976.

63. Chang HJ, Clark RD, Bachman H. The phenotype of 45,X/46,XY mosaicism: an analysis of 92 prenatally diagnosed cases. Am J Hum Genet 1990; 46:156–167.

64. Sher ES, Addelston MB, Plotnick L, Urban MD, Berkovitz GD. Molecular investigation of two male subjects with short stature and a 45,X/46,X,ring(Y) karyotype. Horm Res 1998; 49:46–50.

65. Wolff DJ, Brown CJ, Schwartz S, Duncan AM, Surti U, Willard HF. Small marker X chromosomes lack the X inacti-

vation center: implications for karyotype/phenotype correlations. Am J Hum Genet 1994; 55:87–95.

66. Migeon BR, Luo S, Stasiowski BA, Jani M, Axelman J, Van Dyke DL. Deficient transcription of XIST from tiny ring X chromosomes in females with severe phenotypes. Proc Natl Acad Sci USA 1993; 90:12025–12029.

67. Turner C, Dennis NR, Skuse DH, Jacobs PA. Seven ring (X) chromosomes lacking the XIST locus, six with an unexpectedly mild phenotype. Hum Genet 2000; 106:93–100.

68. Migeon BR, Luo S, Jani M, Jeppesen P. The severe phenotype of females with tiny ring X chromosomes is associated with inability of these chromosomes to undergo X inactivation. Am J Hum Genet 1994; 55:497–504.

69. Migeon BR, Jeppesen P, Torchia BS, Fu S, Dunn MA, Axelman J. Lack of X inactivation associated with maternal X isodisomy: evidence for a counting mechanism prior to X inactivation during human embryogenesis. Am J Hum Genet 1996; 58:161–170.

70. Yorifuji T, Muroi J, Kawai M, Uematsu A, Sasaki H, Momoi T. Uniparental and functional X disomy in Turner syndrome patients with unexplained mental retardation and X derived marker chromosomes. J Med Genet 1998; 35:539–544.

71. Jacobs P, Baikie AG, Court Brown WM, MacGregor TM, Maclean N, Harnden DG. Evidence for the existence of the human "superfemale." Lancet 1959; II:423–425

72. Jacobs P, Harnden DG, Court Brown WM, Baikie AG. Trisomic condition of a large chromosome. Lancet 1960; II:368.

73. Hogge WA, Vick DJ, Schnatterly PA, MacMillan RH. Bilateral renal agenesis and Mullerian anomalies in a 47,XXX fetus. Am J Med Genet 1989; 33:242–243.

74. Lin HJ, Ndiforchu F, Patell S. Exstrophy of the cloaca in a 47,XXX child: review of genitourinary malformations in triple-X patients. Am J Med Genet 1993; 45:761–763.

75. Hoang MP, Wilson KS, Schneider NR, Timmons CF. Case report of a 22-week fetus with 47,XXX karyotype and

multiple lower mesodermal defects. Pediatr Dev Pathol 1999; 2:58–61.

76. Robinson A, Bender BG, Linden MG. Summary of clinical findings in children and young adults with sex chromosome anomalies. In: Evans JA, Hamerton JL, Robinson A, eds. Children and Young Adults with Sex Chromosome Aneuploidy. New York: Wiley-Liss, 1991:225–228.

77. Tungphaisal S, Jinorose U. True 47,XXX in a patient with premature ovarian failure: the first reported case in Thailand. J Med Assoc Thai 1992; 75:661–665.

78. Wu RC, Kuo PL, Lin SJ, Liu CH, Tzeng CC. X chromosome mosaicism in patients with recurrent abortion or premature ovarian failure. J Formos Med Assoc 1993; 92:953–956.

79. Witek A, Skalba P, Zieba M. Pituitary tumor in a woman with a 47,XXX karyotype—case report. Med Sci Monit 2001; 7:304–307.

80. Holland CM. 47,XXX in an adolescent with premature ovarian failure and autoimmune disease. J Pediatr Adolesc Gynecol 2001; 14:77–80.

81. Castillo S, Lopez F, Tobella L, Salazar S, Daher V. The cytogenetics of premature ovarian failure. Rev Child Obstet Ginecol 1992; 57:341–345.

82. Fitzgerald PH, Donald RA, McCormick P. Reduced fertility in women with X chromosome abnormality. Clin Genet 1984; 25:301–309.

83. Gekas J, Thepot F, Turleau C, Siffroi JP, Dadoune JP, Wasels R. Chromosomal factors of infertility in candidate couples for ICSI: an equal risk of constitutional aberrations in women and men. Hum Reprod 2001; 16:82–901.

84. Harmon RJ, Bender BG, Linden MG, Robinson A. Transition from adolescence to early adulthood: adaptation and psychiatric status of women with 47,XXX. J Am Acad Child Adolesc Psychiatry 1998; 37:286–291.

85. Rovet J, Netley C, Bailey J, Keenan M, Stewart D. Intelligence and achievement in children with extra X aneuploidy: a longitudinal perspective. Am J Med Genet 1995; 60:356–363.

86. May KM, Jacobs PA, Lee M, Ratcliffe S, Robinson A, Nielsen J. The parental origin of the extra X chromosome in 47, XXX females. Am J Hum Genet 1990; 46:754–761.

87. MacDonald M, Hassold T, Harvey J, Wang LH, Morton NE, Jacobs P. The origin of 47,XXY and 47,XXX aneuploidy: heterogeneous mechanisms and role of aberrant recombination. Hum Mol Genet 1994; 3:1365–1371.

88. Ferguson Smith MA, Lennox B, Mack WS, Stewart JSS. Klinefelter's syndrome: frequency and testicular morphology in relation to nuclear sex. Lancet 1957; II:475–476.

89. Bojesen A, Juul S, Gravholt CH. Prenatal and postnatal prevalence of Klinefelter syndrome: a national registry study. J Clin Endocrinol Metab 2003; 88:622–626.

90. Ratcliffe S. Long-term outcome in children of sex chromosome abnormalities. Arch Dis Child 1999; 80:192–195.

91. Tanner JM. Normal growth and techniques of growth assessment. Clin Endocrinol Metab 1986; 15:411–451.

92. Becker KL. Clinical and therapeutic experiences with Klinefelter's syndrome. Fertil Steril 1972; 23:568–578.

93. Kamischke A, Baumgardt A, Horst J, Nieschlag E. Clinical and diagnostic features of patients with suspected Klinefelter syndrome. J Androl 2003; 24:41–48.

94. Jacobs PA, Hassold TJ, Whittington E, Butler G, Collyer S, Keston M. Klinefelter syndrome: an analysis of the origin of the additional sex chromosome using molecular probes. Ann Hum Genet 1988; 52:93–109.

95. Thomas NS, Collins AR, Hassold TJ, Jacobs PA. A reinvestigation of non-disjunction resulting in 47,XXY males of paternal origin. Eur J Hum Genet 2000; 8:805–808.

96. Winter JSD. Androgen therapy in Klinefelter syndrome in adolescence. In: Evans JA, Hamerton J, Robinson A, eds. Children and Young Adults with Sex Chromosome Aneuploidy. New York: Wiley-Liss, 1991:235–245.

97. Manning MA, Hoyme HE. Diagnosis and management of the adolescent boy with Klinefelter Syndrome. Adolesc Med 2002; 13:367–374.

98. Visootsak J, Aylstock M, Graham Jr JM. Klinefelter syndrome and its variants: an update and review for the primary pediatrician. Clin Pediatr (Phila) 2001; 40:639–651.

99. Abramsky L, Chapple J. 47,XXY (Klinefelter syndrome) and 47,XYY: estimated rates of and indication for postnatal diagnosis with implications for prenatal counseling. Prenat Diagn 1997; 17:363–368.

100. R Ron-el, Friedler S, Strassburger D, Komarovsky D, Schachter M, Raziel A. Birth of a healthy neonate following the intracytoplasmic injection of testicular spermatozoa from a patient with Klinefelter's syndrome. Hum Reprod 1999; 14:368–370.

101. Ron-el R, Strassburger D, Gelman-Kohan S, Friedler S, Raziel A, Appelman Z. A 47,XXY fetus conceived after ICSI of spermatozoa from a patient with non-mosaic Klinefelter's syndrome: case report. Hum Reprod 2000; 15:1804–1806.

102. Friedler S, Raziel A, Strassburger D, Schachter M, Bern O, Ron-el R. Outcome of ICSI using fresh and cryopreserved–thawed testicular spermatozoa in patients with non-mosaic Klinefelter's syndrome. Hum Reprod 2001; 16:2616–2620.

103. Rives N, Joly G, Machy A, Simeon N, Leclerc P, Mace B. Assessment of sex chromosome aneuploidy in sperm nuclei from 47,XXY and 46,XY/47,XXY males: comparison with fertile and infertile males with normal karyotype. Mol Hum Reprod 2000; 6:107–112.

104. Cruger D, Toft B, Agerholm I, Fedder J, Hald F, Bruun-Petersen G. Birth of a healthy girl after ICSI with ejaculated spermatozoa from a man with non-mosaic Klinefelter's syndrome. Hum Reprod 2001; 16:1909–1911.

105. Poulakis V, Witzsch U, Diehl W, de Vries R, Becht E, Trotnow S. Birth of two infants with normal karyotype after intracytoplasmic injection of sperm obtained by testicular extraction from two men with nonmosaic Klinefelter's syndrome. Fertil Steril 2001; 76:1060–1062.

106. Bergere M, Wainer R, Nataf V, Bailly M, Gombault M, Ville Y. Biopsied testis cells of four 47,XXY patients: fluorescence in-situ hybridization and ICSI results. Hum Reprod 2002; 17:32–37.

107. Rosenlund B, Hreinsson JG, Hovatta O. Birth of a healthy male after frozen thawed blastocyst transfer following intracytoplasmic injection of frozen thawed testicular spermatozoa from a man with nonmosaic Klinefelter's syndrome. J Assist Reprod Genet 2002; 19:149–151.

108. Kitamura M, Matsumiya K, Koga M, Nishimura K, Miura H, Tsuji T. Ejaculated spermatozoa in patients with non-mosaic Klinefelter's syndrome. Int J Urol 2000; 7:88–92.

109. Foresta C, Galeazzi C, Bettella A, Stella M, Scandellari C. High incidence of sperm sex chromosomes aneuploidies in two patients with Klinefelter's syndrome. J Clin Endocrinol Metab 1998; 83:203–205.

110. Hennebicq S, Pelletier R, Bergues U, Rousseaux S. Risk of trisomy 21 in offspring of patients with Klinefelter's syndrome. Lancet 2001; 357:2104–2105.

111. Yamamoto Y, Sofikitis N, Kaponis A, Georgiou J, Giannakis D, Mamoulakis C. Use of a highly sensitive quantitative telomerase assay in intracytoplasmic sperm injection programmes for the treatment of 47,XXY non-mosaic Klinefelter men. Andrologia 2002; 34:218–226.

112. Mroz K, Carrel L, Hunt PA. Germ cell development in the XXY mouse: evidence that X chromosome reactivation is independent of sexual differentiation. Dev Biol 1999; 207:229–238.

113. Jacobs PA, Brunton M, Melville MM, Brittain RP, McClemont WF. Aggressive behaviour, mental subnormality, and the XYY male. Nature 1965; 208:1351–1352.

114. Jacobs PA, Price WH, Court Brown WM, Brittain RP, Whatmore PB. Chromosome studies on men in a maximum security hospital. Ann Hum Genet 1968; 31:339–358.

115. Beckwith J, King J. The XYY syndrome: a dangerous myth. New Sci 1974; 64:474–476.

116. Hamerton JL. Human population cytogenetics: dilemmas and problems. Am J Hum Genet 1976; 28:107–122.

117. Beckwith J, Miller L. The XYY male: the making of a myth. Harv Mag 1976; 79:30–33.

118. Witkin HA, Mednick SA, Schulsinger F, Bakkestrom E, Christiansen KO, Goodenough DR. Criminality in XYY and XXY men. Science 1976; 193:547–555.

119. Philip J, Lundsteen C, Owen D, Hirschhorn K. The frequency of chromosome aberrations in tall men with special reference to 47,XYY and 47,XXY. Am J Hum Genet 1976; 28: 404–411.

120. Schiavi RC, Owen D, Fogel M, White D, Szechter R. Pituitary–gonadal function in XYY and XXY men identified in a population survey. Clin Endocrinol 1978; 9:233–239.

121. Fryns JP, Kleczkowska A, Kubien E, Van den Berghe H. XYY syndrome and other Y chromosome polysomies. Mental status and psychosocial functioning. Genet Couns 1995; 6: 197–206.

122. Hunter H. XYY males. Some clinical and psychiatric aspects deriving from a survey of 1,811 males in hospitals for the mentally handicapped. Br J Psychiatry 1977; 131:468–477.

123. Robinson DO, Jacobs PA. The origin of the extra Y chromosome in males with a 47,XYY karyotype. Hum Mol Genet 1999; 8:2205–2209.

124. Linden MG, Bender BG, Robinson A. Sex chromosome tetrasomy and pentasomy. Pediatrics 1995; 96:672–682.

125. Carr DH, Barr ML, Plunkett ER. An XXXX sex chromosome complex in two mentally defective females. Can Med Assoc J 1961; 84:131–137.

126. Kesaree N, Woolley PV. A phenotypic female with 49 chromosomes, presumably XXXXX. J Pediatr 1963; 63:1099–1103.

127. Muldahl S, Ockey CH. The "double male" a new chromosome constitution in Klinefelter's syndrome. Lancet 1960; II: 492–493.

128. Court Brown WM, Harnden DG, Jacobs PA, Maclean N, Mantle DJ. Abnormalities of the sex chromosome complement in man. Spec Rep Ser Med Res Counc No. 305, 1964.

129. Casey MD, Segall LJ, Street DRK, Blank CE. Sex chromosome abnormalities in two state hospitals for patients requiring special security. Nature 1966; 209:641–642.

130. Casey MD, Blank CE, Street DRK, Segall LJ, McDougall JH, Mcgrath PJ. YY chromosomes and anti-social behaviour. Lancet 1966; II:859–860.

131. Sorensen K, Nielsen J, Jacobsen P, Rolle T. The 48,XXYY syndrome. J Ment Defic Res 1978; 22:197–205.

132. Benn PA, Sugarman M, Greco MA, Harris G, Deguire GB, Hsu LY. Prenatal diagnosis of 49,XXXYY. Prenat Diagn 1982; 2:309–312.

133. Barr ML, Shaver EL, Carr DH. An unusual sex chromatin pattern in three mentally deficient subjects. J Ment Defic Res 1959; 3:87.

134. Fraccaro M, Kaijser J, Lindsten J. A child with 49 chromosomes. Lancet 1960; II:899–902.

135. Borghgraef M, Fryns JP, Smeets E, Marien J, Van den Berge H. The 49,XXXXY syndrome. Clinical and psychological follow-up data. Clin Genet 1988; 33:429–434.

136. Townes PL, Ziegler NA, Lenhard LW. A patient with 48 chromosomes (XYYY). Lancet 1965; 1:1041–1043.

137. Kyriakakos A, Sansaricq C, Perle MA, Barnabe C. A nine year old boy with bone and joint abnormalities and a unique genetic tetrasomy Y. Am J Hum Genet 1995; 57:A95.

138. Shanske A, Sachmechi I, Patel DK, Bishnoi A, Rosner F. An adult with 49,XYYYY karyotype: case report and endocrine studies. Am J Med Genet 1998; 80:103–106.

139. DesGroseilliers M, Lemyre E, Dallaire L, Lemieux N. Tetrasomy Y by structural rearrangement: clinical report. Am J Med Genet 2002; 111:401–404.

140. Das GP, Shukla A, Verma IC. Phenotype of 49,XXYYY. Clin Genet 1993; 43:196–199.

141. Frey-Mahn G, Behrendt G, Geiger K, Sohn C, Schafer D, Miny P. Y chromosomal polysomy: a unique case of 49,XYYYY in amniotic fluid cells. Am J Med Genet 2003; 118A:184–186.

142. Hassold T, Pettay D, May K, Robinson A. Analysis of nondisjunction in sex chromosome tetrasomy and pentasomy. Hum Genet 1990; 85:648–650.

143. de la Chapelle A, Hortling H, Niemi M, Wennstrom J. XX sex chromosomes in a human male. Acta Med Scand 1964; 175:25–38.

144. Goodfellow PN, Lovell-Badge R. SRY and sex determination in mammals. Annu Rev Genet 1993; 27:71–92.

145. Capel B. New bedfellows in the mammalian sex-determination affair. Trends Genet 1995; 11:161–163.

146. Haqq CM, Donahoe PK. Regulation of sexual dimorphism in mammals. Physiol Rev 1998; 78:1–33.

147. Ferguson-Smith MA. X–Y chromosomal interchange in the aetiology of true hermaphroditism and of XX Klinefelter's syndrome. Lancet 1966; II:475–476.

148. de la Chapelle A , Koo GC, Wachtel SS. Recessive sex-determining genes in human XX male syndrome. Cell 1978; 15:837–842.

149. Andersson M, Page DC, de la Chapelle A. Chromosome Y-specific DNA is transferred to the short arm of X chromosome in human XX males. Science 1986; 233:786–788.

150. Simpson E, Chandler P, Goulmy E, Disteche CM, Ferguson-Smith MA, Page DC. Separation of the genetic loci for the H-Y antigen and for testis determination on human Y chromosome. Nature 1987; 326:876–878.

151. Palmer MS, Sinclair AH, Berta P, Ellis NA, Goodfellow PN, Abbas NE. Genetic evidence that ZFY is not the testis-determining factor. Nature 1989; 342:937–939.

152. McElreavey K, Cortes LS. X–Y translocations and sex differentiation. Semin Reprod Med 2001; 19:133–139.

153. Cotinot C, Pailhoux E, Jaubert F, Fellous M. Molecular genetics of sex determination. Semin Reprod Med 2002; 20:157–168.

154. Abusheikha N, Lass A, Brinsden P. XX males without SRY gene and with infertility. Hum Reprod 2001; 16:717–718.

155. Lim HN, Berkovitz GD, Hughes IA, Hawkins JR. Mutation analysis of subjects with 46,XX sex reversal and 46,XY gonadal dysgenesis does not support the involvement of SOX3 in testis determination. Hum Genet 2000; 107:650–652.

156. Boucekkine C, Toublanc JE, Abbas N, Chaabouni S, Ouahid S, Semrouni M. Clinical and anatomical spectrum in XX sex reversed patients. Relationship to the presence of Y specific DNA-sequences. Clin Endocrinol (Oxf) 1994; 40:733–742.

157. Lopez M, Torres L, Mendez JP, Cervantes A, Perez-Palacios G, Erickson RP. Clinical traits and molecular findings in 46,XX males. Clin Genet 1995; 48:29–34.

158. Vilain E. Anomalies of human sexual development: clinical aspects and genetic analysis. Novartis Found Symp 2002; 244:43–53.

159. Harley VR. The molecular action of testis-determining factors SRY and SOX9. Novartis Found Symp 2002; 244:57–66.

160. Marshall Graves JA. The rise and fall of SRY. Trends Genet 2002; 18:259–264.

161. Tiepolo L, Zuffardi O. Localization of factors controlling spermatogenesis in the non fluorescent portion of the human Y chromosome. Hum Genet 1976; 34:119–124.

162. Ma K, Sharkey A, Kirsch S, Vogt P, Keil R, Hargreave TB. Towards the molecular localisation of the AZF locus: mapping of microdeletions in azoospermic men within 14 subintervals of interval 6 of the human Y chromosome. Hum Mol Genet 1992; 1:29–33.

163. Vogt P, Chandley AC, Hargreave TB, Keil R, Ma K, Sharkey A. Microdeletions in interval 6 of the Y chromosome of males with idiopathic sterility point to disruption of AZF, a human spermatogenesis gene. Hum Genet 1992; 89:491–496.

164. Vogt PH, Edelmann A, Kirsch S, Henegariu O, Hirschmann P, Kiesewetter F. Human Y chromosome azoospermia factors (AZF) mapped to different subregions in Yq11. Hum Mol Genet 1996; 5:933–943.

165. Foresta C, Moro E, Ferlin A. Y chromosome microdeletions and alterations of spermatogenesis. Endocr Rev 2001; 22:226–239.

166. Rozen S, Skaletsky H, Marszalek JD, Minx PJ, Cordum HS, Waterston RH. Abundant gene conversion between arms of palindromes in human and ape Y chromosomes. Nature 2003; 423:873–876.

167. Sun C, Skaletsky H, Rozen S, Gromoll J, Nieschlag E, Oates R. Deletion of azoospermia factor a (AZFa) region of human Y chromosome caused by recombination between HERV15 proviruses. Hum Mol Genet 2000; 9:2291–2296.

168. Blanco P, Shlumukova M, Sargent CA, Jobling MA, Affara N, Hurles ME. Divergent outcomes of intrachromosomal recombination on the human Y chromosome: male infertility and recurrent polymorphism. J Med Genet 2000; 37:752–758.

169. Kamp C, Hirschmann P, Voss H, Huellen K, Vogt PH. Two long homologous retroviral sequence blocks in proximal Yq11 cause AZFa microdeletions as a result of intrachromosomal recombination events. Hum Mol Genet 2000; 9: 2563–2572.

170. Kuroda-Kawaguchi T, Skaletsky H, Brown LG, Minx PJ, Cordum HS, Waterston RH. The AZFc region of the Y chromosome features massive palindromes and uniform recurrent deletions in infertile men. Nat Genet 2001; 29:279–286.

171. Repping S, Skaletsky H, Lange J, Silber S, Van Der Veen F, Oates RD. Recombination between palindromes P5 and P1 on the human Y chromosome causes massive deletions and spermatogenic failure. Am J Hum Genet 2002; 71:906–922.

172. Foresta C, Moro E, Ferlin A. Prognostic value of Y deletion analysis. The role of current methods. Hum Reprod 2001; 16:1543–1547.

173. Kleiman SE, Bar-Shira MB, Yogev L, Paz G, Yavetz H. The prognostic role of the extent of Y microdeletion on spermatogenesis and maturity of Sertoli cells. Hum Reprod 2001; 16:399–402.

174. Krausz C, Quintana-Murci L, McElreavey K. Prognostic value of Y deletion analysis: what is the clinical prognostic value of Y chromosome microdeletion analysis? Hum Reprod 2000; 15:1431–1434

175. deKretser D, Baker HWG. Infertility in men: recent advances and continuing controversies. J Clin Endocrinol Metab 1999; 84:3443–3450.

176. Hultborn R, Hanson C, Kopf I, Verbiene I, Warnhammar E, Weimarck A. Prevalence of Klinefelter's syndrome in male

breast cancer patients. Anticancer Res 1997; 17: 4293–4297.

177. Scheike O. Male breast cancer. Acta Pathol Microbiol Scand [A] 1975; 251:3–35.

178. Langlands AO, Maclean N, Kerr GR. Carcinoma of the male breast: report of a series of 88 cases. Clin Radiol 1976; 27: 21–25.

179. Evans DB, Crichlow RW. Carcinoma of the male breast and Klinefelter's syndrome: is there an association? CA Cancer J Clin 1987; 37:246–251

180. Price WH, Clayton JF, Wilson J, Collyer S, De Mey R. Causes of death in X chromatin positive males (Klinefelter's syndrome). J Epidemiol Community Health 1985; 39:330–336.

181. Radakovic B, Jukic S, Bukovic D, Ljubojevic N, Cima I. Morphology of gonads in pure XY gonadal dysgenesis. Coll Antropol 1999; 23:203–211.

182. Iezzoni JC, Kap-Herr C, Golden WL, Gaffey MJ. Gonadoblastomas in 45,X/46,XY mosaicism: analysis of Y chromosome distribution by fluorescence in situ hybridization. Am J Clin Pathol 1997; 108:197–201.

183. Sultana R, Myerson D, Disteche CM. In situ hybridization analysis of the Y chromosome in gonadoblastoma. Genes Chromosomes Cancer 1995; 13:257–262.

184. Uehara S, Funato T, Yaegashi N, Suziki H, Sato J, Sasaki T. SRY mutation and tumor formation on the gonads of XP pure gonadal dysgenesis patients. Cancer Genet Cytogenet 1999; 113:78–84.

185. Uehara S, Hashiyada M, Sato K, Nata M, Funato T, Okamura K. Complete XY gonadal dysgenesis and aspects of the SRY genotype and gonadal tumor formation. J Hum Genet 2002; 47:279–284.

186. Salo P, Kaariainen H, Petrovic V, Peltomaki P, Page DC, de la Chapelle A. Molecular mapping of the putative gonadoblastoma locus on the Y chromosome. Genes Chromosomes Cancer 1995; 14:210–214.

187. Midro AT, Wojtukiewicz M, Bielawiec M, Sawicka A. XYY syndrome and acute myeloblastic leukemia. Cancer Genet Cytogenet 1987; 24:363–365.

188. Gilgenkrantz S. XYY males and leukemia. Cancer Genet Cytogenet 1988; 30:337–338.

189. Tanaka S, Fukue H, Kanaya M, Mizunuma M, Watanabe H, Fujii M. Dysgerminoma and gonadoblastoma in a phenotypic female with 45,X/47,XYY mosaicism. Nippon Sanka Fujinka Gakkai Zasshi 1989; 41:769–772.

190. Rudnik-Schoneborn S, Schuler HM, Schwanitz G, Hansmann M, Zerres K. Further arguments for non-fortuitous association of Potter sequence with XYY males. Ann Genet 1996; 39:43–46.

191. Sandlund JT, Krance R, Pui CH, Hancock M, Crist WM, Filatov LV. XYY syndrome in children with acute lymphoblastic leukemia. Med Pediatr Oncol 1997; 28:6–8.

192. Palanduz S, Aktan M, Ozturk S, Tutkan G, Cefle K, Pekcelen Y. 47,XYY karyotype in acute myeloid leukemia. Cancer Genet Cytogenet 1998; 106:76–77.

193. Linden MG, Bender BG, Robinson A. Genetic counseling for sex chromosome abnormalities. Am J Med Genet 2002; 110:3–10.

194. Sagi M, Meiner V, Reshef N, Dagan J, Zlotogora J. Prenatal diagnosis of sex chromosome aneuploidy: possible reasons for high rates of pregnancy termination. Prenat Diagn 2001; 21:461–465.

195. Christian SM, Koehn D, Pillay R, MacDougall A, Wilson RD. Parental decisions following prenatal diagnosis of sex chromosome aneuploidy: a trend over time. Prenat Diagn 2000; 20:37–40.

196. Meschede D, Louwen F, Nippert I, Holzgreve W, Miny P, Horst J. Low rates of pregnancy termination for prenatally diagnosed Klinefelter syndrome and other sex chromosome polysomies. Am J Med Genet 1998; 80:330–334.

197. Hall S, Marteau TM, Limbert C, Reid M, Feijoo M, Soares M. Counseling following the prenatal diagnosis of Klinefelter syndrome: comparisons between geneticists and obstetricians in five European countries. Community Genet 2001; 4: 233–238.

198. Marteau TM, Nippert I, Hall S, Limbert C, Reid M, Bobrow M. Outcomes of pregnancies diagnosed with Klinefelter syndrome: the possible influence of health professionals. Prenat Diagn 2002; 22:562–566.

17

Expanded Newborn Screening and Phenylketonuria (PKU)

RICHARD HILLMAN

Division of Medical Genetics, University of
Missouri, Columbia, Missouri, U.S.A.

I. THE CHILD AT BIRTH

The infant before birth can be thought of as undergoing continuous dialysis through the placenta. Thus, most disorders of small molecule metabolism are of very little consequence until the time of birth. Intermediates in metabolism, which accumulate after birth, are removed before birth through the mother's blood stream. Most products needed for normal development that are reduced by a metabolic error e.g. tyrosine in infants with phenylketonuria (PKU) are provided through the placenta by the mother. There is a period of time after birth when intermediates in metabolism, which are toxic to the infant, have not yet accumulated to the point where

Table 1   Examples and Frequency of Disorders Screened by
Newborn Screening Programs

PKU	1:12,000 overall
	Higher in Causcasians than in
	African-Americans
Galactosemia	1:60,000
	Does not seem to have ethnic specificity
Congenital hypothyroidism	1:3,000 to 1:4,000
Maple syrup urine disease	1:70,000 to 1:150,000
	Except in old order Mennonites where
	it is 1:150

they may cause irreversible damage but elevated enough to
ensure their detection and identification as abnormal. This
time interval is the period when newborn screening by substrate level is possible. Newborn screening by enzymatic
assay (e.g., in galactosemia) and for low or high hormone
levels (hypothyroidism or congenital adrenal hyperplasia)
must also be accomplished during this predamage window
of opportunity. Table 1 gives representative examples and
frequencies of disorders screened by newborn screening
programs.

II. TIMING OF NEWBORN SCREENING

Because newborn screening for PKU nationwide has been in
place for the longest, the best understanding of screening is
for this disorder. It is clear that at least 24 hr of protein feeding is required before serum concentrations of phenylalanine
(the measured substrate) are certain to be elevated. Only in
some infants, concentrations are elevated before that time.
Because many infants are sent home from the hospital before
they have been fed protein for 24 hr, it has been recommended
that these infants should have their screening repeated later.
The period before a child may be damaged by elevated phenylalanine concentrations is uncertain and depends on the
degree of elevation. It is generally assumed, without much
data, that a period of up to one month of age is safe before diet

is instituted. The goal in most programs is to start the diet before 10 days of age.

The window of opportunity for successful treatment of other newborn diseases is less certain. Hypothyroid screening can be confused by the surge in thyroid stimulating hormone (TSH) concentrations in the 24 hr after birth and by variations in total thyroxine (T4) and TSH concentrations in premature infants (1). An unexpected number of hypothyroid infants have been identified on repeat screens suggesting that second screening for this disease should be carried out between 2 and 4 weeks after birth. There is no reason why screening for galactosemia should not be accurate immediately after birth (it is an enzyme assay). The usual problem with galactosemia screening is obtaining the result before the child becomes ill. The greatest unknown at present is the timing of screening for the 40 or 50 disorders that can be identified by expanded newborn screening by tandem mass spectroscopy (MS) (Table 2). It is assumed that timing similar to that for PKU will be acceptable but only now is any data accumulating to support that view.

III. HISTORY OF NEWBORN SCREENING

In 1954, Bickel and coworkers (2) demonstrated that a phenylalanine-restricted diet could prevent mental retardation in children with PKU. The need for a relatively noninvasive and safe test for phenylalanine in the newborn was not met until 1963. Guthrie and Susi (3) developed a bacterial assay for phenylalanine that required only a minimal amount of blood collected on a filter paper from a newborn's heel. This assay had the additional advantage that it could be dried and then mailed to a central laboratory for analysis. Routine newborn screening became a reality in Massachusetts in 1962 (4). It soon became almost universal in the United States and in most other developed nations.

The addition of hypothyroidism to newborn screening using the same filter paper blood spot used for PKU began in the 1970s (5). Testing for sickle cell disease and other

Table 2 Classes of Disorders Identified by Expanded Newborn Screening

Amino acid disorders	In addition to PKU and maple syrup urine disease, a variety of other disorders of amino acid metabolism may be detected. Some of these disorders lead to neonatal death. Others cause delays in development.
Fatty acid disorders	In addition to MCAD (Medium Chain Acyl-CoA Dehydrogenase Deficiency), screening by tandem MS can detect other deficiencies in fatty acid metabolism. These disorders may cause problems in maintaining blood glucose levels and are reported to be associated with sudden death in otherwise normal appearing infants. The low blood sugars can lead to developmental problems.
Short chain fatty acid disorders	These disorders result from the inability to fully metabolize amino acids and fatty acids, including propionic acidemia. These disorders can produce severe acidosis in the newborn period and are sometimes mistaken for infection. They also may cause developmental problems in later life.
Other disorders where organic acids are accumulated	In addition to all of the problems mentioned above, many other problems with metabolism in which organic acids can be measured in the blood will be detected. Because many of these diseases are individually rare, tandem MS is the only measure currently available to detect many of these disorders before they become clinically evident.

hemoglobinopathies soon followed. Gradually, screening has come to all of the states in this nation and in several countries worldwide and includes other diseases such as galactosemia, other amino acid disorders, congenital adrenal hyperplasia due to 21-hydroxylase deficiency, and cystic fibrosis. Because, as noted below, there are no national standards in the United States, each state determines which tests will be done and only PKU and congenital hypothyroidism are tested for in every state.

The biggest change in newborn screening nationwide is now underway. Led by the commercial firm Neogen and North Carolina (6), the use of tandem MS to diagnose a variety of diseases of newborn intermediate metabolism has led to the possibility of greatly expanding the range of diseases that can be diagnosed. Because of the association of disorders of fatty acid metabolism with cases of sudden infant death, there has been great pressure from parents' groups to rapidly expand the availability of this testing. Unfortunately, this call for expansion of newborn screening comes at a time of economic downturn when states nationwide are having difficulty in financing this move. Nonetheless, we may expect to have expanded newborn screening in most of the United States and other developed countries in the near future.

IV. ARCHITECTURE OF A SCREENING PROGRAM

In the United States of America, since there is no National Health Plan, each state and district has the right to determine which screening tests are required, where the tests can be done, and the cost and mechanism of paying for them. (The rules in other countries are quite varied, but generally the cost of newborn screening is absorbed by the government). Extended newborn screening is not yet included in mandated screening in most states and is largely available on demand and payment through private laboratories. Thus, in most states expanded newborn screening is available only to those who can pay. In Missouri, expanded newborn screening is not yet covered by all insurance and is paid by check directly when the sample is sent.

Discussions of the needs of a newborn screening program were extensively held in the early years of screening programs. Strangely, this discussion has been largely absent during the recent rush for extended newborn screening and needs to be reviewed. Probably the United States National Academy of Sciences (NAS) provided the best outline of what a screening program should be in 1975 (7).

The NAS recommended, in part, that a specific rationale should be defined for screening. It should be stated that the goal would be medical intervention, family planning, or research. It is interesting that the newborn screening legislation in Missouri and, I believe, most of the rest of the United States still state that the reason for newborn screening is to prevent mental retardation, even though the goals are now much broader. Because the expanded newborn screening done by tandem MS tests for as many as 40 or 50 different diseases, no single rational can be given for screening. Usually, the pressure to increase screening has come from parents of children who have died unexpectedly and where a disease has been identified postmortem, which could have been screened for. Thus, the rationale is mostly to prevent sudden death rather than to prevent disabilities.

The NAS report stated that population screening for medical intervention should only be performed in an integrated program capable of information dispersal, screening, retrieval of persons with positive tests, diagnosis, counseling, medical management, and outcome evaluation. It is assumed that the mechanism in place for PKU screening can be applied to the more extensive program. However, at this time, private companies do much of the screening and the State mechanism, even when capable, is not in the loop. Centers or individual doctors who have expertise for many of these diseases have not been identified and treatment centers within the physical reach of many patients have not been found. Adequate literature explaining the screening programs has not been distributed to either health care workers or to families. At present, a phone call to our office saying that the "PKU" test is abnormal could mean any of the tests done is out of line. A call saying that an extended screen is abnormal may or may not be specific for a disease. Fortunately in Missouri there are four centers to which a patient may be referred, but even then, a family may have to travel 4 or 5 hr to be seen. Distances in areas even less settled than ours can be extreme.

The NAS report states that the test should have minimal false positives and false negatives in order to maximize specificity and sensitivity. Interestingly, this had not been evaluated when PKU was first screened for in the 1960s (it took several years) and has certainly not been done for many of the diseases that can now be screened for by tandem MS. Statistics on false positives and negatives will have to be collected over a long period of time for these mostly rare diseases in order to have adequate numbers to study.

A new wrinkle has entered as potential problems for screening programs in the United States, i.e., HIPAA regulations concerning privacy. Screening data are only available in theory to the patient (or family) and the designated physician. Unfortunately, in many centers the responsible physician is difficult to identify, the newborn's last name may have changed, and it may require law enforcement help to locate an address. In addition the infant may present at an emergency center without the necessary information. New legislation is needed to allow data from the State laboratories to be reviewed by identifiable qualified individuals. Data from private laboratories are subject to the privacy rules and not necessarily available to the treating health care worker.

Finally, mechanisms will be required for states, provinces, or other governments to certify the quality of laboratories located in other jurisdictions. One of the reasons that newborn screening had been centralized in State laboratories in the USA was to centralize quality control. The local governments now will have to make some effort to obtain a means of acceptable national certification.

V. METHODS OF COLLECTING SAMPLES

Virtually, in all screening programs whole blood is collected on standard thickness filter paper as first described by Guthrie and Susi (3). This has many advantages. Firstly, the blood can be collected by heel-stick and thus is relatively noninvasive. Secondly, the filter paper can be attached to standardized forms, which allow the automation of the screening process and for ready identification of the sample source. Thirdly, the filter paper can be marked with standard sample sizes (circles) allowing the collection by relatively untrained individuals. Lastly, dried samples can be more easily and cheaply shipped to laboratories.

The greatest problem with filter paper samples is poor collection. An ongoing program of training of hospital personnel is required to maintain the quality of the samples. Another problem has been heat. Galactose-1-phosphate uridyltransferase is heat sensitive and can be destroyed in poorly shipped samples. In states or countries where the summer temperature is high, heat inactivation is the commonest cause of false positive results.

VI. METHODS OF ANALYZING SAMPLES

The original Guthrie method for phenylalanine, a bacterial inhibition assay, continues to be used in most state screening programs. In this assay, a phenylalanine analog, which inhibits bacterial growth, is added to the culture plate. When a filter paper circle saturated with blood is placed on the plate, growth around the circle depends on the concentration of phenylalanine in the sample. Thus, the size of the growth circle can be measured and correlated with phenylalanine concentrations. Similar tests for other amino acids have been developed, but are not widely used. Guthrie's method has been replaced in some programs with a fluorescent assay, still using the filter paper circle. It seems destined to be replaced in the future with a tandem MS method (see discussion below).

Galactosemia is identified in two ways. First, an assay can measure either the concentration of galactose or a combination of galactose and galactose-1-phosphate. More commonly, an enzyme assay for galactose-1-phosphate uridyltransferase (GALT) activity is done (8). It is the assay that is heat sensitive. Immunoassays for thyroxine (T4) and/or TSH are used to assess congenital hypothyroidism (1). A similar assay for 17-hydroxyprogesterone is used to test for congenital adrenal hyperplasia (only the 21-hydroxylase form of this disease is screened for) (9). An immunoassay can also be used for trypsinogen as a screen for cystic fibrosis.

The most exciting change in newborn screening has come from the development of tandem mass spectrometry using a

Guthrie blood spot as a source of screening. This method allows the screening of many amino acid disorders and most disorders of fatty acid metabolism in a single assay. The sample is chemically ionized in the first mass spectrometer that determines the molecular weight of the compounds present (usually only compounds with molecular weights $< 500 \mu$). The compounds then pass through a second ionization chamber that breaks them down into distinctive fragments that can be identified by a second mass spectrometer in order to distinguish different compounds with the same molecular weight. No small part of the success of this method has come from the advancement in computer technology that has allowed the analysis and correlation of the huge amount of data generated.

VII. FALSE POSITIVES AND NEGATIVES

False positive screening tests cause anxiety in families. They also increase the effective cost of newborn screening because they lead to repeated testing, visits to medical facilities, and lost time for screening personnel. The proportion of false positive results is dependent on which disease is being screened, the cut-off value used by the laboratory to report positive and borderline results, and the season of the year with regard to galactosemia. For premature infants, the number of false positive tests increases. For tests of hormonal function, false positive tests occur most frequently during the hormonal surge in the first 24 hr of life. False positive results for most newborn screening collectively account for 10 reports for every sample that is a true positive. In the summertime, carriers for the disease cause many of the positive tests for galactosemia. Carriers are less likely to be detected in the winter. Setting the cut-off to help eliminate false negative results, i.e., to prevent missing any cases increases the number of false positives. Perhaps for this reason, false negative test results are fortunately much less common. However, the identification of many cases of hypothyroidism missed by initial screening and rare cases of PKU has led to a call for children to be screened a second time. The use of tandem MS to provide ratios of compounds, i.e., phenylalanine to tyrosine and leucine to alanine, will hopefully decrease the incidence of false positive and negative results.

VIII. PKU—THE BEST-STUDIED EXAMPLE OF NEWBORN SCREENING

Phenylketonuria has the longest history for newborn screening and is the best studied. Lessons learned from PKU can be applied to most screening programs (10,11).

A. Interpretation of a Positive Result

Scriver and Kaufman (10) list five frequent causes of positive screening tests for high phenylalanine levels (Table 3). The purpose of this chapter is not to review the biochemistry of this disorders, but instead to point out the need to do follow-up studies to rule out conditions other than PKU while at the same time starting treatment as if the patients had classical PKU. If one of the other disorders is present, then treatment can be changed. The treatment and the outcome for the patients with these various disorders are different and the families must be prepared for the future. It must be remembered that PKU itself is an enzyme deficiency that does not go away.

B. Need for Long-Term Treatment Facilities

Treatment with diet for classical PKU is almost universally successful in the early years of life if managed by a team accustomed to treating this disorder. Development is usually quite normal. As with many children with chronic illness and much adult contact, at age 4 or 5, the IQ will often test in the

Table 3   Causes of Positive Screening Tests for Phenylalanine Levels

1. Transient hyperphenylalaninemia
2. Persistent non-PKU hyperphenylalaninemia
3. PKU
4. Three disorders of tetrahydrobiopterin synthesis
5. Dihydropteridine reductase deficiency

superior range. However, treatment must continue throughout life in patients with classical PKU. One of the saddest experiences for a clinician taking care of patients with PKU is to meet a patient previously known to him/her who has been off diet for several years. Figure 1 shows the frontal view of a typical child with classical PKU. The PKU patient will have noticeably lost intelligence and often has a history of depression or severe mood swings. Although patients successfully restarted on diets can regain some intellectual function, particularly short-term memory, they do not seem to return to the level they had previously attained. We recently managed to have several teenagers who had taken their college boards while out of control of diet (phenylalanine >12 mg%) to retake them after their serum phenylalanine levels were lower and found the scores to be near the normal range. Their board

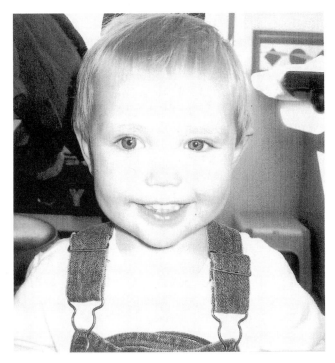

Figure 1 Frontal view of a successfully treated (diet controlled) 2-year-old white male with classical PKU.

scores were 30% better on the average with lower phenylalanine concentrations. We have also had the negative experience of patients with good board scores admitted to good
colleges and then fail after taking themselves off diet. Thus,
PKU is the best example of the success of newborn screening
but emphasizes that screening for diseases in the newborn
period commits clinicians to a lifetime of caring for these
patients. Table 2 shows classes of disorders identified on
extended newborn screening.

IX. CASE DESCRIPTIONS OF PKU

A. The Treated Patient with PKU

The diet of a treated patient with PKU is extremely limited.
The average classical PKU patient will tolerate only about
200–250 mg of phenylalanine per day. In real dietary terms,
a slice of bread contains 100–150 mg of phenylalanine and
meat and normal dairy products are way above daily allowan-
ces except in quantities too small to satisfy. In order to reduce
the phenylalanine intake to acceptable levels and maintain
adequate nutrition, the patients are totally dependent on synthetic milk substitutes that contain little or no phenylalanine.
A PKU individual is limited in a fast food restaurant to a little
salad and a few French fries (a small order of French fries
contains about 115 mg of phenylalanine). Nonetheless, most
children can maintain this diet in the early years of life.

On diet and with regular blood levels of phenylalanine in
the acceptable range, PKU children have IQs appropriate for
their age. In fact, probably due to their constant exposure to
adults, at age 4–5 years, most PKU children test in a superior
range. Usually, by age 8 years or more, their performance in
school is appropriate for their age and social situation. Although
learning problems have been described in PKU children on diet,
it is unclear whether the frequency of these problems is higher
in the PKU children than their non-PKU siblings.

B. The Treated Patient Who Goes Off Diet

One of the great tragedies in medicine was the belief, still mentioned in some textbooks, that PKU children can be taken off

diet at age 5 or later. What is abundantly clear from many international studies is that the IQ steadily declines with time, perhaps 1–2 IQ points per year. What is also clear to families and health care workers is that an acute rise in phenylalanine levels can lead to the loss of short-term memory and striking problems in learning. In recent years, as the PKU population is aging, it is also clear that psychiatric problems, depression, and mood swings in our experience are also frequent in patients who go off diet. A few older patients have experienced life threatening neurological problems. Diet and monitoring phenylalanine levels are for the entire life of the patient.

C. The Child of a Woman with PKU

A mother without PKU who is carrying a PKU infant removes the excess phenylalanine from the child until the time of birth. A mother with PKU, who is off diet, actually infuses excess phenylalanine into her fetus with or without PKU. The phenylalanine levels in the unborn infant are about 1.5 times higher than those in the mother. Seventy-five to 90% of children born to inadequately treated women with PKU have microcephaly while only about 1% of these babies born to PKU mothers will actually have inherited PKU. They may also have congenital heart disease, other birth defects, and growth retardation. In addition, there is a higher than normal incidence of neonatal death. Although head size increases after birth and becomes closer to the normal range, the children are mostly severely developmentally delayed. Mothers who are maintained on diet to lower their phenylalanine levels during pregnancy can have normal infants. In most cases, it is best to get the serum phenylalanine maintained in a treatment range before the mother becomes pregnant. Therefore, close medical management is needed for the mother and her developing fetus.

REFERENCES

1. Fischer DA. Thyroid disorders. In: Rimoin DL, Connor JM, Pyeritz RE, Korf BR, eds. Emery and Rimoin's Principles

and Practice of Medical Genetics. 4th ed. Edinburgh: Churchill Livingstone, 2002:2183–2202.

2. Bickle H, Gerrard JW, Hickmans EM. Influence of phenylalanine intake on the chemistry and behavior of a phenylketonuric child. Acta Pediatr 1954; 43:64–77.

3. Guthrie R, Susi A. A simple phenylalanine method for detecting phenylketonuria in large populations of newborn infants. Pediatrics 1963; 32:338–343.

4. MacCready RA, Hussey MG. Newborn phenylketonuria detection program in Massachusetts. Am J Public Health 1964; 54: 2075–2081.

5. Dussault JH, Coulombe P, Laberge C, Letarte J, Guyda H, Khoury K. Preliminary report on a mass screening program for neonatal hypothyroidism. J Pediatr 1975; 86:670–674.

6. Chace DH, Naylor EW. Expansion of newborn screening programs using tandem mass spectrometry. Mental Retardation Dev Disability Res Rev 1999; 5:150–154.

7. Genetic Screening: Principles and Research. Washington, DC: National Academy of Sciences, 1975.

8. Holton JB, Walter JH, Tyfield LA. Galactosemia. In: Scriver CR, Beaudet AL, Valle D, Sly WS, eds. The Metabolic Molecular Bases of Inherited Disease. 8th ed. New York: McGraw-Hill, 2001:1553–1587.

9. New MI, Wilson RC. Genetic disorders of the adrenal gland. In: Rimoin DL, Connor JM, Pyeritz RE, Korf BR, eds. Emery and Rimoin's Principles and Practice of Medical Genetics. 4th ed. Edinburgh: Churchill Livingstone, 2002:2277–2314.

10. Scriver CR, Kaufman S. Hyperphenylalaninemia: phenylalanine hydroxylase deficiency. In: Scriver CR, Beaudet AL, Valle D, Sly WS, eds.The Metabolic Molecular Bases of Inherited Disease. 8th ed. New York: McGraw-Hill, 2001:1667–1724.

11. Meryash DL, Levy HL, Guthrie R, Warner R, Bloom S, Carr JR. Prospective study of early neonatal screening for phenylketonuria. New Eng J Med 1981; 304:294–296.

18

Fetal Alcohol Syndrome

MARGARET P. ADAM and H. EUGENE HOYME

Department of Pediatrics, Division of Medical
Genetics, Stanford University School of Medicine,
Stanford, California, U.S.A.

I. INTRODUCTION

The possible teratogenic effects of alcohol on the developing fetus have been suspected for centuries and admonitions against pregnant women drinking alcohol or strong drink date back to biblical times. It was recognized during the "gin epidemic" (a period between 1720 and 1751 in which alcohol consumption increased because of the low price of gin) in London that the children of women who were drinking distilled liquors were born weak and sickly (1). In 1899, Sullivan, describing a controlled, patient-matched study of the offspring of women inmates of Liverpool prison, observed: "Maternal inebriety is a condition peculiarly unfavorable to the vitality and to the normal development of offspring. Its

665

gravity in this respect is considerably greater than that of paternal alcoholism. (There is) a tendency to stillbirths and abortions, and a high rate of epilepsy in the surviving children. This influence of alcohol is ... in part due to a direct toxic action on the embryo" (2). This study was largely ignored, and there is little evidence to suggest that historical figures or physicians knew about the direct toxic effects of alcohol on the developing fetus. The first description in the modern medical literature of a distinctly recognizable pattern of malformation associated with maternal alcohol abuse was reported by Lemoine et al. (3) in France in 1968 and independently by Jones et al. (4) in the United States in 1973. Since that time, substantial progress has been made in developing specific criteria for defining and diagnosing this condition.

Maternal alcohol consumption during pregnancy represents a significant population burden. This can be conceptualized as an excess of various "bad" outcomes of pregnancy caused by current drinking patterns within the population. Those excesses per year for the United States are estimated in Table 1.

Discounting the personal and emotional burden of maternal alcohol consumption, the financial burden alone is overwhelming. Estimates for the state of New York are approximately US$ 155 million per year. If these data are extrapolated to the entire population of the United States, and corrected for inflation, a rough estimate of the annual

Table 1 Excesses of Unfavorable Outcomes Caused by Drinking During Pregnancy

Outcome	No drinking	Current drinking	Excess
Spontaneous abortions	600,000	630,000	30,000
FAS	0	6,000	6,000
All congenital malformations	200,000	230,000	30,000
Growth retardation	120,000	132,000	12,000
Mental retardation	120,000	140,000	20,000

Source: Ref. 2.

costs of the harmful effects of maternal alcohol consumption on the developing fetus approaches US$ 4 billion (2).

II. DEFINITION/TERMINOLOGY

The adverse effects of alcohol on the developing human represent a spectrum of structural anomalies and behavioral and neurocognitive disabilities, most accurately termed "fetal alcohol spectrum disorders" (FASD) (5). The fetal alcohol syndrome (FAS) denotes a specific pattern of malformation, which includes the following: confirmed history of maternal alcohol abuse during pregnancy, prenatal onset of growth deficiency (including length and/or weight) that persists postnatally, a specific pattern of minor anomalies of the face, and neurocognitive deficits. Although children at the severe end of the spectrum of FASD are easily diagnosed by an experienced clinician, much controversy remains about the diagnosis of children with some, but not all, of the features of full-blown FAS. The need for a term to describe these children who have a "forme fruste" of FAS led to the term "suspected fetal alcohol effects." This term was not originally intended to be a diagnostic category, but rather it was a population-based term which served as a reminder to clinicians that certain abnormalities (compatible with some, but not all, of the features of FAS) observed in a particular patient could be associated with in utero alcohol exposure. Unfortunately, the term "fetal alcohol effect" (FAE) began to be applied to patients with a variety of problems based solely on either suspected or confirmed maternal alcohol use during pregnancy. Because this term was used so frequently, some health agencies began to accept FAE as a medical diagnosis for which patients could become eligible for educational and financial services (6).

In 1980, the Fetal Alcohol Study Group of the Research Society on Alcohol noted a wide range of effects of alcohol on the developing fetus, with FAS at one end of the spectrum. They proposed that "possible fetal alcohol effects" be used to refer to patients who had disabilities that were thought to be related to prenatal alcohol exposure but who did not meet the diagnostic criteria of FAS (7). However, this definition remained problematic because, in any given case, it could not be proved or disproved. In addition, the term FAE allowed for wide interpretation by clinicians, making it clinically useless. For example, it could be applied to any structural, learning, or behavioral problem in an exposed child, regardless of the underlying diagnosis or lack thereof. Such diagnostic imprecision led to frustration among health care providers, parents, and guardians alike. This frustration led clinicians to either disregard alcohol as a contributing factor to any of their patients' problems or to overdiagnose alcohol's contribution to such problems, in turn hampering efforts to elucidate the real magnitude of alcohol-related birth defects (ARBD).

Because the term FAE had gained acceptance by health care agencies, tremendous pressure began to be exerted on clinicians by parents, foster parents, and schools to make this diagnosis. Although the positive results of making this diagnosis are well known, the consequences of misdiagnosis have often been overlooked. For example, inaccurate diagnosis of an alcohol-related disability may lead to stigmatization of mothers of labeled children, although it may be unclear that prenatal alcohol exposure lead to their child's problems. It can also lead to inaccurate and potentially damaging labeling by schools and social service agencies. Finally, once a diagnosis of an alcohol-related disability has been made, the search for other causes of a patient's symptoms is often abandoned. Therefore, an inaccurate diagnosis can result in the lack or premature termination of diagnostic studies to determine the etiology of the disabilities.

In 1995, Aase et al. (6) argued that the term FAE be eliminated because of the above-mentioned ambiguities. The authors pointed out that the individual known effects of in utero exposure to alcohol are those that as a composite make up FAS, i.e., each component of FAS, such as growth retardation or neurocognitive deficits, is nonspecific and it is only the combination of all components that allows the definition of FAS. As a further example, the authors observed that the facial features of FAS encompass a group of minor anomalies or structural variants that can be found as isolated characteristics in normal individuals and families. As such, they can be thought of as representing polygenic traits inherited in a multifactorial pattern. Therefore, the significance of these variations from normal lies only in their association with one another into a specific pattern that can be recognized as a specific syndrome. Since the term FAE does not allow for such a consistently recognized pattern, it cannot be applied to a specific individual. Aase et al. (6) suggested that the term FAE be used only in population or animal studies in which the independent variable is maternal alcohol use during pregnancy.

III. DIAGNOSTIC CRITERIA

Although many papers in the literature attempt to define the findings necessary to make a diagnosis of FAS and alcohol-related effects, there are two major published sets of diagnostic criteria that are currently used in evaluating and categorizing children prenatally exposed to alcohol. The first set of criteria was published by the Institute of Medicine of the National Academy of Sciences in 1996 after the U.S. Congress mandated a study on FAS. The Institute of Medicine study group developed five diagnostic categories for FAS and alcohol-related effects.

The first category is termed "FAS with confirmed maternal alcohol exposure" (Figs. 1 and 2). Along with confirmed alcohol exposure, it requires that the patient exhibit all three of the following:

1. Characteristic minor facial anomalies, including short palpebral fissures and abnormalities in the premaxillary area (flattened philtrum, thin upper lip, and maxillary hypoplasia).

2. Evidence of growth retardation, including either low birth weight for gestational age, decelerating weight over time not due to nutrition, or disproportionate low weight to height.

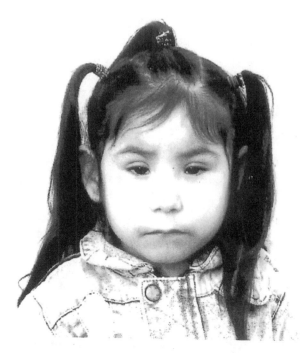

Figure 1 Native American child with FAS. Note short palebral fissues, smooth philtrum, and thin upper lip.

3. Evidence of CNS neurodevelopmental abnormalities, defined as either decreased head size at birth, structural brain abnormalities (for example, microcephaly, cerebellar hypoplasia, or complete or partial agenesis of the corpus callosum), or signs of neurologic abnormalities on examination (for example, poor eye–hand co-ordination or impaired fine motor skills).

The second category is termed "FAS without confirmed maternal alcohol exposure," and also requires characteristics 1–3 above. The third category is "partial FAS with confirmed maternal alcohol exposure." This category is reserved for patients who have documented in utero alcohol exposure, some of the typical facial anomalies of FAS, and evidence of either growth retardation or CNS neurodevelopmental abnormalities, as defined above.

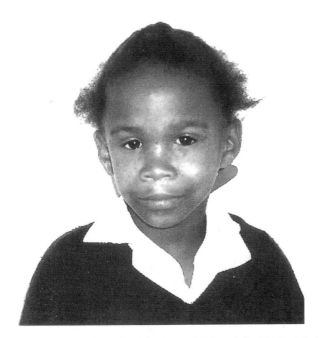

Figure 2 South African child with FAS. Note short palebral fissues, smooth philtrum, and thin upper lip.

Categories four and five fall into the realm of alcohol-related effects. Alcohol-related effects encompass two clinical conditions in which a history of maternal alcohol use must be documented, and there is some evidence, in the form of human or animal studies, that links maternal alcohol consumption to the observed outcomes. The fourth category is termed "alcohol-related birth defects." This includes a heterogeneous list of structural malformations which have been described in concert with prenatal alcohol exposure, such as certain congenital heart defects and skeletal, renal, and ocular abnormalities. The fifth category is termed "alcohol-related neurodevelopmental disorder" (ARND). This category requires the presence of CNS neurodevelopmental abnormalities as described in number 3 above and/or behavioral and cognitive abnormalities, such as learning difficulties or poor impulse control (8).

There are several problems with the Institute of Medicine diagnostic criteria for FAS and alcohol-related effects as currently written. Firstly, they are somewhat vague. For example, the degree of growth deficiency or the exact facial dysmorphology required for each category is not defined. In addition, there are no guidelines on which components of the "complex pattern of behavioral or cognitive difficulties" are suggestive of FAS and how best to assess these abnormalities. Secondly, the family and genetic history of the patient is not adequately addressed. Thirdly, ARBD and ARND are not practically defined in a clinical sense.

Because of these concerns, Astley and Clarren (9) sought to develop a more objective set of diagnostic criteria, which were published in 2000. These diagnostic criteria are commonly referred to as the "Washington Criteria" because they were formulated by reviewing the medical records of 1014 patients diagnosed with FAS through the Washington State Fetal Alcohol Syndrome Diagnostic and Prevention Network. This set of criteria retains the four commonly accepted key diagnostic features for FAS, including growth deficiency, the characteristic FAS facial phenotype, central nervous system damage/dysfunction, and alcohol exposure in utero. The degree to which each of these four factors is present in any given patient is ranked on a four-point Likert scale, with 1 representing the complete absence of the feature and 4 representing a classic presentation of the feature. From this, each patient is assigned a four-digit diagnostic code, with each digit corresponding to the degree to which each of the four main features of FAS is present. This results in 256 possible combinations, ranging from 1111 to 4444, which are collapsed into 22 diagnostic categories, termed A through V. The authors of this system point out that since a number of categories differ by only the amount of alcohol exposure, there are nine unique diagnostic outcomes. These diagnostic outcomes range from "no cognitive/behavioral or sentinel physical findings detected" to "FAS" (9).

While this system appears to be extremely accurate in placing each patient into a specific diagnostic category within the spectrum of alcohol associated abnormalities, the myriad of diagnostic categories is confusing and the system is impractical for routine use. In order to use this system properly, the

University of Washington published a 111-page manual to aid practitioners. The manual is equipped with instructions, case definitions, normal anthropometric charts, a pictorial scale for ranking lip thinness and philtrum smoothness, and a New Patient Information Form for recording developmental history and exposures. It also comes equipped with an instructional CD-ROM. While this may be useful for the practitioner who evaluates a majority of patients prenatally exposed to alcohol, it is time consuming to learn for the physician with a more diverse practice.

The Washington Criteria also suffer from problems similar to the Institute of Medicine Criteria. For example, the Washington Criteria places much emphasis on the "encephalopathy" and "neurobehavioral disorder" present in a patient. These two findings are not specific to the prenatal effects of alcohol on fetal development. In addition, the family and genetic background of the patient is not adequately integrated into the criteria. Such a structured system also has the potential for overdiagnosis of alcohol-related disabilities.

One advantage of the Washington Criteria is the attempt to define the facial phenotype of FAS in an objective manner. Astley and Clarren (9) have created a pictorial "lip/philtrum guide" to aid in the objective assessment of the structure of the upper lip and philtrum (Fig. 3). This guide depicts five categories, ranging from normal to those observed in classical FAS. In order to use the guide for the diagnosis of FAS, the upper lip thinness and the philtrum smoothness are assessed separately by comparing the patient's face to the guide. A rank of 1 is considered completely normal while a rank of 5 is most suggestive of FAS. Medical practitioners who evaluate patients with in utero exposure to alcohol should be encouraged to use this objective lip/philtrum guide even if they do not employ the full diagnostic system proposed by Astley and Clarren.

An ideal diagnostic system for FASD would accurately diagnose affected individuals by minimizing the false positive and false negative rates, by precisely defining diagnostic categories, by taking genetic and family history into account, by utilizing a multidisciplinary approach (including a careful

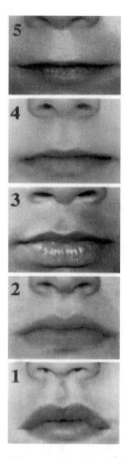

Figure 3 Lip/philtrum guide. Plates 4 and 5 are compatible with FASD. (Reproduced with permission from the University of Washington FAS Diagnostic and Prevention Network, Astley and Clarren, 1999.)

behavioral and neuropsychological assessment) and by creating straightforward, understandable, and practical terminology that can be easily applied in local clinical settings. Both the Institute of Medicine diagnostic criteria and the Washington diagnostic criteria have advantages and disadvantages with respect to these characteristics. Therefore, investigators in the field of FASD continue to revise the currently available diagnostic systems with these ideals in mind.

IV. EPIDEMIOLOGY

Estimates of the prevalence of FAS have been difficult to determine because of differences in study populations and modes of data collection. In general, three methods have been used in an attempt to delineate the prevalence of this condition. These three methods include retrospective record collection and review, clinic-based studies, and active case ascertainment and diagnosis in specific populations (10). Retrospective studies have used special registries and reviews of birth certificates in an attempt to identify those patients with features that could be consistent with FAS. This method tends to result in higher prevalence rates. Clinic-based studies generally involve screening for alcohol use in a group of pregnant women and then evaluating their children at or after birth. Data using this method can either be obtained retrospectively or prospectively. Retrospective clinic-based studies tend to give higher estimates for the prevalence of FAS. When clinic-based studies are performed prospectively, they tend to give lower rates; however, prospective clinic-based studies appear to be more accurate for determining maternal alcohol use. The third method involves seeking referrals for all children who may have FAS within a specific population. It is thought that this method gives the most accurate rate, as strict diagnostic criteria can be applied uniformly to a group of patients within the specific population. However, when this method is applied to high-risk populations, it may overestimate the risk in the general population (8,10,11).

The estimated prevalence of FAS in the United States has ranged from 0.0/1000 children to 10.7/1000 children depending on which of the above methods is used and which population is being studied (10). However, in 1995, Abel calculated the birth prevalence of FAS as 0.97/1000 using data from a number of prospective studies in a variety of locations throughout the United States. This is currently the generally accepted prevalence rate within the United States. Obviously, this number varies substantially depending on alcohol consumption rates within given subpopulations (12).

V. DRINKING PATTERNS AND ALCOHOL TERATOGENICITY

Prior to discussing proposed mechanisms of alcohol teratogenicity, it is appropriate to discuss patterns of alcohol consumption among all women in the Unites States, regardless
of pregnancy status. In order to do so, levels of alcohol use
must be defined. A standard drink is often defined as one-half
ounce of alcohol. Among the general population, consuming
an average of 0–3 standard drinks per week is considered
light drinking. Moderate drinking is defined as consuming
an average of 4–13 drinks per week and heavy drinking is
defined as 14 or more drinks per week. A 1991 U.S. National
Survey of 1099 women who were 21 years or older found that
58.4% had consumed alcohol in the past year. Of the women
who reported drinking alcohol, 23.7% reported drinking six
or more drinks per drinking occasion (13). In general, young
women tend to report the highest rates of drinking, with rates
declining as women age (8).

It is estimated that pregnant women consume substantially less amounts of alcohol than nonpregnant women in
the general population. A number of surveys of drinking habits
among pregnant women conducted in the late 1980s to mid-
1990s found that approximately 15–20% of pregnant women
reported drinking any amount of alcohol during their pregnancies (8). Similarly, it was estimated that approximately 86% of
pregnant women abstained from alcohol use during pregnancy
in 1996 and 1997 (14). Because of this fact, many authors have
lowered their cutoff definitions for light, moderate, and heavy
drinking when applying them to pregnant women. Unfortunately, precise definitions of levels of drinking for pregnant
women vary depending on the survey or study being done,
which makes scientific research on the effects of alcohol
consumption on human fetal development difficult.

In general, there appears to be a positive correlation
between increasing alcohol consumption and adverse postnatal outcome in humans. A recent rat model of FAS did not find
a simple dose–response curve, but that adverse outcome
depended on how rapidly the dose of alcohol was administered

and how long the blood alcohol levels were above a toxic threshold (15). This, in part, supports human findings that binge drinking and drinking earlier in pregnancy appear to be associated with the highest risks of adverse outcomes to offspring (16). In addition, there appears to be a positive correlation between the duration of drinking, the parity of the woman, and poorer outcome in the fetus (7). This has been supported by a miniature swine model of FAS, in which greater anomalies were found in the offspring of miniature swine that were multiparous and that had been exposed to alcohol for a longer duration (up to 2.5 years) prior to breeding (17).

VI. MECHANISMS OF TERATOGENESIS

Many mechanisms of teratogenesis have been proposed for ethanol, and it is likely that there is no single mechanism by which alcohol exerts its adverse effects on the developing fetus. As with any teratogenic exposure, the timing of exposure, the dosage, the presence of other confounding factors (such as poor nutrition or polysubstance abuse), and the genetic background of the exposed individual all play a role in the ultimate outcome. In a small twin study by Streissguth and Dehaene in 1993 (18), five out of five monozygotic twin pairs were concordant for FAS, whereas only seven out of 11 dizygotic twin pairs were concordant for FAS. This provides some evidence for possible genetic factors which may either predispose certain individuals to or protect them from the adverse effects of alcohol in utero.

One of the proposed genetic susceptibility factors for FAS is the activity of the enzyme alcohol dehydrogenase (ADH), which catalyzes the oxidation of ethanol to acetaldehyde. There are at least four classes of ADH enzymes in humans, of which class I ADH appears to be the most important (19). Class I ADH isoenzymes are heterodimers composed of some combination of either alpha, beta, or gamma subunit chains. The gene which encodes the beta chain, *ADH2*, has three common alleles, known as *ADH2*1*, *ADH2*2*, and *ADH2*3*. Each of these alleles has a different affinity for alcohol and a different rate of maximum catalysis. McCarver et al. in 1997 (19) proposed that the *ADH2*3* allele protected against ARBD in an African-American population, possibly related to its increased catalytic activity. In 2000, Jacobson et al. (20) reported that a group of African-Americans with the *ADH2*3* allele drank less amounts of alcohol less frequently than a group of African-Americans without the *ADH2*3* allele. Studies on the effects of the *ADH2*2* allele have been more controversial, with some studies reporting a protective effect against alcoholism and FAS (21–23) and some studies reporting no effect on alcohol consumption (24). Thus, the role of the alleles of *ADH2* in susceptibility remains controversial.

Because of the cognitive and neurobehavioral abnormalities observed in patients with FAS, much research has been conducted as to the effects of alcohol on the developing brain in both animals and humans. In 2000, Ikonomidou et al. (15) demonstrated that alcohol can act as a trigger for neuronal apoptosis in rat brains through blockade of the N-methyl-D-aspartate (NMDA) glutamate receptors and activation of the $GABA_A$ receptors. In rats, the affected neurons appeared to be most sensitive to these effects during synaptogenesis, which is a period of time when the brain undergoes significant growth. In humans, synaptogenesis occurs primarily between the sixth month of gestation to several years after birth. Ikonomidou et al. (15) concluded that even transient alcohol exposure during critical times in brain development can lead to the death of millions of neurons through these two mechanisms. They suggested that this can explain the findings of reduced brain mass and neurobehavioral abnormalities described in patients with FAS (15). Their observations also provide evidence that there is no safe period of time during pregnancy for alcohol consumption.

Retinoic acid has also been implicated in the pathogenesis of FAS (25). It is a potent morphogen, normally synthesized from retinol through the actions of ADH and critically important in early fetal development. Because alcohol is a competitive inhibitor of ADH, it has been postulated that in utero exposure to alcohol can cause a deficiency of retinoic acid (25).

The term "vitamin A" is used to describe a group of compounds, both naturally occurring and synthetically derived, known as retinoids. The naturally occurring alcohol form of vitamin A is retinol. There are multiple similarities between the fetal embryopathy associated with alcohol consumption and those seen in both vitamin A toxicity and vitamin A deficiency. For example, humans with in utero vitamin A deficiency can have prenatal and postnatal growth deficiency, microcephaly, mental retardation, and congenital heart defects, most commonly ventriculoseptal defects (VSD) and atrioseptal defects (ASD). Likewise, prenatal vitamin A toxicity can be manifested by mandibular/maxillary hypoplasia, microcephaly, and congenital heart defects (ASD, VSD, and conotruncal malformations) similar to patients with FAS. However, these patients often have microtia/anotia, micrognathia, and microphthalmia, as well.

Ethanol exposure in quail embryos, for example, can mimic vitamin A deficiency. This can be corrected by the addition of retinoic acid. Supplemental retinoic acid can also prevent the adverse effects of alcohol on neurite extension in cultured neuroblastoma cells. However, data from rat embryos have demonstrated that microsomal retinol oxidation was not affected by alcohol. Therefore, the effects of alcohol on retinol metabolism are somewhat controversial. It is unlikely that all the effects seen in FAS can be explained by alcohol's alteration in a single step of retinol metabolism (25). Further research is needed to elucidate the interaction of ethanol on retinol metabolism.

In addition, it has been proposed that alcohol exerts adverse effects on the glial cells of the brain or on glial–neuronal interactions. Initial postmortem pathologic studies of the brains of children who had been exposed to heavy amounts of alcohol in utero demonstrated a number of abnormalities, such as aberrant neural and glial tissue partially incorporating the pia matter and migrational defects of neural and glial cells (26). More modern techniques of head MRI have demonstrated that some patients with FAS have agenesis or hypoplasia of the corpus callosum and anterior commissure, which are areas of the brain formed by neuroglial cells. Guerri et al. (27) have reported that prenatal alcohol exposure markedly affects the morphology of radial glia cells (the main precursors of astrocytes) in culture and significantly decreases the expression of glial fibrillary acidic protein (GFAP), which is an astrocyte marker. This suggests that alcohol has an adverse effect on astroglial development. Furthermore, there is evidence that alcohol can adversely affect protein signaling and trafficking in the brain and other tissues (27).

Similarly, neuronal migration is mediated in part by the action of cell adhesion molecules (CAMs), which aid in cell–cell and cell–matrix signaling. In particular, the L1 cell adhesion molecule, which is located on the surfaces of long axons and on postmitotic neuronal growth cones, has been implicated in the process of neuronal outgrowth. It has been found that patients with CRASH syndrome (corpus callosum hypoplasia, mental retardation, adducted thumbs, spasticity, and hydrocephalus) have genetic defects in L1. These patients have a similar phenotype to patients with FAS (28). Based on this similarity, Bearer et al. (29), in 1999, decided to investigate the possible effects of alcohol on L1-mediated neuronal outgrowth in the cerebellum of rats. They were able to demonstrate that cerebellar granule cells exposed to alcohol inhibited L1-mediated neuronal outgrowth (29). Therefore, it appears that alcohol can disrupt brain growth and development on many levels.

It has been recognized that in utero alcohol exposure can be associated with holoprosencephaly, a developmental field defect in which there is failure of the embryonic forebrain to undergo midline cleavage in order to form the two cerebral hemispheres (30). The embryonic forebrain gives rise to the cephalic premigratory and migratory neural crest, which populate midfacial structures. Therefore, abnormalities in the premigratory and migratory neural crest result in a range of facial dysmorphology, from cyclopia to midface hypoplasia. It is hypothesized that neuronal death in this region leads to deficient tissue for midfacial development, thus contributing to many of the facial features present in FAS, such as the smooth philtrum and thin upper lip.

Mutations in many different genes have been found to cause holoprosencephaly. Mutations in the gene *Sonic*

Hedgehog (SHH) have been found to account for 3.7% of all cases of holoprosencephaly and about 17% of cases of familial holoprosencephaly (30–32). The Sonic Hedgehog protein is a signaling molecule that initiates a cascade of events that eventually leads to activation and transcription of a group of target genes. The pattern of *Shh* expression in vertebrates is largest in the developing head region (33). In the mouse, gene expression of *Shh* has been found, among other places, in the notochord and floorplate of the neural tube. In addition, disruption of the *Shh* gene expression in the mouse has been found to cause cyclopia with absence of the ventral neural tube cells (30). More recently, in 2002, Ahlgren et al. (33) demonstrated a marked downregulation of *Shh* in chick embryos exposed to alcohol at embryonic stage 9–10, with resultant cranial neural crest cell death and decreased size of the frontonasal mass. This effect could be rescued by administration of Shh protein. In addition, they found similar craniofacial phenotypes in chick embryos treated with antibodies that block Shh signaling. Therefore, data from Ahlgren et al. (33) support the theory that alcohol causes neural crest cell death, possibly by inhibiting the Sonic Hedgehog pathway, therefore leading to many of the craniofacial and neurodevelopmental abnormalities observed in FAS.

VII. DIFFERENTIAL DIAGNOSIS AND PHENOCOPIES OF FAS

It is important for clinicians to remember that children with other genetic and dysmorphic syndromes are born as frequently to women who abuse alcohol as they are to other women in the general population. Therefore, a diagnosis of FAS should not automatically be assigned to a child with disabilities just because his or her mother drank alcohol during the pregnancy. Since the phenotype of FAS is caused by increased cell death and migrational abnormalities in the fetal brain with resultant deficiency in the frontonasal prominence of the embryo, any genetic condition or teratogen that causes deficiency of the frontonasal prominence can

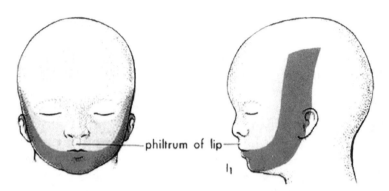

philtrum of lip

Figure 4 Hatched areas of the face, including the philtrum, are derived from cephalic neural crest in the frontonasal prominence of the embryo, thus explaining the finding of a smooth philtrum and thin upper lip in a number of malformation syndromes. (Reproduced from *Clinically Oriented Embryology. 3rd ed.*, W.B. Saunders Co.)

lead to a similar facial phenotype (Fig. 4). Fetal alcohol syndrome should therefore be thought of as a diagnosis of exclusion.

Fetal alcohol syndrome shares many common features with velocardiofacial syndrome (VCFS). Patients with VCFS can have short palpebral fissures, malar hypoplasia, microcephaly, and learning disabilities. However, patients with VCFS also can have a broad nasal root with bulbous nasal tip, deficiency of the alae nasi, hypocalcemia, and long and slender fingers. Although patients with FAS can have congenital heart defects, patients with VCFS have a higher prevalence of congenital heart defects, most commonly of the conotruncal type. Velocardiofacial syndrome is caused by a microdeletion on chromosome 22q11, which can be confirmed with a fluorescence in situ hybridization (FISH) analysis using a probe specific to this deleted region.

Fetal alcohol syndrome also shares many features with Williams syndrome. Patients with Williams syndrome can have mild prenatal growth deficiency with microcephaly, short palpebral fissures, long smooth philtrum, and learning and behavioral problems. In contrast to patients with FAS, patients with Williams syndrome also can have periorbital fullness, stellate irises, hallux valgus, hypercalcemia, a distinctive "cocktail party" personality, and congenital heart defects, most commonly supravalvular aortic stenosis and peripheral pulmonary artery stenosis. Williams syndrome is caused by a microdeletion of chromosome 7q11, which can be detected by FISH analysis.

A third phenocopy of FAS is the blepharophimosis syndrome, in which patients can have short palpebral fissures with lateral displacement of the inner canthi. Mental retardation and cardiac defects are variable features of this syndrome. There appears to be two forms of this condition, both of which are inherited in an autosomal dominant fashion. Type I is associated with premature ovarian failure with resultant female infertility. This form appears to be completely penetrant within families. Type II does not appear to affect female fertility and is associated with incomplete penetrance. Both forms are due to mutations in the gene which encodes the transcription factor, FOXL2. Commercial genetic testing is currently available for both types of this syndrome (34,35).

Aarskog syndrome is another entity that can be confused with FAS, as patients with Aarskog syndrome can have ptosis, smooth philtrum, midface hypoplasia, and mild mental retardation. However, these patients also have hypertelorism, shawl scrotum, and brachydactyly. This condition is inherited in an X-linked fashion, with females often having a milder phenotype compared to males. The etiology of this condition is currently under investigation but no genetic testing is available at this time.

Noonan syndrome can also mimic some features of FAS. In particular, patients with Noonan syndrome can have short stature, ptosis, and mild mental retardation. However, these patients can be distinguished from patients with FAS by their other dysmorphic features, which include webbed neck, low posterior hairline, shield chest, cryptorchidism, and pulmonic stenosis. Noonan syndrome is an autosomal dominant condition and approximately 50% of patients with Noonan syndrome have been found to have mutations in the *protein-tyrosine phosphatase, nonreceptor type 11 (PTPN11)* gene on chromosome 12q24.1. This gene encodes a protein that appears to be important in several intracellular signal transduction pathways that control a wide variety of developmental processes (36). Mutation analysis for the *PTPN11* gene is now available clinically.

Dubowitz syndrome is characterized by prenatal growth deficiency, mental retardation, microcephaly, short palpebral fissures, and ptosis, which can be suggestive of FAS. However, patients with Dubowitz syndrome can also manifest an eczema-like skin eruption, limb anomalies, cryptorchidism, and ocular abnormalities. This condition is inherited in an autosomal recessive fashion. The etiology of this condition is currently unknown (11).

Cornelia de Lange syndrome, also known as Brachmann–de Lange or simply as de Lange syndrome, also shares some features with FAS. Patients with Cornelia de Lange syndrome can have prenatal onset growth deficiency, mental retardation, long philtrum, and thin upper lip. However, they also have synophrys, downturned angles of the mouth, and various limb defects, most commonly micromelia. Most cases appear to be sporadic, although autosomal dominant inheritance has been suggested. The etiology of this condition is unknown, and no genetic testing is available.

This list of conditions that have features in common with FAS is certainly not exhaustive, but it illustrates the need to consider other genetic syndromes and etiologies for patients with dysmorphic features, developmental or behavioral abnormalities, and a history of prenatal alcohol exposure. It also emphasizes the need to pursue further genetic testing in patients who do not fit into the classical FAS phenotype.

VIII. MANAGEMENT OF FAS

The management of FASD is multidisciplinary. Because of the history of growth deficiency associated with FAS, the patient's growth and nutrition should be monitored. In addition, the patient should be evaluated for any other birth defects (such as congenital heart defects, renal anomalies, and visual and hearing deficits), and these conditions should be addressed as needed. The child should be referred for early interventional services as early as possible after the diagnosis is made, in order to maximize the patient's developmental potential and minimize secondary disabilities. As part of the early intervention services, a developmental assessment or educational evaluation should be performed, and physical therapy, occupational therapy, and speech therapy should be considered for patients who have evidence of gross motor, fine motor, or speech delay, respectively. A variety of classroom interventions have been suggested to be helpful in children with FASD and should be considered in the school setting (see section on "Prognosis"). A diagnosis of FAS may prompt recognition of a previously hidden alcohol problem in the mother and community resources to address this issue should be implemented as well.

It is important to realize that many children with FAS live in an environment compounded by poverty, lack of appropriate emotional support, unstable home situations, and inadequate educational services. This can lead to a host of emotional and behavioral problems that can be misinterpreted as due to the patient's underlying diagnosis. Therefore, it is important to evaluate each patient's home situation to determine if further community support of the family can improve the social situation.

Furthermore, as mentioned in the section on "Drinking Patterns and Alcohol Teratogenicity," it is often the case that the youngest child will be the most severely affected member of the family. Therefore, the youngest child may be the first child in the family diagnosed with this condition. It is imperative that the older siblings of the index case be evaluated for signs and symptoms of FAS so that appropriate interventions for them can also be initiated (1,11).

IX. PROGNOSIS

Patients with prenatal alcohol exposure are at risk for learning disabilities that can result in school failure. While

FAS is among the most common causes of mental retardation, most patients fall within the mild mental retardation category. Reported IQ scores of patients with FAS have ranged from 16 to 105, with an average of 66 (11). It has been postulated that patients with FAS have problems in higher level cognitive processes, such as learning and memory.

In a study by Mattson and Roebuck in 2002 (37), a battery of five tests to evaluate learning and memory were administered to 19 patients with FAS, 16 patients with heavy prenatal exposure to alcohol who did not meet the diagnostic criteria for FAS, and a group of control children. All subjects were aged 8–16 years. They found that alcohol-exposed children learned less information on all tests and approached a learning plateau sooner than the control children. In addition, immediate memory deficits and delayed verbal recall were greater in the alcohol-exposed group as compared to the control group. Alcohol-exposed children appeared to have better retention of verbal as opposed to nonverbal information. There appeared to be no significant difference between the outcomes of the group of children diagnosed with FAS and those children exposed to alcohol who did not meet the formal diagnostic criteria for FAS.

The authors also found that the rate of learning acquisition varied depending on the test that was administered. They postulated that inconsistent attention or delayed utilization of learning strategies may account for some of these differences. In addition, it was found that children with prenatal alcohol exposure had difficulty in encoding new information; this difficulty was overcome somewhat through repeated opportunities at learning the new material. These data, therefore, suggest that alcohol-exposed children may benefit from repeated learning experiences and this should be incorporated into their educational planning (37). Even in patients whose IQs fall within the normal range, a variety of cognitive deficits have been described, including higher rates of perseveration, difficulties in self-regulation and planning abilities, inefficient information processing, and problems completing tasks that require complex attention and memory (16). They are at higher risk for severe behavioral problems and psychiatric disorders, which in turn may affect their ability to live independently, hold a job, and maintain personal relationships (11).

X. PREVENTION

Methods of preventing alcohol consumption during pregnancy can be classified into three categories: primary prevention, secondary prevention, and tertiary prevention. Primary prevention consists of disseminating information about the adverse effects of alcohol in pregnancy widely to the population at large. This is typically achieved through mass media educational efforts and targeted educational tactics, such as placing the surgeon general's warning label about alcohol consumption during pregnancy on alcohol bottles or posting it in bars. Although this is the least expensive of the three types of prevention, it is also the least effective in changing drinking behaviors.

Secondary prevention consists of disseminating information about FASD to a targeted high-risk population known to drink more heavily than women in the general population, such as women with polysubstance abuse problems or women who smoke cigarettes during pregnancy. This method of prevention relies on being able to identify high-risk populations and is more expensive than primary prevention.

Tertiary prevention is the most expensive, but most effective, method of preventing the birth of children with FASD. This consists of targeting alcoholic women or women who have had previous children with FAS and enrolling them in educational and support programs to address their alcohol problems. The National Organization on Fetal Alcohol Syndrome (NOFAS) is a nonprofit organization that provides educational and supportive resources for families with children who have FAS. This organization can be accessed through their website at www.nofas.org. The website contains information about FAS, various support groups, and newsletters (11).

XI. CONCLUSION

Fetal alcohol spectrum disorder represents a recognizable spectrum of disabilities in some individuals exposed to maternal alcohol abuse during pregnancy. It represents a completely preventable group of disorders. Although the specific teratogenic dose of alcohol during pregnancy is not defined, human and animal studies have demonstrated that alcohol consumption during pregnancy is dangerous to the developing fetus. Women who drink steadily during pregnancy and women who binge drink to the point of intoxication are at highest risk for having the most severely affected children. Since the teratogenic dose of alcohol is not known, practitioners should recommend that women abstain from alcohol use during pregnancy. However, it should be emphasized that women who have several drinks prior to knowing they are pregnant are at low risk for FAS and other alcohol-related adverse outcomes in the spectrum of FASD.

Although patients who meet the full diagnostic criteria for FAS are easy to diagnose, patients with partial features of FAS and a maternal history of alcohol use are difficult to classify. Practitioners should remember that FAS is a diagnosis of exclusion, and other genetic and teratogenic causes for a patient's features should be ruled out prior to assigning an alcohol-related diagnosis. In addition, when evaluating a patient with features of FASD, it is important to assess other family members for more subtle features of FAS. Once a diagnosis of FASD is made, appropriate educational and support resources should be identified for the patient and his or her family.

REFERENCES

1. Abel E. *Gin Lane*: did Hogarth know about fetal alcohol syndrome? Alcohol Alcohol 2001; 36:131–134.

2. Fetal alcohol syndrome and fetal alcohol effects. The Wisconsin Fetal Alcohol Syndrome Surveillance System. http://www.wisc.edu/fasscreening/background.htm 2005.

3. Lemoine P, Harrousseau H, Borteryu JP, Menuet JC. Les infants de parents alcooliques: anomalies observees: a propos de 127 cas. Ouest Med 1968; 8:476–482.

4. Jones K, Smith DW, Ulleland CN, Streissguth AP. Pattern of malformation in offspring of chronic alcoholic mothers. Lancet 1973; 1:1267–1271.

5. Barr HM, Streissguth AP. Identifying maternal self-reported alcohol use associated with fetal alcohol spectrum disorders. Alcohol Clin Exp Res 2001; 25:283–287.

6. Aase JM, Jones KL, Clarren SK. Do we need the term "FAE"? Pediatrics 1995; 95:428–430.

7. Rosett HL. A clinical perspective of the fetal alcohol syndrome. Alcohol Clin Exp Res 1980; 4:119–122.

8. Stratton K, Howe C, Battaglia F. Fetal Alcohol Syndrome: Diagnosis, Epidemiology, Prevention, and Treatment. Washington, DC: National Academy Press, 1996:74–79, 82–89, 104–107.

9. Astley SJ, Clarren SK. Diagnosing the full spectrum of fetal alcohol-exposed individuals: introducing the 4-digit diagnostic code. Alcohol Alcohol 2000; 35:400–410.

10. Warren KR, Calhoun FJ, May PA, Viljoen DL, Li T-K, Tanaka H, Marinicheva GS, Robinson LK, Mundle G. Fetal alcohol syndrome: an international perspective. Alcohol Clin Exp Res 2001; 25(May suppl):202S–206S.

11. Thackray HM, Tifft C. Fetal alcohol syndrome. Pediatr Rev 2001; 22:47–55.

12. Abel EL. Update on incidence of FAS: FAS is not an equal opportunity birth defect. Neurotoxicol Teratol 1995; 17:437–443.

13. Wilsnack RW, Vogeltanz ND, Wilsnack SC, Harris TR. Gender differences in alcohol consumption and adverse drinking consequences: cross-cultural patterns. Addiction 2000; 95: 251–265.

14. Rolater S, Winslow EH, Jacobson AF. One drink too many. Am J Nurs 2000; 100:64–66.

15. Ikonomidou C, Bittigau P, Ishimaru MJ, Wozniak DF, Koch C, Genz K, Price MT, Stefovska V, Horster F, Tenkova T, Dikranian K, Olney JW. Ethanol-induced apoptotic neurode-

generation and fetal alcohol syndrome. Science 2000; 287: 1056–1060.

16. Olson CH, Streissguth AP, Sampson PD, Barr HM, Bookstein FL, Thiede K. Association of prenatal alcohol exposure with behavioral and learning problems in early adolescence. J Am Acad Child Adolesc Psychiatry 1997; 36:1187–1194.

17. Dexter JD, Tumbleson ME, Decker JD, Middleton CC. Fetal alcohol syndrome in Sinclair (S-1) miniature swine. Alcohol Clin Exp Res 1980; 4:146–151.

18. Streissguth AP, Dehaene P. Fetal alcohol syndrome in twins of alcoholic mothers: concordance of diagnosis and IQ. Am J Med Genet 1993; 47:857–861.

19. McCarver DG, Thomasson HR, Martier SS, Sokol RJ, Li T-K. Alcohol dehydrogenase-2*3 allele protects against alcohol-related birth defects among African Americans. J Pharmacol Exp Ther 1997; 283:1095–1101.

20. Jacobson SW, Chiodo L, Jester J, Carr L, Sokol R, Jacobson J, Li T-K. Protective effects of ADH2*3 in African American infants exposed prenatally to alcohol [abstr]. Alcohol Clin Exp Res 2000; 24(suppl 5):28A.

21. Viljoen DL, Carr LG, Foroud TM, Brooke L, Ramsay M, Li T-K. Alcohol dehydrogenase-2*2 allele is associated with decreased prevalence of fetal alcohol syndrome in the mixed-ancestry populations of the Western Cape Province, South Africa. Alchol Clin Exp Res 2001; 25:1719–1722.

22. Tanaka F, Shiratori Y, Yokosuka O, Imazeki F, Tsukada Y, Omata M. High incidence of ADH2*1/ALDH2*1 genes among Japanese alcohol dependents and patients with alcoholic liver disease. Hepatology 1996; 23:234–239.

23. Muramatsu T, Wang ZC, Fang YR, Hu KB, Yan H, Yamada K, Higuchi S, Harada S, Kono H. Alcohol and aldehyde dehydro-genase genotypes and drinking behavior of Chinese living in Shanghai. Hum Genet 1995; 96:151–154.

24. Vidal F, Perez J, Panisello J, Toda R, Gutierrez C, Richart C. Atypical liver alcohol dehydrogenase in the Spanish popula-tion: its relation with the development of alcoholic liver disease. Alcohol Clin Exp Res 1993; 17:782–785.

25. Zachman RD, Grummer MA. The interaction of ethanol and vitamin A as a potential mechanism for the pathogenesis of fetal alcohol syndrome. Alcohol Clin Exp Res 1998; 22:1544–1556.

26. Clarren SK, Alvord EC, Sumi SM, Streissguth AP, Smith DW. Brain malformations related to prenatal exposure to ethanol. J Pediatr 1978; 92:64–67.

27. Guerri C, Pascual M, Renau-Piqueras J. Glia and fetal alcohol syndrome. Neurotoxicology 2001; 22:539–599.

28. Bearer CF. L1 cell adhesion molecule signal cascades: targets for ethanol developmental neurotoxicity. Neurotoxicology 2001; 22:625–633.

29. Bearer CF, Swick AR, O'Riordan MA, Cheng G. Ethanol inhibits L1-mediated neurite outgrowth in postnatal rat cerebellar granule cells. J Biol Chem 1999; 274:13264–13270.

30. Cohen MM, Shiota K. Teratogenesis of holoprosencephaly. Am J Med Genet 2002; 109:1–15.

31. Roessler E, Belloni E, Gaudenz K, Jay P, Berta P, Scherer SW, Tsui L-C, Muenke M. Mutations in the human *Sonic Hedgehog* gene cause holoprosencephaly. Nat Genet 1996; 14:357–360.

32. Roessler E, Belloni E, Gaudenz K, Vargas F, Scherer SW, Tsui L-C, Muenke M. Mutations in the C-terminal domain of *Sonic Hedgehog* cause holoprosencephaly. Hum Mol Genet 1997; 6: 1847–1853.

33. Ahlgren SC, Thakur V, Bronner-Fraser M. *Sonic Hedgehog* rescues cranial neural crest from cell death induced by ethanol exposure. Proc Natl Acad Sci USA 2002; 99:10476–10481.

34. Jones KL. Smith's Recognizable Patterns of Human Malformation. 5th ed. Philadelphia, PA: W.B. Saunders Company, 1997: 232–233.

35. Online Mendelian Inheritance in Man. http://www.ncbi.nlm.nih.gov/omim/, 2003.

36. Allanson JE. Noonan syndrome. GeneReviews, 2002. http://www.geneclinics.org.

37. Mattson SN, Roebuck TM. Acquisition and retention of verbal and nonverbal information in children with heavy prenatal alcohol exposure. Alcohol Clin Exp Res 2002; 26:875–882.

19

Prevalence and Genetic Epidemiology of Developmental Disabilities

COLEEN A. BOYLE

National Center on Birth Defects
and Developmental Disabilities, Centers
for Disease Control and Prevention,
Atlanta, Georgia, U.S.A.

KIM VAN NAARDEN BRAUN

Oak Ridge Institute for Science
and Education, United States
Department of Energy, Oakridge,
Tennessee, U.S.A.

MARSHALYN YEARGIN-ALLSOPP

National Center on Birth Defects
and Developmental Disabilities, Centers
for Disease Control and Prevention,
Atlanta, Georgia, U.S.A.

I. INTRODUCTION

Developmental disabilities (DDs) include a broad spectrum of physical, cognitive, psychological, sensory, and speech and language impairments resulting from neurological damage or dysfunction, and are typically identified between birth and age 18 years. About 17% of U.S. children have been reported to have one or more of a wide range of DDs (1). Data from the Centers for Disease Control and Prevention's Metropolitan Atlanta Developmental Disability Surveillance

693

Program, an ongoing, population-based monitoring program, have indicated that about 2% of school-age children have a serious DD, which is defined as one that requires lifelong care and special services (2). Lifetime medical and direct nonmedical (e.g., special education) costs and productivity losses for some of these DDs have been calculated recently; for mental retardation (MR), the average lifetime cost per person has been estimated at US $800,000 (in 2000 dollars) (3).

Genetic factors play a major role in the etiology of many DDs. In this chapter, we highlight what is known about the prevalence of two of the most serious DDs—MR and autism—and review the contribution of genetic factors in both disorders. We focus on the unique role that epidemiology and population-based studies have played in identifying genetic risk factors and causes of MR and autism. Throughout the discussion, we highlight some of the major methodological challenges in furthering our knowledge of the influence of genetic factors in the etiology of MR and autism through epidemiology. Many of the methodological factors that we discuss in reference to these two disorders will have relevance to other DDs not discussed (e.g., cerebral palsy and epilepsy). Finally, we conclude with some thoughts about future epidemiologic approaches that might be helpful in furthering our understanding of the role of genetic factors in the etiology of autism and MR.

II. MENTAL RETARDATION

Mental retardation is a group of heterogeneous disorders with varying underlying etiologies. The primary feature of MR is a deficit in general cognitive or intellectual functioning with onset up to 18 years of age. Mental retardation is measured as a standardized intelligence quotient (IQ), through individually administered psychometric tests (4). An IQ of 70 or lower reflects a score of two standard deviations below the population mean score of 100 and is felt to reflect performance in the mentally retarded range. While IQ tests are designed to measure verbal communication, reasoning, and performance on tasks of motor and spatial capabilities, they do not capture other aspects of a person's functioning. As a result, the American Association of Mental Retardation

(AAMR) has suggested that adaptive functioning (a person's ability to perform activities of daily living and social functioning) be taken into consideration when determining the level of MR (4).

A. Prevalence of Mental Retardation

Epidemiologic studies of MR have generally used an IQ of 70 to define MR. This is because standardized intelligence testing represents a systematic and objective way to assess cognitive functioning across populations. Much has been written and debated about the biases and shortcomings of intelligence testing in eliciting the underlying construct of intelligence (5). The important point of this debate regarding prevalence is whether these shortcomings affect subgroups of the population differently so that they might be over-represented or under-represented in the prevalence. This could be true especially for those with milder deficits, for whom the impacts of social circumstances and cultural experiences are most pronounced.

Severity of MR is defined similarly in the ICD-10 and DSM-IV, with an $IQ<20$ indicating profound MR, an IQ of 20–34 indicating severe MR, 35–49 for moderate MR, and 50–70 for mild MR (6,7). While this broad classification might have utility for clinical applications, for research purposes, severity is usually categorized into two groups—mild (defined as above) and severe (which is $IQ<50$). While the AAMR definition uses adaptive functioning to further define severity, few researchers use adaptive functioning as part of their case definition of MR.

Prevalence (the proportion of the population with disease at a specific point in time) is used rather than incidence (the number of people who develop the disease or disorder in the population over a specific time period) to measure the frequency of MR in the population (8) because most cases of MR are of prenatal origin. Thus, children are born with the disorder, even though the manifestation of the disorder might not occur for months or years after the causal event. Denominators have also varied with some studies using the birth population as the denominator (yielding birth prevalence): however, the majority of studies use the current population (and the resulting period prevalence). To understand the contribution of genetics to the etiology of MR, birth prevalence would be more applicable because current prevalence would be influenced by factors such as migration and death. Even the birth population and corresponding birth prevalence may underestimate the contribution of genetics to MR. Many conditions, e.g., chromosomal abnormalities, have a high fetal or infant death rate.

There are several excellent recent reviews of the prevalence of MR (9–11). Rates for severe MR are similar across studies, with the majority of the studies in the 3–4 per 1000 range. There are fewer studies on the prevalence of mild MR and the rates of mild MR have been quite variable, from 5.0 to 80.5 per 1000. This variation is believed to be a function of case ascertainment methods and case definition (10). Figure 1 shows a clustering of studies for severe MR, around 3–4 per 1000, with some indication of a lower rate in several recent studies; a similar downward shift is not evident for mild MR. Why there appears to be a downward trend in severe MR is unclear, but Leonard and Wen (11) suggest that this is due to a more restrictive definition of severe MR in at least one study.

About one-fifth of children with MR have at least one other DD—primarily cerebral palsy and epilepsy (2,12). The likelihood of an associated DD is greater for children with more severe MR than for those with mild MR (45% vs. 12%). It has been suggested that the epidemiology of MR varies according to the severity of MR, with social factors contributing more to the etiology of mild MR and biologic (e.g., genetic) factors involved with severe MR (13). Because there is considerable overlap in the characteristics between mild and severe MR, other approaches to subclassifying MR have also been examined. Drews et al. (14) classified MR according to the presence or absence of other disabilities, and showed that social factors (e.g., maternal education) were strongly associated with MR without disabilities independent of the severity. Croen et al. (15) used a different categorization— MR of known and MR of unknown etiology—and found some of the same associations; maternal education associated with MR of unknown etiology independent of severity level.

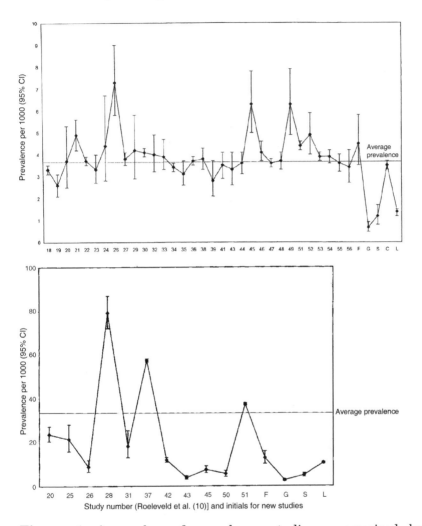

Figure 1 A number of prevalence studies summarized by Roeleveld et al. (10) for severe mental retardation (upper) and mild retardation (lower) in children from 1960 to 2002 are shown. The numbers on the horizontal axis correspond to earlier studies while letters correspond to more recent studies. (From Ref. 11.)

More males than females are identified with MR, particularly with mild MR, with prevalence rate ratios ranging from 1.4 to 1.7 (2,10,12). X-linked genetic conditions could be responsible for some of the excess—a recent review identified

178 X-linked conditions associated with MR (16,17). Chelly and Mandel (18) estimated that 13% to 21% of MR in males is due to X-linked mutations. Additionally, there might be selective factors resulting in more referral, testing, and identification of male children (19), although the one study to examine this issue found this not to be the case (20).

Age at diagnosis varies with the severity of MR. Typically, children with more severe MR are diagnosed at younger ages; however, prevalence peaks at 10–14 years of age, remains stable into the 20s, and declines thereafter (10). The initial rise in prevalence is due to delays in identification, particularly for mild MR; the decline in early adulthood could reflect a number of factors: higher mortality rates for individuals with severe MR, lack of services for individuals beyond school age, and the assimilation of individuals with good adaptive skills into the community (10). The rates of MR have also been shown to vary by race and ethnicity, with African-, Hispanic-, and Asian-Americans reported to have higher rates than Caucasian-Americans (12,15). Similarly, Leonard and Wen (11) found higher rates in the Australian indigenous populations. Yeargin-Allsopp et al. (21) showed that some of this excess was due to differences in social factors among these populations—unmeasured confounding could also contribute, as well as differences in underlying risk factors, e.g., a higher prevalence of preterm birth in African-American children (22).

B. Genetics and Epidemiology of Mental Retardation

The genetic causes of MR have not been identified from epidemiologic studies, but rather from genetic studies of clinical populations with similar phenotypes or from family studies (23). Of note, new technologies including fluorescence in situ hybridization, subtelomeric screening, and other molecular techniques (24) have played a key role in identifying many genetic causes of MR. Likewise, the study of MR has led to many of the key discoveries in genetic mechanisms and patterns of inheritance—including the identification of dynamic mutations (e.g., fragile X syndrome), and genomic imprinting and uniparental disomy identified from the study of Angelman and Prader–Willi syndromes (25).

Epidemiology has been useful in determining the prevalence of individual mutations and understanding the range of phenotypic expression in specific genetic mutations (26). Additionally, population-based studies have been useful in understanding the recurrence risks for MR due to specific genetic factors, as well as for MR of unknown etiology—information that is particularly useful in genetic counseling. Because the majority of MR is of unknown etiology, epidemiology has been used to pursue causes of the remaining undefined cases.

In examining etiology (both genetic and otherwise), most investigators have classified cases according to the most probable time of onset of the disorder (see Refs. 27, 28 for examples of detailed classification schemes), using the following developmental sequence: (1) prenatal (arising before birth), (2) perinatal (arising during the period from birth through the first month of life), (3) postnatal (occurring after the first month of life and before 18 years of age), and (4) unknown. In examining the contribution of genetic causes to MR, we have focused on recent studies because of the rapid development and improvement in technologies to detect genetic defects. However, the most recent population-based studies are from the mid-1990s, so it is likely that the proportion of MR attributable to genetic causes is somewhat higher than what is presented here. For example, the recent discovery that Rett syndrome is caused by mutations in the MECP2 gene was only published in 1999 and would not be included in these epidemiologic studies (29). Similarly, recent studies found subtelomeric deletions in 7% of clinically referred children with moderate to severe MR and 0.5% of children with mild MR of unknown etiology, suggesting that such subtle submicroscopic changes might play an important etiologic role in MR (30,31).

Table 1 shows the more recent population-based studies of the etiology of MR. These studies indicate that prenatal etiologies—including genetic and environmental (primarily teratogens, e.g., alcohol or infections), dominate the known causes of MR and account for 12–59% of all MR (27,28,32–34). This proportion increases with the severity of MR; 25–70% of the

Table 1 Epidemiologic Studies that Used Multiple Sources of Case Ascertainment and Examined the Contribution of Genetic Disorders to the Prevalence of Mental Retardation

Reference/ location/ population size	No. of cases: total/SMR/ MMR	Prevalence per 1,000: total/SMR/ MMR	Evaluation methods	Etiology (%), pre-/peri-/postnatal/ unknown	Genetic (%)	M/F ratio
Ref. 32/ Sweden/ $N = 14{,}138$	SMR = 64	SMR = 4.5	Medical records	SMR = 66/6/5/23	Down syndrome, SMR = 13	1.7:1
Ref. 27/ Georgia/ NR	Total = 715, SMR = 206, MMR = 509	NR	Medical records	Total = 12/6/4/78, SMR = 25/11/7/57, MMR = 7/4/2/87	Total = 7, SMR = 17, MMR = 3 Down syndrome, Total = 5, SMR = 12, MMR = 2	NR

Ref. 28/ Taiwan/ $N = 423{,}000$	Total = 11,892, SMR = 4400, MMR = 7492	Total = 20.8	Medical records, parent interview, cytogenetic and molecular studies	Total = 55/10/3/32, SMR = 70/11/5/14, MMR = 47/9/2/43	Total = 21, SMR = 37, MMR = 11, Down syndrome, Total = 13	1.4:1
Ref. 33 Norway/ $N=30{,}037$	Total = 185	Total = 6.2, SMR = 2.7, MMR = 3.5	Parent interview, Chromosomal analysis, FISH	Total = 59/4/3/34[a], SMR = 70/4/5/22, MMR = 51/5/1/43	Total = 35, SMR = 48, MMR = 25, Down syndrome, Total = 10	1.3:1
Ref. 34/ New South Wales/NR	Total = 429, SMR = 280, MMR = 114	NR	Parent interview, genetic evaluation	Total = 32/8/5/56[b]	Total = 29, Down syndrome, Total = 15	1.4:1

SMR, severe mental retardation; MMR, mild mental retardation; NR, not reported.
[a]Unknown includes biopathological, undetermined + unspecified.
[b]Includes "well recognized clinical group without a known etiology + "unknown diagnosis."

population case series in the studies annotated in Table 1 identified an underlying prenatal etiology for severe MR. In contrast, for mild MR, the proportion was less (7–51%) due to prenatal causes. The wide range in proportions reported has to do with a number of factors: the completeness of the case ascertainment, particularly for mild MR, the methods used to determine the underlying etiology, and whether cases with a suspected genetic etiology (e.g., family history or presence of associated medical conditions) were included in the known cause category.

To illustrate the first issue, the completeness of case ascertainment, all studies relied on multiple sources to identify cases—however, some studies (32,33) used only traditional medical or social service providers. While these records would have provided complete ascertainment for severe MR, they would have missed many children with mild MR. When schools, in addition to medical and social service providers (27,28) necessary to identify children with mild MR (35), are included, then a comparable proportion of children are identified in the case series with mild MR (about two-thirds) and severe MR (about one-third). Those that did not use schools had a distribution that was more skewed to severe MR.

Regarding the second factor affecting the proportion of known cases, the approaches used to determine etiology varied widely. Several studies relied on existing medical record information (27,32) and had lower proportions with known etiologies. Others used more extensive evaluations including medical records, interviews of parents to obtain a medical and family history, and selected cytogenetic and molecular analyses to identify specific genetic etiologies (28,33). Finally, some studies (28) included within the prenatal/genetic category cases with an unknown etiology, but with a family history of MR, while others classified such a child's disorder in the unknown cause category.

Because of its large size (nearly 12,000 case children), extensive diagnostic evaluation and broad case ascertainment methods (schools as well as traditional sources), the study by Hou et al. (28) probably represents the best epidemiologic study of the specific types of genetic causes of MR. Overall,

20.7% of MR in that study was due to known genetic causes. This was higher for severe (36.5%) than mild MR (11.4%). Chromosomal disorders accounted for the majority (16%) of the genetic etiologies, with most of these due to Down syndrome (13% of all cases). Among all studies in Table 1, Down syndrome accounted for 5–15% of case children with MR. Fragile X syndrome (by molecular diagnosis) was identified in 2.0% of the children; single gene disorders in 2.0%; contiguous gene disorders (Prader–Willi, Angelman, Williams, and Kallmann syndromes) in 0.8%; and other genetic disorders in 0.5% (e.g., muscular dystrophy, mucopolysaccharidosis). Interestingly, an additional 18% had a family history of MR, suggesting an underlying genetic etiology, although the authors note that environmental factors for such cases could not be ruled out.

C. Recurrence of Mental Retardation

Most recurrence risk estimates for MR are based on studies conducted done more than 10 years ago and, therefore, included some individuals with MR for whom we now have a known genetic cause (36–39). In addition, most of these studies were hospital- or clinic-based, thus including families with serious cases or those already experiencing recurrence. As a result, recurrence risk estimates based on these populations are more likely to overestimate the risk of recurrence. Another important factor that has not been considered in these studies is family size, which can be influenced by the presence of a child with MR and thus limit recurrence. Despite these methodologic problems, it is worthwhile to review the main factors on which recurrence risk estimates are hypothesized to differ.

Previous studies have examined recurrence risks for MR by severity, sex, and the presence of comorbidities. Many studies have shown that families with individuals with mild MR have a higher risk for recurrence than those with severe MR and that the presence of comorbidities decreases the chance for recurrence (36,38). While MR is more prevalent in males, there is conflicting evidence as to whether boys with MR are more likely to have affected siblings. More specifically, it is hypothesized that, due to X-linked MR, brothers of males with MR could be at higher risk for having MR than sisters (37,38,40,41). It is necessary to know the baseline prevalence of the disorder in the population under study to interpret population-based recurrence risk estimates meaningfully. A high recurrence risk might simply reflect a high prevalence in the population. Only Herbst and Baird (38) reported the baseline prevalence and found the recurrence risk for non-specific MR as 37 per 1000, which was approximately eight times the baseline prevalence of the population under study (4.6 per 1000). This study found that there was no increased risk for brothers of males with nonspecific MR, but that the risk of recurrence was greater for subsequent siblings of individuals with mild MR.

D. Other Epidemiologic Approaches to Examining the Causes of Mental Retardation

Beyond prevalence studies to examine the occurrence of specific genetic factors in MR prevalence and recurrence risk, a few epidemiologic case–control studies have tried to identify the contribution of a number of demographic, maternal, and medical risk factors as potential risk factors (14,15). Such studies, while not examining specific genetic markers, can highlight what additional role genetic factors can play in MR, particularly in the large group with unknown etiology, and what subgroups of the population might be the most likely to yield results in future clinical research. A recent study by Croen et al. (15) reported a number of demographic and social factors linked to mild and severe MR of unknown etiology that may suggest an underlying biologic or genetic insult. For example, older maternal age (30+ years) and male gender are associated with mild and severe MR of unknown etiology. X-linked genetic factors and increased chromosomal problems in offspring of older mothers may further contribute to MR.

E. Conclusions

Much of the etiology of MR remains unknown. Epidemiology can continue to play an important role by characterizing the importance of genetic causes of MR on a population level and by characterizing the range of phenotypes associated with specific genetic disorders. Further, epidemiologic case–control studies can help further elucidate subgroups of the population in which genetic factors could be particularly important.

III. AUTISM

The core clinical features of the children with autism initially described by Leo Kanner included functional impairments in three areas: social interactions, communication, and restrictive or repetitive patterns or behaviors (42). While the field of autism has advanced considerably since these initial observations, these features remain the defining characteristics of autism. What has changed with refinement of knowledge is the level of impairment that is necessary to characterize autism. The children initially described by Kanner had severe impairments in each of the three areas of functioning. We now have a better appreciation that autism varies greatly in presentation and severity (43,44). This variation presents methodologic challenges in conducting epidemiologic studies of autism. Similar to MR, it has been challenging for researchers to create phenotypic groupings of autism that will facilitate the epidemiologic study of this disorder.

There are no standardized tests for the diagnosis of autism (unlike for MR). Instead, the diagnosis is based on clinical observations of behaviors that are consistent with the diagnostic criteria for autism (45). The current diagnostic criteria include those of the American Psychiatric Association's Diagnostic and Statistical Manual, fourth edition (7) and the International Classification for Disease, 10th edition (6). These classifications (which are similar between systems) include criteria for autistic disorder; Asperger disorder; and pervasive developmental disorder, not otherwise specified (PDD-NOS). These three disorders comprise a continuum of conditions referred to as autism spectrum disorders (ASDs). Asperger disorder is used to describe children with higher intellectual functioning who have the behavioral features of autism without the language impairments. PDD-NOS is a default category for children who do not meet the criteria for autistic disorder.

Structured diagnostic instruments, such as the Autism Diagnostic Observation Schedule-General (ADOS-G) and the Autism Diagnostic Interview-Revised (ADI-R) have been developed for use in diagnostic assessments (46–48). Extensive training and ongoing monitoring for clinical reliability are necessary for the proper use of these instruments. While these instruments have improved the validity and reliability of the diagnosis of autism, they are still based on having a skilled practitioner examine specific behaviors in the child and elicit accurate historical descriptions of such behaviors from the child's parents.

A. Prevalence of Autism and Autism Spectrum Disorders

The methodology used in prevalence studies of autism has generally involved a process of case finding followed by one of case confirmation (49,50). There have been a number of methods of case finding. The most comprehensive involves total population screening using the schools or pediatric well-child care visits as the vehicles for screening. The advantage of this methodology is that children who have not yet been diagnosed will come to the examiner's attention. However, the process is labor intensive and has been done only in relatively small populations, which has limited the number of children identified with autism (43). Other methods used in case finding have targeted *at-risk* populations by focusing on programs and clinics specifically for children with DDs. Sources targeted have included special education programs, specialty diagnostic clinics, and other service programs for children with DDs. Methods used to identify children at such sources have varied from asking providers to identify children with possible autism to a comprehensive review of all service provider records. An advantage of the *at-risk* approach is that large populations can be targeted, but its success is dependent on the quality and comprehensiveness of diagnostic and treatment services in the community, as well as the extent of detail that is recorded in the individual records.

Methods used in the second phase, case confirmation, have also been variable (44,49). The most comprehensive method has been the clinical evaluation of the child using the ADOS-G or ADI-R (described previously), or both, to assess the presence of various behaviors of autism. As with case finding techniques, the complexity and costs of this approach have generally limited its use in larger population studies. A second approach has been an expert review based on available diagnostic record information on the child. While this approach has resource advantages and potentially allows for a developmental perspective of the child's behavior, it is dependent on the quality of the records. Finally, some have relied on a diagnosis as provided by the service provider. However, because the diagnosis of autism varies widely, this approach needs to be used with caution, keeping in mind methodologic factors that might explain specific trends in the data.

There has been much current debate about the prevalence of autism (also referred to as classic autism or autistic disorder) and ASDs, and whether the prevalence has increased over time. The first epidemiologic studies examining the prevalence of autism did not appear in the scientific literature until the late 1960s and early 1970s (51–54). Since these earlier investigations, there have been an increasing number of population-based prevalence studies (55–84). However, these vary in terms of their methods, case definitions, and population size; hence, comparisons of temporal trends in rates of autism are difficult (Table 2).

The first population-based study reported a prevalence of 4.5 per 10,000; the other studies using the same criteria (Kanner's), with the exception of one U.S. study, reported similar prevalence rates (51–55,58). Three studies used Rutter's criteria, similar to Kanner's criteria, and showed that prevalence rates differed considerably (1.9, 3.0, and 16 per 10,000 children) (56,57,60). The Diagnostic and Statistical Manual of Mental Disorders III (DSM-III) (85) first used the term pervasive developmental disorders, which broadened the criteria, differentiating between autism and schizophrenia

Table 2 Summary of Autism Prevalence Studies

Author	Year published	Country	Time period studied	Age range studied	Number of children in population	Criteria used	Methodology used	Prevalence rate (PR) for autism/ other ASD	IQ <70(%)
Lotter	1966	England	1964	8–10	78,000	Kanner	Case enumeration and direct exam	4.5/–	84
Brask	1970	Denmark	1962	2–14	46,500	Kanner	Case enumeration	4.3/–	NR
Treffert	1970	U.S.A.	1962–1967	3–12	899,750	Kanner	Case enumeration	0.7/2.4	NR
Wing and Gould	1979	England	1970	0–14	35,000	Kanner	Case enumeration and direct exam	4.6/15.7	70
Hoshino et al.[a]	1982	Japan	1977	0–17	234,039	Kanner	Case enumeration and direct exam	5.0/–	NR
Ishi and Takahashi	1983	Japan	1981	6–12	35,000	Rutter	Case enumeration and direct exam	16.0/–	NR
Bohman et al.	1983	Sweden	1979	0–20	69,000	Rutter	Case enumeration and direct exam	3.0/2.6	NR

McCarthy et al.	1984	Ireland	1978	8–10	65,000	Kanner	Case enumeration and direct exam	4.3/–	NR
Gillberg	1984	Sweden	1980	4–18	128,584	DSM-III	Case enumeration and direct exam	2.0/1.9	80, 77
Steinhausen et al.	1986	Germany	1982	0–14	279,616	Rutter	Case enumeration and direct exam	1.9/–	44
Steffenberg and Gillberg	1986	Sweden	1984	< 10	78,413	DSM-III	Case enumeration and direct exam	4.5/2.2	88
Matsuishi et al.	1987	Japan	1983	4–12	32,834	DSM-III	Case enumeration and direct exam	15.5/–	NR
Burd et al.	1987	U.S.A.	1985	2–18	180,986	DSM-III	Case enumeration and direct exam	1.2/2.1	NR
Bryson et al.	1988	Canada	1985	6–14	20,800	DSM-III	Case enumeration and direct exam	10.1/–	76
Tanoue et al.	1988	Japan	1977–1985	3–7	95,394	DSM-III	Case enumeration	13.8/–	NR

(Continued)

Table 2 Summary of Autism Prevalence Studies (*Continued*)

Author	Year published	Country	Time period studied	Age range studied	Number of children in population	Criteria used	Methodology used	Prevalence rate (PR) for autism/ other ASD	IQ <70(%)
Cialdella and Mamelle	1989	France	1986	3–9	135,180	DSM-III	Case enumeration	5.1/5.2	NR
Sugiyama and Abe	1989	Japan	1979–1984	2–5	12,263	DSM-III	Population screen and direct exam	13.0/–	38
Ritvo et al.	1989	U.S.A.	1984–1988	8–12	184,822	DSM-III	Case enumeration and direct exam	4.0/–	NR
Gillberg	1991	Sweden	1988	4–13	78,106	DSM-III-R	Case enumeration and direct exam	7.0/2.4	82,80
Fombonne and Mazaubrun[a]	1992	France	1985	9–13	274,816	ICD-10	Case enumeration and direct exam	4.9/–	87
Honda et al.	1996	Japan	1994	1.5–6	8,537	ICD-10	Population screen and direct exam	21.1/–	50
Fombonne et al.	1997	France	1992–1993	8–9	325,347	ICD-10	Case enumeration and direct exam	5.4/10.9	88

Arvidsson et al.	1997	Sweden	1994	3–6	1,941	ICD-10	Population screen and direct exam	31.0/15.0	100
Webb et al.	1997	Wales	1992	3–15	73,300	DSM-III-R	Case enumeration and direct exam	7.2/–	NR
Sponheim and Skjeldae	1998	Norway	1992	3–14	65,688	ICD-10	Case enumeration and direct exam	3.8/1.4	64
Kadesjö et al.	1999	Sweden	1992	6.7–7.7	826	ICD-10	Case enumeration and direct exam	60.0/60.0	60
Baird et al.	2000	England	1998	1.5–8	16,235	ICD-10	Population screen and direct exam	30.8/27.1	40
Powell et al.	2000	England	1995	1–4	29,200	DSM-III-R or DSM-IV	Case enumeration	9.6/10.6	NR
Kielinen et al.	2000	Finland	1996	5–18	152,732	DSM-IV	Case enumeration	12.2/1.2	73
Magnusson and Saemundsen	2001	Iceland	1997	5–14	43,153	ICD-10	Population screen and direct exam	8.6/4.6	95,65
Chakrabarti and Fombonne	2001	England	1998	2.5–6.5	15,500	DSM-IV	Population screen and direct exam	16.8/45.8	24,70

(Continued)

Table 2 Summary of Autism Prevalence Studies (*Continued*)

Author	Year published	Country	Time period studied	Age range studied	Number of children in population	Criteria used	Methodology used	Prevalence rate (PR) for autism/ other ASD	IQ <70(%)
Fombonne et al.[b]	2001	U.K.	1999	5–15	12,529	DSM-IV	Population screen and direct exam	26.1	44,4
Bertrand et al.	2001	U.S.A.	1998	3–10	8,996	DSM-IV	Case enumeration and direct exam	40.0/67.0	49,58
Croen et al.	2002	U.S.A.	1987–1999	0–21	4,600,000	DSM-III-R or DSM-IV	Case enumeration	11.0/–	NR
Yeargin-Allsopp et al.[b]	2003	U.S.A.	1996	3–10	290,000	DSM-IV	Case enumeration and direct exam	34	64,68[c]

[a] The prevalence rate that is provided represents an average prevalence rate.
[b] The prevalence study provided overall rate only.
[c] Sixty-four percent had MR based on IQ data and 68% had cognitive impairment based on IQ and developmental tests.

and describing onset at younger than 30 months of age. Studies using DSM-III criteria yielded rates from 1.2 to 15.5 per 10,000 children (59,61–68). Three studies using DSM-III-Revised (86) criteria reported rates of 7.0, 9.6, and 11.0 per 10,000 children (69,78,84). DSM-IV and ICD-10 criteria are consistent; however, recent studies using either criterion have yielded disparate prevalence rates (70–84,87).

There have been only a few studies of trends in autism prevalence in the same population. The prevalence was determined for two French birth cohorts (children born in 1972 and 1976); no change in prevalence (5.1 and 4.9 per 10,000 children) occurred over that short period of time (70). In Sweden, the prevalence of autism was determined for two time periods, 1962–1976 and 1975–1984 and was reported to increase from 4.0 to 11.6 per 10,000 children (59,69). The Swedish investigators offered a possible explanation for the increase. Rates of autism in children with mild MR remained relatively stable, while the rates increased in children with severe MR (IQ < 50) and in children with normal intelligence (IQ > 70). Swedish investigators have suggested that changes in overall prevalence are influenced by improved ability to identify children with autism who have very low, as well as, normal to high functioning. A third study examined trends in autism occurrence and reported the incidence in preschool children in two areas of the United Kingdom from 1991 to 1996 and found the rates increased for classic autism by 18% per year, but a much larger increase than that seen for other ASDs (78). The investigators attributed this increase in incidence to better awareness among clinicians rather than to true changes in the occurrence of autism.

Because of the lack of recent prevalence data for the United States, there has been considerable attention paid to trends in service provider data that show an increase in the numbers of children receiving services for autism. However, these data are limited because (1) the diagnosis of autism has not been consistently applied over time and (2) the numbers of individuals receiving services do not represent a true prevalence rate. In addition, such data depend on other sources of services within a community and are community-specific for a range of factors. Data from the California Department of Developmental Services (CADDS) from 1987 to 1998 showed a 273% increase in the number of individuals receiving autism services (2778–10,360), whereas the number receiving services related to a diagnosis of other DDs increased only 44% (88). During the same time period, the number of individuals with a diagnosis of other pervasive developmental disorders receiving CADDS services increased nearly 200-fold. Also, in 1998, the individuals with autism were younger and higher functioning than those receiving services in 1987. An updated CADDS report in 2003 showed an increase from 10,360 cases of autism in 1998 to 20,377 in 2002, a 97% increase in just 4 years (89). U.S. Department of Education data also indicate that the number of children with autism served under the Individuals with Disabilities Education Act (IDEA), Part B (children aged 3–21 years), increased from 4795 to about 53,000, a more than 500% increase in services from the 1991–1992 school year to the 1998–1999 school year (90).

    Because of the lack of data in the United States about the prevalence of autism and the concern resulting from the service provider data, the Centers for Disease Control and Prevention (CDC) initiated a number of prevalence studies. The first, conducted in Brick Township, NJ, included an intensive case identification phase using schools and service providers and case verification (clinical examinations, psychological examinations, and administration of the ADOS-G). The prevalence of autistic disorder was found to be 40 per 10,000 children (95% confidence interval [CI]: 28–56) and the prevalence for ASDs was 67 per 10,000 children (95% CI: 51–87) (83). The prevalence of autism in Brick Township was higher than most previously published rates.

    In a second effort, the CDC conducted a population-based study to determine the prevalence of autism in five counties of metropolitan Atlanta; this was the largest study of autism conducted in the United States, with a base population of 290,000 children (85). Children with autism were identified through screening and abstraction of records at multiple medical and educational sources, with expert review to determine autism case status. A total of 987 children who displayed behaviors consistent with the DSM-IV criteria for autistic disorder, PDD-NOS, or Asperger disorder, were identified. The prevalence for autism was 3.4 per 1000 children. Overall, the prevalence was comparable for children of African-American and Caucasian-American ancestry. A total of 68% of children had cognitive impairment. As severity of cognitive impairment increased, the male to female ratio decreased from 4.4–1.3. About 40% of children with autism were identified only at school sources. Schools were the most important source for information on African-American children, children of younger mothers, and children of mothers with less than 12 years of education. Clearly, the rate of autism found in this study was higher than the rates from studies conducted in the United States during the 1980s and early 1990s, but the rate is consistent with the Brick investigation and several recent non-U.S. studies that used intensive case finding. Based on the data from these studies, the CDC concluded that autism is not a rare condition and is an extremely important public health problem.

It remains uncertain whether the higher rates of autism are due to a true increase in prevalence or whether recent reports of a possible increase are due to methodologic issues, greater awareness of the conditions, or better availability of services. However, there appear to be more children with autism today than in the past and continued monitoring of the prevalence of autism might shed some light on the contribution of each of these factors.

B. Genetics of Autism

Over the past three decades, evidence from studies using various methodologies has strongly indicated genetic factors in the etiology of autism. Twin- and family-based studies, molecular and chromosomal findings, and the association of autism with other known genetic disorders have provided convincing support for genetic susceptibility in the etiology of autism (Table 3). In addition to the role of genetic effects, a wide spectrum of nongenetic influences ranging from environmental exposures to obstetrical complications have been

Table 3 Evidence for Genetic Contribution to ASD Etiology

Twin studies Reference	Concordance-MZ Twin pairs (N)	(%)	Concordance-DZ Twin pairs (N)	(%)	Diagnostic criteria
91	4	36	0	0[a]	Ref. 42; Ref. 158
92	22	96	4	24	DSM-III
93	10	91	0	0[a]	DSM-III-R
94	15	60	0	0[b]	ICD-10; ADI, ADOS

Family studies Reference	% Recurrence	Ratio to prevalence[c]	Diagnostic criteria
142	2.8	47–70	Ref. 158
143	2.0	33–50	DSM-III
144	5.9	98–148	DSM-III
101	3.0	50–75	–
145	4.5	75–113	DSM-III
146	3.0	50–75	DSM-III
147	4.5	75–113	DSM-III
148	2.6	43–65	DSM-III
149	2.9	48–73	ICD-10, DSM-III-R, ADI and ADOS

Co-morbidity with known genetic disorders[d]

Reference	Co-morbidity
150	Fragile X
151	Fragile X
107	Fragile X
108	Fragile X

106	Fragile X
152	Neurofibromatosis type 1
111	Neurofibromatosis type 1
153	Tuberous sclerosis
109	Tuberous sclerosis
154	Tuberous sclerosis
114	Down syndrome
115	Down syndrome

Genome scans and linkage studies[e]

Reference	Chromosome	Multipoint maximum LOD score[f]
155	7q	2.5
122	1p	2.2
125	13p21.3	3.0
	13p12.3	2.3
	7q	2.2
156	1q	2.2
126	2q	2.4
155	2q	3.7
124	16p	3.0
127	16p	-
	X	2.6
157	X	2.5

[a]10 dizygotic twin pairs were studied.
[b]20 dizygotic twin pairs were studied.
[c]At the time of the majority of these studies the accepted prevalence for autism was 4-6/10,000.
[d]Listed are the most commonly reported co-morbidities.
[e]Includes LOD scores of greater than or equal to 2.0.
[f]LOD scores are listed for overall ASD only, not sub-typed ASD.

hypothesized as contributing to the etiology of autism. The potential influences of these nongenetic factors provide further support of the complex, multifactorial nature of the etiology of autism. Conceptual advances in genetic epidemiologic methods have made it possible to discuss options for future research to elucidate the specific roles of genetic and nongenetic factors and their interactions.

C. Twin Studies

In 1977, Folstein and Rutter (91) reported their results from the first twin study providing compelling evidence of a strong genetic component to the etiology of autism. From this study, two main findings emerged. First, they showed a significant difference in the concordance of autism between monozygotic (MZ) and dizygotic (DZ) twins, 36% and 0%, respectively (91). Additional twin studies by other investigators with larger sample sizes have provided even higher concordance rates ranging from 60% to 96% for MZ twins compared with a consistently low concordance of autism among DZ twins (0–24%) (Table 3) (92–94). While these works provide compelling evidence of genetic factors in autism, the fact that MZ twins do not have 100% concordance indicates the presence of interacting environmental factors (95).

Folstein and Rutter's seminal work also showed within MZ twins that the concordance for autism extended to behavioral and cognitive characteristics beyond classic autism, suggesting genetic factors in a broader phenotype and the possibility of genetic heterogeneity (91). These findings were supported and further refined by Bailey et al. (94) and Le Couteur et al.(96) who identified the broader phenotype as including behaviors such as emotional or social difficulties that resemble autism, but are less severe. Le Couteur et al. (96) investigated this broader phenotype further and found that the clinical phenotypic variation within MZ twins was as great as that found between unrelated twin pairs.

Because of the sex differences seen in the prevalence of autism, it is important to consider the potential confounding and modifying effects of sex when evaluating results from twin studies. Because autism is more common in males, male siblings of affected female twins will increase the DZ concordance rate compared with female siblings of affected females or affected male twins (97). Of the twin studies on autism discussed in this chapter, with the exception of Ritvo et al. (92) all examined same sex twin pairs. Interestingly, the studies using same sex twin pairs found 0% DZ concordance and Ritvo et al. (92) found 24% DZ concordance for autism. Upon further investigation, however, the finding of Ritvo et al. was not attributable to a differential increase in autism among male siblings of affected females.

While findings from twin studies have provided much of the empirical basis for the belief that there is a strong genetic component to the etiology of autism, Greenberg et al. (98) posited that twinning itself is an important risk factor for autism. These authors suggested that MZ twins are at a higher risk of autism as a result of the shared physical environment and the competition for limited intrauterine resources. From an epidemiologic perspective, Hallmayer et al. (99) pointed out that Greenberg et al. focused only on multiplex affected sibships and did not quantify the increased risk of autism in twins in the population. Hallmayer et al. (99) supported their contradictory opinion of no increase in the prevalence of twins among those with autism with evidence from population-based studies in Western Australia, California, and Sweden.

D. Family Studies

Family studies have consistently shown that the rate of autism in siblings ranges from 2% to 6% (Table 3). The increased risk for autism among siblings of affected children is meaningful only in relation to the population prevalence of autism. While current population-based prevalence rates are higher than those reported at the time of the family studies presented in this chapter, by applying the accepted prevalence at the time these family studies were conducted (approximately 4–6 per 10,000), the recurrence risk estimates range from 30 to 150 times greater than the population prevalence (if current population rates are applied, i.e., 2–4 per 1000, recurrence risks are 5–30 times greater) (100,101). The 4:1 male to female ratio in autism prevalence has implications for understanding recurrence risk estimates. The risk of autism for siblings of male cases has been shown to be about half that of siblings of female cases, indicating that the estimates of 2–6% increased risk for subsequent siblings with autism may not be uniform across gender (102).

As discussed previously, family studies are limited to study samples generally selected from clinics or recruited from voluntary and advocacy organizations. The issues of family size and the phenomenon of stoppage limit the opportunity for recurrence. Population-based sampling is most effective at reducing selection bias and often results in the most generalizable findings. The problem of inconsistent case definitions is pervasive across most studies on autism (e.g., prevalence, twin, and family). The lack of a standard case definition makes comparison of results difficult and could account for some of the differences in results. In addition, a number of studies have included cases with comorbidities that could also be associated with characteristics that overlap with the broader autism phenotype. More homogeneous groupings of autism based on distinct phenotypic subgroups could lead to uncovering various etiologies (103). Spiker et al. (104) provided evidence for genetic recurrence among siblings using cluster analyses for a continuous severity gradient rather than small behaviorally discrete subgroups. Both Lord et al. (103) and Spiker et al. (104) advocated using a continuous measure of broader phenotype expression to allow for greater statistical power to identify underlying biological mechanism(s) for the etiology of ASDs. Despite these methodologic challenges, the majority of family studies have reported similar findings, lending support to the argument of a strong genetic basis for autism.

E. Comorbid Conditions with Known Genetic Etiology

Autism is associated with several genetic disorders. Careful examination of the physiological pathways underlying these comorbid genetic disorders may improve our understanding of the pathogenesis of autism, may point to pleiotropy of specific known genes, or may help identify closely linked alleles or the chromosomal location of a gene, or a combination thereof (105). The two most frequent comorbid conditions associated with autism are Fragile X syndrome and tuberous sclerosis. Genes have been identified for both of these conditions (106). Given the consistently reported 4:1 male to female ratio in autism, the initial evidence of a strong association between autism and Fragile X syndrome located on the X chromosome has been encouraging. With the advent of DNA techniques, the Fragile X gene (FMR1 at Xq27.3) has been shown to be present in approximately 4% of individuals with autism (107,108). The frequency of tuberous sclerosis, measured by mutations in one of two tumor-suppressor genes, TSC1 (chromosome 9q34) or TSC2 (chromosome 16p13), is also notable and has been identified in approximately 1–3% of the population with autism (109). Prader–Willi and Angelman syndromes, untreated phenylketonuria (PKU), Down syndrome, and neurofibromatosis are examples of additional genetic disorders with known genetic etiologies that are associated with autism (110–115). Given the low prevalence of these comorbid genetic disorders, it is unlikely that their co-occurrence with autism is coincidence. While known associations exist between autism and various genetic disorders, all of these conditions do not account for a significant fraction of autism in the population.

In addition to the comorbidities of chromosomal origin (i.e., Fragile X and Down syndromes) mentioned above, a number of studies have reported aberrations in chromosome 15 to be associated with autism. Studies have reported the frequency of 15q11–q13 chromosome abnormalities, specifically, in individuals with autism to range from 1–2% (116–118). Many genes in the 15q11–q13 region are imprinted and are either maternally or paternally expressed. The majority of genes in this region associated with autism are maternally duplicated (119). Herzing et al. (120) reported the frequency of maternally derived 15q11–q13 duplications at approximately 0.5–3.0% of individuals with autism. These findings support the importance of one or more imprinted genes in this region and the need for further chromosome 15 investigations for finding the etiology of autism. Some of the previously mentioned comorbidities with a known genetic etiology are also associated with varying severities of MR in addition to autism. It is suggested that a diagnosis of autism is an artifact due to the difficulty in diagnosing a child with MR. Yet, these comorbidities remain, even as the diagnostic criteria for autism evolve and methods to apply those criteria improve.

F. Genome Scans and Candidate Genes

Identification of the gene(s) that cause autism might help identify underlying neurological pathways and mechanisms, assist in identification of environmental risks, and develop pharmaceutical treatments and other protective interventions. To this end, genome-wide scans and candidate gene studies have been conducted in efforts to identify the responsible genes. Over the past 5 years, genetic studies have produced promising findings supporting the notion that multiple genes are involved in the etiology of autism, with several genes potentially interacting with weak or moderate effects. Latent-class analyses of twin and family data for complex autism phenotypes have been conducted, and, as a result, Pickles et al. (121) have suggested that 2–10 loci might be operating in such a manner that the expression of one gene is altered or suppressed by other loci. Risch et al. (122) also conducted latent-class analyses and posited that up to 15 distinct loci could be involved in autism, with the interaction of three genes being the best model. While others have suggested that up to 100 different genes might be involved, this variability is likely to reflect clinically heterogeneous study populations that were assumed to be homogeneous.

While no specific genes for autism have been identified to date, chromosomal regions have been identified based on genome-wide scans and linkage studies. Log-odds, more commonly known as LOD scores, represent the statistical method used in linkage studies to determine whether two loci are linked (i.e., in close enough proximity to be inherited together). Traditionally a LOD score of 2.0 or greater is suggestive of a potential association (123). Table 3 presents studies that have identified regions on chromosomes 1, 2, 7, 13, 16, and X as yielding multipoint maximum LOD scores of greater than or equal to 2.0 suggestive of potential associations. While none of the identified regions have been replicated by other studies, regions identified by different investigators have overlapped. This provides further support for the importance of a particular region. For example, the finding by the International Molecular Genetic Study of Autism Consortium (IMGSAC) of linkage on chromosome 7q (124) was found at a different, but overlapping region by Barrett et al. (125). Similar scenarios occurred for the 2q chromosomal region between Buxbaum et al. (126) and the IMGSAC and regions on the 16p chromosome by Lui et al. (127) and the IMGSAC. As previously mentioned, the phenotypic heterogeneity of study populations between studies may be significant and may account for the lack of replication of findings. Therefore, it is quite powerful when different studies identify overlapping regions on the same chromosome. The validity of these and other findings from linkage analyses will be strengthened in future research by controlling for the bias introduced by clinical heterogeneity.

Initial efforts to define more homogeneous subgroups in families with autism have focused on linkage analyses between autism and the candidate region on chromosome 15q11–q13. While much discussion has ensued about an association between autism and the chromosome 15q11–q13 region, evidence from linkage studies has been inconsistent and LOD scores have not exceeded 2.0 (128,129). Shao et al. (130) and Nurmi et al. (131) conducted principle components factor analyses to identify more homogeneous phenotypic subgroups of autism and examined their association with this chromosomal region. Shao et al. (130) found that by the analysis of families sharing high scores on the factor of "repetitive behaviors/stereotypical patterns" (a domain on the ADI-R), LOD scores increased from 1.5 to 4.7. Nurmi et al. (131) saw a similar trend for families with "savant skills", with an increase in LOD scores from 0.6 to 2.6. Based on these results, the investigators concluded that analyses using homogeneous subgroups may be powerful for mapping disease-susceptibility genes in complex traits.

G. Conclusions

While genetic factors appear to play a dominant role in the etiology of autism, from all available evidence, a simple mode of inheritance is not clear and a multifactorial mechanism of genetic and nongenetic factors is most likely responsible for autism etiology. The suggested temporal trends in autism prevalence have also fueled discussion about the role of nongenetic factors in the etiology of autism. A wide range of nongenetic factors has been posited as risk factors for autism including pregnancy complications (132,133), twinning (98), vaccination for measles, mumps and rubella (MMR) (134–136), and xenobiotics (137). While some of these factors, such as the MMR vaccine, have received much publicity as a cause of autism in a portion of children, currently the epidemiologic evidence is weak or in support of no association between these factors and autism. In addition to increased movement toward identification of a gene using genomic scanning and cytogenetic testing methods, epidemiologic methods can also be applied to help understand this complex disorder by examining the potential role(s) of a single gene, gene–gene, or gene–environment interactions across a continuous measure of autism severity and at multiple levels of analysis (parents and children).

IV. GENETIC EPIDEMIOLOGY FOR TESTING MULTIFACTORIAL MODELS IN MENTAL RETARDATION AND AUTISM

Traditionally, case–control study designs have been used to study the associations between genetic variants and specific disorders, with the variant allele being the exposure. However, application of the case–control study design to evaluate a potential genetic association raises the problem of population stratification bias, defined by confounding attributable to differences in genetic backgrounds between cases and controls (138). While adjustment for factors possibly related to differing allelic distributions is possible using information on ethnicity, social background, and geographical origin of the parents, these factors are also often related to the disorder under study for other reasons (139). Without adequate adjustment of these systematic differences between cases and controls, this bias can obscure identification of a weak association of genes with modest effects. Some argue that the effects of population stratification bias are not a major threat to the validity of results from case–control studies of polymorphisms and disease risk (140). Using hypothetical simulations of the effects of ethnicity on the association between a genetic factor and disease risk, Wacholder et al. (141) suggested that in well-designed case–control studies in the United States, the risk ratio is biased less than 10% when ignoring the role of ethnicity. Aside from the presence or magnitude of population stratification bias, using nonrelated subjects in a case–control study requires large, and often unrealistic, sample sizes to detect interactions.

An alternative study design that minimizes population stratification bias and provides more power to detect interactions and a broad range of genetic mechanisms is the case–parent triad design (139). The case–parent triad uses biological family members of cases as controls, matching the cases and controls on their genetic descent, while controlling for a number of environmental factors (e.g., socioeconomic status). Unlike case–control studies, this design requires availability of DNA samples from all members of the triad: both parents and the affected child. The case–parent triad can be viewed as a matched case–control study and, therefore, can be easily analyzed using conditional logistic regression methods. Taking this design a step further, Ahsan et al. (139) have suggested that conceptualizing and sampling the case–parent triad as a case–cohort study provides an exposure odds measure of effect that is generalizable to the source population from which the cases and controls were drawn. The authors point out the added feature of the case–cohort design is that the cross-product ratio (ratio of exposure odds for cases relative to controls) equals the relative risk estimates from a cohort study on the same population (139).

Newschaffer et al. (100) recently suggested that expansion of the case–parent triad design to include controls and their parents (a case–parent/control–parent design) might be best suited to estimating and testing the full combination of genetic and environmental effects of interest in DD research. This design, while more complex, allows for estimations of genetic and environmental effects at both the parent and child levels, including all possible interactions. A genetic effect operating at the parental level could be a genotype important in the mother because, for example, it influences intrauterine environment during pregnancy and that same gene in the child could not be associated at all with autism risk. The case–parent/control–parent design also would allow estimation of the interaction of genetic effects at the parent or child level with environmental exposure at either level (100).

At least three outstanding issues remain with the case–parent/control–parent study design: (1) sample size, (2) phenotypic heterogeneity, and (3) consistency of case definition. As previously mentioned, large sample sizes are needed to detect both statistical and biological interaction and, while the case–triad and case–parent/control–parent designs require smaller sample sizes than traditional case–control studies, these sample sizes remain substantial. It is well documented that controls are less likely to participate in studies requiring sensitive information such as biologic sampling. As a result, for studies that require DNA samples, participation bias could ensue from requiring this type of information from a control population. It would be important here, as with any epidemiologic study, to examine whether there are any systematic differences between individuals who participate and those who refuse. This potential obstacle might require extensive resources to overcome and might result in a compromised sample size.

As discussed previously, the wide variability in behavioral characteristics present in individuals with autism and milder autistic-like behavioral problems pose difficulties in isolating associations between distinct phenotypes and specific genetic variants. Similar challenges in case definition are evident for MR. Until a standard case definition (i.e., diagnostic criteria) is consistently applied, the strength of inferences made from both genetic and epidemiologic studies will be weakened by potentially inconsistent and uncomparable results. The over-riding challenge in understanding the etiology of these DDs, which permeates the outstanding issues, is that of conceptualizing and operationalizing specific hypotheses for testing gene–environment interactions using population-based data and epidemiologic methods.

ACKNOWLEDGMENTS

The authors would like to acknowledge the valuable comments of Drs. Muin Khoury, Sonja Rasmussen, and Craig Newschaffer on early drafts of the chapter. Also, Tanya Karapurkar contributed significantly to the development of the autism prevalence table.

REFERENCES

1. Boyle CA, Decoufle P, Yeargin-Allsopp M. Prevalence and health impact of developmental disabilities in U.S. children. Pediatrics 1994; 93:399–403.

2. Boyle CA, Yeargin-Allsopp M, Doernberg NS, Holmgreen P, Murphy CC, Schendel DE. Prevalence and selected developmental disabilities in children 3–10 years of age: the Metropolitan Atlanta Developmental Disabilities Surveillance Program, 1991. MMWR 1996; 45(SS-2):1–14.

3. Honeycutt AA, Grosse SD, Dunlap LJ, Scheudel DE, Chen H, Brann E, al Homsi G. Economic costs of mental retardation, cerebral palsy, hearing loss, and vision impairment. In: Altman BM, Barnartt SN, Hendershot GE, Larson SA, eds. Using survey data to study disability: results from the National Health Interview Survey. Amsterdam: Elsevier; 2003:207–228.

4. American Association on Mental Retardation. Mental Retardation: Definitions, Classification, and Systems of Support.

Washington DC: American Association on Mental Retardation, 1992.

5. Zigler E. The definition and classification of mental retardation. Ups J Med Sci Suppl 1987; 44:9–18.

6. American Psychiatric Association. Diagnostic and Statistical Manual of Mental Disorders (DSM-IV). 4th ed. Washington, DC: American Psychiatric Association, 1994.

7. World Health Organization. The International Classification of Mental and Behavior Disorders: Clinical Descriptions and Diagnostic Guidelines. Geneva: WHO, 1992.

8. Rothman KF, Greenland S. Modern Epidemiology. Philadelphia: Lippincott–Raven, 1998.

9. Kiely M. The prevalence of mental retardation. Epidemiol Rev 1987; 9:194–218.

10. Roeleveld N, Zielhuis GA, Gabreels F. The prevalence of mental retardation: a critical review of recent literature. Dev Med Child Neurol 1997; 39:125–132.

11. Leonard H, Wen X. The epidemiology of mental retardation: challenges and opportunities in the new millennium. Ment Retard Dev Disabil Res Rev 2002; 8:117–134.

12. Murphy CC, Yeargin-Allsopp M, Decoufle P, Drews CD. The administrative prevalence of mental retardation in 10 year-old children in metropolitan Atlanta, 1985–1987. Am J Public Health 1995; 85:319–323.

13. Susser MW. Community Psychiatry: Epidemiology and Social Themes. New York: Random House, 1968.

14. Drews CD, Yeargin-Allsopp M, Decoufle P, Murphy CC. Variation in the influence of selected sociodemographic risk factors for mental retardation. Am J Public Health 1995; 85: 329–334.

15. Croen LA, Grether JK, Selvin S. The epidemiology of mental retardation of unknown cause. Pediatrics 2001; 107. http://www.pediatrics.org/cgi/content/full/107/6/e86.

16. Lubs H, Chiurazzi P, Arena J, Schwartz C, Tranebjaerg L, Neri G. XLMR genes: update 1998. Am J Med Genet 1999; 83:237–247.

17. Chiurazzi P, Hamel BC, Neri G. XLMR genes: update 2000. Eur J Hum Genet 2000; 9:71–81.

18. Chelly J, Mandel JL. Monogenic causes of X-linked mental retardation. Nat Rev 2001; 2:669–680.

19. Nance WE, Engel E. One X and four hypotheses: response to Lehrke's theory of X-linkage of major intellectual traits. Am J Ment Defic 1972; 76:623–625.

20. Mercer JR. Labeling the Mentally Retarded. Berkeley, CA: University of California Press, 1973.

21. Yeargin-Allsopp M, Drews CD, Decoufle P, Murphy CC. Mild mental retardation in black and white children in metropolitan Atlanta: a case–control study. Am J Public Health 1995; 85:324–328.

22. Mervis CA, Decoufle P, Murphy CC, Yeargin-Allsopp M. Low birth weight and the risk for mental retardation later in childhood. Paediatr Perinat Epidemiol 1995; 9:455–468.

23. Couvert P, Bienvenu T, Aquaviva C, Poirier K, Moraine C, Cenfrot C, et al. MECP2 is highly mutated in X-linked mental retardation. Hum Mol Genet 2001; 10:941–946.

24. Battaglia A, Carey JC. Diagnostic evaluation of developmental delay/mental retardation: an overview. Am J Med Genet 2003; 117C:3–14.

25. State MW, Bryan KH, Dykens E. Mental retardation: a review of the past 10 years. Part II. J Am Acad Child Adolesc Psychiatry 1997; 36:1664–1671.

26. Crawford DC, Meadows KL, Newman JL, Taft LF, Scott E, Leslie M, et al. Prevalence of the fragile X syndrome in African–Americans. Am J Med Genet 2002; 110:226–233.

27. Yeargin-Allsopp M, Murphy CC, Cordero JF, Decoufle P, Hollowell JG. Reported biomedical causes and associated medical conditions for mental retardation among 10-year-old children, metropolitan Atlanta, 1985 to 1987. Dev Med Child Neurol 1997; 39:142–149.

28. Hou W, Wang TR, Chuang SM. An epidemiological and aetiological study of children with intellectual disability in Taiwan. J Intellect Disabil Res 1998; 42:137–143.

29. Amir RE, Van den Veyver GJC, Wan M, Tran CQ, Francke U, Zoghbi HY. Rett syndrome is caused by mutations in X-linked MECP2, encoding methyl-CpG-binding protein 2. Nat Genet 1999; 23:185–188.

30. Knight SJL, Regan R, Nicod SW, Horsley A, Kearney L, Homfray T, Winter RM, Bolton P, Flint J. Subtle chromosomal rearrangements in children with unexplained mental retardation. Lancet 1999; 354:1676–1681.

31. Baker E, Hinton L, Callen DF, Altree M, Dobbie A, Eyre HJ, Sutherland GR. Study of 250 children with idiopathic mental retardation reveals nine crytic and diverse subtelomeric chromosome anomalies. Am J Med Genet 2002; 107:285–293.

32. Fernell E. Aetiological factors and prevalence of severe mental retardation in children in a Swedish municipality: the possible role of consanguinity. Dev Med Child Neurol 1998; 40: 608–611.

33. Stromme P. Aetiology in severe and mild mental retardation: a population-based study of Norwegian children. Dev Med Child Neurol 2000; 42:76–86.

34. Partington M, Mowat D, Einfeld S, Tonge B, Turner G. Genes on the X chromosome are important in undiagnosed mental retardation. Am J Med Genet 2000; 92:57–61.

35. Yeargin-Allsopp M, Murphy CC, Oakley GP, Sikes RK. A multiple source method for studying the prevalence of developmental disabilities in children: the Metropolitan Atlanta Developmental Disabilities Study. Pediatrics 1992; 89: 624–629.

36. Costeff H, Weller L. The risk of having a second retarded child. Am J Med Genet 1987; 27:753–766.

37. Bundey S, Thake A, Todd J. The recurrence risks for mild idiopathic mental retardation. J Med Genet 1989; 26: 260–266.

38. Herbst DS, Baird PA. Sibs risks for nonspecific mental retardation in British Columbia. Am J Med Genet 1982; 13: 197–208.

39. Bundey S, Carter CO. Recurrence risks in severe undiagnosed mental deficiency. J Ment Defic Res 1974; 18:115–134.

40. Turner G, Collins E, Turner B. Recurrence risk of mental retardation in sibs. Med J Austral 1971; 1:1165–1166.

41. Bundey S, Webb TP, Thake A, Todd J. A community study of severe mental retardation in West Midlands and the importance of fragile X chromosome in its aetiology. J Med Genet 1985; 22:258–266.

42. Kanner L. Autistic disturbances of affective contact. Nerv Child 1943; 2:217–250.

43. Gillberg W, Wing L. Autism: not an extremely rare disorder. Acta Psychiatr Scand 1999; 99:399–406.

44. Wing L, Potter D. The epidemiology of autistic spectrum disorders: is the prevalence rising? Ment Retard Dev Disabil Res Rev 2002; 8:151–161.

45. Filipek PA, Accardo PJ, Baraned GT, Cook EH, Dawson G, et al. The screening and diagnosis of autistic spectrum disorders. J Autism Dev Disord 1999; 29:439–484.

46. Lord C, Rutter M, Goode A, Heemsbergen J, Jordan H, Mawhood L, Schopler E. Autism diagnostic observation schedule: a standardized observation of communicative and social behavior. J Autism Dev Disord 1989; 19:185–212.

47. Lord C, Rutter M, Le Couteur A. Autism diagnostic interview-revised: a revised version of a diagnostic interview for caregivers of individuals with possible pervasive developmental disabilities. J Autism Dev Disord 1994; 24:659–667.

48. Lord C, Risi S. Frameworks and methods in diagnosing autism spectrum disorders. Ment Retard Dev Disabil Res Rev 1998; 4:90–96.

49. Fombonne E. The epidemiology of autism: a review. Psychol Med 1999; 29:769–786.

50. Boyle CA, Bertrand J, Yeargin-Allsopp M. Surveillance of autism. Infants Young Child 1999; 12:75–78.

51. Lotter V. Epidemiology of autistic conditions in young children. Some characteristics of the parents and children. Soc Psychiatry 1966; 1:124–137.

52. Brask B. In: Nordic Symposium on the Comprehensive Care of Psychotic Children. Oslo, Norway: Barnepsykiatrisk, 1972.

53. Treffert D. Epidemiology of infantile autism. Arch Gen Psychiatry 1970; 22:431–438.

54. Wing L, Gould J. Severe impairments of social interaction and associated abnormalities in children: epidemiology and classification. J Autism Dev Disord 1979; 9:11–29.

55. Hoshino Y, Kumashiro H, Yashima Y, Tachibana R, Watanabe M. The epidemiological study of autism in Fukushima-ken. Folia Psychiatr Neurol Jpn 1982; 36(2):115–124.

56. Ishi T, Takahashi O. The epidemiology of autistic children in Toyota, Japan: prevalence. Jpn J Child Adolesc Psychiatry 1983; 24:311–321.

57. Bohman M, Bohman I, Bjorck P, et al. Childhood psychosis in a northern Swedish county: some preliminary findings from an epidemiological survey. In: Schmidt M, Remschmidt H, eds. Epidemiological Approaches in Child Psychiatry. Vol. II. New York: Thieme-Stratton, 1983:164–173.

58. McCarthy P, Fitzgerald M, Smith M. Prevalence of childhood autism in Ireland. Ir Med J 1984; 77:129–130.

59. Gillberg C. Infantile autism and other childhood psychoses in a Swedish urban region: epidemiological aspects. J Child Psychol Psychiatry 1984; 25:35–43.

60. Steinhausen H, Gobel D, Breinlinger M, et al. A community survey of infantile autism. J Am Acad Child Adolesc Psychiatry 1986; 25:186–189.

61. Steffenburg S, Gillberg C. Autism and autistic-like conditions in Swedish rural and urban areas: a population study. Br J Psychiatry 1986; 149:81–87.

62. Matsuishi T, Shiotsuki Y, Yoshimura K, et al. High prevalence of infantile autism in Kurume City, Japan. J Child Neurol 1987; 2:268–271.

63. Burd L, Fisher W, Kerbeshian J. A prevalence study of pervasive developmental disorders in North Dakota. J Am Acad Child Adolesc Psychiatry 1987; 26:704–710.

64. Bryson S, Clark B, Smith IM. First report of a Canadian epidemiological study of autistic syndromes. J Child Psychol Psychiatry 1988; 29:433–446.

65. Tanoue Y, Oda S, Asano F, et al. Epidemiology of infantile autism in the Southern Ibaraki, Japan. J Autism Dev Disord 1988; 18:155–167.

66. Cialdella P, Mamelle N. An epidemiological study of infantile autism in a French Department Rhone: a research note. J Child Psychol Psychiatry 1989; 30:165–176.

67. Sugiyama T, Abe T. The prevalence of autism in Nagoya, Japan: a total population study. J Autism Dev Disord 1989; 19:87–96.

68. Ritvo E, Freeman B, Pingree C, et al. The UCLA-University of Utah epidemiological study of autism: prevalence. Am J Psychiatry 1989; 146:194–245.

69. Gillberg C. Outcome in autism and autistic-like conditions. J Am Acad Child Adolesc Psychiatry 1991; 30:375–382.

70. Fombonne E, du Mazaubrun C. Prevalence of infantile autism in four French regions. Soc Psychiatry Psychiatr Epidemiol 1992; 27:203–210.

71. Honda H, Shimizu Y, Misumi K, et al. Cumulative incidence and prevalence of childhood autism in children in Japan. Br J Psychiatry 1996; 169:228–235.

72. Fombonne E, du Mazaubrun C, Cans C, et al. Autism and associated medical disorders in a French epidemiological survey. J Am Acad Child Adolesc Psychiatry 1997; 36: 1561–1569.

73. Arvidsson T, Danielsson B, Forsberg P., et al. Autism in 3–6 year-old children in a suburb of Goteborg, Sweden. Autism 1997; 1:163–171.

74. Webb E, Thompson W, Morey J, et al. A prevalence study of Asperger syndrome and high functioning autism. J Intellect Disabil Res 2000; 44:513.

75. Sponheim E, Skjeldal O. Autism and related disorders: epidemiological findings in a Norwegian study using ICD-10 diagnostic criteria. J Autism Dev Disord 1998; 28:217–228.

76. Kadesjö B, Gillberg C, Hagberg B. Brief report. Autism and Asperger syndrome in seven-year-old children. J Autism Dev Disord 1999; 29:327–332.

77. Baird G, Charman T, Baron-Cohen S, et al. A screening instrument for autism at 18 months of age: a 6-year follow-up study. J Am Acad Child Adolesc Psychiatry 2000; 39:694–702.

78. Powell JE, Edwards A, Edwards M, Pandit BS, Sungum-Paliwal SR, Whitehouse W. Changes in the incidence of childhood autism and other autistic spectrum disorders in preschool children from two areas of the West Midlands, UK. Dev Med Child Neurol 2000; 42:624–628.

79. Kielinen M, Linna S, Moilanen I. Autism in northern Finland. Eur Child Adolesc Psychiatry 2000; 19:162–167.

80. Mágnússon P, Saemundsen E. Prevalence of autism in Iceland. J Autism Dev Disord 2001; 31:53–163.

81. Chakrabarti S, Fombonne E. Pervasive developmental disorder in preschool children. JAMA 2001; 285:3093–3099.

82. Fombonne E, Simmons H, Ford T, Meltzer H, Goodman R. Prevalence of pervasive developmental disorders in the British nationwide survey of child mental health. J Am Acad Child Adolesc Psychiatry 2001; 40(7):820–827.

83. Bertrand J, Mars A, Boyle C, et al. Prevalence of autism in a United States population: the Brick Township, New Jersey, investigation. Pediatrics 2001; 108:1155–1161.

84. Croen L, Grether J, Hoogstrate J, Selvin S. The changing prevalence of autism in California. J Autism Dev Disord 2003; 33(2):223–226.

85. American Psychiatric Association. Diagnostic and Statistical Manual of Mental Disorders. 3rd ed. Washington, DC: American Psychiatric Association, 1987:87–92.

86. American Psychiatric Association. Diagnostic and Statistical Manual of Mental Disorders [Revised]. 3rd ed. Washington, DC: American Psychiatric Association, 1987.

87. Yeargin-Allsopp M, Rice C, Karapurkar T, Doernberg N, Boyle C, Murphy C. The prevalence of autism in a US metropolitan area. JAMA 2003.

88. California Department of Developmental Services. Changes in the Population of Persons with Autism and Pervasive

Developmental Disorders in California's Developmental Services System: 1987–1998. A Report to the Legislature. Sacramento, CA: California Department of Developmental Services, March 1999.

89. California Department of Developmental Services. Autistic Spectrum Disorders: Changes in the California Caseload; an Update: 1999–2002. Sacramento, CA: California Department of Developmental Services, April 2003.

90. U.S. Department of Education. Office of Special Education Programs, Data Analysis System (DANS). Number of children served under IDEA by disability and age group, during the 1989–90 through 1998–1999 school years. Cited by: US Department of Education. Twenty-second Annual Report to Congress on the Implementation of the Individuals with Disabilities Education Act. Washington, DC: US Department of Education; 2000; II-20.

91. Folstein S, Rutter M. Infantile autism: a genetic study of 21 twin pairs. J Child Psychol Psychiatry 1977; 18:291–321.

92. Ritvo ER, Freeman BJ, Mason-Brothers A, et al. Concordance for the syndrome of autism in 40 pairs of afflicted twins. Am J Psychiatry 1985; 142:74–77.

93. Steffenburg S, Gillberg C, Hellgren L, Andersson L, Gillberg L, Jakobsson G, Bohman M. A twin study of autism in Denmark, Finland, Iceland, Norway, and Sweden. J Child Psychol Psychiatry 1989; 30:405–416.

94. Bailey A, Le Couteur A, Gottesman I, Bolton P, Simonoff E, Yuzda E, Rutter M. Autism is a strongly genetic disorder: evidence from a British twin study. Psychol Med 1995; 25:63–77.

95. Piven J, Folstein S. The genetics of autism. In: Bauman ML, Kemper TL, eds. The Neurobiology of Autism. Baltimore, MD: Johns Hopkins University Press, 1997.

96. Le Couteur A, Bailey A, Goode S, Pickles A, Robertson S, Gottesman I, Rutter M. A broader phenotype of autism: The clinical spectrum in twins. J Child Psychol 1996; 36:785–801.

97. Lauritsen MB, Ewald H. The genetics of autism. Acta Psychiatr Scand 2001; 103:411–427.

98. Greenberg DA, Hodge SE, Sowinski J, Nicoll D. Excess of twins among affected sibling pairs with autism: implications for the etiology of autism. Am J Hum Genet 2001; 69: 1062–1067.

99. Hallmayer J, Glasson EJ, Bower C, Petterson B, Croen L, Grether J, Risch N. On the twin risk in autism. Am J Hum Genet 2002; 71:941–946.

100. Newschaffer CJ, Fallin D, Lee NL. Heritable and nonheritable risk factors for autism spectrum disorders. Epidemiol Rev 2002; 24:137–153.

101. Smalley SL, Asarnow RF, Spence MA. Autism and genetics: a decade of research. Arch Gen Psychiatry 1988; 45:953–961.

102. Ritvo ER, Spence MA, Freeman BJ, et al, Evidence for autosomal recessive inheritance in 46 families with multiple incidences of autism. Am J Psychiatry 1985; 142:187–192.

103. Lord C, Leventhal BL, Cook EH. Quantifying the phenotype in autism spectrum disorders. Am J Med Genet 2001; 105: 36–38.

104. Spiker D, Lotspeich LJ, Dimiceli S, Myers RM, Risch N. Behavioral phenotypic variation in autism multiplex families: evidence for a continuous severity gradient. Am J Med Genet 2002; 114:129–136.

105. Lamb JA, Parr JR, Bailey AJ, Monaco AP. Autism, in search of susceptibility genes. Neuromolecular Med 2002; 2:11–28.

106. Dykens E, Volkmar FR. Medical conditions associated with autism. In: Volkmar C, ed. Handbook of Autism and Pervasive Developmental Disorders. New York, NY: Wiley, 1997: 388–410.

107. Oberle I, Rousseau F, Heitz D, Kretz C, Devys D, Hanauer A. Instability of a 550-base pair DNA segment and abnormal methylation in fragile X syndrome. Science 1991; 252: 1097–1102.

108. Cohen IL, Sudhalter V, Pfadt A, Jenkins EC, Brown T, Vietze PM. Why are autism and the fragile X syndrome associated? Conceptual and methodological issues. Am J Hum Genet 1991; 48:195–202.

109. Smalley SL, Tanguay PE, Smith M, Gutierrez G. Autism and tuberous sclerosis. J Autism Dev Disord 1992; 22:339–355.

110. Page T. Metabolic approaches to the treatment of autism spectrum disorders. J Autism Dev Disord 2000; 30:463–469.

111. Williams PG, Hersh JH. Brief report: the association of neurofibromatosis type 1 and autism. J Autism Dev Disord 1998; 28:567–571.

112. Steffenburg S, Gillberg CL, Steffenburg U. Autism in Angelman syndrome: a population-based study. Pediatr Neurol 1996; 28:131–136.

113. Folstein SE, Rutter ML. Autism: familial aggregation and genetic implications. J Autism Dev Disord 1998; 18:3–30.

114. Rasmussen P, Borjesson O, Wentz E, Gillberg C. Autistic disorders in Down syndrome: background factors and clinical correlates. Dev Med Child Neurol 2001; 43:750–753.

115. Kent L, Evans J, Paul M, Sharp M. Co-morbidity of autistic spectrum disorders in children with Down syndrome. Dev Med Child Neurol 1999; 41:153–158.

116. Schinzel AA, Brecevic L, Bernasconi F, Binkert F, Berthet F, Wuiloud A, et al. Intrachromosomal triplication of 15q11–q13. J Med Genet 1994; 31:798–803.

117. Schroer RJ, Phelan MC, Michaelis RC, Crawford EC, Skinner SA, Cuccaro M, et al. Autism and maternally derived aberrations of chromosome 15q. Am J Med Genet 1998; 76:327–336.

118. Veenstra-VanderWeele J, Gonen D, Leventhal BL, Cook EH. Mutation screening of the UBE3A/E6-AP gene in autistic disorder. Mol Psychiatry 1999; 4:64–67.

119. Sutcliffe JS, Nurmi EI. Genetics of childhood disorders: XLVII. Autism, part 6: duplication and inherited susceptibility of chromosome 15q11–q13 genes in autism. J Am Acad Child Adolesc Psychiatry 2003; 42:253–256.

120. Herzing LB, Cook EH, Ledbetter DH. Allele-specific expression analysis by RNA-FISH demonstrates preferential maternal expression of UBE3A and imprint maintenance within 15q11–q13 duplication. Hum Mol Genet 2002; 11:1707–1718.

121. Pickles A, Bolton P, Macdonald H, Bailey A, Lecouteur A, Sim CH, Rutter M. Latent class analysis if recurrence risks for phenotypes with selection and measurement error: a twin and family history study of autism. Am J Hum Genet 1995; 57:717–726.

122. Risch N, Spiker D, Lotspeich L, Nouri N, Hinds D, Hallmayer J, et al. A genomic screen of autism: evidence for a multilocus etiology. Am J Hum Genet 1999; 65:493–507.

123. Thompson MW, McInnes RR, Willard HF. Genetics in Medicine. 5th Phildelphia, PA: WB Saunders Co., 1991:435.

124. International Molecular Genetic Study of Autism Consortium. A full genome screen for autism with evidence for linkage to a region on chromosome 7q. Hum Mol Genet 1998; 7:571–578.

125. Barrett S, Beck JC, Bernier R, et al. An autosomal genomic screen for autism. Collaborative linkage study of autism. Am J Med Genet 1999; 88:609–615.

126. Buxbaum JD, Silverman JM, Smith CJ, Kilifarski M, Reichart J, Hollander E, et al. Evidence of a susceptibility gene for autism on chromosome 2 and genetic heterogeneity. Am J Hum Genet 2001; 68:1514–1520.

127. Liu J, Nyholt DR, Magnussen P, et al. A genome wide screen for autism susceptibility loci. Am J Hum Genet 2001; 69: 327–340.

128. Salmon B, Hallmayer J, Rogers T, Kalaydijeva L, Peterson PB, Nicholas P, et al. Absence of linkage and linkage disequilibrium to chromosome 15q11–q13 markers in 139 multiplex families with autism. Am J Med Genet 1999; 88:551–556.

129. Cook EH, Courchesne RY, Cox NJ, Lord C, Gonen D. Linkage-disequilibrium mapping of autistic disorder, with 15q11–13 markers. Am J Hum Genet 1998; 62:1077–1083.

130. Shao Y, Cuccaro ML, Hauser ER, Raiford KL, Menold MM, Wolpert CM, et al. Fine mapping of autistic disorder to chromosome 15q11–q13 by use of phenotypic subtypes. Am J Hum Genet 2003; 72:539–548.

131. Nurmi EL, Dowd M, Tadevosyn-Leyfer O, Haines JL, Folstein SE, Suton JS. Exploratory subsetting of autism

families based on savant skills to improve evidence of genetic linkage to 15q11–q13. J Am Acad Child Adolesc Psychiatry 2003; 42:856–863.

132. Gillberg C, Gillberg JC. Infantile autism: a total population study of nonoptimal, pre-, peri- and neonatal conditions. J Autism Dev Disord 1983; 13:153–166.

133. Deykin EY, MacMahon B. Pregnancy, delivery, and neonatal complications among autistic children. Am J Dis Child 1980; 134:860–864.

134. Wakefield AJ, Murch SH, Anthony A, Linnell J, Casson DM, Malik M, Berelowitz M, Dhillon AP, Thomson MA, Harvey P, Valentine A, Davies SE, Walker-Smith JA. Ileal-lymphoid-nodular hyperplasia, non-specific colitis, and pervasive developmental disorder in children. Lancet 1998; 351:637–641.

135. Chen RT, DeStefano F. Vaccine adverse events: causal or coincidental? Lancet 1998; 351:611–612.

136. Taylor B, Miller E, Farrington CP, Petropoulos MC, Favot-Mayaud I, Li J, Waight PA. Autism and measles, mumps, and rubella vaccine: no epidemiological evidence for a causal association. Lancet 1999; 353:2062–2029.

137. Edelson SB, Cantor DS. Autism: xenobiotic influences. Toxicol Ind Health 1998; 14:553–563.

138. Khoury MJ. Case–parental control methods in the search for disease susceptibility genes. Am J Hum Genet 1994; 55: 414–415.

139. Ahsan H, Hidge SE, Heiman GA, Begg MD, Susser ES. Relative risk for genetic associations: the case–parent triad as a variant of case–cohort design. Int J Epidemiol 2002; 31: 669–678.

140. Wacholder S, Rothman N, Caporaso N. Counterpoint: bias from population stratification is not a major threat to the validity of conclusions from epidemiological studies of polymorphisms and cancer. Cancer Epidemiol Biomarkers Prev 2002; 11:505–512.

141. Wacholder S, Rothman N, Caporaso N. Population stratification in epidemiologic studies of common genetic variants and

cancer: quantification of bias. J Natl Cancer Inst 2000; 92:1151–1158.

142. August GJ, Stewart MA, Tsai L. The incidence of cognitive disabilities in the siblings of autistic children. Br J Psychiatry 1981; 138:416–422.

143. Minton J, Campbell M, Green WH, Jennings S, Samit C. Cognitive assessment of siblings of autistic children. J Am Acad Child Adolesc Psychiatry 1982; 21:256–261.

144. Baird TD, August GJ. Familial heterogeneity in infantile autism. J Autism Dev Disord 1985; 15:315–317.

145. Ritvo ER, Jorde LB, Mason-Brothers A, et al. The UCLA-University of Utah epidemiologic survey of autism: recurrence risk estimates and genetic counseling. Am J Psychiatry 1989; 146:1032–1036.

146. Piven J, Gayle J, Chase GA, et al. A family history study of neuropsychiatric disorders in the adult siblings of autistic individuals. J Am Acad Child Adolesc Psychiatry 1990; 29: 177–183.

147. Jorde LB, Hasstedt SJ, Ritvo ER, Mason-Brothers A, Freeman BJ, Pingree C. Complex segregation analyses in autism. Am J Hum Genet 1991; 49:932–938.

148. Szatmari P, Jones MB, Tuff L, Bartolucci G, Fisman S, Mahoney W. Lack of cognitive impairment in first-degree relatives of children with pervasive developmental disorders. J Am Acad Child Adolesc Psychiatry 1993; 32:1264–1272.

149. Bolton P, Macdonald H, Pickles A, et al. A case control study of family history study of autism. J Child Psychol Psychiatry 1994; 35:877–900.

150. Brown WT, Jenkins EC, Cohen IL, et al. Fragile X and autism: a multicenter survey. Am J Med Genet 1986; 23: 341–352.

151. Folstein SE, Piven J. Etiology of autism: genetic influences. Pediatrics 1991; 87:767–773.

152. Folstein SE, Rutter ML. Autism: familial aggregation and genetic implications. J Autism Dev Disord 1988; 18:3–30.

153. Gillberg C. The treatment of epilepsy in autism. J Autism Dev Disord 1991; 21:61–77.

154. Baker P, Piven J, Sato Y. Autism and tuberous sclerosis complex: prevalence and clinical features. J Autism Dev Disord 1998; 28:279–285.

155. International Molecular Genetic Study of Autism Consortium. A genome-wide screen for autism: strong evidence for linkage to chromosomes 2q, 7q, 16p. Am J Hum Genet 2001; 659:570–581.

156. Auranen M, Nieminen T, Majun S, Vanhala R, Peltonen L, Jarvela I. Analyses of autism susceptibility gene loci on chromosomes 1p, 4p, 6q, 7q, 13q, 15q, 16p, 17q, 19q, and 22q in Finnish multiplex families. Mol Psychiatry 2000; 5:320–322.

157. Shao Y, Wolpert CM, Raiford KL, Menold MM, Donnelly SL, Ravan SA. Genomic screen and follow-up for autistic disorder. Am J Med Genet 2002; 8:99–105.

158. Rutter M. Brain damage in childhood: concepts and findings. J Child Psychol Psychiat Allied Disciplines 1977; 18:1–21.

20

Neuropsychiatric Aspects of Genetic Disorders

BARBARA Y. WHITMAN

Department of Pediatrics, Cardinal Glennon
Children's Hospital, St. Louis, Missouri, U.S.A.

I. INTRODUCTION

Individuals with genetic disorders demonstrate an increased
vulnerability for developing complex, difficult, and challenging behaviors as well as frank psychiatric illness (1–5).
Although actual prevalence estimates vary across studies, it
is generally accepted that mental retardation, emotional,
behavioral, and psychiatric disorders are three to four times
commoner in those with genetic abnormalities compared with
the general public (6–8). Furthermore, neuropsychiatric concerns are not limited to those genetic disorders with mental
retardation. Learning disabilities and increased behavior,
emotional and interpersonal difficulties are documented in a

wide range of disorders such as Turner syndrome, cystic
fibrosis, and Tourette syndrome (9–12). For many, the consequences of such disorders are severer than in other populations as they can seriously disrupt, and even prevent, those
affected from being included in family and community life.
Moreover, the burden these disorders impose on both family
and professional care-providers significantly extends the morbidity impact.

Not only are neuropsychiatric disturbances more frequent in some genetic conditions, but also many of these concerns resist or respond differently and unpredictably to
established treatment protocols. For many, management
demands a multimodal treatment approach, usually over an
extended period of time (13). Meeting these complex needs
is too often hampered by a lack of accessible, affordable, and
effective mental health treatment services. While lack of services is not restricted to this population, this lack is magnified
for those dually affected with neuropsychiatric problems and
genetic disorders. This chapter will first provide an overview
of neuropsychiatric concerns associated with a number of
genetic disorders, followed by a model for determining treatment needs, and finally will discuss current research trends
aimed at developing a better understanding of the genetic
basis of these disorders.

II. AN OVERVIEW OF NEUROPSYCHIATRIC
CONCERNS ASSOCIATED WITH SELECTED
GENETIC DISORDERS

It is obvious to many observers that individuals with genetic
disorders carry an increased risk of neuropsychiatric disturbances. As O'Brien (14) points out, the majority of genetic
syndromes produce physical distress, neurologically mediated
emotional dyscontrol, sensory and perceptual impairment,
distorted drives and motivation, and (altered) responses from
the child's social environment that have a profound and
enduring impact on behavior. Until recently, however, most
studies treated those affected as a singular population

focusing on behavioral concerns primarily as they correlated with IQ scores (3,15,16). Recent advances in molecular and cytogenetic techniques have allowed for earlier identification of many children affected with genetic disorders and the recognition that a characteristic cognitive and behavior pattern or "behavior phenotype" often accompanies the physical phenotype or pattern of dysmorphology associated with many genetic syndromes. Investigations over the past 2 decades delineating syndrome specific behavioral phenotypes have documented behavioral commonalities across syndromes as well as unique syndrome specific neuropsychiatric outcomes (17). These differences seem to suggest that the effect of genes on behavioral function is substantial with very real differences in the resulting neuropsychiatric picture depending on the underlying genetic disturbance. Tables 1 and 2 compare the neuropsychiatric profiles of a number of genetic syndromes (18).

Self-injury, defined as actual or potential tissue damage (19,20), is one of the more dramatic behaviors associated with many genetic disorders. Once established, self-injurious behavior (SIB) is perhaps the most persistent and refractory of all neuropsychiatric manifestations, which, along with outer directed aggression, causes the most management problems. Since self-injury is relatively rare in the "normal" population, a closer examination of this neuropsychiatric aspect of many genetic syndromes is in order.

A. Self-Injurious Behavior

SIB is a particularly problematic behavior in several different genetic syndromes that frequently requires an urgent medical and psychiatric referral and request for psychotropic medication. As with other neuropsychiatric concerns, SIB prevalence rates vary across studies, primarily depending on the genetic heterogeneity of the sample. In a sample of 2,412 persons with mental retardation living in Queensland, Australia, Sigafoos et al. (21) documented a 4% prevalence rate while Griffin et al. (22) reported a 14% rate. However, a very different prevalence picture emerges from studies of specific genetic

Table 1 Cognitive Features of Specific Genetic Syndromes.

Syndrome/ prevalence	Intelligence	Language Receptive	Expressive	Visuospatial abilities	Memory Short term	Long term	Cognitive strengths	Learning disability
Down 1:1,000	MR: Moderate–Severe	Equal to IQ	↓↓	Equal to IQ	↓	→	Pragmatic language	Uneven profile
Fragile X (male) 1:2,000	MR: Mild–Severe	→	↓↓	→	→	Equal to IQ		Uneven profile
Fragile X (female) 1:4,000	Borderline MR—Mild in 50%	Equal to IQ	Equal to IQ	Equal to IQ	Both equal to IQ			Mild to moderate
Rett 1–10,000–15,000	MR—Severe	↓↓	↓↓	↓↓	→	→		+
Prader–Willi 1:10,000–12,000	Borderline MR: Mild–Moderate	→	→	↑For 15q deletion only		Equal to IQ	Jigsaw puzzles (15q deletion subjects)	+ Mild uneven profile
Angelman 1:12,000	MR: Severe	→	none	↓↓	→			+
Williams 1: 10,000	Borderline MR: Mild–Moderate	→	← (Better than IQ)	↓↓	Both equal to IQ	Both equal to IQ	Language skills	+
Velo-Cardio-Facial 1:5,000	Normal MR: Mild	Equal to IQ	Equal to IQ	Equal to IQ	Both equal to IQ		Language skills	+ Moderate
Smith–Magenis 1:25,000	MR: Moderate	Equal to IQ	→	→	→	Equal to IQ	Visual learning	+ Moderate
Turner 1:2,500 females	Usually normal	Equal to IQ	Equal to IQ	→	Both equal to IQ			± Variable but usually mild

Table 2 Psychopathology in Specific Genetic Syndromes

Syndrome	Anxiety	Depression	Hyper-activity	Aggression	Autistic features	Psychoses	Other behavioral features
Down	Not inherent	In adult-hood	+	+	Rarely	Rarely	Early dementia
Fragile X (male)	++	+	++	Rarely	++	–	Hypersensitive to stimuli, sleep problems
Fragile X (female)	++	+	+	Rarely	+ Asperger?	–	Avoidance disorder
Rett	–	–	–	–	+ Mainly in infancy	–	Loss of purposeful movement, develop hand stereotypies
Prader–Willi	++	+	+	+	+Infant Asperger?	+	Lack of satiety, food foraging, skin-picking, sleep problems
Angelman	–	–	+	–	+	–	Frequent smiling, inappropriate outbursts of laughter
Williams	+	In adult-hood	+	+	+	–	Loquacious behavior, hypersensitive to sound
Velo-Cardio-Facial	+	+	+	–	–	++	Increased prevalence of schizophrenia and bipolar disorders
Smith–Magenis	–	–	++	+	–	–	Self-injury, sleep problems
Turner	+	+	++	Rarely	Rarely	–	Immature personality, social, and self-esteem difficulties

Key: – absent; + present; ++ marked; – not characteristic.
Source: Adapted from Ref. 18.

disorders. For example, hyperphagia is considered the cardinal symptom of Prader-Willi syndrome but Einfeld et al. (23) found that self-injury in the form of skin-picking was far more problematic in this syndrome (89% vs. 72%). Eighty-five percent of children with Lesch–Nyhan syndrome exhibited "compulsive" SIB including lip, mouth, or finger biting; head banging; hitting ears and face; and attempting to trap fingers in wheelchair spokes. Thirty-nine to 49% of girls with Rett syndrome demonstrated self-injury, particularly to the hands. Other syndromes routinely associated with self-injury behavior include Cornelia de Lange, Smith-Magenis, fragile X, cri du chat, Aicardi, and Joubert (24). Self-injury appears to correlate with increasing age, peaking in late adulthood, and increased severity with increased cognitive impairment. Prevalence rates are higher among those in institutions; however, this may be in part due to a population skewed to those with the severest cognitive impairments.

Specific genetic disorders appear to carry an increased vulnerability for self-injury. Paralleling other concerns, the severity of self-injury varies between syndromes, and may significantly vary among those with the same syndrome. For instance, most persons with Prader–Willi syndrome spot-pick at "available" sores with consequences no more serious than cosmetic, although infection and cellulitis can occur. Others maintain large open wounds. However, those who attempt to hide their skin-picking engage primarily in rectal picking and can inflict sufficient injury to incur more serious consequences such as chronic ulceration and incontinence requiring surgical diversion to allow healing. Those with Lesch–Nyhan syndrome frequently exhibit mild injuries from biting and chewing fingers and hands; however, severer forms may include hand to head banging, hand to object banging, head banging alone, hair-pulling, and scratching.

One of the more puzzling aspects of SIB is why individuals continue, and even escalate, obviously painful behaviors. In milder forms, self-injury often is meant to serve a function, and may serve different functions at different times (25). These include communication, social contact, terminating social contact, alleviating boredom or stress, or, as a response to pain. The resulting environmental response, however, may serve a conditioning or reward function, so that future episodes of self-injury are directed toward obtaining the environmental response rather than in service of the original purpose. Thus, the adult with Prader–Willi syndrome left with too much unstructured time may, out of boredom, begin skin-picking. The resulting, often unsightly, sore or lesion precipitates an anxious reaction with increased attention from staff seeking to prevent further picking damage. However, the increased attention may be so rewarding that it creates the opposite effect. Thus, episodes of skin-picking increase in number and severity to obtain more attention, rather than serving its initial function of alleviating boredom.

By contrast, when self-injury is particularly severe and unremitting, there often appears to be an organic basis for the behavior. For instance, some children with Lesch–Nyhan syndrome may show an episodic nature to their SIB, manifesting such behavior intensely for a few weeks followed by a period of a few weeks remission (24,26). Many of the children try to avoid hurting themselves and are unable to do so, leading to speculations of abnormal causative brain mechanisms.

Several neurochemical abnormalities have been causally implicated in self-injury, including dopamine and serotonin. Others propose that for many individuals, such injury, rather than feeling painful, paradoxically precipitates a release of beta-endorphins ultimately resulting in relative analgesia and a rewarding mood state, similar to a "runner's high". To the extent that such a mechanism is operating, genetics may serve to increase an individual's vulnerability to self-injury, and environmental factors may stimulate the initial behavioral incident, nonetheless, the resulting neurochemical rewards may provide the principle sustaining factor.

B. Neuropsychiatric Dimensions of Genetic Disorders: A New Model

Coupling the findings from behavior phenotype research with those from the fields of psychiatric genetics, psychosocial influences, neurodevelopment, and neurology (e.g., functional brain imaging) allows emergence of a new model for examining and understanding the neuropsychiatric aspects of genetic conditions. The resulting conceptual framework seeks to link genetics with brain function, cognition, and ultimately behavior (see Fig. 1) while raising a different set of questions than that driven by previous research findings (see Fig. 2). From this perspective, many previous findings seem superficial, at best, prompting a re-examination of our present understanding of the neuropsychiatric aspects of genetic disorders.

At the heart of this re-examination is an effort to define the altered paths of brain development resulting from specific genetic disturbances (neurodevelopmental variants) and the specific impact of these variants on cognition and behavior. While our present technology allows a more in-depth examination of brain functioning than previously possible, such a specific micro level of analysis is still in the future. Thus, most of our present understanding is anchored at the two endpoints of the model. Those working from the genetics and developmental perspective start with a known genetic disorder and seek to trace the impact of that genetic disorder through to the "behavioral phenotype" (27,28). This work requires identifying both the cardinal characteristics of the disorder (e.g., the hyperphagia associated with Prader–Willi syndrome) along with secondary features, which may be

| Alteration of Genetic Status |
| Abnormalities in Genetic Code for Brain Development |
| Abnormal Mechanisms of Brain Development |
| Structural and Functional Abnormalities of Brain |
| Cognitive and Neurologic Abnormalities |
| Behavioral Syndrome |
| Specific Intervention |

Figure 1 Conceptual framework linking genetics to brain function.

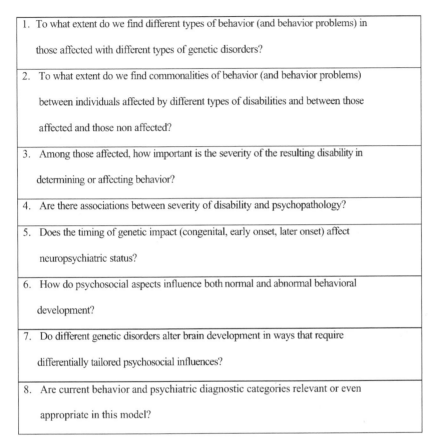

1. To what extent do we find different types of behavior (and behavior problems) in those affected with different types of genetic disorders?

2. To what extent do we find commonalities of behavior (and behavior problems) between individuals affected by different types of disabilities and between those affected and those non affected?

3. Among those affected, how important is the severity of the resulting disability in determining or affecting behavior?

4. Are there associations between severity of disability and psychopathology?

5. Does the timing of genetic impact (congenital, early onset, later onset) affect neuropsychiatric status?

6. How do psychosocial aspects influence both normal and abnormal behavioral development?

7. Do different genetic disorders alter brain development in ways that require differentially tailored psychosocial influences?

8. Are current behavior and psychiatric diagnostic categories relevant or even appropriate in this model?

Figure 2 Questions raised relating genetic factors to brain function.

present in the majority of affected individuals or features that may be shared by other disorders (17). By necessity, the focus is on small numbers of subjects with uncommon (usually single gene) disorders and unusual patterns of deficits (e.g., fragile X, Prader–Willi syndrome, Smith-Magenis syndrome).

By contrast, those working in the behavioral sciences start with a defined neuropsychiatric disorder such as schizophrenia and with the aid of family, adoption, and twin studies combined with quantitative genetic methods work "backward" toward the probable genetic origins (29,30). From this vantage point, evidence for genetic influence has been found for nearly all behavioral disorders that have been investigated including autism, depression, anxiety and panic disorders, language disorders, antisocial personality, eating disorders, and Tourette syndrome (31). However, not all behavioral disorders are influenced to the same degree by genetic factors (32). Recent research suggests that, in addition to overall intelligence, there is also strong genetic influence on specific cognitive dimensions including information processing, electroencephalographic evoked potentials, and cerebral glucose metabolism. Autism and autism spectrum disorders are prototypic of this approach.

C. Autism and Autistic Spectrum Disorders

Autism and autistic spectrum disorders (ASD) constitute a group of behaviorally defined, complex neurodevelopmental disorders with onset prior to the age of 2.5 to 3 years although behavioral symptoms may be evident prior to the age of 1 year. The cardinal features of these disorders include striking deficits in four areas: verbal and nonverbal language, communicative use of language, social interactions, and the range of interests and activities (33). Level of cognitive ability is not a defining feature of autism; however, about two-thirds of persons with a primary diagnosis of autism have cognitive impairments (34). In addition, males are affected more often than females (3:1) (35). Prevalence rates range from 0.02 to 1%, with evidence of a recent and relatively steep increase in occurrence (36,37).

The characteristics of the 11 children first described by Kanner (38) in 1943 are essentially unchanged in today's more sophisticated autistic diagnostic schema; however, not all affected children exhibit all characteristic features. Children who have relatively normal language development, but exhibit deficits of social interaction and range of interests and activities are considered to have Asperger syndrome. Those who exhibit "some" symptoms of autism and are clearly "not normal," or whose symptoms are "atypical" usually are placed into the diagnostic category "Pervasive Developmental

Disorder—Not Otherwise Specified." These disorders are termed "ASD" with an implicit assumption of least to most severe.

Although Kanner's original description attributed etiology to neurobiological origins, until recent family and twin studies documented that autism is both familial and heritable (38), these assertions were largely ignored. The tremendous heterogeneity of behavioral expression along with an apparent complex mode of inheritance suggests that autism most likely results from the action of several genes. Current estimates postulate the involvement of at least two, and perhaps ten or more genes (39). However, not all cases of autism will have the same genetic origin. While many chromosome abnormalities have been reported in autism, three separate chromosomal regions involving chromosomes 2, 7, and 15 are more commonly involved and offer the most consistent candidate sites, although most autistic subjects have normal chromosome study results. In addition, both ASD and specific autistic features (particularly stereotypies) are associated with many other medical, metabolic, or genetic disorders (e.g., fragile X, Rett, tuberous sclerosis, and myotonic dystrophy).

The neuropsychiatric impact of autism is pervasive. In addition to the core language, social, behavioral, and cognitive deficits previously outlined, children with autism frequently present with attention deficits including hyperactivity and impulsivity, tics, sensory and motor deviances, mood disorders, compulsive-sameness oriented-explosive symptom cluster, and SIB (40). Approximately 25–30% of autistic subjects will develop seizures.

All young children with autism and ASD are language impaired, but their language disorders vary. There may be an initial concern that the child with autism is hearing impaired due to an early failure of responsive orientation to sound from parental vocalizations coupled with delays in vocalization. As many as 50% of children with autism fail to develop functional speech (41). While those with the greatest cognitive impairment are least likely to develop speech, cognition is not the only determinative factor. Among those children who do develop speech, the emergence of verbal skills is frequently delayed and may be deviant in form. Echoing, absent or abnormal use of pronouns (e.g., "pick you up" instead of "pick me up") and a lack of inflection with no variation in tone are frequently observed (42). Nonverbal language may also be impaired with an avoidance of eye-contact, a failure to point even when needing to express a need, and oddities of tactile functioning (avoidance of hug, clothing textural preferences, and extreme food dislikes) often impact the ability of the younger child to develop goal directed or effective interactions. Further, difficulties with language are not limited to the expressive realm. Receptive abilities may be delayed and may remain literal and concrete. The progression from "my dog," to "my dog the Labrador retriever," to the more abstract concept of "dogs including labradors, dachshunds, cocker spaniels," to "dogs as an example of a more general concept of animals" may not take place. Instead, dogs may remain "my dog—not my dog," or even the more elementary "dog—not dog."

Social deficits also vary in severity. At the most severe, affected individuals may appear to be both completely unaware of, and unresponsive to, others in the environment. The previously described failure of the younger child to visually or vocally interact is evidence that these deficits are present even in infancy. Those more mildly affected may display problems of social perception (detecting and recognizing social cues, e.g., facial expressions, emotional tone, and body language), social cognition (understanding social and emotional cues and their implications), and social performance (initiating and sustaining appropriate and reciprocal social behavior) (43). A biologically based failure to develop a theory-of-mind or the ability to attribute mental states to oneself and others and to make sense of and predict behavior on the basis of these mental states is one proposed explanation for these abnormalities. The data used to support this theory includes: (1) the majority of children with autism do not show a clear understanding of how physical objects differ from thoughts about objects; (2) do not understand the difference between brain functions (make you move and do things) and mind functions (thinking, dreaming, and wishing); (3) cannot make appearance–reality distinctions, that is to tell the difference between what an object looks like and what they know it really is (e.g., a red candle shaped like an apple), they cannot say "it looks like, but it really is . . . ."; (4) when presented with a mixed list of words, they have difficulty in identifying and using mental-state words (think, know, and pretend) but have no difficulty in identifying physical state words; (5) have a restricted range of spontaneously used mental and emotional state words; (6) fail to develop pretend play; (7) fail to understand when others are "pretending"; (8) are unaware that the eye region of the face may indicate what a person is thinking or what a person wants; (9) cannot make accident–intention distinctions; (10) cannot deceive or understand deceiving such as how to answer "how do I look in this dress"; (11) have extreme difficulty in understanding metaphor, sarcasm, and irony where meaning is inferential rather than literal; and (12) fail to understand and adhere to unwritten rules of speech (e.g., turn-taking). At the same time, most children with autism are unimpaired in logical reasoning about the physical world and are unimpaired at understanding how physical representations work even though they cannot understand mental representations of the same objects. At the theoretical level, it is difficult to distinguish theory-of-mind from language disabilities. In addition, many higher functioning individuals with autism succeed on theory-of-mind test items, yet exhibit the full range of social deficits attendant to autism (44). Similar difficulties are noted for other explanatory theories such as central coherence and executive (dys)function theories.

An emerging research methodology uses film clips varying in the amount and type of social interaction coupled with eye-tracking technology to compare spontaneous viewing patterns of both normal and autistic individuals (45). Those with autism exhibit consistent failures of social monitoring, including focusing on mouths rather than eyes and looking primarily at background physical elements and objects rather than people. These findings suggest that social failures begin at the most basic level of a failure to attend to and detect crucial social and communicative clues leading to an inability to collect usable social information. Since many of the behavioral difficulties seen in children with autism directly result from the core language and social deficits, early diagnosis followed by an intensive intervention program is critical to optimize outcomes for those affected.

III. ASSESSING AND MANAGING NEUROPSYCHIATRIC DYSFUNCTION

It may seem both obvious and simplistic to say that neuropsychiatric assessment starts with an accurate description and history of the presenting problem; however, obtaining that description is far from simple. Reporting bias and imprecise measurement tools that focus on only a small segment of behavior and qualities of the individual impact the accuracy of the data. For instance, many IQ tests fail to detect or account for speech and language deficits. While speech and language deficits can be separately measured, the interplay between speech and language deficits, uneven cognitive abilities, and behavior is more difficult to demonstrate. Moreover, when assessing psychiatric concerns, intellectual and verbal impairments may limit the affected individual's ability to reliably report fears, anxieties, depression, and psychotic symptoms. A diagnosis of an anxiety disorder in a nonverbal individual may require an inferential leap based on interpreting behavior that appears fearful or anxious. Similarly, an individual with a significant cognitive impairment may not be able to describe a delusion in the same way as another individual. Therefore, third party reports are frequently used as diagnostic data. Often these third party reports originate from inadequately compensated, frequently under-educated and -supervised care-giving staff with high rates of turnover, thus compromising the quality of diagnostic behavior observations on which behavioral descriptions and ultimately treatment may be based. At the same time, these reports may not reveal that the caregiver is handling the person in such a way that behaviors are further aggravated. Bias may also occur when there is a failure to recognize an individual's developmental level leading to erroneous labeling of a "developmental age appropriate" behavior as a neuropsychiatric disruption. Further, many of the most problematic behaviors associated with genetic disorders (e.g., SIB) fall outside the usual diagnostic schemas.

A particularly useful framework for both assessment and treatment planning separately considers three factors: predisposing factors, precipitating factors (or environmental antecedents to behavior), and perpetuating factors (25). Viewed this way, even quite severe and at first sight perplexing problems become more amenable to understanding and consequently to treatment and management (14). Predisposing factors are those characteristics that impact the affected person's perception of the environment including genetic status, medical and personal history, severity of cognitive limitations, and the presence and severity of sleep disturbances. Precipitating or antecedent factors are those environmental factors that set the stage for obtaining positive or provoking negative behavioral responses, such as interpersonal environment, environmental change, expectations, level of imposed stress, and types and level of support. Perpetuating and maintaining factors serve to maintain behavioral problems.

A. Predisposing Factors

As we have discussed, genetic status and the accompanying medical concerns provide a substrate that predisposes the affected person to a particular pattern of challenging behaviors. As with nonaffected individuals, personal history shapes perceptions and drive emotional and behavioral reactions to the environment. Sleep quality is an additional factor impacting behavior; poor sleep quality is known to affect mood and behavior, cognitive function and educational performance, family functioning, and even physical development. The extent of sleep disturbance associated with many genetic disorders is only beginning to be appreciated (e.g., Prader–Willi syndrome, Smith–Magenis syndrome). Sleep disturbances are roughly categorized as: sleeplessness leading to insufficient quantity of sleep, excessive day time sleepiness, episodic disturbance of sleep through awakenings, parasomnias (episodic disturbances of sleep including related movement or vision disturbance), and abnormal sleep architecture (timing and depth of sleep). Until recently, routine inquiry regarding sleep issues was not usually included in conventional history taking protocols. However, a number of known causes of sleep disturbance are frequently associated with specific genetic disorders. These include: upper airway obstruction and apnea, disturbed circadian rhythms, medical and psychiatric disturbance, medication effects, underlying central nervous system deviancies, and seizure disorders. Thus, screening for sleep disturbance recently has become a critical part in assessing etiology and treatment for challenging behaviors in this population.

B. Precipitating Factors

One characteristic, which is frequently described in individuals with genetic disorders, is an inability to be flexible or "go with the flow". While most obvious in those with autism, this characteristic of neurological rigidity is common to many disorders. As a result, there is an increased need for structure and routine in daily living. For many, even the simplest disruption of a daily schedule can be sufficiently stressful to precipitate a behavioral outburst. Larger changes such as changes in family structure, a change in living setting, staff changes, and chronic disruption of routine can be extremely stressful, precipitating multiple episodes of behavioral dysregulation. The death of a close family member can create an extended period of grief that may not be recognizable as such to the individual but will be reflected in behavioral disruption over an extended period of time that clearly dates from the point of loss. Frequently, the behavior is exacerbated by staff and other caregivers that hold an expectation that the individual "should be over it by now". Other acute traumas and acute medical conditions may also serve as precipitants. It is important to identify these during an assessment. While it may not be possible to replace the loss, it may provide caregivers and staff with a different understanding of the behavioral cause and allow them to better provide needed supports.

C. Perpetuating Factors

An insensitive or delayed approach to understanding the precipitating factors behind a neuropsychiatric disturbance often results in a suboptimal response to the disturbance which subsequently becomes incorporated as both a precipitating and perpetuating force in the continuation of the disturbance. Thus, continued administration of a medication that has precipitated an abnormal behavioral response clearly perpetuates the unwanted side effect to the consternation of all concerned. Similarly, inappropriate staff responses may further escalate a behavior and lead to further inappropriate staff responses. Often by the time help is sought, these spiraling factors have become self-sustaining, often masking the original precipitants. A careful assessment should be able to identify these factors and incorporate an alteration of these factors into a treatment plan.

D. Treatment

Treatment considerations and planning for neuropsychiatric difficulties in those with genetic disorders parallel that for the general population (46). However, unlike the general population, many affected individuals live and operate in a protective and more restricted environment. As a result, treatment frequently employs environmental alteration and contingency management as a method for change. Such environmental interventions are infrequent and improbable in a nonaffected population. Moreover, this population does not differ in the need for psychotherapy and adjunctive medication support. Historically, however, treatment has been weighted toward environmental interventions and medication with an under-utilization of individual and group psychotherapy. As individuals achieve greater community integration and participation, the needs for more comprehensive treatments including psychotherapy are being recognized.

The promise of an increased understanding of the altered neurological linkages between specific gene disturbance and behavioral outcomes is a basis for designing more effective developmental programming, behavioral support, and intervention strategies for affected individuals. There are, however, inherent pitfalls. Foremost among these is an inadvertent promotion of "a self-fulfilling prophecy." Once a condition is recognized as carrying a predisposition for a set of behaviors, parents and caregivers anticipating emerging problems may inadvertently promote them. A similar danger is the principle of "therapeutic nihilism". This response to the recognition and description of the phenotype uncritically and erroneously accepts that all behaviors are a function of the phenotype and are therefore inevitable, and by implication, not worth treating. It is clear that, among those syndromes with a well-defined behavior phenotype, there remains considerable "within syndrome" variability. Not all affected individuals develop all aspects of the phenotype. On a given dimension such as memory, there exists a range of abilities across individuals; similarly, for a given behavior such as self-injury there exists a range of severity. Furthermore, some behaviors are directly related to the severity of the cognitive impact and the developmental level of the individual rather than the syndrome itself. For example, an imaginary friend in a child of 9 years whose cognitive ability is at the level of a five year old would be considered behavior well within the normal range; the same behavior in an adult whose cognitive ability may be at the level of a 10 year old could signify psychopathology. Thus, having a genetic disorder may increase the risk or predispose an individual toward particular types of problematic behavior but the development of these behaviors is not inevitable, nor is genetics the only influence. Any influence on behavior for those nonaffected is equally likely as an influence on those with genetic disorders. Therefore, a comprehensive asessment must consider a number of factors in addition to the underlying genetic disorder.

REFERENCES

1. Gustavson KH, Harberg B, Harberg G, Sars K. Severe mental retardation in a Swedish county. I. Epidemiology, gestational age, birth weight and associated CNS handicaps in children born in 1959–1970. Acta Paediatr Scand 1977; 66:373–379.

2. Achenbach TM, McConaughy SH, Howell CT. Child/adolescent behavioral and emotional problems: implications of cross-informant correlations for situational specificity. Psychol Bull 1987; 101:213–232.

3. Borthwick-Duffy SA. Epidemiology and prevalence of psychopathology in people with mental retardation. J Consult Clin Psychol 1994; 62:17–27.

4. Steffenburg S, Gilberg C, Steffenburg U. Psychiatric disorders in children and adolescents with mental retardation and active epilepsy. Arch Neurol 1996; 53(9):904–912.

5. Breau LM, Camfield CS, Symons FJ, Bodfish JW, MacKay A, Finley GA, et al. Relation between pain and self-injurious behavior in nonverbal children with severe cognitive impairments. J Pediatr 2003; 142(5):498–503.

6. Einfeld SL, Tonge BJ. Population prevalence of psychopathology in children and adolescents with intellectual disability. II. Epidemiological findings. J Intellect Disabil Res 1996; 40: 99–109.

7. Jacobson JW. Dual diagnosis services: history, progress and perspectives. In: Bouras N, ed. Psychiatric and Behavioral Disorders in Developmental Disabilities and Mental Retardation. Cambridge: Cambridge University Press, 1999:329–358.

8. Voelker R. Putting mental retardation and mental illness on health care professionals' radar screen. JAMA 2002; 288(4): 433–435.

9. Powell MP, Schulte T. Turner syndrome. In: Cecil R, Goldstein S, eds. Handbook of Neurodevelopmental and Genetic Disorders in Children. New York, NY: The Guilford Press, 1999.

10. Rovet J, Buchanan L. Turner syndrome: a cognitive neuroscience approach. Tager-Flusberg H, ed. Neurodevelopmental Disorders. Cambridge, MA: The MIT Press, 1999:223–249.

11. Britto MT, Garrett JM, Dugliss MA, Daeschner CW Jr, Johnson CA, Leigh MW, et al. Risky behavior in teens with cystic fibrosis or sickle cell disease: a multicenter study. Pediatrics 1998; 101(2):250–256.

12. McMahon WM, Carter AS, Fredine N, Pauls DL. Children at familial risk for Tourette's disorder: child and parent diagnoses. Am J Med Genet 2003; 121B:105–111.

13. O'Brien G. The clinical relevance of behavior phenotypes. In: O'Brien G, ed. Behavior Phenotypes in Clinical Practice. Vol. 157. London: Mac Keith Press, 2002:1–12.

14. O'Brien G. Introduction: different disabilities, different behaviours—same management? In: Gillberg C, O'Brien G, eds. Developmental Disability and Behavior. Vol. 149. London: Mac Keith Press, 2000:1–11.

15. Dykens EM. Maladaptive behavior and dual diagnosis in persons with genetic syndromes. In: Burack JA, Hodapp RM, Zigler EF, eds. Handbook of Mental Retardation and Development. Cambridge: Cambridge University Press, 1998:542–562.

16. Tager-Flusberg H. An introduction to research on neurodevelopmental disorders from a cognitive neuroscience perspective. Neurodevelopmental Disorders. Cambridge, MA: The MIT Press, 1999:3–24.

17. Steinhausen HC, Von Gontard A, Spohr A, Hauffa HB, Eiholzer U, Backes M, et al. Behavioral phenotypes in four mental retardation syndromes: fetal alcohol syndrome, Prader–Willi syndrome, fragile X syndrome and tuberosis sclerosis. Am J Med Genet 2002; 111:381–387.

18. Moldavsky M, Lev D, Lerman-Sagie T. Behavioral phenotypes of genetic syndrome: a reference guide for psychiatrists. J Am Acad Child Adolesc Psychiatry 2001; 40(7):749–761.

19. Clarke D. Self-injurious and aggressive behaviors. In: O'Brien G, ed. Behavioural Phenotypes in Clinical Practice. Vol. 157. London: Mac Keith Press, 2002:16–30.

20. Oliver C, Murphy GH, Corbett JA. Self-injurious behavior in people with mental handicap: a total population study. J Ment Defic Res 1987; 31:146–162.

21. Sigafoos J, Elkins K, Kerr M, Attwood T. A survey of aggressive behaviour among a population of persons with intellectual disability in Queensland. J Intellect Disabil Res 1994; 38: 369–381.

22. Griffin JC, Williams DE, Stark MT, Altmeyer BK, Mason M. Self-injurious behavior: a state-wide prevalence survey of the extent and circumstances. Appl Res Ment Retard 1986; 7:105–116.

23. Einfeld SL, Smith A, Durvasula S, Florio T, Tonge BJ. Behavior and emotional disturbance in Prader–Willi syndrome. Am J Med Genet 1999; 82(2):123–127.

24. Deb S. Self-injurious behavior as part of genetic syndromes. Br J Psych 1998; 172(5):385–388.

25. Clarke D. Psychopharmacology of severe self-injury associated with learning disabilities. Br J Psych 1998; 172(5):389–394.

26. Udwin O, Dennis J. Psychological and behavioural phenotype in genetically determined syndrome: a review of research findings. In: Yule W, O'Brien G, eds. Behavioural Phenotypes. Vol. 138. London: MacKeith Press, 1995:90–208.

27. Asherson PJ, Curran S. Approaches to gene mapping in complex disorders and their application in child psychiatry and psychology. Br J Psychiatry 2001; 179:122–128.

28. McGuffin P, Riley B, Plomin R. Toward behavioral genomics. Science 2001; 291(5507):1232–1239.

29. Karayiorgou M, Gogos JA. Dissecting the genetic complexity of schizophrenia. Mol Psychiatry 1997; 2(3):211–223.

30. Brzustowicz LM, Hodgkinson KA, Chow EW, Honer WG, Bassett AS. Location of a major susceptibility locus for familial schizophrenia on chromosome 1q21-q22. Science 2000; 288(5466): 678–682.

31. Plomin R, Owen MJ, McGuffin P. The genetic basis of complex human behaviors. Science 1994; 264:1733–1799.

32. Rutter M. The interplay of nature, nurture, and developmental influences: the challenge ahead for mental health. Arch Gen Psych 2002; 59(11):996–1000.

33. American Psychological Association. Diagnostic and Statistical Manual of Mental Disorders. 4th ed. Washington, DC: American Psychiatric Association, 1994.

34. Smalley SL, Asarow RF, Spence MA. Autism and genetics. A decade of research. Arch Gen Psychiatry 1988; 45(10):953–961.

35. Howlin P, Asgharian A. The diagnosis of autism and Asperger syndrome: findings from a survey of 770 families. Dev Med Child Neurol 1999; 41:834–839.

36. Hillman RE, Kanafani N, Takahaski TN, Miles JH. Prevalence of autism in Missouri: changing trends and the effect of a comprehensive state autism project. Missouri Med 2000; 97(5): 159–163.

37. Fombonne E. The epidemiology of autism: a review. Psychol Med 1999; 29:769–786.

38. Kanner L. Autistic disturbances of affective contact. Nerv Child 1943; 2:217–250.

39. Santangelo SL, Folstein SE. Autism: a genetic perspective. In: Tager-Flusberg H, ed. Neurodevelopmental Disorders. Cambridge, MA: The MIT Press, 1999:431–447.

40. Cuccaro ML, Shao Y, Bass MP, Abramson RK, Ravan SA, Wright HH, et al. Behavioral comparisons in autistic individuals from multiplex and singleton families. J Autism Dev Disord 2003; 33(1):87–91.

41. Hellings JA. Treatment of comorbid disorders in autism: which regimens are effective and for whom? MedGenmed 2000; 2(1) available at http//www.medscape.com/viewarticle/430507.

42. Lord C, Rutter M. Autism and pervasive developmental disorders. In: Rutter M, Taylor E, Hersov L, eds. Child and Adolescent Psychiatry: Modern Approaches. 3rd ed. Oxford: Blackwell, 1994:569–591.

43. Lord C, Paul R. Language and communication in autism. In: Cohen DJ, Volkmar FR, eds. Handbook of Autism and

Pervasive Developmental Disorders. 2nd ed. New York: Wiley, 1997:195–225.

44. Constantino JN, Pryzbeck T, Friesen D, Todd RD. Reciprocal social behavior in children with and without pervasive developmental disorder. J Dev Behav Pediatr 2000; 21:2–11.

45. Klin A, Volkmar FR. Autism and other pervasive developmental disorders. In: Goldstein S, Reynolds CR, eds. Handbook of Neurodevelopmental and Genetic Disorders in Children. New York: The Guilford Press, 1999:247–274.

46. Klin A, Jones W, Schultz R, Volkmar F, Cohen D. Visual fixation patterns during viewing of naturalistic social situations as predictors of social competence in individuals with autism. Arch Gen Psychiatry 2002; 59(9):809–816.

21

Behavioral Genetics and Developmental Disabilities

STEPHEN A. PETRILL

Department of Biobehavioral Health,
The Pennsylvania State University,
University Park, Pennsylvania, U.S.A.

I. INTRODUCTION

While some instances of developmental disabilities are isolated cases within families, many other developmental disabilities display a familial pattern of transmission. Children with mild mental impairment have been shown to have siblings with general intelligence scores significantly below the average of the population, near the 26th percentile (1). Similarly, quarter of first-degree relatives of children with communication disorders also report communication disorders (2). Siblings and parents of children with reading disabilities have been shown to perform significantly more poorly on measures of reading than parents and siblings of nonreading-disabled children (3).

What is the etiology of the familial aggregation of general cognitive, communication, and reading disorders? The purpose of this chapter is to examine the genetic and environmental etiology of developmental disabilities from a behavioral genetic perspective. Specifically, the chapter will first present the assumptions and methods of the behavioral genetic approach. Next, the behavioral genetic literature concerning general cognitive deficits, communication disorders, and reading disability will be discussed. The chapter will then discuss the implications of these results, not only for our understanding of developmental disabilities, but also for our understanding of the environments associated with these developmental disabilities.

II. THE BEHAVIORAL GENETIC APPROACH

A. Assumptions

Behavioral genetic approaches examining developmental disabilities hinge on two key assumptions. First, the approach assumes that most developmental disabilities are *dimensional* as opposed to categorical. Taking general cognitive ability, for example, mild mental impairment is defined as a cognitive ability score falling below the first standard deviation. However, these individuals are selected by virtue of falling on the lower tail of the larger population distribution of general cognitive ability. Similarly, communication disorders and reading disorders are thought to represent the lower tail of communication and reading ability. Of course, there are cases where developmental disabilities are outside of this normal distribution, in many cases through the result of a major gene or chromosomal abnormality (such as Down's syndrome) or a severe form of environmental deprivation or insult (such as severe environmental neglect or closed head injury). While these kinds of developmental disabilities are important and merit intensive study, it is also the case that many instances of developmental disability arise through no identifiable genetic or environmental cause. These kinds of cases may represent the lower end of a continuum of ability.

A second assumption is that the continuum of ability in general cognitive ability, communication ability, and reading can rise though either major genetic or major environmental mechanisms or through the result of many genes and environments of small effect size that operate as probabilistic risk and protective factors. Major genetic or chromosomal abnormality-based mechanisms have been found for many forms of mental retardation (e.g. Fragile X, Prader–Willi Syndrome) as discussed elsewhere in this volume. In these cases, the gene or chromosomal abnormality is both necessary and sufficient for the disorder. However, in the case of late-onset-dementia and reading disability, for example, quantitative trait loci have been found that are much smaller in effect size (4). These genetic mechanisms are neither necessary nor sufficient to cause these disorders, and operate in concert with other, yet undiscovered, genes and environments in a complex, nonlinear system. In this case, a large number of genetic and environmental differences are operating in a group of individuals that lead to differences in a particular outcome. As depicted in Fig. 1, the total variance in a measured outcome is influenced by normally distributed differences in genetic and environmental factors. In other words, what make people different from one another are differences in their genetic and environmental backgrounds. Behavioral genetic approaches are designed to quantify the relative importance of these normally distributed genetic and environmental influences.

What is particularly powerful about the behavioral genetic approach is that it allows one to empirically test the veracity of these assumptions. If developmental disabilities of unknown etiology represent a different population than unselected cognitive, communication, and reading ability, then we should see some discontinuity in their genetic and environmental etiology. If this is the case, then we have not yet discovered other genes or environmental markers that are related to disability. In contrast, if developmental disabilities

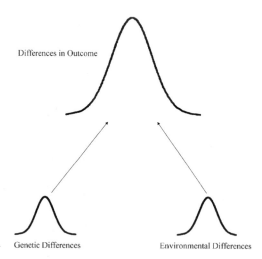

Figure 1 Genetic and environmental influences on measured outcomes.

of unknown etiology represent the lower tail of the distribution of ability, then we should see continuity between the genetic and environmental influences in developmental disability as well as in the unselected population. In this case, we have not yet identified other genetic and environmental markers that are related to ability, both at the high end, average, and low end.

B. Behavioral Genetic Methods

So, how do behavioral genetic studies examine this issue? Behavioral genetic approaches accomplish this quantification by comparing the resemblance of family members that differ in their genetic relatedness. For example, identical twins share 100% of the same genes while fraternal twins share 50% on average. Biological parents share 50% of their additive genes with their children while adoptive parents share 0% of the same genes with their adoptive children. If identical twins are no more similar to one another on a particular outcome than fraternal twins, or adoptive children are as similar to their adoptive parents as biological children are related to their biological parents, then there is strong evidence for a shared family environmental influence on that outcome. What makes family members similar is assumed to be some set of environmental influences that are shared by family members. If, on the other hand, identical twins are more similar to each other than fraternal twins, or biologically related family members are more similar to one another than adoptive family members, then genetic influences are assumed. Finally, identical twins, although identical genetically, are not identical in their outcome measures. These differences are presumably due to some nonshared environmental experiences, as well as due to measurement error. What is important is that these genetic and environmental influences can coexist with one another. The question is not *whether* nature or nurture influence developmental disabilities, but *how* nature and nurture together result in developmental disability.

When studying the behavioral genetic etiology of disability, what one is most interested in is examining why a group of children selected for low cognitive, language, or reading ability possess a mean level of functioning that is different from the unselected population. Using reading disability as an example, Fig. 2 depicts the means of a group of identical and fraternal twins, called probands, selected below a certain cutoff on a measure of reading. These groups may or may not have identical proband means. Thus, one always tests whether identical and fraternal proband means are significantly different. Once this step has been completed, the means of the cotwins (the other siblings) of the proband twins are examined. If there is no familial relationship, then we would expect the mean of the cotwins to be equal to the unselected sample mean. To the extent that there is familial resemblance, then the cotwin means should be closer to the cutoff. If genetic similarity among twins is influencing similarity in reading disability, then the identical cotwins should regress less to the population mean than the fraternal cotwins.

This method, called the DeFries–Fulker regression method (5,6), provides three important statistics, group

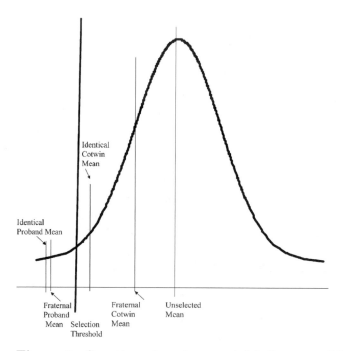

Figure 2   Genetic and environmental influences of disability.

heritability (h^2g), group shared environment (c^2g), and group nonshared environment (e^2g). Group heritability refers to the proportion of the mean difference between a selected group and the unselected population that is due to genetic differences between the groups. Group shared environment and group nonshared environment refer to the proportion of the mean difference between the developmental disability and unselected groups due to shared and nonshared environmental differences, respectively.

This DeFries–Fulker approach can also be used to investigate whether the magnitude of genetic and environmental influences in developmental disability are similar to those found in the unselected population. For example, one can compare the h^2g of reading disability to the h^2 of unselected reading ability. If the results are similar, we can conclude that the genetic environmental influence processes underlying developmental disability are the same as those in the unselected population. These results suggest continuity between developmental disability and the unselected population. If the results for developmental disability groups are different, then we conclude that there are genetic and/environmental influences that are unique to developmental disability. These results suggest discontinuity between developmental disability and the unselected population.

III. BEHAVIORAL GENETIC FINDINGS

What is striking about the behavioral genetic data is that the results vary as a function of the developmental disability that is studied. These findings will be discussed, in turn, along with an examination of the longitudinal course and relationships among different developmental disabilities.

A. Mild Mental Impairment

In unselected samples, the genetic influences on general cognitive ability increase from 30% in infancy, to 50% in early childhood, to 80% in adulthood, and declining to 70% in old age (see Ref. 7). Several studies have examined the genetic and environmental influences on mild mental impairment in early childhood (8,9), adulthood (10), and old age (11) as presented in Table 1. Studies in infancy suggest that the genetic influences on mild mental impairment may be greater than in the unselected sample, suggesting discontinuity. In adulthood, studies suggest continuity between low general cognitive ability and the unselected sample. The group heritability of low cognitive ability (selected no higher than the 10 percentile across all studies listed above) is consistent with what one would expect in the unselected sample in these ages. In the oldest-old, the h^2g of low general cognitive ability was $h^2g = 0.00$ in a sample of 351 pairs of twins 80 years of age or older (11). This discontinuity in the very old, assuming it is not sample-specific, may be due to the heterogeneity of low general cognitive ability in a gerontological sample of this kind (stable low ability, subclinical dementia, and terminal drop).

Table 1 Group Heritability (h2g) Estimates in Studies of Mild
Mental Impairment

Study	Sample age	h2g
Petrill et al. (8)	14 months	0.55
	20 months	0.75[a]
	24 months	0.65[a]
	36 months	0.25
Saudino et al. (10)	65.6 years (average)	0.77[a]
		0.82[a] (replication[b])
Petrill et al. (11)	80[b]years	0.00

[a]*Note*: $p < 0.05$.
[b]*Note*: The replication study involved a second assessment where 52% of the twins
were in both groups.

Longitudinal genetic studies of general cognitive ability
have been largely confined to early childhood. In this case,
the proband twin is selected at one age and their cotwin's
score is examined at a later age. These studies suggest that
while there is moderate correlation between cognitive skills
at different ages, the extent to which they do correlate is
due largely to genetic influences. In other words, stability in
low cognitive ability groups is largely due to genetics.
Instability in low cognitive ability groups is due to the
nonshared environment, and error (8).

B. Communication Disorders

There are four types of communication disorders described in
DSM-IV. These are communication disorders, expressive language (verbalizing thoughts), mixed receptive (understanding
others' spoken language), expressive language disorder, and
phonologic (articulation) and stuttering (speech interrupted
by repeated or prolonged sounds, syllables, or words (see Ref.
12). These subtypes of communication problems are comorbid
and behavioral genetic studies suggest that expressive and
receptive disorders share a common genetic etiology, but different genetic factors appear to be operating between articulation
disorders and other communication problems (13).

Currently, there are about one dozen studies that have examined communication disorders and language from a quantitative perspective (see Ref. 14, for a review). Some of the most intriguing research has emerged from a large population-based twin study in infancy and early childhood based in the United Kingdom. This study, called the Twins Early Development Study (TEDS), involves a representative sample of around 10,000 pairs of twins born in 1994, 1995, and 1996 in England and Wales (see Ref. 15). All children are screened at ages 2, 3, and 4 using parental rating instruments for language delay, cognitive delay, and behavioral problems. At age 4, 400 families with twins who demonstrate language or cognitive delays and 300 control twins. These 700 twin pairs were tested in their homes using standardized measures. In addition to the results on mild mental impairment described above (9), this study has also examined communication disorders. The results of this study suggest that vocabulary delay in 2- and 3-year-olds is strongly influenced by genetic factors ($h^2g = 0.73$), and has a higher heritability than the normal range of vocabulary ability (16). Similar results were found when examining the same sample at 4 years of age (17).

More importantly, TEDS has begun to examine the longitudinal course of communication delays as well as the relationship between communication delays and cognitive delays. In a series of papers, Eley et al.(18,19) suggested that not only are verbal delays highly heritable, but that they are more heritable than nonverbal delays and general cognitive delays. Similar to the result found for general cognitive delays, the stability of verbal delays in early childhood, especially persistent language delays, was due largely to genetic influences while instability was due to the nonshared environment (and error) (20).

C. Reading Disability

Another important behavioral genetic investigation of developmental disabilities has involved the study of reading disability. Reading disability not only accounts for 80% of all

children with a diagnosed learning disorder, but also it affects
10% of all children (12). A seminal set of studies has emerged
from the Colorado Learning Disabilities Research Center (see
Ref. 21 for a review). This study has involved a set of families
ascertained from 27 school districts across the state of Colorado. Twin pairs are selected where at least one pair has a
school history of reading problems. These twins are then
assessed on an extensive battery of psychometric and experimental measures. A control group of twin pairs where neither
pair has a history of reading problems is also assessed using
the same battery. The current sample consists of approximately 1031 twin pairs, 618 pairs selected for reading disability, and 413 control twin pairs.

Gayan and Olson (22) presented univariate and bivariate
analyses of reading disability across several measures of
orthography, phonology, and fluency. The results of this study
suggested that roughly half of the mean difference between
reading-disabled twins and the unselected population was
due to genetics. This study also suggested that shared family
environment was also important to reading disability as well.
Bivariate analyses suggested that not only the comorbidity
between different kinds of reading deficits (e.g. orthographic,
phonological, etc.) is due largely to genetic influences but also
due in part to the shared environment. These results are
largely consistent with studies of reading in unselected
samples, which suggest moderate genetic influences and some
evidence for the shared environment (23,24).

IV. CONCLUSIONS

Taken together, these studies present a complex picture of
the genetics and environment of developmental disabilities.
On one hand, the heritability of disability, particularly
with respect to general cognitive disability in childhood,
adolescence, and adulthood, as well as reading disability
appears to be of the same magnitude as the genetic influences
found in the unselected range of ability for general cognitive
ability and reading. In contrast, the magnitude of genetic

influences appears to be greater for general cognitive disability and communication disorders in early child. Finally, the magnitude of genetic influences is lower in old age for general cognitive ability. Thus, it appears that the genetic continuity of disability varies not only as a function of the outcome, but also as a function of the age of the sample. This picture is complicated by the comorbidity between language and cognitive ability and the likely comorbidity between these outcomes and reading disability.

There are several important conclusions that one can draw from these data. First, behavioral genetic studies of developmental disability suggest that genes operate as risk factors, not as determinants of outcomes. Even in those cases where the h^2g is higher or lower in the disability group than in the unselected sample, these genes, although perhaps somewhat different genes than in the unselected sample, are still likely to be of small effect size working probabilistically. Second, given the degree of comorbidity and the degree of genetic overlap among different subtypes of developmental disability, it is likely that particular kinds of disabilities do not occur in genetic isolation from one another. Thus, it should not be surprising to find DNA markers that are common across different kinds of developmental disability, as well as between developmental disability and attention/behavior problems.

Another important implication involves gene–environment (GE) processes. Because of the high heritability of developmental disabilities, it is likely that many "environmental" measures associated with developmental disability may be a substantial genetic component (see Ref. 25 for a more general discussion). In other words, because developmental disabilities possess a genetic component, the probability of experiencing environments associated with developmental disability may, in part, be a function of the genes associated with developmental disability.

Several theoretical models have been developed to explain the ways in which genes and environments can correlate with one another. Scarr and McCartney (26) described three types of GE correlation. *Passive* GE correlation is found when a child is provided an environment that is correlated with parents' (and hence, the child's) genes. An example of passive GE correlation is number of books in the home (25). Parents with more education and higher cognitive performance scores provide more books for their children. Their biologically related children are not only exposed to more books, but are also provided with some of the parents' genes that are contributing to higher cognitive test performance scores. Thus, a passive GE correlation exists between child cognitive outcomes and the number of books in the home. *Evocative* GE correlation is a second type, and is found when an environment is provided to an individual by others as a reaction to his or her genetically influenced behavior. For example, parents might provide books to their children to read as a function of a child's interest or skill in reading, which in turn, could operate in part as a function of genetic variance in reading ability (27).

Finally, *active* GE correlation occurs when a child seeks out environments based upon his or her genetically influenced characteristics. Scarr and McCartney (26) proposed that these effects become increasingly salient over the course of development as children gain more control over situations and experiences that are more likely to be compatible with their genetically influenced characteristics. In the case of developmental disabilities, it may be that those with poorer reading, communication, or cognitive skills seek out less enriching environments. Additionally, as children move through school they may become increasingly able to select the environments that are associated with their outcomes.

This leads us to perhaps the most important point—that the presence of genetic influences on developmental disabilities does not relegate the environment to a secondary role. The environment is important. However, what is also important is understanding why children with developmental disabilities experience certain environments. In some cases, these are completely independent from genes. In this case, it is possible that these environments operate in a manner similar to major genes and QTLs. Namely, some environmental influences will have profound effects while others are likely to be small in effect size, especially when examining environmental influences across the range of ability. In other cases, the probability of coming into contact with an environment will be influenced by the GE processes described above. If genes are important to developmental disabilities, then genetically sensitive designs are essential to the systematic study of how genes and environments work together in developmental outcomes.

REFERENCES

1. Nichols PL. Familial mental retardation. Behav Genet 1984; 14: 161–170.

2. Felsenfeld S. Nature and nurture during middle childhood. In: DeFries JC, Plomin R, Fulker DW, eds. Nature and Nurture During Middle Childhood. Oxford: Blackwell, 1994:102–119.

3. DeFries JC, Vogler GGP, LaBuda MC. Colorado family reading study: an overview. In: Fuller JL, Simmel EC, eds. Perspectives in Behavior Genetics. Hillsdale, NJ: Erlbaum, 1986:29–56.

4. Plomin R. Genetics, genes, genomics, and g. Mol Psychiatry 2003; 8:1–5.

5. Defries JC, Fulker DW. Multiple regression analysis of twin data. Behav Genet 1985; 15:467–473.

6. DeFries JC, Fulker DW. Etiology of deviant scores versus individual differences. Acta Genetica Med Gemellol Twin Res 1988; 37:205–216.

7. Petrill SA. The case for general intelligence: a behavioral genetic perspective. In: Sternberg R, Grigorenko E, eds. The General Factor of Intelligence: How General is It? Mahwah, NJ: Erlbaum, 2002; 281–298.

8. Petrill SA, Saudino KJ, Cherny SS, Emde RN, Hewitt JK, Fulker DW, Plomin R. Exploring the genetic etiology of low general cognitive ability from 14 to 36 months. Dev Psychol 1997; 33(3):544–548.

9. Spinath FM, Harlaar N, Ronald A, Plomin R. Substantial genetic influence on mild mental impairment in early childhood. Amer J Mental Retardation 2004; 109(1):34–43.

10. Saudino KJ, Plomin R, Pedersen NJ, McClearn GE. The etiology of high and low cognitive ability during the second half of the life span. Intelligence 1994; 19:359–371.

11. Petrill SA, Johansson B, Pedersen NL, Berg S, Plomin R, Ahern F, McClearn GE. Low cognitive functioning in non-demented 80+ year old twins is not heritable. Intelligence 2001; 29:75–83.

12. Plomin R. Genetic factors contributing to learning and language delays and disabilities. Child Adolescent Psychiatric Clinics North America 2001; 10:259–277.

13. Bishop DVM, North T, Donlan C. Genetic basis of specific language impairment: evidence from a twin study. Dev Med Child Neurol 1995; 15:184–187.

14. Stromswold K. The heritability of language: a review and metaanalysis of twin, adoption, and linkage studies. Language 2001; 77:647–723.

15. Trouton A, Spinath FM, Plomin R. Twins early development study (TEDS): a multivariate longitudinal genetic investigation of language, cognition, and behavior problems in childhood. Twin Res 2002; 5:444–448.

16. Dale PS, Simonoff E, Bishop DVM, Eley TC, Oliver B, Price TS, Purcell S, Stevenson J, Plomin R. Genetic influence on language delay in two-year-old children. Nature Neurosci 1998; 1:324–328.

17. Viding E, Spinath FM, Price TS, Bishop DVM, Dale PS, Plomin R. Genetic and environmental influence on language impairment in 4-year-old same-sex and opposite-sex twins. J Child Psychol Psychiatry 2004; 45(2):315–325.

18. Eley TC, Bishop DVM, Dale PS, Oliver B, Petrill SA, Price TS, Purcell S, Saudino KJ, Simonoff E, Stevenson J, Plomin R. Genetic and environmental origins of verbal and performance components of cognitive delay in 2-year-olds. Dev Psychol 1999; 35:1122–1131.

19. Eley TC, Dale PS, Bishop DVM, Price TS, Plomin R. Longitudinal analysis of genetic and environmental components of cognitive delay in preschoolers. J Educational Psychol 2001; 93:698–707.

20. Bishop DVM, Price TS, Dale PS, Plomin R. Outcomes of early language delay: II etiology of transient and persistent language difficulties. J Speech Language Hearing Res 2003; 46:561–575.

21. DeFries JC, Alarcon M. Genetics of specific reading disability. Mental Retardation Dev Disabilities Res Rev 1996; 2:39–47.

22. Gayan J, Olson RK. Genetic and environmental influences on orthographic and phonological skills in children with reading disabilities. Dev Neuropsychol 2001; 20(2):483–507.

23. Byrne B, Delaland C, Fielding-Barnsley R, Quain P, Samuelsson S, Hoien T, Corley R, DeFries JC, Wadsworth S, Willcutt E, Olson RK. Longitudinal twin study of early reading development in three countries: preliminary results. Ann Dyslexia 2002; 52:49–73.

24. Wadsworth SJ, Corley RP, Hewitt JW, DeFries JC. Stability of genetic and environment influences on reading performance at 7, 12, and 16 years in the Colorado Adoption Project. Behav Genet 2001; 31(4):353–359.

25. Plomin R, Bergeman CS. The nature of nurture: genetic influence on "environmental" measures. Behav Brain Sci 1991; 14: 373–427.

26. Scarr S, McCartney K. How people make their own environments: a theory of genotype-environment effects. Child Dev 1983; 54:424–435.

27. Scarborough HS. (1991). Antecedents to reading disability: preschool language development and literacy experiences of children from dyslexic families. Reading and Writing 1991; 3: 219–233.

22

Attention Deficit–Hyperactivity Disorder

MARK L. WOLRAICH and MELISSA A. DOFFING

University of Oklahoma Health Sciences Center,
Child Study Center, Oklahoma City,
Oklahoma, U.S.A.

I. INTRODUCTION

The Diagnostic and Statistical Manual of Mental Disorders, fourth edition (DSM-IV) defines attention deficit–hyperactivity disorder (ADHD) as "a persistent pattern of inattention and/or hyperactivity–impulsivity that is more frequent and severe than is typically observed in individuals at a comparable level of development." Therefore, it is a developmental disorder of inattention and/or hyperactivity–impulsivity, meaning children with the disorder may have difficulty filtering external stimuli, inhibiting motor impulses, anticipating events, and adjusting behavior based on feedback about misconduct.

Contrary to the popular media perspective, ADHD is not a new disorder but has had multiple name changes from hyperkinetic impulse disorder (1), to minimal brain dysfunction (2), to attention deficit disorder with and without hyperactivity (3) before now becoming ADHD. Attention deficit–hyperactivity disorder has been studied extensively, beginning in the early 1900s. However, the diagnosis remains controversial. This is due in part because the common behavioral and academic problems associated with children affected with ADHD may have several underlying causes. The symptoms may arise for several reasons: true ADHD, a condition that mimics ADHD, ADHD complicated by a condition that commonly occurs with ADHD, or normal activity for the child's age. Best practice guidelines for diagnosis and treatment of ADHD published by experts in pediatrics (4,5) and mental health (6) are now available to physicians. Greater uniformity in the diagnosis, treatment, and management processes may help reduce some of the existing controversy about caring for these children with such a complicated symptom complex. This chapter discusses the history of the diagnosis, etiology, prevalence, prognosis, current guidelines for evaluation and diagnosis, and available treatments.

II. HISTORICAL PERSPECTIVE OF ADHD

A German physician, Heinrich Hoffmann, first described the symptoms associated with ADHD in the literature in 1848 (7). His stories of the behaviors of Fidgety Phil and Johnny Head-In-Air provide evidence that the symptoms of ADHD have been puzzling parents and health care providers for many years. Attention deficit–hyperactivity disorder is the most common behavior disorder in children (8,9), yet it has also been one of the most difficult conditions to define. The diagnostic criteria for ADHD have undergone many changes over the years.

The primary focus of the disorder in 1902 was on conduct. Children who displayed symptoms associated with

ADHD were believed to have a "deficit in moral control" (10). Still (10) proposed the patterns of restlessness, inattentiveness, and overaroused behaviors were the result of the child's inability to internalize rules and limits. He suggested that the children had likely experienced brain damage but that the behavior could also arise from hereditary and environmental factors (10).

The connection to brain damage was given more consideration after the 1917 worldwide influenza epidemic with encephalitis, where some children exhibited the residual symptoms of restlessness, inattention, impulsivity, easy arousability, and hyperactivity (11,12). Soon after in 1937, stimulant medication (Benzedrine) was found to improve the behaviors of children displaying these core symptoms (13). Methylphenidate was released for treatment in 1957 (1). Clements (2) described the disorder as a neurological condition suspected of being caused by brain damage and called minimal brain dysfunction.

Evidence of brain damage was difficult to identify in most of the children manifesting the behaviors of ADHD; therefore, the name and focus of the disorder switched to more behaviorally descriptive terms best categorized by the psychiatric classification system (3,14–16). Classification in DSM-II focused on hyperactivity (14) and was called the hyperkinetic reaction of childhood disorder. In 1980, in DSM-III, the focus shifted to inattention (3) because of research by Dr. Douglas and her colleagues (17,18) that identified inattention as the more significant component of the disorder. The diagnosis included the deployment of three dimensions (inattention, impulsivity, and hyperactivity) and two subtypes (attention deficit disorder with and without hyperactivity). This was followed by DSM-IIIR (15), which retained the focus on inattention, impulsivity, and hyperactivity, but eliminated all dimensions and subtypes. Most recently, in the DSM-IV (16), subtypes were reinstituted (the predominantly inattentive, the predominantly hyperactive–impulsive, and the combined type) defining two dimensions (inattention and hyperactivity–impulsivity). DSM-IV also added the requirement of dysfunction in more than one setting, further emphasizing the need for information from multiple sources.

III. ETIOLOGY

A unitary cause of ADHD has not been identified. Roughly 20% of children who have ADHD also have a diagnosis that can be associated with an organic etiology (see Table 1). Attention deficit–hyperactivity disorder is a heterogeneous disorder with multifactorial etiologies. The most common cause has been genetic transmission. Research has not consistently shown food allergies, too much television, poor home life, poor parenting, or poor schools to cause ADHD. However, these issues may exacerbate ADHD symptoms and impairment.

Evidence for a genetic link has been provided by studies involving adoption, twins, siblings, and parents. Twin studies show a heritability of 0.75 (75% of the variance in phenotype can be attributed to genetic factors). If the child has an identical twin, the twin has a greater than 50% chance of developing ADHD (19) and first degree relatives of individuals with ADHD have a greater risk than controls (20–22). Adoptive relatives of children with ADHD are less likely to have the disorder (23,24).

Neuroimaging, neuropharmacology, and neurophysiology studies have raised some possible biological basis for

Table 1 Diagnoses that May Predispose a Child to Develop Attention Deficit–Hyperactivity Disorder

---

Prenatal alcohol/drug use
Prematurity
Low birth weight
Birth complications
Central nervous system infections
Central nervous system trauma
Genetic disorders
  Klinefelter syndrome
  Turner syndrome
  Fragile X syndrome
  Williams syndrome
  Neurofibromatosis type I
  Inborn errors of metabolism
Tourette syndrome

ADHD. Magnetic resonance imaging (MRI) and positron emission tomography (PET) studies have demonstrated a reduced size of the basal ganglia, cerebellar vermis, and frontal lobes in ADHD subjects versus controls. The following areas are thought to regulate attention: (1) the basal ganglia helps inhibit automatic responses, (2) the vermis is thought to regulate motivation, and (3) the prefrontal cortex helps one filter out distractions (19,25,26). A recent longitudinal study found persistent decreases in overall brain volume in all regions reflected in smaller cerebellar and total cerebral volumes (27), and these differences were the same whether or not the individuals had been treated with stimulant medications. Functional studies such as positron emission tomography, single photon emission computed tomography (SPECT), and functional magnetic resonance imaging (fMRI) have shown striatal hypoperfusion in individuals with ADHD compared to control individuals. These advances in research are not yet of clinical utility because of the wide variation of size and function in both individuals with and without ADHD such that the degree of overlap makes any of the assessments inaccurate for individual clinical evaluation.

On a neurotransmitter level, it is clear that the functions relate to the dopamine and norepinephrine systems in the same areas of the brain identified by anatomical studies (28–30). Specific gene associations have been identified in a portion of individuals with ADHD. These include the dopamine transporter gene (DAT1), the D4 receptor gene (DRD4), and the human thyroid receptor-β gene (31–34). Dopamine can inhibit or intensify the activity of other neurons. If the dopamine transporter gene is affected, the transporter can recycle dopamine before it has a chance to bind to the dopamine receptor. If the dopamine receptor gene is affected, the receptor can become less sensitive to dopamine. Because the behaviors related to ADHD are also improved by medications primarily affecting the norepinergic system, this system has also been implicated in behaviors characteristic of ADHD (35,36). The marker genes currently explain only a small number of individuals with ADHD.

Insults and traumatic injuries to the brain can also result in the behaviors characteristic of ADHD. There is a higher incidence of ADHD as well as learning disabilities among children who are born premature (37). Exposures in utero, particularly to alcohol, cause ADHD symptomatology that in its severe form is manifested in fetal alcohol syndrome. Exposures such as to lead or infections such as meningitis in young children can also result in similar behavioral symptoms (38).

IV. PREVALENCE

Researchers have noted the symptoms of ADHD in every nation and culture studied (39). Prevalence estimates for ADHD vary depending on the diagnostic criteria used, the population studied, and the number of sources required to make the diagnosis (40). The prevalence, reported in the DSM-IV, is 3–5% of school-aged children. It is important to note that this prevalence rate is based on studies utilizing criteria prior to that of DSM-IV. The male to female ratio varies crossculturally from 1:1 to 10:1. The difference may be explained in part because males tend to exhibit more hyperactive and impulsive behaviors and are more aggressive, leading to earlier referral because of behavioral problems. Females display more internalizing behaviors (inattentive subtype) and if diagnosed, are diagnosed later with academic difficulties.

Determining the true prevalence of ADHD is a challenging task. Because of this challenge, it has been a main source of controversy in the popular press. Many are concerned that too many children are being diagnosed as having ADHD and being treated with stimulant medication. Two features of the disorder are major contributors to the challenge. First, the diagnosis is dependent on the presence of specific behaviors that are observed and reported by the child's caregivers. Since no specific biologic markers (lab tests or image studies) exist, the diagnosis must rely on the subjective judgment of those caregivers. Second, there is no clear demarcation between appropriate behavior and inappropriate behavior. Unlike schizophrenia where a child may have hallucinations, the behaviors in ADHD are not atypical until the frequency of the behaviors is abnormally high. The judgments are subjective because no clear normative criteria are present about what frequency of any given behavior is normal for any given age not like the assessment of intelligence where there are clear normative guidelines for what tasks can be accomplished at what age. Therefore, the behaviors follow a more normal distribution and a defined cut point has to be set in establishing diagnostic criteria.

The changes in diagnostic criteria over time have further complicated the process of determining the true prevalence of ADHD. The most recent change from only one subtype in DSM-IIIR to three subtypes in DSM-IV is likely to increase the prevalence rates (41,42). Besides the challenges in making accurate diagnosis, studies of prevalence rates are dependent on the sample studied. The rates are different when one examines a mental health clinic-referred sample versus a primary care sample versus a community/school sample.

Given the challenges, it is not surprising that there are varying rates. The prevalence has ranged from 4% to 12% (median 5.8%). Rates are higher in community samples (10.3%) compared with school samples (6.9%) and higher in males (9.2%) than females (3.0%) (40). As with other neurodevelopmental disorders, ADHD is more common in males and has ratios of 5–1 for predominately hyperactive/impulsive type and 2–1 for predominately inattentive type (41,42).

V. PROGNOSIS

It was once thought that children grew out of ADHD. It is now known that 70–80% of children who have ADHD will continue to experience difficulties through adolescence and adulthood (43). The symptom presentation usually changes through a child's lifetime (see Table 2). In summary, over time hyperactive core symptoms decrease, however, inattentive symptoms persist. Some children may learn to adapt by building on their strengths to minimize their impairment. The

Table 2 Attention Deficit–Hyperactivity Disorder: Symptoms and Presentation

Life stage	Symptoms	Possible presentation
Preschool child	Hyperactivity	Motoric hyperactivity
	Impulsivity	Aggressiveness
Elementary school child	Inattention	Underachievement
	Distractibility	Lack of motivation
	Frustration	Class clown
	Boredom	Difficulty following class rules
	Poor social skills	
Older school-aged child	Poor organizational skills	Difficulty completing homework assignments
Teenager/college age student	Difficulty learning from mistakes	Increased social problems
Adults		Trouble with long-term projects
		Car accidents
		Trouble juggling demand of marriage/family and work
		Trouble interacting with colleagues
		Difficulty keeping a job
		Difficulty managing money

majority continue to struggle, with their impairment presenting in different ways. The ultimate outcome is dependent on the severity of the symptoms, presence (or absence) of coexisting conditions, social circumstances, intelligence, socioeconomic status, and treatment history (43). Some negative outcomes have been associated with adolescents and adults with ADHD. Adolescents with ADHD have higher rates of school failure, motor accidents, substance abuse, and encounters with law officials; adults with ADHD may achieve lower socioeconomic status and have more marital problems (41).

VI. CURRENT GUIDELINES FOR EVALUATION AND DIAGNOSIS

Despite extensive research into the disorder, there is no single test to diagnose ADHD. An evaluation for ADHD is indicated if a caregiver, teacher, or physician expresses concern that symptoms of inattention, hyperactivity, or impulsivity are causing significant impairment in a child's academic, psychological, or social performance. Many other diagnoses may present with similar symptoms or be present along with ADHD (Table 3). It is important to do a thorough evaluation and consider these issues. The correct diagnosis will determine the course of treatment, guide treatment monitoring, link treatment to prognosis, and determine if special educational services or treatment for coexisting diagnoses are required.

Reviewing the child's behavior, academic, psychosocial, developmental, birth, medical, and family history, looking for signs and symptoms of other disorders instead of, or in addition to, ADHD is essential to making the correct diagnosis. Laboratory evaluation is unnecessary unless indicated by history. It is essential to gather information from the primary care givers, teachers, and the child. This information comes in various forms, direct interviews, behavior rating scales, medical records, school grades, and previous testing results including psychoeducational testing. Where possible, it is also helpful to obtain information from other observers, such as coaches, scout leaders, and grandparents. Thorough medical

Table 3 Differential Diagnosis for Attention Deficit–
Hyperactivity Disorder

Developmental disorder	Medical	Psychosocial
Learning disability	Anemia	Adjustment disorder
Mental retardation	Lead intoxication	Mood disorder
Pervasive developmental	Medications	Depression
disorder	Asthma	Manic depression
	Antiepileptic	Psychotic disorder
	Allergy	Anxiety
	Seizure disorder	Substance abuse disorder
	Sensory deficits	
	Hearing	
	Vision	
	Sleep apnea	
	Substance abuse	
	Thyroid disease	

and neurological exams are warranted. Direct observations of a child's behavior in the classroom can provide some of the most objective information if it is available, but it is labor intensive and therefore has to be limited to small samples of time (16,44). Observations in the physician's office are frequently not useful because they do not correlate well with the child's behavior in the classroom. The environment of the physician's office is usually novel, which in some children may create more anxiety and worsen symptoms but for other children the same situation may improve their behavior.

To ensure the most accurate diagnosis, the evaluation should include assessing for the specific criteria as listed in the DSM-IV (16). The criteria include the inappropriately often occurrence of at least six of nine core behaviors in at least one of the two dimensions of inattention or hyperactivity–impulsivity. These core behaviors are presented in Table 4. Not only must the requisite number of core symptoms be present, they must be developmentally inappropriate for the child's age and they must cause significant impairment in the child's academic and psychosocial performance. Other criteria include the following: symptoms must be present for at

Table 4 DSM-IC Core Behaviors for Attention Deficit–
Hyperactivity Disorder

Inattention dimension
  Careless mistakes
  Difficulty sustaining attention
  Seems not to listen
  Fails to finish tasks
  Difficulty organizing
  Avoids tasks requiring sustained attention
  Loses things
  Easily distracted
  Forgetful
Hyperactivity–Impulsivity Dimension
Hyperactivity
  Fidgeting
  Unable to stay seated
  Moving excessively (restless)
  Difficulty engaging in leisure activities quietly
  "On the go"
  Talking excessively
Impulsivity
  Blurting answers before questions completed
  Difficulty awaiting turn
  Interrupting/intruding upon others
To be considered as having the symptoms in each dimension, a child must
  display the "often" occurrence of at least six to nine of the dimension's
  behaviors. They must be:
  (1) Inappropriately "often" for the development level of the child
  (2) Onset before 7 years of age
  (3) Present for at least 6 months
  (4) Present in two or more settings (e.g., home, school, or work)
  (5) Evidence for significant clinical impairment in social, academic, or
      occupational functioning

least 6 months, the symptoms need to have started before the age of 7 years, and the symptoms must not be the result of another mental disorder. The individual must have impairment in more than one setting due to the core behaviors. The DSM-IV criteria define three subtypes of ADHD: primarily inattentive type (at least six of nine inattentive core symptoms present), primarily hyperactive–impulsive type (at least six of nine hyperactive–impulsive symptoms present), and combined type (at least six of nine inattentive and at least six of nine hyperactive–impulsive symptoms present).

Possible presentations of ADHD throughout one's life-cycle are listed in Table 2. The degree of functional impairment will indicate whether an affected individual will require medication management as a teenager and ultimately as an adult. The information concerning core symptomatology and impairment are best obtained directly from multiple sources. Parents and teachers are usually the best resources. Direct interviews and rating scales are frequently used. It is important to include all 18 core ADHD symptoms in the information gathered from home and school, and using rating scales is an effective way this can be accomplished. Children behave differently in different environments. This fact may lead to discrepancies between parent, teacher, and physician observations and should not be surprising. The varying environments are why it is important to have information about the child in multiple settings when making the diagnosis.

The requirement of the age of 7 years is included to reflect the biologic basis for the condition starting in childhood. The exact age is not necessarily based on strong empirical evidence, and there is some debate that some children with the inattentive subtype may not present until an older age, when they have a greater need to be able to concentrate. The requirement for at least 6 months duration reflects the chronic nature of the condition. The most important aspect of the diagnosis is the concept that the core symptoms impair the patient's ability to function. There are individuals who have many of the core symptoms, but because of their strengths (such as above average intelligence), they are able to compensate well enough to prevent the symptoms from causing significant dysfunction.

Research indicates 50% or more children with ADHD will have a comorbid condition accompanying the ADHD symptoms. One extensive review shows the following percentages for some of the most common comorbid disorders: 35% oppositional defiant disorder, 25% conduct disorder, 18% depression, 26% anxiety disorder, and 12% learning disorders (40). Other common comorbid disorders are: mood disorder, substance use disorder, tic/Tourette disorder, developmental co-ordination disorder, motor dysfunction, language disorder, and sleep disorder. Young children most commonly have complications such as developmental co-ordination disorder, reading and writing problems, or tic disorder, whereas older children and adults may have comorbid symptomatology related to depression, substance abuse disorder, and antisocial disorder. Therefore, an important aspect of evaluating a child for ADHD includes assessing for possible comorbid conditions. Family history, social history, direct interview, rating scales, physical exam, and neurological exam will aid in identifying coexisting conditions.

VII. TREATMENTS

Treating ADHD requires communication and commitment from the clinicians, parents, educators, and the child. As for any chronic illness, education of the child and his family is the first step in treatment. It is important the child, family, and teacher gain an understanding about the condition and can clarify many misconceptions raised in the popular press. Accepting ADHD as a chronic condition, a child has from birth and is not caused by a "bad child" or "bad parenting," helps the team focus on ways to deal with improving impairments instead of focusing on negative performances. Each child may present with different impairments and thus require different interventions. The clinician should be able to provide information to the child, family, and teacher about the current knowledge of the diagnostic process, etiology, treatment, medications, parenting techniques, teaching tips, social skills, learning issues, and how these affect the child growing up with ADHD, the family members living with a child with ADHD, and the classroom with a child with ADHD. This information can be provided through a variety of resources, including trained staff, handouts, suggested reading lists, internet web sites, local and national support groups, and community programs such as parent training classes. Understanding ADHD and the impact it has on a child's life at home, school, and in leisure activities is the first step in providing a way to cope with the condition and one step closer to helping minimize impairment so a child may reach his or her full potential. Educated families are better able to work as partners with clinician in maintaining an effective treatment program. When a family is invested in the treatment plan, there is an increased chance of adherence to the regimen (6). This investment requires educating the family about their options and taking their opinions and lifestyle into account.

Stimulant medications are one of the two first line evidence-based treatments used for ADHD with selective norepinephrine reuptake inhibitors, antidepressants, and antihypertensives as second-line treatments. The primary medical management is stimulant medication. Stimulants (dextroamphetamine, methylphenidate, mixed salts of amphetamine, and pemoline) have been the most extensively studied and are considered the first line of medicine management for ADHD because of both their efficacy and safety (45). There have been over 300 studies with 6000 subjects demonstrating their short-term efficacy (46). The initial stimulant is likely to be effective in about 70% of children with 80–90% if more than one is tried. The medications often offer immediate and dramatic improvement to a child's symptom complex. The benefits while taking stimulants are well documented and include reducing the core symptoms of ADHD as well as improving behavior, academic productivity and accuracy, parent–child interaction and aggression, they do not improve cognitive abilities or academic skills. These improvements do not remain once the medication is discontinued. Evidence from the National Institute of Mental Health (NIMH) multimodal therapy of ADHD supports efficacy for at least 24 months (47), but longer term studies that are less well designed provide equivocal results (43).

Side effects of medications are usually mild and can be controlled by modifying the dose and distribution time (see Table 5). It is not usually necessary to discontinue the medication due to side effects. A list of stimulant medication is given in Table 5 with dosage information (pemoline, a stimulant used for ADHD in the past, is known to cause liver toxicity in rare cases and is now prescribed infrequently). Unlike most medications in children, stimulant effectiveness is not based on an mg/kg basis. Current recommendations are to start at the lowest dose possible and titrate up based on information gathered from parents and teachers about medication effectiveness.

Initial medication titration can be accomplished in weekly intervals by phone or office visit. Screening for side effects, and attainment of target goals gives the best measurement of medication effectiveness. Once the best dose is determined (the dose where the child is having maximum success in achieving target goals and having the fewest side effects), monitoring can be stretched to monthly and ultimately quarterly office visits. However, with each monthly refill request, it is helpful to check on adherence, impairment, and side effects. Second-line medications include selective norepinephrine reuptake inhibitors (atomoxetine), antidepressants (imipramine and desipramine), alpha adrenergics (clonidine and guanfacine), and buproprion. Adequate studies to evaluate the use of such medications for ADHD are considerably more limited than the information available on stimulant medications and the potential side effects can be more serious. Atomoxetine is a selective norepinephrine reuptake inhibitor. Phase 3 trials demonstrated promising effects. The side effects include appetite suppression, drowsiness, and nausea. The tricyclic antidepressants (imipramine and desipramine) have strong evidence of efficacy but have more significant side effects with dry mouth and possible cardiac arrhythmias and have a fairly narrow margin of safety. The antihypertensive medications, while appearing to work clinically, have very limited rigorous evidence of efficacy and the evidence is also limited for buproprion.

Behavioral therapy can be another important component to managing ADHD. Behavior modification is the most frequently employed psychosocial intervention, and the one with the strongest scientific evidence for its efficacy. Techniques shown to be effective involve contingency reinforcement, including token economies, time outs, and earning or losing

Table 5 Medications for Treating Attention Deficit–Hyperactivity Disorder

Medication	Brand name	Starting dosage recommendations	Dosing intervals	Onset	Duration (hr)	Maximum dose
Stimulants						
Mixed salts of amphetamine	Adderall	2.5–5 mg	QD–BID	20–60 min	6	40 mg
Dextroamphetamine	Dexedrine/Dextrostat	2.5 mg	BID–TID	20–60 min	4–6	40 mg
	Dexedrine Spansule	5 mg	QD–BID	60+ min	6+	40 mg
Methylphenidate	Concerta™	18 mg	QD	20–60 min	12	54 mg
	Methylin™	5 mg	BID–TID	20–60 min	3–5	60 mg
	Methylin™ SR	20 mg	QD–BID	1–3 hr	2–6	60 mg
	Ritalin®	5 mg	BID–TID	20–60 min	3–5	60 mg
	Ritalin-SR®	20 mg	QD–BID	1–3 hr	2–6	60 mg
	Metadate ER®	10 mg	QD		6–8	60 mg
Selective norepinephrine reuptake inhibitor (atomoxetine)	Strattera	0.5 mg/kg increasing to 1.2–1.4 mg/kg	QD	Initial effects are usually seen by the end of the first week		
Antidepressants						
Tricyclics (require baseline ECG)	Imipramine	50 mg	TID			5 mg\kg\day
	Desipramine	2 mg\kg\day	BID–TID			
Burpropion	Wellbutrin	50 mg	BID–TID	4 weeks		100 mg
	Wellbutrin SR	100 mg	QD–TID			150 mg
α-Adrenergic agonist	Clonidine	0.05 mg	QD–TID	0.3		

privileges (48). Social skills therapy tries to address the deficit that many children with ADHD have in social situations, but because of the difficulty that the children have in generalizing what they learn, there is limited evidence for its efficacy unless the training takes place in actual situations with other children. Family therapy may be helpful, particularly on issues such as sibling relationships, but the evidence for its efficacy is weak. Play and cognitive therapy have not been found to be efficacious treatments for children with ADHD (48).

Children with ADHD can receive services from their public schools based on the Rehabilitation Act (Section 504) for milder cases and the Individuals with Disabilities Education Act (IDEA) for more severe cases (49). Section 504 encourages accommodations to be provided for the child when necessary. These modifications could include preferential seating, reduced assignments, clear–direct rules, and a classroom behavioral program. The IDEA applies for children whose impairment significantly affects their academic performance or who have a learning disability and thus qualify for special education services. Examples of other services that may be needed include occupational therapy, physical therapy, speech therapy, assistive technology, and individual therapy. The school and parents should determine the extent and type of services needed and list them in the child's individualized education plan (IEP). A daily report card can also be used effectively in the school setting as an additional type of behavioral therapy as well as a useful method for monitoring medication effects. Two to three specific goals for home and school are selected and an appropriate reward system is created to help parents and teachers provide feedback to the child concerning his/her behavior. Daily report cards help establish daily communication between teachers and parents as well as provide an excellent mechanism to monitor therapy goals and medication management.

Some families may be uncomfortable beginning treatment with stimulants and prefer to use behavioral methods first. However, often they will not be sufficient alone to bring the functioning of a child with ADHD to a normal range (50). Parent satisfaction is usually high when behavioral therapy is used and combining both stimulant medications and behavioral intervention can lower the dose of medication required to reach optimal treatment outcomes (51). Therefore, a multimodal approach is frequently the best choice of treatment.

There are several options of treatments that have been recommended for patients with ADHD, such as broad groups of diets, dietary supplements, alternative medications, exercises, and biofeedback. The three main diets recommended have been the Feingold diet, the oligoantigenic or elimination diet, and a restricted sugar diet. The Feingold diet was proposed by an allergist, Ben Feingold, Ph.D., who suggested that some children with ADHD have allergic-type reaction to certain dietary elements (additives, preservatives, food dyes, and salicylate compounds) (52). Although his clinical impression was that a number of children with hyperactivity had this problem, subsequent blinded studies found very few children responded adversely when challenged with dyes or additives (around 1% of the children studied) (53). Additionally, strict adherence to this diet can provide inadequate vitamin C. Current recommendations have dropped the natural salicylate restrictions so that the low vitamin C should no longer be a problem.

The oligoantigenic or elimination diets are similar to the Feingold diet in that they propose that some children may have adverse reactions to specific foods and dietary ingredients. The diet restricts additives, dyes, and preservatives, but it also initially limits the patient's diet to two meats, two vegetables, two fruits, and two carbohydrates. If the child responds positively after several weeks, other foods are gradually reintroduced, one at a time, in order to determine which foods adversely affect the patient's behavior. About five studies have examined this intervention with blinding and controlled conditions and although some effects were demonstrated, methodological weaknesses, such as problems with blinding in the studies, preclude making a definitive conclusion about its efficacy (54).

Sugar was first believed to adversely affect behavior based on several studies finding an association between worse behavior and increased sugar intake. Those discussing sugar have usually referred to refined and added sugars as the offending agents (usually sucrose or fructose). However, findings from 23 rigorous studies showed no association between sugar and behavior (55). The main side effect of trying to modify sugar intake is the difficulty in having the children comply so that pursuing compliance usually increases the parent–child conflicts.

The dietary supplements recommended for treating children with ADHD include essential fatty acids (linoleic and linolenic acids), megavitamins, zinc, antioxidants, and herbs. There is no clear evidence that these supplements benefit the children, and it is not known if there is any physical risk (56). Megavitamins consist of large quantities (at least 10 times the recommended daily allowance) of most vitamins. There is no clear evidence for their efficacy, and there is a physical side effect of elevated liver function tests (57,58). Zinc has been recommended for treatment based on the finding that some patients have zinc deficiency, and herbal compounds (chamomile, kava hops, lemon balm, valerian root, and passionflower) because of their sedative properties. Again, these treatments have not been studied rigorously. Antioxidants (melatonin, *Ginkgo biloba*, and Pycnogenol®) have also been recommended; however, there have been no scientific studies of their effects on patients with ADHD and their potential side effects are unknown (56). Antifungal therapy based on the hypothesis that children treated on multiple occasions with broad-spectrum antibiotics, such as for otitis media, have alterations in their intestinal flora that make them susceptible to the growth of *Candida* and the absorption of *Candida* toxins that produce behavioral disturbances. Children are treated with antifungal agents (nystatin or ketonazole) and eliminating sugar and foods made with molds and yeast from the diet (56). No studies have been completed to assess efficacy. Some nootropic medications are cerebral metabolic enhancers (piracetam and dimethylaminoethanol) and have been recommended for use with patients with ADHD without rigorous studies of their efficacy (56).

EEG biofeedback works on the premise that the EEG brain wave pattern reflects the behavior of individuals, thus if you change their EEG pattern with the suppression of the theta activity and enhancement of β-wave production, their behavior will change. Individuals can be trained to control these activities. Sensory integration, developed by Jean Ayres, M.D., is based on the theory that improvement in the ability to integrate the senses improves the ability to behave and pay attention. It consists of exercises to improve the integration of the senses. Neither EEG biofeedback nor sensory integration has support from randomized controlled trials that demonstrate their efficacy (59).

VIII. CONCLUSIONS

It is important to understand that ADHD is a complex chronic illness for which there is no cure. However, there are treatments available that have scientific support that symptoms can be effectively managed. Ongoing management is required to minimize the extent of impairment. Although there is no curative treatment, this does not mean the condition will be life long. In order to treat ADHD effectively, one must understand how it can impact children, families, schools, and communities. Children with ADHD must overcome many challenges in order to succeed. Every child should be given a chance to reach his or her maximum potential. Many people with this condition have learned to build on their strengths and become successful adults.

REFERENCES

1. Laufer M, Denhoff E. Hyperkinetic behavior syndrome in children. J Pediatr 1957; 50:463–474.

2. Clements SD. Minimal Brain Dysfunction in Children: Terminology and Identification. Washington, DC: U.S. Department of Health, Education, and Welfare, 1966.

3. American Psychiatric Association. Diagnostic and Statistical Manual for Mental Disorders. 3rd ed. Washington, DC: APA, 1980.

4. American Academy of Pediatrics. Clinical practice guideline: diagnosis and evaluation of the child with attention-deficit/ hyperactivity disorder. Pediatrics 2000; 105:1158–1170.

5. American Academy of Pediatrics. Clinical practice guideline: treatment of the school-aged child with attention-deficit/ hyperactivity disorder. Pediatrics 2001; 108:1033–1044.

6. Pliszka SR, Greenhill LL, Crimson ML. The Texas children's medication algorithm project: Report of the Texas Consensus Conference Panel on medication treatment of childhood attention-deficit/hyperactivity disorder. J Am Acad Child Adolesc Psychiatry 2000; 39:920–927.

7. Hoffman H. Der Struwewelpeter. Frankfurt, Germany: Literarische Anstalt von Rütten und Löning, 1848:11–15.

8. Olfson M. Diagnosing mental disorders in office-based pediatric practice. J Dev Behav Pediatr 1992; 13:363–365.

9. Shaywitz BA, Shaywitz SE. Attention deficit disorder: current perspectives. In: Kavanagh JF, Truss TJ, eds. Learning Disabilities: Proceedings of the National Conference. Parkton, MD: York Press, 1988:369–523.

10. Still GF. The Coulstonian lectures on some abnormal physical conditions in children. Lancet 1902; 1:1008–1012.

11. Hohman LB. Post-encephalitic behavior disorder in children. Johns Hopkins Hosp Bull 1922; 33:372–375.

12. Ebaugh FG. Neuropsychiatric sequelae of acute epidemic encephalitis in children. Am J Dis Child 1923; 25:89–97.

13. Bradley C. The behavior of children receiving benzedrine. Am J Psychiatry 1937; 94:577–585.

14. American Psychiatric Association. Diagnostic and Statistical Manual for Mental Disorders. 2nd ed. Washington, DC: APA, 1967.

15. American Psychiatric Association. Diagnostic and Statistical Manual of Mental Disorders. 3rd ed., revised. Washington, DC: APA, 1987.

16. American Psychiatric Association. Diagnostic and Statistical Manual of Mental Disorders. 4th ed. Washington, DC: APA, 1994.

17. Douglas VI. Differences between normal and hyperkinetic children. In: Conners C, ed. Clinical Use of Stimulant Drugs in Children. Amsterdam: Excerpta Med, 1974:12–23.

18. Douglas VI, Peters KG. Toward a clearer definition of the attention deficit of hyperactive children. In: Hale G, Lewis M, eds. Attention and the Development of Cognitive Skills. New York: Plenum Press, 1979.

19. Barkley RA. Attention-deficit hyperactivity disorder. Sci Am 1998; 279:66–71.

20. Biederman J, Farone SV, Keenan K, Knee D, Tsuang MT. Family-genetic and psychosocial risk factors in DSM-III attention deficit disorder. J Am Acad Child Adolesc Psychiatry 1990; 29:526–533.

21. Morrison JR, Stewart MA. A family study of the hyperactive child syndrome. Biol Psychiatry 1971; 3:189–195.

22. Cantwell DP. Psychiatric illness in the families of hyperactive children. Arch Gen Psychiatry 1972; 27:414–417.

23. Alberts-Corush J, Firestone P, Goodman JT. Attention and impulsivity characteristics of the biological and adoptive parents of hyperactive and normal control children. Am J Orthopsychiatry 1986; 56:413–423.

24. Morrison JR, Stewart MA. The psychiatric status of the legal families of adopted hyperactive children. Arch Gen Psychiatry 1973; 28:888–891.

25. Zametkin AJ, Ernest M. Problems in the management of attention-deficit–hyperactivity. N Engl J Med 1990:40–46.

26. Shaywitz BA, Fletcher JM, Pugh KR, Klorman R, Shaywitz SE. Progress in imaging attention deficit hyperactivity disorder. Ment Retard Dev Disabil Res Rev 1999; 5:185–190.

27. Castellanos FX, Lee P, Sharp W. Developmental trajectories of brain volume abnormalities in children and adolescents with attention-deficit/hyperactivity disorder. J Am Med Assoc 2002; 288:1740–1748.

28. Aylward EH, Reiss AL, Reader MJ, Singer HS, Brown JE, Denckla MB. Basal ganglia volumes in children with attention

deficit–hyperactivity disorder with normal controls. J Child Neurol 1996; 11:112–115.

29. Castellanos FX, Giedd JN, Marsh WL. Quantitative brain magnetic resonance imaging in attention deficit–hyperactivity disorder. Arch Gen Psychiatry 1996; 53:607–616.

30. Filipek PA, Semrud-Clikeman M, Steinggard RJ, Renshaw PF, Kennedy DN, Biederman J. Volumetric MRI analysis comparing subjects having attention deficit–hyperactivity disorder with normal controls. Neurology 1997; 48:589–601.

31. Hauser P, Zametkin AJ, Martinez P. Attention deficit–hyperactivity disorder in people with generalized resistance to thyroid hormone. N Engl J Med 1993; 328:992–1001.

32. Cook EH Jr, Stein MA, Krasowski MD. Association of attention deficit disorder and the dopamine transporter gene. Am J Hum Genet 1995; 56:993–998.

33. Gill M, Daly G, Heron S, Hawi Z, Fitzgerald M. Confirmation of an association between attention deficit–hyperactivity disorder and a dopamine transporter polymorphism. Mol Psychiatry 1997; 2:311–313.

34. Swanson JM, Sunohara GA, Kennedy JL. Association of the dopamine receptor D4 (DRD4) gene with a refined phenotype of attention deficit–hyperactivity disorder (ADHD): a family-based approach. Mol Psychiatry 1998; 3:38–41.

35. Pliszka S, McCracken JT, Maas J. Catecholamines in attention-deficit hyperactivity disorder: current perspectives. J Am Acad Child Adolesc Psychiatry 1996; 35:264–272.

36. Michelson D, Allen A, Busner J. Once-daily atomoxetine treatment for children and adolescents with attention deficit hyperactivity disorder: a randomized, placebo-controlled study. Am J Psychiatry 2002; 159:1896–1901.

37. Goldson E. Developmental consequences of prematurity. In: Wolraich M, ed. Disorders of Development and Learning. Hamilton, Ont.: BC Decker, 2003:345–360.

38. Tuthill RW. Hair lead levels related to children's classroom attention-deficit disorder. Arch Environ Health 1996; 51:214–220.

39.   Scahill L, Schwab-Stone M. Epidemiology of ADHD in school-age children. Child Adolesc Psychiatr Clin N Am 2000; 9: 541–555.

40.   Brown RT, Freeman WS, Perrin JM. Prevalence and assessment of attention-deficit/hyperactivity disorder in primary care settings. Pediatrics 2001; 107:e43.

41.   Baumgaertel A, Wolraich ML, Dietrich M. Comparison of diagnostic criteria for attention deficit disorders in a German elementary school sample. J Am Acad Child Adolesc Psychiatry 1995; 34:629–638.

42.   Wolraich ML, Hannah JN, Pinnock TY, Baumgaertel A, Brown J. Comparison of diagnostic criteria for attention deficit hyperactivity disorder in a countywide sample. J Am Acad Child Adolesc Psychiatry 1996; 35:319–323.

43.   Ingram S, Hechtman L, Morgenstern G. Outcome issues in ADHD: adolescent and adult long-term outcome. Ment Retard Dev Disabil Res Rev 1999; 5:243–250.

44.   Perrin JM, Stein MT, Amler RW. Diagnosis and evaluation of the child with attention-deficit/hyperactivity disorder. Pediatrics 2000; 105:1158–1170.

45.   Perrin JM, Stein MT, Amler RW. Clinical practice guideline: treatment of the school-aged child with attention-deficit/hyperactivity disorder. Pediatrics 2001; 108:1033–1044.

46.   Wigal T, Swanson JM, Regino R. Stimulant medications for the treatment of ADHD: efficacy and limitations. Ment Retard Dev Disabil Res Rev 1999; 5:215–224.

47.   Arnold LE, Jensen P, Hechtman L, Hoagwood K, Greenhill L, for the MTA Cooperative Group. Do the MTA treatment effects persist? New follow-up at 24 months. Proceedings of the Annual Meeting of the American Academy of Child and Adolescent Psychiatry, New York, Oct 2000.

48.   Pelham WEJ, Wheeler T, Chronis A. Empirically supported psycho-social treatments for attention deficit hyperactivity disorder. J Clin Child Psychol 1998; 27:190–205.

49.   Davila RR, Williams ML, MacDonald JT. Memorandum on clarification of policy to address the needs of children with attention deficit disorders within general and/or special education. In:

Parker HC, ed. The ADD Hyperactivity Handbook for Schools. Plantation, FL: Impact Publications Inc., 1991: 261–268.

50. Jensen PS, Hinshaw SP, Swanson JM. Findings from the NIMH multimodal treatment study of ADHD (MTA): implications and applications for primary care providers. J Dev Behav Pediatr 2001; 22:60–73.

51. Pelham W, Gnagy E, Greiner A. Behavioral versus behavioral and pharmacological treatment in ADHD children attending a summer treatment program. J Abnorm Child Psychol 2000; 28:507–525.

52. Feingold B. Why Your Child is Hyperactive. New York: Random House, 1975.

53. Wender EH. The food additive-free diet in the treatment of behavior disorders: a review. J Dev Behav Pediatr 1986; 7:35–42.

54. Wolraich ML. Attention deficit hyperactivity disorder: current diagnosis and treatment, Oct 28, 2000. Available at: http://www.medscape.com/Medscape/CNO/2000/AAP/public/Conference.cfm?conference_id=84.

55. Wolraich ML, Wilson DB, White JW. The effect of sugar on behavior or cognition in children: a meta-analysis. J Am Med Assoc 1995; 274:1617–1621.

56. Baumgaertel A. Alternative and controversial treatments for attention-deficit/hyperactivity disorder. Pediatr Clin N Am 1999; 46:977–992.

57. Arnold LE. Megavitamins for MBD: a placebo-controlled study. J Am Med Assoc 1978; 20:24.

58. Haslam R, Dalby J, Rademaker A. Effects of megavitamin therapy on children with attention deficit disorders. Pediatrics 1984; 74:103–111.

59. Goldstein S, Goldstein M. Managing Attention Deficit Hyperactivity Disorder in Children: A Guide for Practitioners. 2nd ed. New York: John Wiley & Sons Inc., 1998.

23

Cerebral Palsy

BURRIS DUNCAN

Department of Pediatrics, University of
Arizona College of Medicine, Tucson,
Arizona, U.S.A.

I. INTRODUCTION

Cerebral palsy (CP) is a movement disorder or a deficit in motor function due to a nonprogressive insult to the central nervous system (CNS) that occurs at a time when the brain is in a rapid state of development. Since the CNS insult does not change over time, CP is classified as a static encephalopathy: however, the peripheral effects of the nerve damage do change and progress over time. The insult to the CNS may be due to a wide range of different problems that include, but are not limited to, intrauterine or neonatal infections, exposure to toxins such as maternal use of illicit drugs, hypoxic episodes at the time of birth or shortly thereafter, trauma, genetic and metabolic abnormalities. It is estimated that approximately 70–80% of these insults occur prenatally and prematurity is the most frequent antecedent cause of CP. Prematurity predisposes the infant to hypoxic–ischemic encephalopathy, intraventricular hemorrhage, and periventricular leukomalacia, each of which has been associated with the occurrence of CP. The improved survival rate for low and very low birth weight infants is associated with an increase in the rate of CP in these two populations.

The neurological manifestations of CP are divided into five different types and characterized by the degree of muscle tone and/or the movement disorder: spastic (increased tone), dyskinetic (an involuntary uncontrolled movement disorder), ataxic, mixed, and hypotonic (abnormally low tone and relatively uncommon). Cerebral palsy is further classified according to the muscle groups involved: quadriplegia (all four extremities are affected), triplegia (three extremities are affected), diplegia (two lower extremities are most affected), monoplegia (one extremity is affected), and hemiplegia (one side of the body is affected).

II. PREVALENCE

Cerebral palsy is the most frequent cause of childhood disability with incidence rates of 2–2.5 per 1000 live births in most developed countries and with variable rates in developing countries dependent on the availability of prenatal services and level of medical practices (1). In the United States, the prevalence in children under 10 years of age is 2.2/1000 and in children between 10 and 17 years of age is 1.2/1000 with a greater prevalence in boys (2.0/1000) than girls (1.5/1000) (2,3).

III. ETIOLOGY

The etiology of CP is multifactorial. The CNS insult may occur at any time antenatally, during the birth process, immediately postnatally, or within the first two or three years of life. An increased incidence of CP is associated with antenatal problems such as genetic abnormalities, abnormal brain development or neuronal migrational problems, intrauterine viral infections, and intrauterine exposure to maternal infections, including infection of fetal membranes, urinary tract infection, and sepsis. A history of birth asphyxia is found in < 10% of children with CP. There is a significant increase in children with CP, who were born prematurely and particularly in newborns weighing < 1000 g. Naulty et al. (4) found a near threefold greater prevalence of CP in these very low birth weight infants. This is a reflection of the vulnerability of the periventricular white matter to relative hypoxia. Neurons that innervate the muscles of the lower extremities wrap closely around the lateral ventricles and are damaged when oxygen levels decline. The result is spastic diplegia, the most common form of CP. Forty-three percent of the low birth weight infants had evidence of brain injury including intraventricular hemorrhage (4). Postnatal problems or conditions that are associated with an increase in the incidence of CP include neonatal meningitis or encephalitis, sepsis, and head trauma. Unfortunately, nonaccidental trauma or child abuse is responsible for CP in a number of children. This problem may be seen with normal newborns but more often is seen in children who were born prematurely or who were born with a disability and are living in a home where the parents are unable to cope (5–7).

IV. CLINICAL PRESENTATION AND EVALUATIONS

The clinical manifestations of CP are diverse and quite variable in their severity. An infant's delay in reaching motor milestones or abnormalities in gross motor function such as increase in tone or abnormal positioning might suggest a diagnosis of CP in the first few months of life. Some of these infants will catch up on their milestones and will normalize their muscle tone with time and should not carry the label of CP. This is especially true with the premature infant who is often a bit developmentally delayed and may also show an increase in muscle tone. Many neurologists will therefore reserve the diagnosis of CP in the questionable infant or toddler until the child is a bit older, and it is obvious that the delay in motor milestones is persistent and the increased tone will not dissipate. The accuracy of the diagnosis of CP can be improved not only by assessing the degree of movement, but also by evaluating the quality of movement and including an assessment of the age when the primitive reflexes are still present and when they disappear. Other less specific signs and symptoms include irritability, a poor or weak cry, inability to suck well, a persistent head lag, cortical thumbs, scissoring, and a lack of interest in their surroundings. The increase in motor tone in the lower extremities leads to an inability to fully abduct the thighs and in toe walking. Crawling is abnormal and is usually a commando crawl where the infant pulls the legs along rather than getting on all fours. Spasticity may be found in isolated muscle groups and is often associated with exaggerated deep tendon reflexes, clonus, and up-going toes or a positive Babinski.

Each of the different types of CP corresponds to an insult in a different area of the CNS (Table 1). The spastic form occurs in ~75% of children with CP. This variety results when the neurological insult involves the pyramidal area of the brain and often the periventricular white matter. Dyskinetic CP is present in approximately 10–15% of children with CP and occurs when the insult involves the extrapyramidal areas. Dyskinetic CP is further subdivided into three different patterns of abnormal movement: athetoid, choreoathetoid,

Table 1 Classification of CP

Types of CP	Percentage	Areas of brain
Spastic	75	Pyramidal areas
Dyskinetic	10–15	Extrapyramidal areas
Athetoid		
Choreoathetoid		
Dystonia		
Ataxic	< 10	Cerebellum
Mixed		Any or all of the above areas

and dystonic. A smaller percent of children have ataxic CP that is secondary to a lesion in the cerebellum and is characterized by an unsteady gait or inability to reach and touch with precision. Some children with CP have a mixture of the above in which insults involve both the pyramidal and the extrapyramidal areas of the CNS.

The severity of CP is based on the ability to ambulate (8). This classification system varies from Level I (able to walk without assistance, but advanced gross motor skills are limited) to Level V (severely limited mobility even with the use of assistive technology) (Table 2). Approximately 75% of children with CP are classified as Level I, II, or III. The vast majority of children who do not sit unaided by 2 years of age or who do not walk by age 7 will typically never walk.

Laboratory tests that are often of value in the evaluation of CP include a head CT scan or MRI and might show dilated ventricles indicative of poor brain growth or atrophy and periventricular leukomalacia. If the arms are completely spared, imaging of the cervical cord and spine is indicated to rule out a cord lesion. If the cause is suspected to be a metabolic disorder, a genetic evaluation should be undertaken. A variety of appropriate tests to assess the myriad of associated findings or comorbidities are mandatory to insure that they are discovered early and treatments instigated. Of special

Table 2 Functional Levels of CP

Level	Ability to ambulate
I	Walks without restrictions; limitations in more advanced gross motor skills
II	Walks without assistant devices; limitations in walking outdoors and in the community
III	Walks with assistive mobility devices; limitations in walking outdoors and in the community
IV	Self-mobility with limitations; children are transported or use power mobility outdoors in the community
V	Self-mobility is severely limited even with the use of assistive technology

concern are evaluations of sensory function such as hearing and vision. Problems are frequently found in these areas, and treatments must be started early to insure that the child's potential is not further compromised.

There are several functional tests that have been standardized, and some of these are specific for the child with CP. For example, the Peabody Developmental Motor Scales (PDMS) was developed in 1983 (9) and is divided into a fine and a gross motor part and is widely used by physical and occupational therapists to assess and monitor the progress of the child with CP. The Gross Motor Functional Measure (GMFM) was developed in 1989 to measure the child's functional gross motor skills (10). Two other assessment tools have been developed and often used to determine functional skills. The Pediatric Evaluation of Disability Inventory (PEDI) was developed in 1990 (11) and measures performance in three domains: self-care, mobility, and social function. The Wee Functional Independence Measure for Children (WeeFIM) was developed in 1991 (12) and assesses ability to self-care, sphincter control, transfer, locomotion, communication, and social cognition. In some centers, a computerized gait analysis is used to assess and monitor the child's gait and is an important tool in helping decide on the most appropriate therapy for the child.

V. ASSOCIATED FINDINGS

Seventy-five percent of children with CP have one or more comorbidities in addition to the motor abnormalities (13). These associated problems may begin very early in life and include feeding difficulties, irritability, and disordered sleep. Between 30% and 50% of children with CP are mentally retarded, with the higher figure seen in children with spastic quadriplegia. Visual problems including strabismus occur in many children, and some have cortical blindness. Hearing impairments depend on the responsible process that caused the CNS insult, i.e., some prenatal infections or ototoxic drugs used in the postnatal period. Communication disorders of receptive and/or expressive speech further isolate these children. Seizure disorders occur in approximately one-half of all children with CP, most commonly in children with spastic quadriplegia. Behavioral problems are also quite common and may develop secondary to the motor disturbances and feelings of being different. Constipation and gastroesophageal reflux are also very common, particularly in the more neurologically involved children. Many children develop difficulty with coordination of oral motor function that often results in aspiration and necessitates feeding through a surgically inserted gastrostomy tube. Drooling is frequently severe enough to present embarrassment and maceration of perioral skin. In addition, child abuse is 3.4 times more frequent in children with disabilities than in their nondisabled peers (7).

VI. MANAGEMENT

The center piece or goal of treatment should be improvement in function and also a recognition by health-care providers, the patient, and the family that the deficits cannot be totally reversed or eliminated. It is absolutely vital that the family and others who are involved with the child not only understand but also accept this premise and that everyone treats the child as normal as possible. The distinction between a "disease" and an illness must be explained and its implication emphasized. The "disease" or condition of CP will not go away. The motor abnormalities must be accepted as "what is," and the child and family must learn to adjust without these problems inciting the child to become "ill." It has been our observation that the most successful families and the most well-adjusted children are those who are given expectations and pushed to reach their highest potential. Misery comes when the child is pitied and waited upon. These children tend to fall further behind, and the families far too often become more and more discouraged and become victims themselves.

The National Center for Medical Rehabilitation Research of the National Institutes of Health has defined disability in several different spheres or dimensions such as the pathophysiology—what is the lesion and where it is located; impairment—degree of spasticity or contractions of joints; functional limitations—ability to ambulate or use of hands; and societal barriers—wheel chair accessibility and health-care availability and affordability. It is important to address each of these areas with the family and, as the child matures, with the involved child, him or herself.

Treatment is frequently directed at the motor dysfunction. The physical and occupational therapists are the care providers who are most involved, but the parents and the siblings should be an integral part of the therapeutic team in a home program designed by the professionals but administered on a daily basis by the family.

Treatment should not be directed exclusively at the major motor difficulties at the expense of the other problems. Each of the comorbidities also demands attention. With such a wide and diverse array of problems, a team of specialists representing each modality is needed. The list is long and may include a general pediatrician, a pediatric neurologist, a clinical geneticist, a pediatric orthopedist and an orthotic specialist, a pediatric pulmonologist, a pediatric gastroenterologist and nutritionist, a pediatric ophthalmologist, physical therapists, occupational therapists, speech therapists and communication specialists, audiologists, feeding therapists, social workers, developmental specialists, psychologists, and educators who have been trained in special education and in vocational training and selective placements.

The pediatric neurologist is needed to help with the evaluation of why the child has CP, to interpret the findings to the parents, and to assist in the management of seizures that so frequently accompany this condition. The clinical geneticist is needed to evaluate for a genetic basis of the CP, including pedigree analysis to identify if other family members are also affected and determine the inheritance pattern, if any; for genetic testing (chromosome, DNA, metabolic and mitochondrial); and for genetic counseling to discuss recurrence risks and testing of other at risk family members. The orthopedist will evaluate the extent of the motor disabilities and work with an orthotist and physical therapist to prescribe medications to decrease muscle tension and to order orthotics, braces, assistive devices, and adaptive equipment, including a wheel chair should those motor devices be deemed necessary to improve function. The orthopedist will also monitor the child for the development of hip dislocation, contractures, and scoliosis and may suggest surgical intervention to improve function. If the child is nonambulatory, osteopenia is not an uncommon complication and may result in pathologic fractures. Many of these children develop pulmonary problems, particularly if the child has progressive scoliosis and hence a pulmonologist is important to maintain and maximize respiratory function. Respiratory infections and/or aspiration are a frequent cause of death in the child who is severely neurologically involved. Feeding issues and drooling are often prominent problems in the young infant, and the child needs a feeding specialist who can direct the parents in proper feeding techniques. Medicines may be necessary to address the drooling. Many children with CP have nutritional problems that often initially manifest as failure to thrive. Esophageal gastric reflux is common and consultation from a gastroenterologist is useful. Protron pump medications may be prescribed and the feeding issues may be severe enough to mandate gastrostomy tube placement with or without a fundoplication. This puts control of intake in the hands of the care provider and often reverses the failure to thrive issue. Constipation is a very frequent problem and is probably related to poor abdominal muscles, relative dysfunction of gastrointestinal motility, a diet limited to a milk-based supplement that is deficient in fiber, and some medications used in the child with CP. Strabismus is a very common finding and may require ophthalmologic treatments. In addition, the child with CP is more susceptible to dental caries, as many are quite resistance to teeth brushing and some have an excessive amount of saliva. Skin breakdown or decubitus ulceration is not infrequent, secondary to a lack of movement and lying in the same position when there is a deficiency of subcutaneous tissue overlying bony prominences.

From the first detection of a delay in developmental milestones and suspicion of a problem in motor function, an array of therapists should be mobilized to assist the child and train

the family to give the child the most appropriate interventions as early as possible. This should maximize the child's
potential of achieving his or her full potential. When the
suspicion is first entertained, social workers and family
counselors should be consulted and dispatched to the child's
home, as there will be numerous questions that will need to
be addressed quickly and thoroughly. Families often feel
guilty and need to be reassured. Families need support, both
emotional and financial.

This multitude of health-care providers demands that
there is a coordinator of the team of specialists and one who
will accept the responsibility of relaying and interpreting
the findings and recommendations to the child and the family.
After carefully considering the recommendations and discussing the options with the specialists, the coordinator should
assume the responsibility of assisting the child and family
in choosing which treatments among those suggested are
truly in the best interest of the child.

The coordinator must periodically review the progress or
lack of it and initiate appropriate referrals in a timely fashion.
Only with this type of continued monitoring and surveillance
can problems be detected as they arise and can therapy be
instituted early to prevent deterioration. Examples of some
orthopedic problems that commonly develop are dislocation
of the hips, contractures, and scoliosis. If detected early, less
invasive therapies can be instituted, assistive devices can be
utilized, and hopefully, surgical intervention can be prevented. A nutritional assessment is an important component
of this review process, but unfortunately it is one aspect that
is too often neglected. These children also need all the usual
anticipatory guidance and well-childcare recommendations,
including immunizations and behavior management, just as
all children do. Of course, children with CP are subject to all
the acute illnesses that children have, but due to their underlying condition, the comorbidities, and their compromised
status, more aggressive therapies are often indicated.

There are some relatively new treatments, some of
which have been well researched and are of considerable
benefit and others that are being promoted but lack scientific

studies that substantiate the benefits being claimed. Those with proven benefits include the use of botulinum toxin to temporarily reduce spasticity (14). The injection of this toxin into selected muscle groups will result in partial paralysis of the muscles. When combined with intensive physical therapy to stretch the muscles and tendons, it provides an attempt to prevent contractures or to decrease their severity. The use of intrathecal baclofen has also been studied extensively and will relieve spasm much more effectively than the oral use of this agent (15). Selective dorsal rhizotomy is a permanent intervention and has been found to be very useful. It will reduce or eliminate spasticity and, when done in conjunction with physical therapy in children with spastic diplegia, has been shown to have a small positive effect on gross motor function (16). There are several less well-studied strategies and some that have not been studied at all. One such modality is "conductive education" in which an instructor leads a group of children through exercises aimed at improving function. One randomized study found this therapy to be no more effective than conventional therapies (17). Intensive passive muscle manipulation or patterning requires a tremendous amount of time and commitment and has not been proven to be effective. The use of astronaut weighed suits designed to improve independent mobility has also not been shown to be effective. Hyperbaric oxygen is being promoted as a means to increase blood circulation to the areas of damaged neurons. A randomized multicentral trial of this approach found no difference between the group that received hyperbaric 100% oxygen and the group that received only slightly pressurized air with the oxygen content of room air (18). In addition, some alternative and complementary therapies such as acupuncture, osteopathic manipulation, and self-hypnosis are under investigation to determine their effectiveness in the treatment of CP (19–22). Families are very eager to find something that will benefit their child and are prey to many of these therapies. It is important not to dash their hopes, but it is also vital that families not be given unrealistic expectations.

There are many useful resources regarding CP, especially with regard to information for physicians and other care providers who manage children with CP. Among the resources, the author has found the book "Health Care Issues and Other Services" by Nickel to be particularly informative (23). This is a guide on children's disabilities and chronic conditions written for medical students and postgraduate medical trainees, as well as for physicians and nurses. The Centers for Disease Control and Prevention has a general guide to CP that is helpful for trainees and for parents who have had no previous exposure to this condition (13).

VII. PROGNOSIS

Cerebral palsy cannot be cured but is not a fatal condition. Whereas the CNS insult is nonprogressive, the effects from the motor deficit and the muscle imbalance between the flexors and extensors may gradually increase resulting in contractures of joint or in scoliosis where the paraspinal muscles on either side of the vertebrae are not in balance. Over time, the motor deficits intensify resulting in a progressive and often in a severely distorted body, particularly in those children whose functional level is IV or V (Table 2).

The degree of disability is closely related to survival, yet 90% of children with CP will live into adulthood. Death is frequently due to pulmonary problems secondary to aspiration pneumonia or to prolonged seizures and perhaps due to problems associated with limited mobility and inanition.

There is great pleasure in caring for children with CP and in helping their families. In general, we have found these children to be very happy and are loved by their families. Even those who are nonverbal find a way to communicate and respond to their environment beyond one's expectation. If the family has raised their child in a "no nonsense" way and pushed him or her to achieve their greatest potential, one cannot help but be impressed and even inspired both by the process and by the outcome.

REFERENCES

1. Stanley F, Blair E, eds. Cerebral Palsies: Epidemiology and Causal Pathways. Alberman E. MacKeith Press, 2000.

2. Postnatal causes of developmental disabilities in children ages 3–10 years. MMWR 1996; 45(6):130–134 (Atlanta, GA, 1991).

3. Newacheck PW, Taylor WR. Childhood chronic illnesses: prevalence, severity, and impact. Am J Public Health 1992; 82: 364–371.

4. Naulty CM, Long LB, Pettett G. Prevalence of prematurity, low birthweight, and asphyxia as perinatal risk factors in a current population of children with cerebral palsy. Am J Perinatol 1994; 11:377–381.

5. Sidebotham P, Heron J. ALSPAC Study Team. Child maltreatment in the "children of the nineties": the role of the child. Child Abuse Negl 2003; 27:337–352.

6. American Academy of Pediatrics: Committee on Child Abuse and Neglect and Committee on Children with Disabilities. Assessment of maltreatment of children with disabilities. Pediatrics 2001; 108:508–512.

7. Sullivan PM, Knutson JF. Maltreatment and disabilities: a population-based epidemiological study. Child Abuse Negl 2000; 24:1257–1273.

8. Palisano R, Rosenbaum P, Walter S, Russell D, Wood E, Galuppi B. Gross motor function classification system for cerebral palsy. Dev Med Child Neurol 1997; 39:214–223.

9. Folio MR, Fewell RR. . Peabody Developmental Motor Scales and Activity Cards. Itasca, IL: Riverside Publishing Company, 1983.

10. Russell DJ, Rosenbaum PL, Cadman DT, Gowland C, Hardy S, Jarvis S. The gross motor functional measure: a means to evaluate the effects of physical therapy. Dev Med Child Neurol 1989; 31:341–352.

11. Fedman AB, Haley SM, Coryell J. Concurrent and constructive validity of the pediatric evaluation of disability inventory. Phys Ther 1990; 70:602–610.

12. Hamilton BB, Granger CV. WeeFim. Buffalo: Research Foundation of the State University of New York, 1991.

13. CDC Resource Page. National Center of Birth Defects and Developmental Disabilities Web Site. Available at: www.cdc. gov/ncbddd/dd/ddcp.htm. Cerebral Palsy. Accessed Oct 22, 2003.

14. Edgar TS. Clinical utility of botulinum toxin in the treatment of cerebral palsy: a comprehensive review. J Child Neurol 2001; 16:37–46.

15. Butler C, Campbell S. Evidence of the effects of intrathecal baclofen for spastic and dystonic cerebral palsy. AACPDM treatment outcomes committee review panel. Dev Med Child Neurol 2000; 42:634–645.

16. McLaughlin J, Bjornson K, Temkin N, Steinbok P, Wright V, Reiner A, Roberts T, Drake J, O'Donnell M, Rosenbaum P, Barber J, Ferrel A. Selective dorsal rhizotomy: meta-analysis of three randomized controlled trials. Dev Med Child Neurol 2002; 44:17–25.

17. Reddihough DS, King J, Coleman G, Catanese T. Efficacy of programmes based on conductive education for young children with cerebral palsy. Dev Med Child Neurol 1998; 40:763–770.

18. Collet JP, Vanasse M, Marois P, Amar M, Goldberg J, Lambert J, Lassonde M, Hardy P, Fortin J, Tremblay SD, Montgomery D, Lacroix J, Robinson A, Majnemer A. Hyperbaric oxygen for children with cerebral palsy: a randomized multicentre trial. Lancet 2001; 357:582–586.

19. Frymann VM, Carney RE, Springhall P. Effect of osteopathic medical management on neurologic development in children. JAOA 1992; 92(6):729–744.

20. Si T, Hu Y-Y. To observe the effect of comprehensive rehabilitation of motor function for cerebral palsy. Nowadays Rehabil 1999; 3(10):1168–1169.

21. Duncan B, Barton L, Edmonds MA, Blashill BM. Parental perceptions of the therapeutic effect of osteopathic manipulation or acupuncture in children with cerebral palsy. J Clin Pediatr 2004; 43(4):349–353.

22. Mauersberger K, Artz UK, Duncan B, Gurgevich S. Can children with cerebral palsy use self-hypnosis to reduce their muscle spasticity? Integr Med 1999; 2:93–96.

23. Nickel RE. Cerebral palsy. In: Nickel RE, Desch LW, eds. The Physician's Guide to Caring for Children with Disabilities and Chronic Conditions. Baltimore: Paul H Brookes Publishing Co., 2000.

24

Diagnostic Evaluation and Treatment of Developmental Disabilities

KATHY ELLERBECK and CHET JOHNSON

Developmental Disabilities Center, University of Kansas Medical Center, Kansas City, Kansas, U.S.A.

EDWARD HOFFMAN

Special Care Pediatrics, P.A., Leawood, Kansas, U.S.A.

I. INTRODUCTION

> As to diseases make a habit of two things—to help, or at least, to do no harm. (*Hippocrates*)

This quote also applies to developmental disabilities which are estimated to affect at least 5–10% of children (1). Thus, developmental delays and/or motor impairments are common clinical problems presenting to the pediatrician and family practitioner. Unfortunately, fewer than half of children with developmental disabilities are identified by school entrance, which precludes their participation in early intervention programs (2,3). There is increasingly strong evidence that early intervention results in significant improvement both in children at increased biological risk, and in children with established developmental disabilities (4,5). Although primary care physicians are uniquely positioned to address developmental problems and promote optimal development, many barriers to providing good quality developmental services exist (6). In 2003, the Commonwealth Fund published a report by Halfon that examined primary health care services that promote infant and young child development in the United States. The report examined developmental services in primary care, dividing the services into four general categories: assessment, education, intervention, and care co-ordination (6). Using this typology, in this chapter we will review research findings and current recommendations for diagnostic evaluation and treatment for children presenting with suspected developmental disability. This chapter will also review some of the barriers to the provision of comprehensive developmental care and their potential solutions.

II. ASSESSMENT SERVICES

Fewer than 30% of primary care providers conduct standardized screening tests at well-child visits. Most primary care providers continue to use informal developmental surveillance as opposed to systematic developmental screening (7). Developmental surveillance involves "eliciting and attending to parents' concerns, making accurate and informative longitudinal observations of children, and obtaining a relevant developmental history" (8). Pitfalls in developmental diagnosis and cognitive obstacles to effective developmental surveillance have been well described (9,10). In 1991, Blasco (9) noted a tendency for both families and physicians to miss or downplay motor developmental delay until late infancy, and to disregard language delays until children were at least 24 months old. Glascoe and Dworkin (10) have shown that the physician's unique experiences, beliefs, and attitudes, and a resultant set of judgment heuristics for sorting information mediate a physician's selection from the array of clinical data. Depending on how information is sorted, physicians may arrive at accurate, or inaccurate, diagnoses.

Given the problems inherent to developmental surveillance, in 2001, the American Academy of Pediatrics' Committee on Children with Disabilities issued a policy statement recommending routine administration of a validated, accurate developmental screening test at each well-child check (11). Several parent report tools meet standards for screening test accuracy, with sensitivity and specificity of at least 70–80%. As noted by Glascoe and Macias, implementing systematic developmental screening in pediatric practice requires a "committed leader who believes in the value of such screening and intervention and can convey enthusiasm to staff" (3).

Although the continuity of the developmental process is well established, discontinuities do exist (4), and contribute to physician fears of unnecessarily worrying parents. It is often difficult for a physician seeing an individual child to know whether or not a delay will persist, and if a disability exists. Because these are such difficult questions to answer, primary care physicians often refer to either child neurologists or developmental pediatricians. Unfortunately, there is often substantial loss of time between parental concern and a visit to a subspecialist. In a study of children presenting to a neurologist with developmental delay, parents were asked at what age they had initially suspected a problem. The mean age reported was approximately 8 months. The child neurologist initially examined the children at a group mean age of 3.58 years, with a mean delay between parental concern and the initial visit to the neurologist of nearly 3 years (12). In a study of 1300 families who had a child diagnosed with autism, the average age at diagnosis was about 6 years, though most parents felt that something was wrong by 18 months, and most had sought medical assistance by the age of 2 years (13).

Parents generally seek to answer the following questions: (1) Is there a developmental disorder, and, if so, what disorder?; (2) What caused it?; (3) What tests are needed?; and

(4) What can be done about it medically and educationally? (14). Primary care physicians can, and should, begin to answer these questions.

A. Beyond Screening: Is There a Developmental Disorder, and If So, What Disorder?

The evaluation of a child with possible developmental disability begins with a thorough history and physical examination. The first step is to determine if there is indeed variation from normal. Each developmental domain needs to be assessed separately. The physician can make a preliminary "neurodevelopmental" diagnosis using screening tools and milestones. The primary care physician can supplement office screening or age equivalent estimates with more specific testing from community early intervention teams to arrive at a more complete and accurate neurodevelopmental diagnosis. Referral to early intervention, however, will not answer the families' second question: "What caused this?" A neurodevelopmental diagnosis (such as global developmental delay or possible autism) is not an etiologic diagnosis.

B. What Caused the Developmental Disorder?

Etiologic diagnosis is important in predicting a child's developmental progress, in allowing knowledgeable surveillance for potential associated health problems, and in genetic evaluation and counseling and prenatal diagnosis (15). Physicians are trained in biomedicine, and with advances in the understanding of pathophysiology and in the technology for diagnosis, they are increasingly able to make an etiologic diagnosis. Previously, classification of the severity of developmental delay/mental retardation was thought to be important from an etiologic point of view (16). More recently, it has been found that diagnostic yield does not differ substantially across categories of degrees of developmental delay (17). The clinician should not rely on the severity of the delay to direct the investigational approach. In a recent cohort of 120 children referred for evaluation of developmental delay/mental retardation, a causal/pathogenetic diagnosis was reached in 80.8%. The high yield was thought to be the result of improved awareness that developmental/genetic factors underlie most cases of developmental delays, and the recognition that more and more developmentally delayed patients may have a syndrome. There has also been improvement in diagnostic testing (17).

Two recent practice parameters from the Quality Standards Subcommittee of the American Academy of Neurology are very helpful in the medical evaluation of children presenting with developmental concerns. The first parameter, "Practice parameter: screening and diagnosis of autism," was published in 2000 (7), and involves a two-level screening process. The first level includes routine developmental surveillance/screening to identify those children at risk for any type of atypical development, using standardized measures. Absolute indications for immediate evaluation are listed. If the child fails formal routine developmental surveillance, he or she is specifically screened for autism. Children who fail the autism screen are then referred to a clinician experienced in the diagnosis of the autistic spectrum disorders (Fig. 1).

Developmental disabilities associated with genetic conditions often present with global developmental delay. Global developmental delay is a subset of developmental disabilities defined as a significant delay in two or more of the following developmental domains: gross/fine motor, speech/language, cognition, social/personal, and activities of daily living (1). The second practice parameter, "Practice parameter: evaluation of the child with global developmental delay," was published in 2003 (1). The algorithm is specific, and, if based on a comprehensive history and physical examination, could be carried out by a primary care physician with targeted subspecialty consultation (Fig. 2).

C. What Tests Are Needed?

In terms of assessment, what is needed is an organized, disciplined, and structured method of analyzing the clinical evidence, so that no specifically treatable possibilities are over-

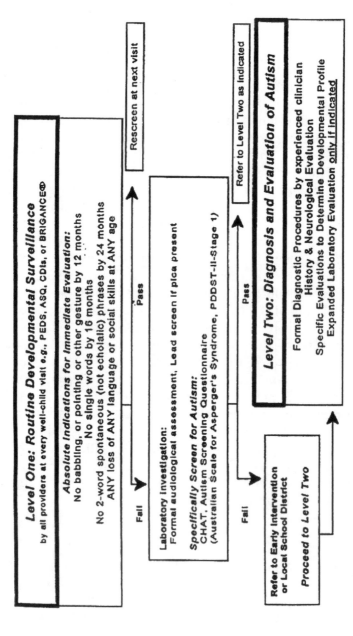

Figure 1 Practice parameter: autistic spectrum disorders (ASD). (From Ref. 7.)

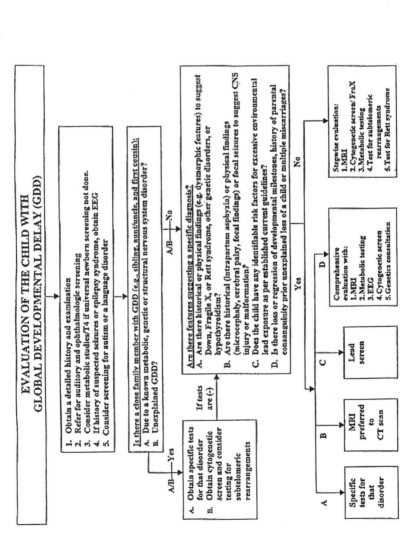

EVALUATION OF THE CHILD WITH GLOBAL DEVELOPMENTAL DELAY (GDD)

1. Obtain a detailed history and examination
2. Refer for auditory and ophthalmologic screening
3. Consider metabolic studies/T4 if universal newborn screening not done.
4. If history of suspected seizures or epilepsy syndrome, obtain EEG
5. Consider screening for autism or a language disorder

Is there a close family member with GDD (e.g., siblings, aunt/uncle, and first cousin):
A. Due to a known metabolic, genetic or structural nervous system disorder?
B. Unexplained GDD?

A/B — Yes

A. Obtain specific tests for that disorder
B. Obtain cytogenetic screen and consider testing for subtelomeric rearrangements

If tests are (−)

A/B — No

Are there features suggesting a specific diagnosis?
A. Are there historical or physical findings (e.g. dysmorphic features) to suggest Down, Fragile X, or Rett syndrome, other genetic disorders, or hypothyroidism?
B. Are there historical (intrapartum asphyxia) or physical findings (microcephaly, cerebral palsy, focal findings) or focal seizures to suggest CNS injury or malformation?
C. Does the child have any identifiable risk factors for excessive environmental lead exposure as per established current guidelines?
D. Is there loss or regression of developmental milestones, history of parental consanguinity prior unexplained loss of a child or multiple miscarriages?

Yes

No

A — Specific tests for that disorder

B — MRI preferred to CT scan

C — Lead screen

D — Comprehensive evaluation with:
1. MRI
2. Metabolic testing
3. EEG
4. Cytogenetic screen
5. Genetics consultation

Stepwise evaluation:
1. MRI
2. Cytogenetic screen/ FraX
3. Metabolic testing
4. Test for subtelomeric rearrangements
5. Test for Rett syndrome

Figure 2 Practice parameter: global developmental delay (GDD). (From Ref. 1.)

looked. One way to approach assessment is to use milestones, screening tools, and/or the evaluations of community early intervention teams to determine a neurodevelopmental diagnosis, and then to use algorithms and targeted subspecialty consultation to arrive at possible etiologic diagnosis (Fig. 3).

Neurodevelopmental Diagnosis	*Etiologic Diagnosis*
Necessary information:	*Necessary information:*

Gross motor age equivalent
Fine motor age equivalent
Visuomotor-problem solving (cognitive) age equivalent
Expressive language age equivalent
Receptive language age equivalent
Social and self help skills age equivalent
	History
	  Attention to prenatal exposures, family history, any history of developmental regression
	Physical examination
	  Attention to dysmorphic features, neurologic exam, growth parameters

Interpretation (possibilities):	*Interpretation (possibilities):*
Isolated delay (1 domain) Global developmental delay (2 or more domains) Motor impairment with or without delays Possible autism	Abnormal neurologic examination Dysmorphic features History suggesting static CNS injury (teratogenic, ischemic, traumatic) History suggesting developmental regression (needs emergent diagnostic assessment)
Needed testing or consultation (possibilities):	*Needed testing or consultation (possibilities):*
More detailed domain assessment(s) Formal psychoeducational testing Systematic screening for autism spectrum disorder Referral to diagnostic assessment team (community EI team and/or hospital-based assessment teams)	MRI of the brain High resolution chromosomes/specific genetic (FISH) probes Metabolic testing Subspecialty consultation
Sources of information (possibilities):	*Sources of information (possibilities):*
Formal screening tools (PEDS, CDI, other) Early intervention team arena assessments Schools Assessment teams (e.g. University-based autism team)	Primary care physician with subspecialty consultation as necessary: Geneticist/metabolic experts Neurologists Developmental pediatricians Other

Figure 3 Diagnostic decision-making.

Using an organized approach to collect information, and following practice parameters for developmental screening and for evaluation of developmental delay, the primary care physician is well positioned to (1) detect developmental disabilities, (2) to begin an etiologic evaluation, and (3) to support families through education and collaboration with early intervention teams.

III. EDUCATION SERVICES

> For any story to make sense, to have meaning for its teller or hearer, it must have a plot. Plot is an organizing feature of narrative, constructing "meaningful totalities out of scattered events—Landsman, 2003 (18)

Based on her qualitative research carried out in a newborn follow-up program, Gail Landsman suggests that most mothers of infants and toddlers diagnosed with risk of disability "employ the scattered events of their children's lives in anticipation of a particular and culturally acceptable ending—that of overcoming (or at the very least minimizing) disability" (18). Once a diagnosis is made, parents often question the diagnosis, treatment and prognosis as the normal process of adjustment to the permanence of the condition and the desire to ensure the best outcomes for their child (19). The AAP Committee on Children with Disabilities has noted that the emphasis of biomedicine on pathophysiology and technical outcomes has resulted in the perception of some families that physicians undervalue their relationships with their patients (19).

Physicians, parents, and providers need to understand the meaning of the diagnosis and the disability to the family. Arthur Kleinman, a psychiatrist and medical anthropologist at the Harvard Medical School, developed a set of eight questions designed to elicit a patient's (or a parent's) "explanatory model" (20). The questions were designed for use in crosscultural medicine and families, physicians, and early interventionists who come from different "subcultures" with their own sets of interests, emotions, and biases. Parents, physicians, and communities negotiate diagnoses, roles, and narratives, often from very different vantage points. Understanding the parents' explanatory model is critically important to adequately supporting the family of the child at risk for developmental disability. Thus, "Kleinman's eight questions" should be carefully considered in relation to developmental delay or disability:

1. What do you call the problem?
2. What do you think has caused the problem?
3. Why do you think it started when it did?
4. What do you think the delay/disability does? How does it work?
5. How severe is the delay/disability? Will it have a short or a long course?
6. What kind of treatment do you think the patient should receive? What are the most important results you hope she/he receives from this treatment?
7. What are the chief problems the delay/disability has caused?
8. What do you fear most about the delay/disability?

Families commonly describe difficulties with getting and/or accepting the diagnosis; confusion over labeling; the need to understand the cause; grief and sorrow; trials of day to day living; stresses imposed by the diagnosis and search for adequate treatments; difficulty knowing long-term prognosis; and social stigma. The adjustment to, and treatment of, developmental disability occurs over a period of years. The primary care physician can be instrumental to making families' lives better. Many families can eventually describe "surviving and transcending" the difficulties posed by developmental disability (21).

A. What Can Be Done About the Disability— Medically and Educationally?

After diagnosis, and education about diagnosis, families want to know what can be done for their child. Primary care physicians are often the "gateway" to early intervention services.

Primary care providers also play a key role in coordinating care for these children who often have complex medical needs.

IV. INTERVENTION SERVICES

Referral for early intervention services should occur for any child suspected to have a neurodevelopmental disorder, whether or not the etiology for the disorder has been determined. The reasoning is twofold. First, families desire appropriate intervention for their child. Second, there is increasingly strong research evidence on the effectiveness of appropriate early intervention.

The field of early intervention for established disabilities has a long history. Prior to the 1970s, legislation and programs to address treatment of disability [e.g., Title V of the Social Security Act of 1935, Public Law (PL) 74–271] and education of the disabled (e.g., Handicapped Children's Early Education Act of 1968, PL 90–538) was limited. Then, in 1975, the Education for All Handicapped Children Act (PL 94–142) guaranteed the right to a free and appropriate education for all school-age children with handicaps. A decade later, the Education of the Handicapped Act Amendments of 1986 (PL 99–457) moved the access to this education down to the age of 3 and also created incentives for states to identify and provide services for infants and toddlers (birth to 2 years) with disability or at risk for disability—a legislative mandate for early intervention.

The conceptual basis for "intervention" has evolved as well. Knowledge in the fields of neuroscience, genetics, and special education has come together as never before. The 1990s were designated the "decade of the brain" (Presidential Proclamation 6158, July 17, 1990), and in the last 15 years our understanding of brain development and processes has expanded exponentially. The importance of appropriate early experiences in driving synaptogenesis and the development of neural networks is now well recognized (5,22). At the same time, excessive synaptic formation, or ineffective synaptic elimination, can be harmful to cognitive functioning, as is the case in fragile X syndrome (23,24) and possibly in at least a subset of children with autism (25,26). Behavioral phenotypes, defined as the constellation of likely behavioral and cognitive characteristics clinically expressed by a specific genetic syndrome have become better delineated. This information can be helpful to early intervention specialists. As more genetic syndromes are linked to an identified gene defect, matching behavioral phenotypes can be better predicted. Hodapp and colleagues have proposed that special educators and parents use behavior phenotypes to guide special education research and intervention efforts, "teaching to the child's strengths" (27,28). As an example, knowing that a child with Down syndrome typically has a relatively stronger visual memory than auditory memory can translate to use of sign language in early communication intervention.

Interpretation and implementation of early intervention legislation varies between states, but the criteria are developmentally based and are not driven by income or insurance coverage. Thus, the infant or toddler identified with a neurodevelopmental delay or disorder should simply be referred to the state's early intervention program (National Early Childhood Technical Assistance Center—http://www.nectac.org). After the child's third birthday, the child should be referred to the local public school system.

V. CARE COORDINATION

Children with developmental disabilities and their families experience an improved quality of life when their considerable needs (Table 1) are matched by access to appropriate resources. How do families access those resources? Who are the responsible parties? Increasingly, researchers, clinicians, and policy makers are suggesting that family–physician partnerships are critical to good care (29,30).

Pediatricians now generally accept that "every child deserves a medical home." The "medical home" has been an initiative of the American Academy of Pediatrics over the past decade. What is a medical home? What are its characteristics?

A July 2002 AAP policy statement recommends that "the medical care of infants, children, and adolescents ideally should be accessible, continuous, comprehensive, family-centered, coordinated, compassionate, and culturally effective. It should be delivered or directed by well-trained physicians who provide primary care and help to manage and facilitate essentially *all* aspects of pediatric care. The physician... and family... should be able to develop a partnership of mutual responsibility and trust" (29).

Family–physician partnerships are critical for children with disabilities with acute medical problems requiring multi-specialty care or hospitalization. This may be especially true early in the child's life or around the time of assessment and diagnosis, and for minority children and children with less educated parents (31). As the child gets older, medical problems may become less of an issue while developmental, educational, and behavioral challenges become more difficult (Table 1). In order to effectively address these challenges, the family–physician partnership needs to stretch and change its shape and dimensions to add community partners (see Fig. 4). The evolution of the partnership is necessitated by the ever-expanding world of the child. The infant and toddler who has primarily

Table 1 Important Issues for Children with Disabilities

Advocacy
Behavioral and emotional
Dental
Dependent care
Developmental and educational
Financial
Information and resources
Legal—wills, trust, guardianship
Leisure time/recreation
Living arrangements
Medical—including nutrition, vision, hearing...
Occupation
Respite care
Sexuality and intimacy
Transitions
Transportation

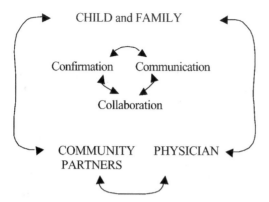

Figure 4 Care coordination and dimensions for a child with developmental disabilities.

interacted with family and childcare providers becomes the pre-school-/school-age child in a school and a community of peers.

Expanding the family–physician partnership to include community partners will challenge the integrity of the partnership. The bonds of mutual respect and trust that have been carefully established must be loosened to allow the inclusion of new players on the team. Either the primary care physician or the early intervention specialist may feel that "two's company, three's a crowd" as each learns how to relate to the other effectively. A real concern and caring for each other can help to carry the day, particularly when "the best interests of the child" remain central to the diverse work of the various parties.

Three guiding tenets will advance the coordination of care. These tenets are:

1. *Communication:* Families of children with disabilities consistently identify their primary needs as (i) information about community resources and finances; and (ii) parent-to-parent support (32). Physicians and nurses need to be able to provide information about various community resources, and with some organizational effort, to keep ready handouts, fliers, and phone numbers that address the other informational needs. Community partners may provide more specific information and linkages to financial counselors, specialized services, and veteran parents.

2. *Collaboration:* The "collaboration of many minds" is often necessary for the optimal planning and implementation of a care plan for a child with disabilities. Included among the "many minds" are the minds of the child, the various family members (including siblings and extended family), educators, social service workers, physicians, and other health care providers. During complex medical procedures or at a school individualized educational plan (IEP) meeting, many minds may be necessary. At other times, such as when a child's medication needs adjustment, involvement of only a few may serve the child well.

3. *Confirmation:* We propose confirmation as an important third tenet, completing and yet extending the care co-ordination relationship. By confirmation, a veteran parent and educator refers to that "brief conversation/follow-up visit to confirm that a resolution had been made or changes had occurred in the situation, or services were in process... Confirmation is a word to replace accountability that has the same kind of function. It is a time taken by the child's partners to assess how the efforts of communication and collaboration have worked" (Donna Beauchamp, 2003, personal communication).

In summary, primary care physicians are being asked to improve the content and quality of their developmental health services for all children. Neal Halfon has devised a model to organize needed services that includes assessment, education, intervention, and care co-ordination (6). This typology is useful in organizing the approach to diagnosis and management of the child who presents with developmental delay or disability. Raising a child with a congenital anomaly or developmental disability is challenging for families. Thoughtful attention to assessment, education, intervention, and care coordination improves life for both our patients and their families.

APPENDIX A

The following three cases illustrate some of the problems and some of the opportunities in the diagnosis and management of children with developmental delay and developmental disability.

1. Assessment and Education

Case in point: Taylor was born with what was thought to be an isolated cleft palate, and was followed in a multidisciplinary cleft palate clinic. As an infant, she had chronic and recurrent otitis media. She had surgical repair of her cleft palate and placement of myringotomy tubes at $10\frac{1}{2}$ months. At 18 months, Taylor's parents and speech pathologist noted that Taylor had very little language, poor joint attention, and limited eye contact. Her hearing was tested and found to be normal. At 24 months, all of Taylor's language was echolalic. By 34 months, Taylor used only occasional spontaneous phrases, but still did not point. She qualified for an early childhood special education program. At the request of the speech pathologist, Taylor's primary care physician referred her to a hospital-based developmental assessment clinic. An interdisciplinary team saw Taylor when she was 40 months. She was found to have moderate delays and was also given a diagnosis of "atypical autism" (pervasive developmental disorder—NOS) by the interdisciplinary assessment team. A developmental pediatrician completed an etiologic assessment. The prenatal history and birth history were unremarkable. The family history was negative for cleft palate. A sibling had a "heart murmur," but no developmental problems. There was depression on the maternal side of the family, and a sibling carried the diagnosis of ADHD. On physical examination, Taylor's height and weight were both at the 5th–10th percentile. Taylor was noted to have several unusual features, including posteriorly rotated ears, inverted nipples, pectus excavatum, a left transverse palmar crease, and several hemangiomas. High-resolution chromosomes and a FISH probe for velocardiofacial syndrome were ordered. The FISH probe was normal, however, Taylor was found to have a 45,X karyotype consistent with a diagnosis of Turner syndrome.

What's the point? Children with birth defects are nearly 27 times more likely to have mental retardation by 7 years of age compared to children without a diagnosed birth defect, regardless of type of defect (33). By 18 months, Taylor was noted to have delays and atypical behaviors that probably could not be accounted for by an isolated cleft palate. The primary care physician could have used milestone lists and/or a parental screening tool to arrive at age equivalent estimates for each developmental domain, and asked the early intervention program to do a more detailed assessment of the child's delays. Given the concerns about abnormal social behaviors, screening for autism using a tool like the M-CHAT was also indicated, and could have helped to support an earlier diagnosis of autism spectrum disorder. Although it was very appropriate to refer the child for subspecialty assessment, the primary care physician might have started with the etiologic determination using the AAN guidelines for evaluation. Given this child's dysmorphic features, high-resolution chromosomes were indicated. The genetic testing revealed that this child had X monosomy, or Turner syndrome. The diagnosis was important for the child's physicians, therapists, and family. The child had an echocardiogram, which was normal. She was referred to pediatric endocrinology and is currently receiving growth hormone. Girls with Turner syndrome have been described as having atypical social development and learning differences. Although most girls with Turner syndrome are not diagnosed with an autism spectrum disorder, the diagnoses of Turner syndrome and atypical autism provided the family with some explanation for their child's developmental problems. The family also received support from both the Turner Syndrome Foundation and from a local autism support group.

Primary care physicians have relationships over time with the families of the children they follow, rather than the "snapshot" encounters provided by even very good interdisciplinary birth defect and developmental evaluation teams. Physicians and early childhood specialists often recognize delays, but families may wait months, if not years, for both diagnosis and targeted intervention. Physicians advocate for their patients when they support early intervention and early diagnosis. Referral may well be necessary, but, unfortunately, waits for neurologists, developmental pediatricians, or university-based interdisciplinary assessment teams are often long, delaying treatment and increasing family anxiety.

Physicians can become part of community interdisciplinary assessment teams by not only referring to early intervention, but also by acting as the medical member of community early intervention teams. These federally funded programs exist across the country. Early intervention teams can help physicians to refine the "neurodevelopmental diagnosis," and physicians, using published practice parameters and targeted subspecialty referral, can determine etiologic diagnoses and make appropriate medical recommendations to early intervention providers.

2. Intervention

Case in point: At Casey's 6-month well child visit, his mother expressed concern that his development seemed slower relative to his sister's at that age. His physician scheduled a follow-up visit 2 weeks later to address these concerns. At that visit, the history was reviewed. Casey was born after an uncomplicated term pregnancy. Delivery was by cesarean section for failure of labor to progress. Casey was 7 lb 1 oz at birth. The nursery course lasted an extra day to establish adequate feeding, but there were no concerns at discharge. Casey's mother did not report any other real problems, but noted that Casey's head control seemed to be poor and that he was not consistently rolling over or sitting independently. She also worried that he was a little thin and took a longer time to eat than had his sister. The physical examination was not particularly remarkable except for perhaps decreased muscle tone. Deep tendon reflexes were present, and no abnormal posturing or primitive reflexes were noted. Casey appeared to be socially aware, but did not babble. He could not sit without support, and even with support his head wobbled. He did not reach for the stethoscope or reflex hammer. Casey's mother was appropriately concerned about Casey's delays and anxious about his future. Casey was referred to a developmental pediatrician, but his mother called back to say that the appointment was more than 3 months away and asked what could be done in the meantime. The physician was about to suggest a physical therapy clinic consult when his partner mentioned that the state's early intervention program, "Helping Hands," might be appropriate. The physician asked Casey's mother to call that number, and let him know what happened. He asked to see Casey in follow-up in 6 weeks. At follow-up, Casey, now 8 months of age, still was not sitting independently and was not crawling. He was just beginning to babble. Casey's mother reported that Casey was receiving physical therapy and special infant instruction, and that the therapists were coming to her home. She also spoke positively about a parent group the program sponsored. Her demeanor was decidedly upbeat, although she clearly understood that Casey's development continued to lag. Casey's physical therapist accompanied his mother to the visit. She mentioned that Casey seemed to fatigue more than did the other infants and toddlers that she treated. When Casey was seen at the child development center two months later at age 10 months, "easily fatigued" was noted in the physician's summary letter. Clinically, Casey was almost 50% behind in motor, speech, and cognitive development. He was also noted to be hypotonic.

The developmental pediatrician discussed the concerns and implications with Casey's mother, and ordered several laboratory tests, including: thyroid studies, chromosomes, plasma amino acids, urine organic acids, long-chain fatty acids, serum lactic acid, serum pyruvate, and carnitine levels; a brain MRI was also recommended. The primary care physician called the developmental pediatrician 3 weeks later to say that thyroid studies, chromosomes, urine organic acids, and long-chain fatty acids were normal, but lactic acid, pyruvate, and carnitine levels were slightly abnormal, and the serum amino acids had some "nonspecific elevations." The possibility of a mitochondrial disorder was discussed, and further recommendations made.

What's the point? Physicians traditionally have been trained to diagnose and then to treat according to diagnosis. Etiologic diagnosis is important, but it may be difficult to accomplish. Treatment may be limited to referral for early intervention (EI) services. Although most physicians do believe in the importance of federally funded EI programs, they often delay referring children (34). Although early intervention is usually not "curative," it *is* therapeutic, not only for the child, but for the entire family. Casey's mother partnered with the therapists caring for her son. She learned some of the treatment techniques her child's therapists recommended. While she continued to have some anxiety about the cause of Casey's delays and about his future, her fear was somewhat diminished with support to her family and with the clearly stated goals in Casey's individualized family service plan (IFSP). Casey's mother and her therapists also partnered with the primary care physician. Casey's physical therapist was an astute observer who pointed out fatigability and weakness that might well have been missed by both the primary care physician and the subspecialist. Her observations helped direct the etiologic work-up. Casey was eventually diagnosed with a mitochondrial disorder. Her mother became an ardent advocate for her child, and over the next several years she helped support other families whose children were diagnosed with developmental disability.

3. Coordination of Care

Case in point: Alex's parents called their family physician in April of Alex's sixth grade year "at the end of their rope." They were finding Alex's unpredictable, aggressive behaviors to be unmanageable. They were afraid for Alex and for his 8-year-old sister, Rachel. They were also afraid for themselves. Alex, age 12, had been diagnosed with autism, fragile X syndrome, and moderate mental retardation. Problem behaviors, increasing in frequency over the last couple of years, had been attributed to his developmental disabilities.

Alex had many care coordination partners, including his parents, his sister, his family physician, the special education staff, the school social worker, the school psychologist, the HMO case worker, the behavior specialist at school, and the psychiatrist who had diagnosed autism at age 4. Except for an occasional one-on-one phone encounter, these individuals had never conferenced together around Alex's needs. Ordinarily, Alex's father would have taken the lead to call a meeting, but he had a new job and could not easily get away. The family and Alex's physician agreed that the school social worker would be the best person to get people together. There was general agreement that "a meeting of the minds" was necessary. Alex's psychiatrist, who had only had occasional contact over the last 8 years, joined the group gathered at the school office by conference call. By carefully listening to the description of Alex's behavior over the last 7 months of school, the varied parties agreed that there was something very different about the "Alex" they had known in the fifth grade. The group consensus was that Alex was perhaps experiencing a mental health problem separate from autism and mental retardation, and the psychiatrist suggested that a brief inpatient evaluation would be useful. With the support of the care coordination team, the HMO medical director agreed to a 4-day inpatient psychiatric hospitalization. Alex was diagnosed with a mood disorder and was started on appropriate medication. Alex's family received a brief respite, information about the mood disorder and its management, and family training to protect family members and prevent outbursts of problem behavior. A behavior therapist was brought in to work with Alex and his family in their home. The family physician and psychiatrist kept in close contact with each other, the family, and the school nurse. Two months later, Alex had finished the school year without further incident and had transitioned successfully to a summer program. Alex and the family both reported improvements in Alex's ability to enjoy himself and others at home and in the community.

What's the point? Families often wait until a problem escalates to a crisis before seeking "professional" assistance. Primary care physicians and other care partners need to recognize that most families have already tried many options to solve the problem, and that in crisis the family may seem unreasonable in demanding that "something be done." Recognizing this will help all the partners be patient and come to a good solution.

Problem behaviors often emerge or escalate during adolescence. Behaviors that had previously been difficult but manageable may, with adolescent growth and hormonal changes, become serious to the point where they pose a threat to the safety of the adolescent, other family members, peers, or other members of the community. It is also increasingly evident that persons with developmental disabilities can have significant mental health problems that may or may not be related to the developmental disability.

There are many potential care coordination partners to collaborate for Alex's benefit. However, the number of individuals involved also creates the potential for miscommunication and for fragmentation of care. In this case, the care partners got together with the assistance of technology and a flexible approach to team leadership to work out a plan to help Alex. Their collaboration also made a much stronger case for a short-term inpatient psychiatric evaluation, which in some managed care environments can be very difficult to accomplish.

Mood disorders, like nearly all mental health disorders, are best treated with a multimodal approach that includes medication, behavioral management, family support, and a plan to bring the successes achieved in the hospital to the home and community setting. This combination of services is sometimes referred to as "wraparound" care. All of the partners working together for the well being of the child and the family are involved in the planning, implementation, and follow-up.

REFERENCES

1. Shevell M, Ashwal S, Donley D, Flint J, Gingold M, Hirtz D, et al. Standards Subcommittee of the Child Neurology Society. Practice parameter: evaluation of the child with global developmental delay: Report of the Quality Standards Subcommittee of the American Academy of Neurology and The Practice Committee of the Child Neurology Society. Neurology 2003; 60(3):367–380.

2. Glascoe FP. Evidence-based approach to developmental and behavioural surveillance using parents' concerns. Child Care Health Dev 2000; 26(2):137–149.

3. Glascoe FP, Macias MM. How can you implement the AAP's new policy on developmental and behavioral screening. Contemp Pediatr 2003; 20(4):85–102.

4. Sonnander K. Early identification of children with developmental disabilities. Acta Paediatr Suppl 2000; 89(434):17–23.

5. Shonkoff JP. From neurons to neighborhood: old and new challenges for developmental and behavioral pediatrics. J Dev Behav Pediatr 2003; 24(1):70–76.

6. Halfon N. Building a Bridge from Birth to School: Improving Developmental and Behavioral Health Services for Young Children. Available on online at www.cmwf.org/programs/child/halfon_bridge_564.pdf.

7. Filipek PA, Accardo PJ, Ashwal S, Baranek GT, Cook EH Jr, Dawson C, et al. Practice parameter: screening and diagnosis of autism: Report of the Quality Standards Subcommittee of the American Academy of Neurology and the Child Neurology Society. Neurology 2000; 55(4):468–479.

8. Dworkin PH. Developmental screening—expecting the impossible? Pediatrics 1989; 83(4):619–622.

9. Blasco PA. Pitfalls in developmental diagnosis. Pediatr Clin N Am 1991; 38(6):1425–1438.

10. Glascoe FP, Dworkin PH. Obstacles to effective developmental surveillance: errors in clinical reasoning. J Dev Behav Pediatr 1993; 14(5):344–349.

11. American Academy of Pediatrics. Developmental surveillance and screening of infants and young children (RE0062). Pediatrics 2001; 108(192).

12. Majnemer A, Shevell MI. Diagnostic yield of the neurologic assessment of the developmentally delayed child. J Pediatr 1995; 127(2):193–199.

13. Howlin PM. A diagnosis of autism. A survey of over 1200 patients in the UK [Class II]. Autism 1997; 1:135–162.

14. Rapin I. Physicians' testing of children with developmental disabilities. J Child Neurol 1995; 10(suppl 1):S11–S15.

15. Macmillan C. Genetics and developmental delay. Semin Pediatr Neurol 1998; 5(1):39–44.

16. Aicardi J. The etiology of developmental delay. Semin Pediatr Neurol 1998; 5(1):15–20.

17. Battaglia A, Bianchini E, Carey JC. Diagnostic yield of the comprehensive assessment of developmental delay/mental retardation in an institute of child neuropsychiatry. Am J Med Genet 1999; 82(1):60–66.

18. Landsman G. Emplotting children's lives: developmental delay vs. disability. Soc Sci Med 2003; 56(9):1947–1960.

19. American Academy of Pediatrics. Counseling families who choose complementary and alternative medicine for their child with chronic illness or disability. Pediatrics 2001; 107(3): 598–601.

20. Kleinman A. Culture, illness, and care: clinical lessons from anthropologic and cross-cultural research. Ann Intern Med 1978; 88(2):251–258.

21. Dillon KM. Living with Autism—The Parents' Stories. Boone, NC: Parkway Publishers, Inc., 1995.

22. Ramey CT, Ramey SL. Early experience and early intervention. Am Psychol 1998; 53:109–120.

23. Weiler IJ, Greenough WT. Synaptic synthesis of the Fragile X protein: possible involvement in synapse maturation and elimination. Am J Med Genet 1999; 83(4):248–252.

24. Greenough WT, Klintsova AY, Irwin SA, Galvez R, Bates KE, Weiler IJ. Synaptic regulation of protein synthesis and the Fragile X protein. Proc Natl Acad Sci USA 2001; 98(13): 7101–7106.

25. Courchesne E, Karns CM, Davis HR, Ziccardi R, Carper RA, Tigue ZD, et al. Unusual brain growth patterns in early life in patients with autistic disorder: an MRI study. Neurology 2001; 57(2):245–254.

26. Courchesne E, Carper R, Akshoomoff N. Evidence of brain overgrowth in the first year of life in autism. J Am Med Assoc 2003; 290(3):337–344.

27. Dykens EM, Hodapp RM, Finucane BM. Genetics and Mental Retardation Syndromes: A New Look at Behavior and Interventions. Baltimore, MD: Paul H. Brookes, 2000.

28. Hodapp RM, DesJardin MS, Ricci LA. Genetic syndromes of mental retardation: should they matter for the early interventionist? Infants Young Child 2003; 16(2):152–160.

29. American Academy of Pediatrics. The medical home. Medical homes initiatives for children with special needs project advisory committee. Pediatrics 2002; 110(1):184–186.

30. American Academy of Pediatrics. Family-centered care and the pediatrician's role. Pediatrics Policy Statement. Pediatrics 2003; 112(3):691–696.

31. Weller WE, Minkovitz CS, Anderson GF. Utilization of medical and health-related services among school-age children and adolescents with special health care needs (1994 National Health Interview Survey on Disability [NHIS-D] Baseline Data). Pediatrics 2003; 112(3 Pt 1):593–603.

32. American Academy of Pediatrics. Family pediatrics, supplement to pediatrics. Pediatrics 2003; 111(6):1539–1572.

33. Jellife-Pawlowski LL, Shaw GM, Nelson V, Harris JA. Risk of mental retardation among children born with birth defects. Arch Pediatr Adolesc Med 2003; 157(6):545–550.

34. Sices L. Developmental delay referrals: time and money. Pediatric News, Sep 2003; 57.

25

Complementary and Alternative Medicine for Children with Disabilities

MELINDA F. DAVIS

Department of Pediatrics, University of Arizona
College of Medicine, Tucson, Arizona, U.S.A.

I. INTRODUCTION

Parents of children with disabilities are very likely to use complementary and alternative medicine (CAM) for their children (1–12). CAM is often used for chronic conditions when conventional medicine is not enough, and as a result, children with significant medical needs are at the leading edge of pediatric CAM use in the United States. In this chapter, we will explore the varieties of CAM practices, reasons for CAM use, and offer some recommendations for the integration of validated CAM therapies with traditional medicine.

Children are our most precious assets, so there should be no surprise when parents go to any length to improve their children's lot in life. Parents of children with disabilities will make every effort to reduce their child's impairments, improve functioning, increase their child's integration into the world of children, reduce discomfort, and make life a kinder and more pleasant experience for their children.

Traditional allopathic medicine is the first resort for children with significant disabilities in the United States, first for diagnosis, and then for treatment, if any exists. Some conditions have medical solutions with excellent prognoses, such as cleft lip/cleft palate, scoliosis, and some congenital heart defects. Other conditions may not be repairable, but do not keep the child from engaging in the typical activities in which children participate.

Medicine has taken great strides in the last hundred years, eliminating devastating diseases such as polio and smallpox outright and ameliorating others. Sometimes, a condition can be prevented, such as folic acid for neural tube defects, or the treatment for a disease may be amazingly simple, as vitamin D for rickets, or the avoidance of gluten for celiac disease. This progress gives parents realistic hope for significant gains in many of the remaining conditions. Why should parents whose children have diseases yet uncured or unstopped be less hopeful?

Some conditions remain lifelong and brutal experiences for the child and family. When the child suffers, the parents suffer. Our children are our future, and watching one's child not being able to fulfill his or her role as a child is a grueling and unrelenting experience. Searches for more accurate diagnoses, better treatments, different treatments, devices that might help, are all fair game in the quest to make one's child whole. When one has run the gamut of medical cures and treatments, what then?

Often parents turn to treatments that fall outside the range of allopathic medicine. Complementary and alternative medicine, as defined by the National Center for Complementary and Alternative Medicine (NCCAM), is a group of diverse medical and health care systems, practices, and products that are not currently considered to be part of conventional medicine. Integrative medicine is considered the combination of mainstream medical therapies and validated CAM therapies, that is, for which there is some high-quality scientific evidence of safety and effectiveness (13).

II. CAM USE IN CHILDREN

CAM therapies include such varied and diverse treatments as music therapy, Mormon tea, conductive education, Johrei, and hippotherapy, from traditions as varied as Eastern religion to the American frontier. CAM treatments can be organized according to the mechanisms by which the therapy is believed to work: mind–body interventions, biologically based therapies, manipulative or body-based therapies, and energy therapies (Table 1). In addition to these modalities, there are also complete systems of care or approaches, such as homeopathic medicine, naturopathic medicine, Christian

Table 1 Categories of Complementary and Alternative Medicine

	Mechanism	Examples
Mind–body interventions	Enhance the mind's capacity to affect bodily function and symptoms	Meditation, prayer, mental healing, creative therapies such as art, music, or dance
Biologically based therapies	Biological substances ingested or rubbed on the skin	Herbs, foods, megavitamins
Manipulative and body-based therapies	Manipulation and/or movement of the body	Osteopathic manipulation, chiropractic treatment, massage, hippotherapy
Energy therapies	Energy fields	
Biofield therapies	Effects energy fields that surround the body	Qi gong, Reiki, Therapeutic touch
Bioelectromagnetic-based therapies	Effects energy fields in general	Magnetic fields

Science, Traditional Chinese Medicine (TCM), and Ayurvedic medicine (13).

There has been a heightened interest in pediatric CAM use, as evidenced by numerous surveys of CAM use in children. The surveys have varied widely in location, study design, and sample characteristics.

A. General Samples

The percentage of lifetime pediatric CAM use reported in primary care settings and in household surveys conducted in North America and Europe has ranged from 8% to 24%, with approximately 15% of children receiving some form of CAM therapy at some point in their life. Typically, the percentage of reported CAM use is for lifetime or cumulative use and includes common CAM therapies such as herbs, vitamins, meditation, and massage that do not require visits to a CAM practitioner (14–19).

B. Children with Disabilities

More than a dozen studies have estimated CAM use for children with a range of disabling conditions including asthma (1,3,8–10), those for which care is provided in multidisciplinary clinics (2), arthritis (5,11), cystic fibrosis (12), cerebral palsy (7), and attention-deficit disorder (ADHD) (20). The average rates of CAM use for children with asthma were 58%; conditions seen in multidisciplinary clinics, 58%; cerebral palsy, 56%; autism, 32%; arthritis, 67%; cystic fibrosis, 66%; and ADHD, 64%. The extent of lifetime CAM use for children with special health care needs is dramatically higher than those for children in general.

C. Children with Cancer

Cancer is the only condition that has estimates for pediatric CAM use collected over an extended span of years. Before 1985, only 10% of the families reported using CAM for their child being treated for cancer (21–23); subsequently, CAM use averaged 56%, over a fivefold increase (16,24–32).

While CAM use clearly appears to be increasing in Western culture over time, and children with special health care needs are more likely to receive CAM, it is difficult to interpret the divergent results seen in these pediatric CAM surveys. The reasons for the variability are probably due to survey characteristics (e.g., lifetime CAM use or use during the last year), the situation (where and how the survey was administered), sample characteristics (the type and severity of the child's disability), and random sampling error.

III. REASONS FOR CAM USE

Because of increasing CAM use, and higher use in children with medical problems, it is important to understand why parents use CAM for their children. Reasons respondents have given for using CAM therapies include fear of drug side effects, chronic medical problems that were not improving, belief in the effectiveness of a CAM therapy, or dissatisfaction with conventional medicine (18,33). Almost half of the families surveyed by Hurvitz et al. (6) felt CAM could improve the quality of their child's life.

When allopathic medicine fails or cannot cure, parents continue to search for something that will help their child. These may include a second opinion, a new treatment, a new physician, more therapy, and finally, different treatments. A CAM treatment may be the one that provides relief or may yet be the unknown treatment that restores one's child to health. Cures have been found and there are swings in conventional medical wisdom, as old truths have been overturned. The list of medical successes for disabilities is heartening (34), and gives parents reason to hope their child's disease may be the next.

Many families will use CAM therapies when the traditional arsenal is not enough, and they will go to considerable time and expense to do so. Therapies that do not help are a waste of a family's resources, in time, money, and opportunity costs. For these reasons, it is imperative to test the effectiveness of the CAM therapies that parents use for their children and recommend those with proven effectiveness.

IV. EVIDENCE-BASED CAM THERAPIES

How can we tell if a CAM treatment works for a given condition? CAM therapies are tested using the same methods that are used to test non-CAM treatments. Evidence-based CAM therapies are those with demonstrated effectiveness for specific conditions. There are standards of evidence, with the highest level being multiple consistent randomized controlled trials and the lowest being a series of cases without a control group. The results on the effectiveness of many CAM therapies are still limited, but the number of studies is growing rapidly. Evidence accumulates as additional studies are completed, with more weight given to the more rigorous studies. Unfortunately, a great deal of the information on CAM therapies is still anecdotal or not based on careful research. We agree wholeheartedly with Kemper (35), "In God we trust; everyone else must have data."

What is wrong with trusting word of mouth or studies without a control group? An improvement in a child may be due to other causes such as a placebo effect, natural history, or nonspecific effects of the treatment. Case reports and uncontrolled trials do not have the necessary mechanisms to rule out other possible causes.

The following quote from United Cerebral Palsy (36) succinctly captures the situation that parents confront:

> Innovative therapies are generally characterized by periods (sometimes long periods) of special attention to the person with the disability; the unbridled enthusiasm and support of the person by a hopeful and frustrated parent or other care giver; a change in the environment of the person (going to a clinic—sometimes in another city or country); participating in group sessions with other persons with a similar disability which often includes group self-encouragement; a short-term improvement in

some function; and too often, a longer term return to the previous functional status. Unfortunately, they are also often characterized by a profound feeling of guilt on the part of parents or other care givers who feel that they failed to participate adequately in the home phase of the treatment program when the loss of function returns to its previous level. Sound familiar?

V. RESEARCH ON CAM TREATMENTS

Because parents of children with disabilities will continue to use CAM treatments, it is imperative to measure their effectiveness for each condition. Children have very little say in the medical treatments they receive and professionals need solid evidence upon which to base their advice. Anecdotal reports are not enough. The cumulative weight of evidence from multiple and rigorous studies is needed to come to definitive conclusions. Case studies and anecdotal information are only a good reason to test a treatment, not to use it.

A change that appears to result from a treatment may be due to a variety of causes. Improvements reported in case studies may be due to the natural history of the disease or normal development. Differences seen in uncontrolled trials may be due to specific or nonspecific effects of treatments. Only carefully designed research studies can sort out the causes of any changes observed in treatments. The United Cerebral Palsy Foundation (37) has stated:

> Remember, the history of the treatment of persons with disabilities due to cerebral palsy is filled with 'enthusiastically hailed, revolutionary new approaches,' which are now no longer in use. Keep an open mind; be prudent; be cautious.

Using a CAM therapy can have a variety of costs to the family. There are the costs to the child (time and discomfort) and the costs to the parents (money, time, and effort). The effects of a CAM therapy may be small or even harmful. Finally, there are opportunity costs. For example, if a family is using one CAM therapy, it will not have time or money to use another.

Practitioners need to know what CAM therapies are being used by their patients. If a family is going to use a complementary therapy, encourage the use of CAM treatments that have a proven effect for the child's condition. If there are none, encourage the use of CAM treatments that can be a good experience for the child and the entire family, are unlikely to cause harm, and have a low cost to the child and family. A CAM therapy, even if it does nothing else, may evoke a placebo effect, giving the parents hope and engendering positive feelings about the child.

Parents need to know the benefit they can expect from a CAM therapy so that they can make a personal assessment of the value to their child, and practitioners need to be prepared to talk about the relative merits of CAM therapies. Our children are worth the efforts of good research. Parents never want to give up hope. If a family is going to use unproven treatments, they can be encouraged to use CAM therapies that are low-cost, low-effort and have other benefits for the child.

ACKNOWLEDGMENTS

The author would like to acknowledge the support of NIH grant P50 AT00008.

REFERENCES

1. Andrews L, Lokuge S, Sawyer M, Lillywhite L, Kennedy D, Martin J. The use of alternative therapies by children with asthma: a brief report. J Paediatr Child Health 1998; 34(2): 131–134.

2. Saunders H, Davis MF, Duncan B, Meaney FJ, Haynes J, Barton LL. Use of complementary and alternative medical therapies among children with special health care needs in southern Arizona. Pediatrics 2003; 111(3):584–587.

3. Ernst E. Complementary/alternative medicine for asthma: we do not know what we need to know. Chest 1999; 115(1):1–3.

4. Golomb MR, Hune S, MacGregor DL, deVeber GA. Alternative therapy use by Chinese-Canadian children with stroke and cerebrovascular disease. J Child Neurol 2003; 18(10):714–717.

5. Hagen LE, Schneider R, Stephens D, Modrusan D, Feldman BM. Use of complementary and alternative medicine by pediatric rheumatology patients. Arthritis Rheum 2003; 49(1):3–6.

6. Hurvitz EA, Leonard C, Ayyangar R, Nelson VS. Complementary and alternative medicine use in families of children with cerebral palsy. Dev Med Child Neurol 2003; 45(6):364–370.

7. Levy SE, Hyman SL. Use of complementary and alternative treatments for children with autistic spectrum disorders is increasing. Pediatric Ann 2003; 32(10):685–691.

8. Mazur LJ, de Ybarrondo L, Miller J, Colasurdo G. Use of alternative and complementary therapies for pediatric asthma. Tex Med 2001; 97(6):64–68.

9. Orhan F, Sekerel BE, Kocabas CN, Sackesen C, Adalioglu G, uncer A. Complementary and alternative medicine in children with asthma. Ann Allergy Asthma Immunol 2003; 90(6):581–582.

10. Pachter LM, Cloutier MM, Bernstein BA. Ethnomedical (folk) remedies for childhood asthma in a mainland Puerto Rican community. Arch Pediatr Adolesc Med 1995; 149(9):982–988.

11. Southwood TR, Malleson PN, Roberts-Thompson PJ, Mahy M. Unconventional therapies used for patients with juvenile arthritis. Pediatrics 1990; 85(2):150–154.

12. Stern RC, Candra ER, Doershuk CF. Use of nonmedical treatment by cystic fibrosis patients. J Adolesc Health 1992; 13(7): 612–615.

13. National Center for Complementary and Alternative Medicine. What is complementary and alternative medicine? [accessed March 12, 2004]. http://nccam.nih.gov/health/whatiscam/.

14. Friis B. [Alternative treatment of children—why and how often? A questionnaire study at a pediatric department (Danish)]. Ugeskr Laeger 1987; 149(12):806–808.

15. Kitai E, Vinker S, Sandiuk A, Hornik O, Zeltcer C, Gaver A. Use of complementary and alternative medicine among primary care patients. Fam Pract 1998; 15(5):411–414.

16. Möttönen M, Uhari M. Use of micronutrients and alternative drugs by children with acute lymphoblastic leukemia. Med Pediatr Oncol 1997; 28(3):205–208.

17. Ottolini MC, Hamburger EK, Loprieato JO, Coleman RH, Sachs HC, Madden R, Brasseux C. Complementary and alternative medicine use among children in the Washington, DC area. Ambul Pediatr 2001; 2:122–125.

18. Spigelblatt LS, Laîné-Ammara G, Pless IB, Guyver A. The use of alternative medicine by children. Pediatrics 1994; 94:811–814.

19. Verhoef MJ, Russell ML, Love EJ. Alternative medicine use in rural Alberta. Can J Public Health 1994; 85(5):308–309.

20. Stubberfield TG, Wray JA, Parry TS. Utilization of alternative therapies in attention-deficit hyperactivity disorder. J Paediatr Child Health 1999; 53:450–453.

21. Faw C, Ballentine R, Ballentine L, van Eys J. Unproved cancer remedies. A survey of use in pediatric outpatients. JAMA 1977; 238:1536–1538.

22. Pendergrass TW, Davis S. Knowledge and use of "alternative" cancer therapies in children. Am J Pediatr Hematol Oncol 1981; 3(4):339–345.

23. Copeland DR, Silberberg Y, Pfefferbaum B. Attitudes and practices of families of children in treatment for cancer. A cross-cultural study. Am J Pediatr Hematol Oncol 1983; 5(1):65–71.

24. Friedman T, Slayton WB, Allen LS, Pollock BH, Dumont-Driscoll M, Mehta P, Graham-Pole J. Use of alternative therapies for children with cancer. Pediatrics 1997; 100(6):E1.

25. Bold J, Leis A. Unconventional therapy use among children with cancer in Saskatchewan. J Pediatr Oncol Nurs 2001; 18: 16–25.

26. Fernandez CV, Stutzer CA, MacWilliam L, Fryer C. Alternative and complementary therapy use in pediatric oncology patients in British Columbia: prevalence and reasons for use and nonuse. J Clin Oncol 1998; 16(4):1279–1286.

27. Grootenhuis MA, Last BF, de Graaf-Nijkerk JH, van der Wel M. Use of alternative treatment in pediatric oncology. Cancer Nurs 1998; 21(4):282–288.

28. Kelly KM, Jacobson JS, Kennedy DD, Braudt SM, Mallick M, Weiner MA. Use of unconventional therapies by children with cancer at an urban medical center. J Pediatr Hematol Oncol 2000; 22(5):412–416.

29. McCurdy EA, Spangler JG, Wofford MM, Chauvenet AR, McLean TW. Religiosity is associated with the use of complementary medical therapies by pediatric oncology patients. J Pediatr Hematol Oncol 2003; 25(2):125–129.

30. Neuhouser ML, Patterson RE, Schwartz SM, Hedderson MM, Bowen DJ, Standish LJ. Use of alternative medicine by children with cancer in Washington State. Prev Med 2001; 33(5): 347–354.

31. Sawyer MG, Gannoni AF, Toogood IF, Antoniou G, Rice M. The use of alternative therapies by children with cancer. Med J Aust 1994; 160(6):320–322.

32. Yeh CH, Tsai JL, Li W, Chen HM, Lee SC, Lin CF, Yang CP. Use of alternative therapy among pediatric oncology patients in Taiwan. Pediatr Hematol Oncol 2000; 17(1):55–65.

33. Johnson GA, Bilbao RM, Graham-Brown RA. The use of complementary medicine in children with atopic dermatitis in secondary care in Leicester. Br J Dermatol 2003; 149(3): 566–571.

34. History of Success: March of Dimes Milestones [accessed March 12, 2004]. http://www.marchofdimes.com/aboutus/ 789_4283.asp.

35. Kemper K. The Holistic Pediatrician: A Parent's Comprehensive Guide to Safe and Effective Therapies for the 25 Most Common Childhood Ailments of Infants, Children, and Adolescents. 2nd ed. Harper Collins, 1996.

36. United Cerebral Palsy Foundation. Evaluating the Usefulness of an "Innovative" Clinical Procedure—How Can We Really Know If It Works? [accessed March 12, 2004]. http://www. ucp.org/ucp_generaldoc.cfm/1/4/24/24–6608/86.

37. United Cerebral Palsy Foundation. Alternative and Complementary Medicine [accessed March 12, 2004]. http://www. ucp.org/ucp_generaldoc.cfm/1/4/24/24–6608/128.

Epilogue

Genes for Developmental Disabilities: Results of Computer Search

MERLIN G. BUTLER

Section of Medical Genetics and
Molecular Medicine, Children's Mercy
Hospitals and Clinics, University of
Missouri-Kansas City School of
Medicine, Kansas City, Missouri, U.S.A.

F. JOHN MEANEY

Department of Pediatrics, University
of Arizona College of Medicine,
Tucson, Arizona, U.S.A.

In this book, we have attempted to present what is known currently with respect to the genetics of developmental disabilities and the important aspects of environmental factors in both the cause and the management and treatment of these disorders. Our knowledge base in these areas continues to grow at a phenomenal pace. For example, Inlow and Restifo (2) have recently estimated that new genes for mental retardation are identified at the rate of 1–2 per month. Thus, the identification of specific mutant genes for developmental

863

disabilities, and genes or genetic factors that contribute to the underlying susceptibility to these disorders, is far ahead of our understanding of the complex interaction of genes and environmental exposures that contribute to developmental disturbances and eventually what we observe as a phenotypic outcome. The state of our knowledge in the latter areas is certain to grow tremendously during the first two decades of this century, and we have tried throughout this text to indicate where we expect to see progress along these lines. With respect to the genetics of developmental disabilities, we decided that an examination of the state of our knowledge in a more global sense would be a useful way of summarizing the book.

Any attempt to evaluate the specific genes responsible for developmental disabilities would be futile, as the category includes so many diverse conditions and a vast array of behavioral, cognitive, and other neurodevelopmental phenotypes. Therefore, we decided to focus on mental retardation (MR) as a developmental disability for which there is the continuously updated, easily searchable database for genetic conditions in the form of Online Mendelian Inheritance in Man or OMIM (1) and for which there have been recent attempts at a global approach to our understanding of its genetic etiology.

Inlow and Restifo (2) have produced the most comprehensive recent analysis of the genetics of MR. One purpose of this elegant study was to determine as best as possible how many genes for MR have been identified on a molecular basis and to examine the existing information about the molecular and biological functions of these gene products. In their analysis, Inlow and Restifo (2) used a broad definition of MR to include "progressive disorders with onset of cognitive impairment in childhood and occasionally, as late as adolescence" (p. 836). The OMIM database was used initially to search for human MR genes and disorders that include MR in the phenotypic description. OMIM was accessed online (http://www.ncbi.nlm.nih.gov/entrez/query.fcgi?db=OMIM) on February 21, 2002, to search all fields using the phrase "mental retardation." This search resulted in 1010 entries for which detailed reviews were conducted. These investigators conducted additional OMIM searches of the phrases "cognitive impairment" and "learning disabilities" to encompass milder MR and as a result identified another 38 nonoverlapping entries for further evaluation. Their final source of information included periodic searches of the National Center for Biotechnology PubMed resources, in part to identify MR genes that were missed, for a variety of reasons, by the OMIM search.

The methods of evaluation of the results of these searches are thoroughly explained in Inlow and Restifo (2) and will not be repeated here. The authors' careful analysis of the 1010 OMIM entries for MR revealed a total of 204 human genes involved in the etiology of MR either in its isolated form or as a phenotypic feature of a syndrome. The additional OMIM searches for mild MR and the literature searches yielded an additional 78 genes for a total of 282 genes causing MR in humans (as of September, 2004 the total number of MR genes is 307; Inlow and Restifo, personal communication). Given a number of additional considerations such as gaps in existing databases and problems that result in MR genes being unrecognized, Inlow and Restifo (2) emphasize how difficult it is to predict the number of human genes for MR but suggest this number could easily reach 1000.

We conducted a search of the OMIM database using the phrase "mental retardation" on January 9, 2005. The number of entries is now 1242, representing a 23% increase during the almost three years subsequent to the searches of Inlow and Restifo (2) or roughly 80 entries per year. Given the estimated 1–2 new genes for MR identified each month estimated by Inlow and Restifo (2), it is probably safe to say that we are now about one-third of the way towards the 1000 MR genes that might eventually be identified according to these investigators. But this is cognitive functioning alone, and developmental disabilities cover a vast array of behavioral and other neurological phenotypes that will take many years to decipher. Much work remains before us, and superlative research opportunities for young scientists abound.

REFERENCES

1. Hamosh A, Scott AF, Amberger J, Bocchini C, McKusick VA. Online mendelian inheritance in man (OMIM), a knowledge base of human genes and genetic disorders. Nucleic Acids Res 2005; 33:D514–D517.

2. Inlow JK, Restifo LL. Molecular and comparative genetics of mental retardation. Genetics 2004; 166:835–881.

Glossary

Acrocentric   A type of chromosome with the centromere near one end. The human acrocentric chromosomes (13, 14, 15, 21, and 22) have satellited short arms that carry genes for ribosomal RNA.

Allele   One of the alternative forms of a gene that occupies a given locus.

Amniocentesis   A procedure used in prenatal diagnosis to obtain amniotic fluid and cells of fetal origin to be cultured for analysis. Amniotic fluid is withdrawn from the amniotic sac with a syringe and needle inserted through the abdominal wall and into the uterus.

Amplification   In molecular biology, the production of multiple copies of a sequence of DNA. In cytogenetics, multiple copies of a sequence in the genome are detectable by comparative genomic hybridization (CGH).

Aneuploidy   Any chromosome number that is not an exact multiple of the haploid number. The common forms of aneuploidy in humans are *trisomy* (the presence of an extra chromosome) or *monosomy* (the absence of a single chromosome).

Anticipation The progressively earlier onset and increased severity of certain diseases in successive generations of a family. Caused by expansion of the number of triplet repeats within or associated with the gene responsible for a disease.

Ascertainment The method of selection of individuals for inclusion in a genetic study.

Association In human genetics, describes the situation in which a particular allele is found either significantly more or significantly less frequently in a group of affected individuals than would be expected from the frequency of the allele in the general population from which the affected individuals were drawn.

Assortative mating Selection of a mate with preference for a particular genotype or nonrandom mating.

Assortment The random distribution of different combinations of the parental chromosomes to the gametes. Nonallelic genes assort independently, unless they are linked.

Autosome Any nuclear chromosome other than the sex chromosomes; 22 pairs in the human karyotype.

Banding One of several techniques that stain chromosomes in a characteristic pattern, allowing identification of individual chromosomes and structural abnormalities (e.g., *C, G, Q, R-bands*).

Barr body The sex chromatin as seen in female somatic cells, representing an inactive X chromosome.

Base pair (bp) A pair of complementary nucleotide bases as in double-stranded DNA. Used as the unit of measurement of the length of a DNA sequence.

Bayesian theorem A mathematical method widely used in genetic counseling to calculate recurrence risks. The method combines information from several sources (genetics, pedigree information, and test results) to determine the probability that a specific individual might develop or transmit a certain disorder.

Benign trait A variant with no clinical significance.

Bioinformatics Computational analysis and storage of biological and experimental data, widely applied to genomic and proteomic studies.

Birth defect   An abnormality or anomaly present at birth, not necessarily genetic.

Candidate gene   In a search for a disease gene, a candidate gene is a gene whose product has biochemical or other properties suggesting that it may be the disease gene.

Carrier   An individual heterozygous for a particular mutant allele. The term is used for heterozygotes for autosomal recessive alleles, for females heterozygous for X-linked alleles, or, less commonly, for an individual heterozygous for an autosomal dominant allele but not expressing it (e.g., a heterozygote for a Huntington disease allele in the presymptomatic stage).

Case–control study   An epidemiological method in which patients with a disease (the cases) are compared with suitably chosen individuals without the disease (the controls) with respect to the relative frequency of various putative risk factors.

Cell cycle   The stages between two successive mitotic divisions described in the text. Consists of the G^1, S, G^2, and M stages.

CentiMorgan (cM)   The unit of distance between genes along chromosomes, named for Thomas Hunt Morgan. Two loci are 1 cM apart if recombination is detected between them in 1% of meioses.

Centromere   The primary constriction on the chromosome, a region at which the sister chromatids are held together and where the kinetochore is formed. Required for normal segregation in mitosis and meiosis.

CG (or CpG) island   Any region of the genome containing an unusually high concentration of the dinucleotide sequence 5'-CG-3'.

Chromosome   One of the threadlike structures in the cell nucleus; consists of chromatin and deoxyribonucleic acid (DNA).

Compound heterozygote   An individual, or a genotype, with two different mutant alleles at the same locus.

Deletion   The loss of a sequence of DNA from a chromosome. The deleted DNA may be of any length, from a single base to a large segment of a chromosome.

Differentiation   The process whereby a cell acquires a tissue-specific pattern of expression of genes and proteins and a characteristic phenotype.

Diploid   The number of chromosomes in most somatic cells, which is double the number found in the gametes. In humans, the diploid chromosome number is 46.

Disruption   A birth defect caused by destruction of tissue; may be caused by vascular occlusion, a teratogen, or rupture of the amniotic sac with entrapment.

Dominant   A trait is dominant if it is phenotypically expressed in heterozygotes.

Dominant negative   A disease-causing allele, or the effect of an allele, that disrupts the function of a wild-type allele in the same cell.

Double heterozygote   An individual who is heterozygous at each of two different loci. Contrast with *compound heterozygote.*

Dysmorphism   Morphological developmental abnormalities, as seen in many syndromes of genetic, multifactorial, or environmental origin.

Empiric risk   In human genetics, the probability that a familial trait will occur or recur in a family member, based on observed numbers of affected and unaffected individuals in family studies rather than on knowledge of the causative mechanism.

Epigenetic   The term that refers to any factor that can affect the phenotype without a change in the genotype.

Epistasis   The situation in which an allele of one gene can block the phenotypic expression of all alleles of another gene.

Euchromatin   The major component of chromatin. It stains lightly with G banding, decondensed and lightly stains during interphase. Contrast with *heterochromatin.*

Euploid   Any chromosome number that is an exact multiple of the number in a haploid gamete *(n).* Most somatic cells are diploid *(2n).* Contrast with *aneuploid.*

Exon   A transcribed region of a gene that is present in mature messenger RNA.

Expressivity   The extent to which a genetic defect is expressed. If there is variable expressivity, the trait may vary in expression from mild to severe but is never completely unexpressed in individuals who have the corresponding genotype. Contrast with *penetrance.*

Familial   Any trait that is more common in relatives of an affected individual than in the general population, whether the cause is genetic, environmental, or both.

Fitness (f)   The probability of transmitting one's genes to the next generation as compared with the average probability for the population.

Founder effect   A high frequency of a mutant gene in a population founded by a small ancestral group when one or more of the founders was a carrier of the mutant gene.

Fragile site   Nonstaining gap in the chromatin of a metaphase chromosome, such as the fragile site at Xq27 in the fragile X syndrome.

Frameshift mutation   A mutation involving a deletion or insertion that is not an exact multiple of three base pairs and thus changes the reading frame of the gene downstream of the mutation.

Gamete   A reproductive cell (ovum or sperm) with the haploid chromosome number.

Gene   A hereditary unit; in molecular terms, a sequence of chromosomal DNA that is required for the production of a functional product.

Gene map   The characteristic arrangement of the genes on the chromosomes. Mapping genes to their chromosomal positions has been one purpose of the Human Genome Project.

Genetic counseling   Providing information and assistance to affected individuals or family members at risk for having a disorder that may be genetic; concerning the consequences of the disorder, the probability of developing or transmitting it, and the ways in which it may be prevented or ameliorated.

Genetic heterogeneity   The production of the same or similar phenotypes by different genetic mechanisms.

Genetic lethal A gene or genetically determined trait that leads to failure to reproduce, although not necessarily to early death.

Genome The complete DNA sequence, containing the entire genetic information, of a gamete, an individual, a population, or a species.

Genotype (1) The genetic constitution of an individual, as distinguished from the phenotype. (2) More specifically, the alleles present at one locus.

Germline The cell line from which gametes are derived.

Haploid The chromosome number of a normal gamete, with only one member of each chromosome pair. In humans, the haploid number is 23.

Haplotype A group of alleles in coupling at closely linked loci, usually inherited as a unit.

Hardy–Weinberg law The law is named after the two codiscoverers and relates gene frequency to genotype frequency, used in population genetics to determine allele frequency and heterozygote frequency when the incidence of a disorder is known.

Hemizygous A term for the genotype of an individual with only one representative of a chromosome, or chromosome segment, rather than the usual two; refers especially to X-linked genes in the male but also applies to genes on any chromosome segment that is deleted on the homologous chromosome.

Heritability (h^2) The fraction of total phenotypic variance of a quantitative trait that is due to genotypic differences. May be viewed as a statistical estimate of the hereditary contribution to a quantitative trait.

Heterochromatin Chromatin that stains darkly throughout the cell cycle, even in interphase. Generally thought to be late replicating and genetically inactive. Satellite DNA in regions such as centromeres, acrocentric short arms, and lqh, 9qh, 16qh, and Yqh constitute *constitutive heterochromatin*, whereas the chromatin of the inactive X chromosome is referred to as *facultative heterochromatin*. Contrast with *euchromatin*.

Heterozygote (heterozygous) An individual or genotype with two different alleles at a given locus on a pair of homologous chromosomes.

Housekeeping genes Genes expressed in most or all cells because their products provide basic functions.

Imprinting The phenomenon of different expression of alleles depending on the parent of origin. Prader–Willi and Angelman syndromes are examples.

Inbreeding The mating of closely related individuals (consanguinity). The progeny of close relatives are said to be inbred.

Index case An affected family member who is the first to draw attention to a pedigree of a genetic disorder.

Intron A segment of a gene that is initially transcribed but is then removed from within the primary RNA transcript, by splicing together the sequences (exons) on either side of it.

Inversion A chromosomal rearrangement in which a segment of a chromosome is reversed end to end. If the centromere is included in the inversion, the inversion is *pericentric*; if not, it is *paracentric*.

Karyotype The chromosome constitution of an individual. The term is also used for a photomicrograph of the chromosomes of an individual systematically arranged and paired.

Kb (kilobase) A unit of 1000 bases in a DNA or RNA sequence.

Kindred An extended family.

Knockout mice Mice in which a specific gene has been disrupted or "targeted" by recombinant DNA technology; used as models for investigations of the function and interactions of the normal counterparts of the disrupted genes.

Linkage Genes on the same chromosome are *linked* if they are transmitted together in meiosis more frequently than chance would allow.

Linkage map A chromosome map showing the relative positions of genes and other DNA markers on the chromosomes, as determined by linkage analysis.

Locus The position occupied by a gene on a chromosome. Different forms of the gene (*alleles*) may occupy the locus.

Lod score   A statistical method that tests genetic marker data in families to determine whether two loci are linked. The lod score is the *log*arithm of the *odd*s in favor of linkage. By convention, a lod score of 3 (odds of 1000:1 in favor) is accepted as proof of linkage and a lod score of −2 (100:1 against) as proof that the loci are unlinked.

Loss of heterozygosity (LOH)   Loss of a normal allele from a region of one chromosome of a pair, allowing a defective allele on the homologous chromosome to be clinically manifest. A feature of many cases of retinoblastoma, breast cancer, and other tumors due to mutation in a tumor-suppressor gene.

Lyonization   Terms used for the phenomenon of X-inactivation, which was first described by the geneticist Mary Lyon.

Meiosis   The type of cell division occurring in the germ cells, by which gametes containing the haploid chromosome number are produced from diploid cells. Two meiotic divisions occur: meiosis I and meiosis II. Reduction in chromosome number takes place during meiosis I.

Microdeletion   A chromosomal deletion that is too small to be seen under the microscope.

Missense mutation   A mutation that changes a codon specific for one amino acid to specify another amino acid.

Mitochondrial inheritance   The inheritance of a trait encoded in the mitochondrial genome. Because the mitochondrial genome is strictly maternally inherited, mitochondrial inheritance occurs solely through the female line.

Mitosis   The process of ordinary cell division, resulting in the formation of two cells genetically identical to the parent cell.

Monosomy   A chromosome constitution in which one member of a chromosome pair is missing, as in 45,X Turner syndrome.

Mosaic   An individual or tissue with at least two cell lines differing in genotype or karyotype, derived from a single zygote.

Multifactorial inheritance   The type of non-Mendelian inheritance shown by traits that are determined by a combination of multiple factors, both genetic and environmental.

Mutation   Any permanent heritable change in the sequence of genomic DNA.

Nondisjunction   The failure of two members of a chromosome pair to disjoin during meiosis I or two chromatids of a chromosome to disjoin during meiosis II or mitosis, so that both pass to one daughter cell and the other daughter cell receives neither.

Oligonucleotide   A short DNA molecule (usually 8–50 bp), synthesized for use as a probe or for use in the polymerase chain reaction.

p   In cytogenetics, the short arm of a chromosome (from the French *petit*). In population genetics, the frequency of the more common allele of a pair. In biochemistry, abbreviation of *protein* (e.g., p53 is a protein 53 kDa in size).

Pedigree   In medical genetics, a family history of hereditary condition, or a diagram of a family history indicating the family members, their relationship to the proband, and their status with respect to a particular hereditary condition.

Penetrance   The fraction of individuals with a genotype known to cause a disease who have any signs or symptoms of the disease. Contrast with *expressivity*.

Phenocopy   A mimic of a phenotype that is usually determined by a specific genotype, produced instead by the interaction of some environmental factors with a normal genotype.

Phenotype   The observed biochemical, physiological, and morphological characteristics of an individual as determined by his or her genotype and the environment in which it is expressed.

Pleiotropy   Multiple phenotypic effects of a single gene or gene pair. The terms is used particularly when the effects are not obviously related.

Point mutation   A single nucleotide base-pair change in DNA.

Polygenic   Inheritance determined by many genes at different loci, with small additive effects. Not to be confused with *complex* (*multifactorial*) inheritance, in which environmental as well as genetic factors may be involved.

Polymerase chain reaction (PCR) The molecular genetic technique by which a short DNA or RNA sequence is amplified enormously by means of two flanking oligonucleotide primers used in repeated cycles of primer extension and DNA synthesis with DNA polymerase.

Polymorphism The occurrence together in a population of two or more alternative genotypes, each at a frequency greater than that which could be maintained by recurrent mutation alone. A locus is arbitrarily considered to be polymorphic if the rarer allele has a frequency of 0.01, so that the heterozygote frequency is at least 0.02. Any allele rarer than this is a *rare variant.*

Polyploid Any multiple of the basic haploid chromosome number other than the diploid number; i.e., $3n$, $4n$, and so forth.

Premutation In triplet repeat disorder—for example, fragile X syndrome—a moderate expansion of the number of triplet repeats that has no phenotypic effect but is at increased risk of undergoing further expansion during meiosis and causing full expression of the disorder in the offspring.

Private mutation A very rare mutation, perhaps known only in a single family or single population.

Proband The affected family member through whom the family is ascertained. Also called the *propositus* or *index case.*

Probe In molecular genetics, a labeled DNA or RNA sequence used to detect the presence of a complementary sequence by molecular hybridization; or a reagent capable of recognizing a desired clone in a mixture of many DNA or RNA sequences. Also, the process of using such a molecule.

q In cytogenetics, the long arm of a chromosome; in population genetics, the frequency of the less common allele of a pair.

Random mating Selection of a mate without regard to the genotype of the mate. In a randomly mating population, the frequencies of the various matings are determined solely by the frequencies of the genes concerned.

Recessive A trait that is expressed only in homozygotes or hemizygotes.

Recombination The formation of new combinations of alleles in coupling by crossing over between their loci.

Regulatory gene A gene that codes for an RNA or protein molecule that regulates the expression of other genes.

Restriction fragment length polymorphism (RFLP) A polymorphic difference in DNA sequence between individuals that can be recognized by restriction endonucleases.

Segregation In genetics, the disjunction of homologous chromosomes at meiosis.

Selection In population genetics, the operation of forces that determine the relative fitness of a genotype in the population, thus affecting the frequency of the gene concerned.

Sib, sibling A brother or sister.

Single nucleotide polymorphism (SNP) A polymorphism in DNA sequence consisting of variation in a single base.

Southern blotting A technique devised by the British biochemist, Ed Southern, for preparation of a filter to which DNA has been transferred, following restriction enzyme digestion and gel electrophoresis to separate the DNA molecules by size. Specific DNA molecules can then be detected on the filter by their hybridization to labeled probes.

Sporadic In medical genetics, a disease caused by a new mutation.

Stem cell A type of cell capable of both self-renewal and of proliferation and differentiation.

Structural gene A gene coding for any RNA or protein product.

Syndrome A characteristic pattern of anomalies, presumed to be causally related.

Teratogen An agent that produces congenital malformations or increases their incidence.

Translation The synthesis of a polypeptide from its mRNA template.

Translocation The transfer of a segment of one chromosome to another chromosome. If two nonhomologous chromosomes exchange pieces, the translocation is *reciprocal*.

Triplet repeat (trinucleotide repeat) disorders Diseases caused when the number of repeating units of a trinucleotide in a particular gene expands beyond a threshold and interferes with gene expression or function.

Triploid A cell with three copies of each chromosome, or an individual made up of such cells.

Trisomy The state of having three representatives of a given chromosome instead of the usual pair, as in trisomy 21 (Down syndrome).

Uniparental disomy The presence in the karyotype of two copies of a specific chromosome, both inherited from one parent, with no representative of that chromosome from the other parent. If both homologs of the parental pair are present, the situation is *heterodisomy*; if one parental homolog is present in duplicate, the situation is *isodisomy*.

X inactivation Inactivation of genes on one X chromosome in somatic cells of female mammals, occurring early in embryonic life, at about the time of implantation.

X linkage The distinctive inheritance pattern of alleles at loci on the X chromosome that do not undergo recombination (crossing over) during male meiosis.

Y linkage Genes on the Y chromosome, or traits determined by such genes are Y-linked.

Zygote A fertilized ovum.

Index

Bacterial artificial chromosomes
(BACs), 140
Bardet–Biedl syndrome, 138
allelic heterogeneity, 138
digenic inheritance, 138
genetic heterogeneity, 138
locus heterogeneity, 138
pleiotropy, 138
positional cloning, 138
Barr body, 586
Basal forebrain cholinergic
neurons, 175
Basal ganglia, 787
Beckwith–Wiedemann
syndrome, 432
Behavior phenotype, 745
Behavior, adaptive, 347
Behavioral presentation, 405
Behavioral problems, 610
Behavioral therapy, 797
β-amyloid, 176
Beta-endorphins, 749
Breakpoint, 285
Broader phenotype, 718
Brown's syndrome, 439

CAM. *See* Complementary and
alternative medicine.
Cancer, 854, 860
Cataracts, 234
Catechol-*O*-methyltransferase
(COMT), 393, 406
Central nervous system, 809
Cerebellar peduncles, 254
Cerebellar vermis, 787
Cerebral palsy, 809
Cervical spine, 239
Childhood in PWS, 296
aggressive behavior, 296
dental caries, 296
enamel hypoplasia, 296
malocclusion, 296
serotonin, 296
Chorionic villus, 82

Chromosomal abnormalities, 86
numerical, 87
structural, 87
deletions, 88
duplications, 90
inversions, 93
markers, 87, 95
translocations, 93
Chromosome 15, 21, 148
abnormal, 87
human, 21, 167
marker, 95, 138
Chromosome microdeletions, 324
Clinical consensus criteria for
Angelman syndrome, 320
Clinical features for Alagille
syndrome, 523
cardiac manifestations, 523
facial features, 525
hepatic manifestations, 523
ophthalmologic manifestations,
523
skeletal manifestations, 525
Clinical phenotypes, 500
Coffin–Lowry syndrome, 257
Cognitive profiles, 338, 344
Community samples, 789
Comorbid disorders, 794
Comorbidities, 703
Comparative genomics, 143
Complementary and alternative
medicine (CAM), 851
cancer, 854
therapy, 854
use, 854
COMT gene, 406
Concordance, 77
Confirmation, 839
Consanguinity, 41
Constipation, 341
chronic, 342
Contiguous gene syndrome,
386, 521
Cornelia de Lange syndrome, 684
Counseling strategies, 628